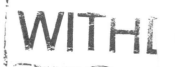

D1579527

Manual of
Clinical
Hematology

Third Edition

Manual of Clinical Hematology

Third Edition

Edited by

Joseph J. Mazza, M.D.
Senior Consultant, Department of Hematology/Oncology,
Marshfield Clinic, Marshfield;
Professor of Clinical Medicine, Department of Medicine,
University of Wisconsin School of Medicine,
Madison, Wisconsin

LIPPINCOTT WILLIAMS & WILKINS
A **Wolters Kluwer** Company
Philadelphia · Baltimore · New York · London
Buenos Aires · Hong Kong · Sydney · Tokyo

Acquisitions Editor: Jonathan W. Pine, Jr.
Developmental Editor: Stacey L. Baze
Production Editor: Melanie Bennitt
Manufacturing Manager: Benjamin Rivera
Cover Designer: Christine Jenny
Compositor: Circle Graphics
Printer: R. R. Donnelley—Crawfordsville

© 2002 by LIPPINCOTT WILLIAMS & WILKINS
530 Walnut Street
Philadelphia, PA 19106 USA
LWW.com

Printed in the USA
First Edition 1988
Second Edition 1995

Library of Congress Cataloging-in-Publication Data

Manual of clinical hematology / edited by Joseph J. Mazza.—3rd ed.
    p. ; cm. — (Perfect bound)
    Includes bibliographical references and index.
    ISBN 0-7817-2981-5
    1. Blood—Diseases—Handbooks, manuals, etc. 2. Hematology—Handbooks, manuals, etc. I. Mazza, Joseph J. II. Series.
    [DNLM: 1. Hematologic Diseases—Handbooks. WH 39 M2935 2002]
  RC636 .M342 2002
  616.1′5—dc21

                                                            2001029916

---

10 9 8 7 6 5 4 3 2 1

*This book is dedicated to all medical residents
for their stimulation and their contributions to medical education.
And to their arduous quest, unceasing dedication,
and relentless pursuit of medical knowledge,
which are so seldom recognized and lauded.*

CONTENTS

CONTRIBUTING AUTHORS

Irit Avivi, M.D.
Professor of Medicine, Department of Hematology and Bone Marrow Transplantation, State of Israel—Ministry of Health, Rambam Medical Center, Haifa, Israel

Edward J. Benz, Jr., M.D.
President, Dana Farber Cancer Institute; Richard and Susan Smith Professor of Medicine, Professor of Pediatrics and Pathology, Harvard Medical School, Boston, Massachusetts

Virgil F. Fairbanks, M.D.
Consultant, Department of Medicine, Mayo Foundation Clinic, St. Mary's Hospital, and Rochester Methodist Hospital; Professor Emeritus, Departments of Internal Medicine, Laboratory Medicine, and Pathology, Mayo Medical School, Rochester, Minnesota

Kenneth A. Foon, M.D.
Professor, Department of Internal Medicine, Division of Oncology, Stanford University Medical Center, Stanford, California

William R. Friedenberg, M.D., F.A.C.P.
Chief, Division of Hematology/Oncology, Department of Medicine, Guthrie Clinic, Robert Packer Hospital, Sayre, Pennsylvania; Clinical Professor, Department of Hematology/Oncology, State University of New York, Upstate Medical University, Syracuse, New York

Dennis A. Gastineau, M.D.
Associate Professor, Divisions of Hematopathology and Transfusion Medicine, Departments of Laboratory Medicine and Pathology, Mayo Medical School, Rochester, Minnesota

Leo I. Gordon, M.D.
Chief, Division of Hematology/Oncology, Department of Medicine, Northwestern Memorial Hospital; Abby and John Friend Professor of Cancer Research, Chief, Division of Hematology/Oncology, Department of Medicine, Northwestern University Medical School, Chicago, Illinois

Jerome L. Gottschall, M.D.
Professor, Department of Pathology, Medical College of Wisconsin; Vice President, Medical Services, Blood Center of Southeastern Wisconsin, Inc., Milwaukee, Wisconsin

John D. Hines, M.D.
Professor, Departments of Medicine and Oncology, Case Western Reserve University School of Medicine; Senior Attending Physician, Department of Hematology/Oncology, MetroHealth Medical Center, Cleveland, Ohio

William G. Hocking, M.D.
Hematologist/Oncologist, Department of Clinical Oncology, Marshfield Clinic, Marshfield, Wisconsin; Associate Clinical Professor, Department of Medicine, University of Wisconsin, Madison, Wisconsin

Neil E. Kay, M.D.
Professor of Medicine, University of Kentucky College of Medicine; Attending Physician, Department of Hematology/Oncology, University of Kentucky Medical Center, Lexington, Kentucky

Robert A. Kyle, M.D.
Consultant, Department of Hematology and Internal Medicine, Mayo Clinic and Mayo Foundation; Professor, Mayo Medical School, Mayo Clinic and Mayo Foundation, Rochester, Minnesota

Hillard M. Lazarus, M.D., F.A.C.P.
Professor of Medicine, Director, Blood and Marrow Transplant Program, Ireland Cancer Center, Case Western Reserve University, University Hospitals of Cleveland, Cleveland, Ohio

Mitchell D. Martin, M.D.
Senior Fellow in Hematology/Oncology, University of Utah Health Sciences Center, Salt Lake City, Utah

Joseph J. Mazza, M.D.
Senior Consultant, Department of Hematology/Oncology, Marshfield Clinic, Marshfield; Professor of Clinical Medicine, Department of Medicine, University of Wisconsin School of Medicine, Madison, Wisconsin

Gordon D. McLaren, M.D.
Consultant and Attending Physician, Department of Hematology/Oncology, VA Long Beach Healthcare System, Long Beach, California; Associate Professor, Department of Medicine, University of California at Irvine, Orange, California

Jay E. Menitove, M.D.
Executive Director and Medical Director, Community Blood Center of Greater Kansas City; Clinical Professor, Department of Internal Medicine, Kansas University School of Medicine and University of Missouri—Kansas City School of Medicine, Kansas City, Missouri

Kenneth B. Miller, M.D.
Director, Bone Marrow Transplantation, Department of Medicine, New England Medical Center; Associate Professor, Department of Medicine, Tufts University School of Medicine, Boston, Massachusetts

Scott Murphy, M.D.
Adjunct Professor of Medicine, Department of Medicine, University of Pennsylvania; Attending Physician, Department of Medicine, Hospital of the University of Pennsylvania, Philadelphia, Pennsylvania

Lawrence D. Petz, M.D.
President and Chief Medical Officer, StemCyte, Inc., Arcadia, California; Emeritus Professor, Departments of Pathology and Laboratory Medicine, UCLA Medical Center, Los Angeles, California

A. Koneti Rao, M.D.
Professor of Medicine and Thrombosis Research, Director, Thromboembolic Diseases, Temple University School of Medicine; Attending Physician, Department of Medicine, Temple University Hospital, Philadelphia, Pennsylvania

George M. Rodgers, M.D., Ph.D.
Staff Physician, Department of Medicine, University Hospital; Professor, Divisions of Hematology and Oncology, Departments of Medicine and Pathology, University of Utah Health Sciences Center, Salt Lake City, Utah

Jacob M. Rowe, M.D.
Director, Department of Hematology and Bone Marrow Transplantation, State of Israel—Ministry of Health, Rambam Medical Center, Haifa, Israel

Sandra F. Schnall, M.D.
Associate, Department of Hematology / Oncology, Bryn Mawr Hospital, Bryn Mawr; Associate, Department of Hematology, Thomas Jefferson University Hospital, Philadelphia, Pennsylvania

Ayalew Tefferi, M.D.
Consultant, Division of Hematology and Internal Medicine, Mayo Clinic and Mayo Foundation; Associate Professor, Department of Medicine, Mayo Medical School, Rochester, Minnesota

Stephan D. Thomé, M.D.
Fellow, Department of Hematology and Medical Oncology, Mayo Clinic; Instructor, Department of Internal Medicine, Mayo Graduate School of Medicine, Rochester, Minnesota

PREFACE

The reward for work well done is the opportunity to do more.
Jonas Salk, M.D.

The incentive to proceed with the third edition of the *Manual of Clinical Hematology* was predicated on the success of the first and second editions. Updating the new edition was a more difficult task, however, given the recent explosion of technology in molecular biology and genetics that has had a direct bearing on the specialties of hematology and immunology, and the importance of maintaining this successful concise format of the text. The update information added to the chapters and the addition of the chapter on transplantation to the text will result in a more comprehensive edition that we hope will be more helpful to the reader in his or her quest to establish a firm foundation in hematology. The added chapter on transplantation procedures in hematologic disorders is in keeping with the current aim of more aggressive approaches to the treatment of hematopoietic malignancies.

We have attempted to retain the intended focus and purpose of the book; that is, to provide a concise clinical text—aimed at students, house staff, and medical practitioners not primarily involved in hematology—that describes common hematologic disorders. This publication is not intended to be an all-inclusive hematology text, but rather an introduction to clinical hematology and a readily available source of information upon which the student and physician can build. It is my fervent wish that the book will provide sufficient motivation and excite the curious student or house staff to seek additional, more detailed information from the more comprehensive reference textbooks of hematology.

Many persons have assisted and contributed to this undertaking. I am first indebted to my colleagues in the field of hematology who have so generously contributed their time and expertise to the contents of the text. I am especially grateful to my colleagues at Marshfield Clinic for allowing me sufficient time away from my practice and supplying me with unlimited library, stenographic, and medical illustration support in reviewing and editing the manuscript. Special acknowledgment is extended to Alice Stargardt for her stenographic expertise and prompt transcription of the many manuscripts prepared for the text; to Julie Seehafer for her help and guidance in preparing the appendices; to Stacey Baze for her editorial assistance; and finally, to my wife, Ginny, for her many years of encouragement and support through all my endeavors.

J.J.M.

Manual of
Clinical
Hematology

Third Edition

1. HEMATOPOIESIS AND HEMATOPOIETIC GROWTH FACTORS

Joseph J. Mazza

Development of the Hematopoietic System

Embryonic Life

1. Clusters of mesenchyme, mesodermal cells, on the yolk sac proliferate and expand during early embryonic life (about 2 weeks), forming the nidus of the embryonic and fetal hematopoietic system.

2. Vascular channels develop, allowing a connection to develop between the yolk sac and embryo, thus increasing the space available for further expansion of the mesodermal cells. In addition, the **primitive embryonic circulatory system** forms, and the endothelial cells derived from the early embryonic hematopoietic precursor cells become the lining cells of these primitive vascular channels.

3. **Proliferation** of the early hematopoietic cells occurs as the embryo grows and becomes a fetus (10–12 weeks). The development of a complex network of vascular channels connects vital organs and tissues, allowing for multiplication of the hematopoietic cells and perfusion by blood and lymph.

4. Differentiation of the hematopoietic precursor cells occurs in the immature reticuloendothelial system, which provides the unique microenvironment for proliferation and differentiation.

Fetal Hematopoiesis

1. During early fetal life, after the tenth week of gestation, and through the entire second trimester of pregnancy, the **liver** and the **spleen** are the major sites for hematopoiesis.

2. As gestation continues into the third trimester, the sites of hematopoiesis gradually shift from the liver and spleen to the **medullary cavities of the bones.**

3. By birth, the medullary cavities of the bones are the major site of hematopoiesis, with virtually every bone contributing in this proliferative process and providing mature functional hematopoietic cells to the peripheral circulation.

4. **Pluripotential cells** remain in the other organs of the reticuloendothelial system as hematopoietic "rest cells." These cells retain the potential to become sites of active hematopoiesis at any time later in life, thus giving rise to extramedullary hematopoiesis.

Hematopoietic Stem Cells

Hematopoietic stem cells make up a unique clone of cells that are capable of differentiating into the multiple cell lines of hematopoietic system. Hematopoietic stem cells are believed to be present in all major organs that make up the reticuloendothelial system, as well as in the peripheral blood.

The stem cell clone must sustain itself by proliferation to continue its differentiation into the specialized hematopoietic cell lines. **Stem cell proliferation** is believed to be under direct influence of hematopoietic growth factors that are present in the local milieu of the reticuloendothelial system:

1. Proliferation and differentiation depend not only on growth factors (glycoprotein) but also on stromal cells and other cells that make up the unique microenvironment of the bone marrow.
2. If and when the uncommitted stem cell compartment has been depleted, hematopoiesis ceases. This may occur following exposure to ionizing radiation or high-dose chemotherapy.

Most **evidence for the existence** of these pluripotential stem cells comes from *in vitro* studies and animal models. Such studies have shown regenerative capabilities of the marrow and hematopoietic system after infusion of certain populations of mononuclear cells following complete hematopoietic ablation (Fig. 1).

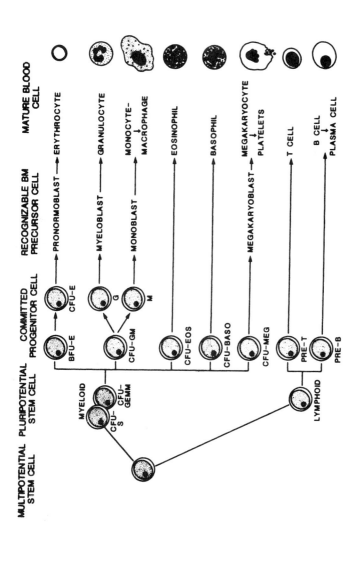

FIG. 1. A model of hematopoietic stem cell differentiation. Illustrated are progenitor cells of increasingly restricted potentiality, which give rise to the maturing cells recognizable in bone marrow preparations as the immediate precursors of peripheral blood elements. BM, bone marrow; CFU, colony-forming unit; S, spleen; GEMM, granulocyte-erythrocyte-monocyte (or macrophage)-megakaryocyte; BFU, burst-forming-unit; EI, erythroid; GM, granulocyte-monocyte (or macrophage); EOS, eosinophil; BASO, basophil; MEG, megakaryocyte. (From Robinson SH. Hematopoiesis. In: Stein JH, ed. *Stein's internal medicine*, 3rd ed. Boston: Little, Brown and Company, 1990, with permission.)

1. Cultured stem cells on agar media grow and differentiate within 5 to 10 days, giving rise to colonies of hematopoietic cells.
2. Given a suspension of mononuclear bone marrow cells, lethally irradiated mice show hematopoietic proliferation in the marrow and spleen.

Only recently have these pluripotential stem cells been identified by surface markers through **cell membrane phenotyping** with monoclonal antibodies (Table 1). Morphologically, they are believed to be similar to large immature lymphocytes and to be diffusely distributed throughout the marrow.

A certain number of the uncommitted pluripotential stem cells will differentiate or become "committed" and give rise to the various myeloid and lymphoid cell lines, thus providing further proliferation and differentiation along the various specific myeloid and lymphoid cell lines.

In early childhood, the medullary cavities of virtually all bones are active sites of hematopoiesis. During adolescence and adulthood, the site of hematopoiesis gradually shifts from the long bones of the skeleton to the more central flat bones (i.e., the skull, vertebrae, ribs, sternum, and pelvis). These flat, more centrally located bones of the skeleton become the major sites of hematopoiesis in the adult.

Kinetics of Hematopoietic Cells

Under normal conditions, all progenitor cells of the various cell lines undergo replication via the cell cycle (i.e., mitosis). Proliferation and differentiation are directly influenced and regulated by low-molecular-weight glycoproteins or hormones that are specific for each lineage of the hematopoietic system (see Appendix Q). These growth factors affect progenitor cells through specific membrane receptors, resulting in activation of the cell and replication and expansion of that precursor cell or lineage (see section entitled **Hematopoietic Growth Factors**). Many factors, in turn, regulate the production and elaboration of the necessary growth factors involved in hematopoiesis. This complex network of various hematopoietic growth factors and hormones, present in the local milieu of the marrow, is currently under careful, extensive investigation and has important therapeutic implications.

Erythropoiesis

Various factors and mechanisms are involved in the regulatory process of production of the new erythrocytes to balance the rate of destruction. In the normal state, the balance of production and destruction is maintained at a remarkably constant rate. Both endocrine and exocrine hormones make important contributions to this dynamic, well-balanced mechanism (Table 2).

The **earliest recognizable erythroid precursor** seen in the bone marrow is a **large basophilic staining cell,** approximately 15 to 20 μm in diameter, which contains a single large, well-defined, round nucleus; ribosomes; mitochondria; and Golgi apparatus (Table 1). As this early precursor cell matures, its nucleus becomes denser and smaller and eventually is extruded into the extracellular matrix of the bone marrow.

As maturation proceeds, the cell becomes progressively smaller and its cytoplasm more eosinophilic, representing increasing amounts of hemoglobin being synthesized from the ribosomes. During **intermediate stages of maturation,** the cytoplasm of the erythroblast is polychromatophilic, indicating the mixture of basophilic cytoplasmic proteins and the eosinophilic hemoglobin. With **further maturation,** hemoglobin synthesis continues, and the cytoplasm becomes entirely eosinophilic. In the **late stages of maturation,** hemoglobin is abundant. Few mitochondria and ribosomes are present in the cytoplasm; a small, dense, well-circumscribed nucleus is apparent.

When the nucleus is extruded, the cell becomes a **reticulocyte,** the last stage of development before it becomes a mature erythrocyte. Shortly thereafter, it acquires a biconcave external contour and specific properties of deformability and pliability. Its diameter is approximately 8 to 9 μm. Most reticulocytes spend 1 to 2 days in the marrow undergoing further maturation before being released into the systemic circulation.

Erythrokinetics

The **turnover rate of circulating erythrocytes** can be calculated easily because the number is constant under normal conditions and their circulating life span is

Table 1. Some immune cell antigens detected by monoclonal antibodies

Antigen designation	Comments
Primary T cell associated	
CD1	Expressed on cortical thymocytes and Langerhans histiocytes
CD2	Present on all T cells (thymic and peripheral) and NK cells
CD3	Expressed by thymocytes, peripheral T cells, and NK cells; surface expression requires coexpression of T-cell receptor
CD4	Expressed on the helper subset of peripheral T cells, single positive medullary thymocytes, and CD4/CD8 double positive thymocytes
CD5	Expressed on all T cells and small subset of B cells
CD6	Expressed on all T cells and subset of myeloid cell precursors
CD8	Expressed on the cytotoxic subset of peripheral T cells, single positive medullary thymocytes, double positive cortical thymocytes, and some NK cells
Primary B cell associated	
CD10	Expressed at high levels on marrow pre-B cells and follicular center B cells; also called CALLA
CD19	Present on marrow pre-B cells and mature B cells but not on plasma cells
CD20	Expressed on marrow pre-B cells after CD19 and mature B cells but not on plasma cells
CD21	EBV receptor; present on mature B cells and follicular dendritic cells
CD22	Present on mature B cells
CD23	Present on activated mature B cells
Primarily monocyte or macrophage associated	
CD13	Expressed on immature and mature monocytes and granulocytes
CD14	Expressed on all monocytes
CD15	Expressed on all granulocytes; also expressed by Reed-Sternberg cells and variants in Hodgkin disease
CD33	Expressed on myeloid progenitors and monocytes
CD117	Found on early myeloid precursors and myeloid leukemic clones
Primarily NK cell associated	
CD16	Present on all NK cells and granulocytes
CD56	Present on all NK cells and a subset of T cells
Primarily stem cell and progenitor cell associated	
CD34	Expressed on pluripotent hematopoietic stem cells and progenitor cells of many lineages
Activation markers	
CD30	Present on activated B cells, T cells, and monocytes
Present on all leukocytes	
CD45	Also known as leukocyte common antigen (LCA)
CD45RO	Expressed on activated memory T cells
CD45RA	Expressed on naïve T cells
Miscellaneous	
CD55	
CD59	Defective in paroxysmal nocturnal hemoglublinura;
CD58	Present on all hematopoietic cells but not lineage specific;
CD40	Expressed on dendritic (antigen-presenting) cells
CD82	

CALLA, common acute lymphoblastic leukemia antigen; CD, cluster designation; EBV, Epstein-Barr virus; NK, natural killer.

Modified from Cotran RS, et al. *Robbins pathologic basis of disease*, 6th ed. Philadelphia: WB Saunders, 1999:654, with permission.

Table 2. Hormones that stimulate erythropoiesis

Growth factors	Other hormones
Stem cell factor	Androgens
Erythropoietin	Corticosteroids
Interleukin-3	Thyroxin
GM-CSF	Prostaglandin E_2
	Growth hormone

GM-CSF, Granulocyte-macrophage colony-stimulating factor.

approximately 120 days. Approximately 20×10^{10} mature erythrocytes are produced and destroyed or undergo hemolysis each day to maintain a normal hemoglobin level.

A small percentage of reticulocytes (1%–2%) are released into the circulation. These cells undergo further maturation in the systemic circulation and the spleen. During that brief period (1–2 days), the reticulocytes lose membrane-coated transferrin and acquire the properties of pliability and reduction in size to make their journey through the peripheral circulatory system more efficient.

Differentiation and maturation from a basophilic erythroblast in the bone marrow occur in approximately 5 to 7 days. Only the early and intermediate-stage erythroblasts (proerythroblasts, basophilic, and polychromatophilic erythroblasts) are capable of undergoing mitosis. Under normal physiologic conditions, approximately 25% of the cells in the bone marrow are erythroid in lineage. All stages of erythroblastic maturation are represented.

During the erythropoiesis, approximately 10% to 15% of the erythroid precursors never completely mature and are destroyed in the bone marrow. Efficient salvage and reutilization of the cellular elements occur during this hemolytic process.

Granulopoiesis

Committed myeloid stem cells further differentiate into three types of granulocytic cells. Under the influence of specific growth factors (hormones) and the appropriate microenvironment, committed stem cells in the marrow eventually rise to neutrophils, eosinophils, and basophils.

The maturation processes of neutrophils, eosinphils, and basophils are similar and probably under the influence of the same growth factors (see section entitled **Hematopoietic Growth Factors**) that stimulate the granulocytic precursor cells.

For **neutrophils,** the process is as follows:

1. The **myeloblast** is the first morphologically recognizable stage of differentiation of the committed granulocyte stem cells. This early precursor cell has a diameter of approximately 15 to 20μm, a low nuclear–cytoplasmic ratio, and no cytoplasmic granules.

2. The **progranulocyte** is the next stage of maturation. This cell is similar in size and appearance to the myeloblast but has numerous small azurophilic, nonspecific granules, called *primary granules,* in the cytoplasm. These primary granules of the neutrophils and their precursors are lysosomal and contain a variety of important enzymes (e.g., myeloperoxidase, acid phosphatase, β-galactosidase, and 5-nucleotidase).

3. At the **myelocyte** stage, secondary or specific granules become apparent in the cytoplasm. They are conspicuous by their increased size and their tinctorial features as compared with the smaller azurophilic primary granules. Secondary cytoplasmic granules contain several potent bactericidal substances (e.g., neuraminidase, lactoferrin, vitamin B_{12}-binding protein).

4. With further maturation, secondary granules become more numerous, the nucleus becomes indented and eventually lobulated, and the nuclear–cytoplasmic ratio increases. Granulocytes also undergo important physical and functional changes, acquiring increased adhesive, motile, and phagocytic properties and becoming less resistant to deformation. These properties allow the more mature granulocytes (band forms and

polymorphonuclear neutrophils) to escape more easily into the marrow sinusoids and eventually into the systemic circulation. These phagocytic cells can exit the systemic circulation and enter the adjacent tissue spaces.

5. Once in the systemic circulation, **mature granulocytes** remain viable for approximately 8 to 12 hours. While in the systemic circulation, many of the granulocytes adhere to the endothelial cells lining the vascular channels. This is referred to as the *marginal compartment* within the systemic circulation. Under certain circumstances, granulocytes can make their way through the walls of the vascular channel and into certain tissues, thus becoming an important component of a host inflammatory response as phagocytic cells. A small but significant percentage of the mature granulocytes remain in the bone marrow as a ready reserve population, called *the marrow storage pool.*

6. Maturation of the committed granulocyte stem cell to a mature neutrophil takes approximately 10 days. Only the early stage forms of maturation are proliferative or undergo mitosis. Metamyelocytes, band forms, and polymorphonuclear neutrophils are postmitotic.

For **eosinphils,** the process is as follows:

1. Other special granulocytes arise from the myeloid stem cell (i.e., eosinophils and basophils) and develop into neutrophils as the result of a similar process of proliferation and differentiation. Although both eosinophils and basophils are phagocytic, they owe their unique function to their special cytoplasmic granules.

2. **Normally, eosinophils make up 2% to 7% of the granulocytes in the peripheral blood.** Their appearance on a peripheral blood smear is conspicuous because of their bright orange-colored **cytoplasmic granules** (secondary). They are able to make their way out of the vascular channels into the tissue, like other granulocytes, and they are responsive to specific chemotactic factors.

3. Eosinophils are **highly specific** in their function and appear to be important cellular components of the host response to parasitic infestation and allergic reactions to foreign antigens (especially in type I reactions). Their numbers also may be increased in some malignant diseases and vasculitis.

4. These large eosinophils cytoplasmic granules are unique in that they contain an arginine-rich alkaline protein called *major basic protein.* This highly alkaline (pH 11) protein is particularly damaging to the cell wall components of many parasites and other microorganisms.

For **basophils,** the process is as follows:

1. Basophils are **specialized granulocytes** that are sparsely present in the peripheral blood (0.5%–1%) compared with other leukocytes. They appear much more frequently in other tissues. Most numerous in the mucosa of the respiratory and gastrointestinal tract, they are indistinguishable from mast cells in these locations.

2. Basophils appear to be the **major cellular element** that participates in **immediate or type I allergic reactions.** Their large, dark-staining eosinphilic cytoplasmic granules are rich in histamine and other mediator substances, which play key roles in this type of allergic response. Basophils may also participate in other types of hypersensitivity reactions (e.g., delayed or type IV response in other species).

Thrombopoiesis

Megakaryocytes are specialized bone marrow cells that differentiate from the myeloid stem cell and are responsible for the production of **platelets.** Platelets are actually cytoplasmic fragments and as such are not complete cellular elements. They are shed from the mature megakaryocytes.

The maturation of megakaryoctyes is believed to occur in three stages:

1. **Basophilic stage.** At this stage, the megakaryocyte is small and contains a diploid nucleus and abundant basophilic cytoplasm.
2. **Granular stage.** Here the nucleus of the megakaryocyte is more polypoid, and the cytoplasm is more eosinophilic and granular.

3. **Platelet-forming or mature stage.** At this point, the megakaryocyte is very large and conspicuous within the bone marrow, with approximately 16 to 32 nuclei. It has an abundance of granular cytoplasm that undergoes the shedding to form platelets.

The maturation of the megakaryoblast is somewhat unique in that the cell is unable to undergo **mitosis,** and the nuclear and cytoplasmic maturation processes do not occur together or on parallel levels. **Proliferation and maturation** appear to be regulated by several hundred factors, interleukin 11 (IL-11), and thrombopoietin, which have only recently been identified and become available for clinical use (see section entitled **Hematopoietic Growth Factors**).

Megakaryocytes may increase in number within the marrow when destruction or sequestration of platelets increases peripherally. Each megakaryocyte is capable of producing thousands of platelets from this unique cytoplasmic shedding process. Individual platelets released into the peripheral blood have life spans of 8 to 10 days. The younger platelets appear larger and less dense in the peripheral circulation than older platelets. The platelet turnover is approximately 35,000 platelets/μL of blood each day.

Lymphopoiesis
Lymphocytes are derived from committed stem cells that originate from the pluripotent hematopoietic stem cell. (Fig. 2) Differentiation depends on a number of cellular as well as hormonal factors in the microenvironment, as with other specialized blood cells derived from this pluripotent stem cell.

Once committed to the lymphoid lineage, this early lymphoid cell further differentiates and gives rise to two major classes of lymphocytes: **B-lymphocytes and T-lymphocytes,** which function cooperatively to form major components of the immune system. These two classes of lymphocytes are distinct subsets and acquire different functions and capabilities as they mature. As they evolve and differentiate, they also become recognizable by a series of membrane "markers" or ligands. Both classes of lymphocytes appear morphologically similar when viewed through the light microscope, however. A third class of lymphocytes, whose role in the immune response has only recently been realized and appreciated, is a small population of non-B, non-T is called null cells.

The **B-lymphocyte** is one of the two major classes of lymphocytes of the immune system:

1. **B-lymphocytes** are referred to as **B cells** because of their functional similarity to lymphocytes that mature in a specialized organ in birds called *the bursa of Fabricius.* Stem cells that migrate to this outpouching of the cloaca proliferate and mature into antibody-producing lymphocytes. Hence, the name *B cells* for bursa cells.

2. The bursa equivalent or analog in more highly evolved species, including humans, has yet to be found. The **bone marrow or fetal liver** may be the organs with the microenvironment necessary for the development of functioning B cells or antibody-producing lymphocytes from uncommitted lymphocytes.

3. **Differentiation into mature B cells** involves a series of complex gene rearrangement steps. The generation of genes necessary for heavy-chain and light-chain production is essential for immunoglobulin production. Maturation culminates with migration of B cells to other lymphoid organs and tissues throughout the body (e.g., spleen, lymph nodes, tonsils, gut, liver), where they remain or circulate freely in the lymph and blood.

4. When **activated or antigenically stimulated,** B-lymphocytes become larger and more metabolically active and undergo blast transformation that culminates in mitotic division. The larger lymphoblastoid cells (12–15 μm in diameter), which become increasingly more efficient in the synthesis and secretion of antibodies, often differentiate into specialized immunoglobulin-producing cells called *plasma cells.*

5. **Plasma cells** are present in the bone marrow, lymphoid organs, and sites of immune response. They are not normally found circulating in blood or lymph. They are believed to be end-stage differentiated cells with little or no capacity to undergo mitosis, plasma cells appear to be the ultimate stage of development for synthesis and secretion of antibody molecules or immunoglobulins.

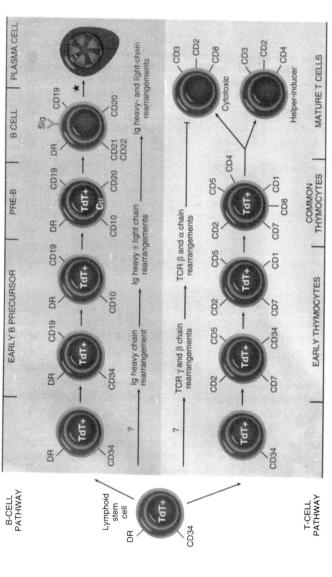

FIG. 2. Schematic illustration of the phenotypic and genotypic changes associated with the differentiation of B cells and T cells. Not shown are some CD4+/CD8+ cells (common thymocytes) that also express CD3. Stages between resting B cells and plasma cells are not depicted. CD, cluster designation; TdT, terminal deoxynucleotidyl transferase; Ig, immunoglobulin; TCR, T-cell receptor. (From Cotran RS, et al. *Robbins pathologic basis of disease,* 6th ed. Philadelphia: WB Saunders, 1999:653, with permission.)

6. B-lymphocytes and plasma cells are the only cells capable of producing immuno-globulins or antibodies.

7. Clones of B cells and plasma cells can expand and contract under the influence of the many regulating factors of the immune system.

The second major class of lymphocyte in the immune system is the **T-lymphocyte**:

1. **T cells,** so named because of their dependence on the thymus gland for their mat-uration and specialized functions, are the second major class of lymphocytes. T cells make up approximately 60% to 70% of the circulating lymphocytes in the peripheral blood and are able to cycle continuously from blood through the lymphoid tissues of the body and return to the blood via the lymphatics.

2. T cells do not synthesize or secrete immunoglobulins. Instead, they secrete pro-teins or hormones called **cytokines (lymphokines),** which function to promote or sup-press the proliferation and differentiation of other T cells, B cells, and macrophages. T cells are the main component of cell-mediated immunity and regulate and coordinate the host immune response.

3. Uncommitted lymphocytes derived from the lymphoid stem cell migrate to the thymus gland, where they undergo **differentiation and maturation** as they pass through the cortical epithelial cells of the thymus. As the lymphocytes (thymocytes) migrate through this unique microenvironment, they acquire and lose antigenic sur-face membrane molecules (Fig. 2). At the final maturation stage, thymocytes differ-entiate into two major subclasses, **helper/effector T lymphocytes** and **suppressor T-lymphocytes,** and are released into the systemic circulation and lymph.

4. Helper T cells and suppressor T cells can be distinguishable by the presence of specific cell-membrane molecules and receptors. These two subtypes of T cells have separate and distinct functions. As the major components of the cell-mediated immune system, they play key roles in regulating and modulating the host immune response.

The **non-B, non-T-lymphocytes (null cells)** are a third, small class of lymphocytes:

1. Non-B, non-T-lymphocytes, or null cells, are **non–antibody-secreting cells** that lack the specific molecules of a thymus-dependent lymphocyte or T cell. **Null cells,** which are larger than average circulating lymphocytes, contain large cytoplasmic granules not seen in the other populations of lymphocytes.

2. Null cells make up only a **small percentage of the circulating lymphocytes** in the blood. They appear to have special unique immunologic function in that they are capable of lysing a variety of tumor- and viral-infected cells through an antibody-mediated mechanism, without overt antigenic stimulation.

3. These large granular lymphocytes are thus called **natural killer (NK) cells.** Their ontogeny and specificity are incompletely understood.

Cluster Differentiation (CD) Antigens
These **surface marker molecules** are cell-membrane proteins (*glycoproteins*) or re-ceptors (*antigens*) that allow identification of multiple cell lines at different stages of maturation (Table 1). Cluster differentiation molecules are present not only on lym-phocytes and other hematopoietic cells but on virtually all cells. Their presence and identification on malignant cells frequently help to provide the necessary information to confirm malignancy of the clone and to determine from what tissue or cell line the malignant clone is derived.

Commercially available catalogs of monoclonal antibodies that correspond to these specific receptors provide information about the phenotype and function of cells.

With perturbation or activation of the cell, these markers or receptors on the surface of various classes and subclasses of lymphocytes **become more numerous and prominent** and tend to cluster on membranes. As lymphocytes undergo matu-ration in the thymus (thymocytes), they acquire and lose surface markers or antigens in the process. Some markers are retained throughout maturation, however, and are present when the T-lymphocytes are released in the peripheral circulation.

T Cells, B Cells, Null Cells, and Macrophages
Along with macrophages (phagocytic antigen-resenting cells), T, B, and null cells all function in concert as a complex immunologic response that provides the host with unique protective mechanisms against invading or foreign antigenic factors that threaten its well-being. Details of the specific functions and identifying molecules of these cellular components of the immune system are beyond the scope of this text, and the reader should refer to larger reference texts on immunology or hematology for more information.

Hematopoietic Growth Factors
Hematopoietic growth factors are a **heterogeneous group of cytokines** that stimulate progenitor cells of the hematopoietic system and induce proliferation and maturation. For the most part, they are **glycoproteins** that are synthesized and elaborated by a variety of cells in the local milieus of the bone marrow (with the exception of erythropoietin). They bind to specific membrane receptors on the surface of the various cells of the hematopoietic system (Fig. 3). These hormones play a critical role in the regu-

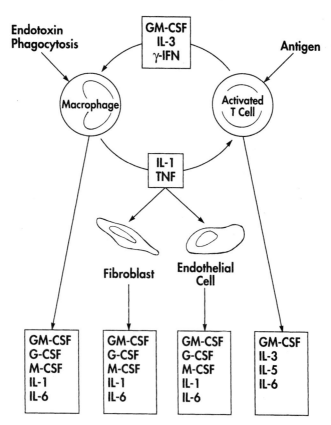

FIG. 3. Regulation of production and cellular sources of colony-stimulating growth factors. IL-3, interleukin-3; γ-IFN, gamma interferon; IL-1, interleukin-1; TNF, tumor necrosis factor; GM-CSF, granulocyte-macrophage colony stimulating factor; G-CSF, granulocyte colony-stimulating factor; M-CSF, macrophage colony-stimulating factor; IL-5, interleukin-5; IL-6, interleukin-6. (From Groopman JE, Molina JM, Scadden DT. Hematopoietic growth factors: biology and clinical applications. *N Engl J Med* 1998; 321:1449–1459, with permission.)

lation of all hematopoietic cells in health and disease. The interaction of the stem cell and progenitor cells with marrow stromal cells is poorly understood, but it is believed that these stromal cells are an important source of a variety of cytokines. By themselves, colony-stimulating factors (CSFs) are not sufficient to maintain hematopoiesis *in vitro*. The cells of the microenvironment of the bone marrow thus appear to play a critical role in the ongoing process of replication and maturation of hematopoietic cells.

Common Characteristic and Properties (Fig. 3)
1. Naturally occurring hormones (all)
2. Low-molecular-weight glycoproteins that must bind to a specific cell membrance ligand to function (most)
3. Variable degree of species specificity
4. Available in purified form through recombinant DNA technology (many)
5. Responsible for the stimulation and release of other growth factors and cytokines that, in turn, induce or suppress production of many other cytokines (some)

Major Hematopoietic Growth Factors
1. **Erythropoietin,** which is **synthesized by the peritubular cells of the kidney** in response to hypoxemia, is always present in minute amounts in human urine. The gene that encodes for this glycoprotein (approximately 30 kDa) is located on chromosome 7 (C7, q11-22). Approximately 10% of endogenous erythropoietin is secreted by the liver. This is responsible for the low-level erythroid activity in anephric persons. The plasma half-life of erythropoietin in anemic patients, which is 6 to 9 hours, shortens with continued therapy. Erythroid response seems to be dose dependent.

2. **Interleukin-3 (IL-3)** is produced by **T-lymphocytes,** and this factor is not lineage specific. The gene that encodes for IL-3 is located on chromosome 5 (C5, q23-31). This factor **appears to stimulate production and renewal of the pluripotent stem cell compartment** and is capable of stimulating pluripotent hematopoietic stem cells to differentiate into all the myeloid cell lines and perhaps lymphocytes. Synergism between Il-3 and granulocyte-macrophage colony-stimulating factor (GM-CSF) and macrophage colony-stimulating factor (M-CSF) has been demonstrated.

3. **Granulocyte-macrophage colony-stimulating factor (GM-CSF)** is synthesized and secreted by a variety of cells in the bone marrow microenvironment: stromal cells, fibroblasts, T cells, and endothelial cells. The gene that encodes for GM-CSF is located on chromosome 5 (C5, q) adjacent to genes that encode for other cytokines. This factor stimulates growth of progenitors for granulocytes, monocytes, and erythrocytes, and often causes eosinophilia as well. It activates granulocytes and monocytes and macrophages and enhances phagocytosis and other functions of these cells. The effect of GM-CSF appears to be dose dependent.

4. **Granulocyte colony-stimulating factor (G-CSF)** is a **potent, low-molecular-weight glycoprotein** that stimulates proliferation and maturation of granulocyte precursors. Stromal cells, monocytes and macrophages, and endothelial cells produce this factor. The gene that encodes for G-CSF is located on chromosome 17 (C17, q11-21). Within 48 hours after administration, the number of circulating granulocytes (neutrophils) dramatically increases. The effect appears to be lineage specific and dose dependent.

5. **Macrophage colony-stimulating factor (M-CSF)** is secreted by stromal cells, macrophages, and fibroblasts. A **heavily glycosylated glycoprotein,** M-CSF exists in a dimer and is encoded for by a gene located on chromosome 5 (C5, q33). It is a potent stimulator of macrophage function and activation, resulting in stimulation and elaboration of other cytokines. M-CSF leads to increased expression of major histocompatibility complex (MHC) class II antigen on macrophages and enhanced cytotoxicity. A slight to modest increase in white blood cells is seen after administration. M-CSF may have important implications for future biotherapy programs in the treatment of cancer.

6. **Interleukin-2 (IL-2) or T-cell growth factor (TCGF)** is synthesized and secreted by activated T cells, primarily helper-T cells (CD 4 and T cells). Primarily, IL-2 leads to the clonal expansion of antigen-specific T cells and the induction of the expression of IL-2 receptors (CD25) on the surface membrane of T cells. This growth factor activates T-cell cytotoxic responses and induces non-MHC restricted cytotoxic lymphocytes. To a lesser degree, it stimulates proliferation of NK cells and B cells.

7. **Interleukin-4 (IL-4) and B-cell stimulating factor (BSF-1),** a **potent growth factor,** is derived from activated T cells and mast cells. The main effect of IL-4 is the induction of proliferation and differentiation of **B cells** and expression of MHC class II antigens on resting B cells. IL-4 also can act on T cells, monocytes and macrophages, mast cells, fibroblasts, and endothelial cells. It may be an important factor in the modulation of host immunity and inflammatory responses *in vitro.*

Other Cytokines that Affect Hematopoiesis

1. **Interleukin-5 (IL-5) or B-cell stimulating factor (BSF-2).** The major source of these growth factors is T cells. This **potent eosinophil differentiation and activation factor** causes a rise in peripheral blood eosinophils. IL-5 stimulates B-cell differentiation and antibody production, and it can induce IL-2 receptor expression and release of soluble Il-2 receptor proteins.

2. **Interleukin-6 (IL-6)** is an important, **multifunctional glycoprotein.** It is produced by lymphoid and nonlymphoid cells and **plays a major role in the mediation of inflammation and immune response.** It is identical to interferon-β2 (IFN-β2) in molecular composition and activities. This growth factor promotes the production of acute-phase proteins and appears to have a stimulating effect on hematopoietic stem cells. It enhances differentiation of B cells and antibody secretion. Apparently, IL-6 is an important growth factor for myeloma cells, and it has been shown to have antiviral activity. This growth factor is also a costimulant of IL-2 production and IL-2 receptor expression of T cells.

3. **Interleukin-7 (IL-7)** is produced by bone marrow stromal cells. Many other tissues express IL-7 (e.g., the spleen, fetal and adult thymus tissue). The human IL-7 gene is located on the long arm of C8, and the gene product (IL-7) is a glycoprotein with a molecular weight of approximately 17 kDa. The receptor molecule for IL-7 appears to be a member of the hematopoietic receptor superfamily. **IL-7 is an important growth and differentiating factor for T cells,** and it may be an important viability factor for immature and nonproliferating thymocytes. This factor, which can stimulate proliferation and differentiation of human T cells, may act synergistically with other lymphokines (IL-2 and IL-6) to stimulate the development of cytolytic T lymphocytes and lymphokine-activated killer cells from CD8 + T cells. Evidence suggests that IL-7 acts synergistically with stem cell factor *in vivo* to stimulate B-cell lineage development. Research has shown that IL-7 stimulates tumoricidal activity of monocytes/macrophages from human peripheral blood, as well as eliciting elaboration of IL-6, IL-1, and tumor necrosis factor alpha (TNF-α).

4. **Interleukin-8 (IL-8)** is a **nonglycosylated protein** with a molecular weight of approximately 8 kDa, is encoded by the long arm of chromosome 4 (C4q). It is produced by a wide variety of cells, and its elaboration can be induced by other proinflammatory molecules or stimuli (e.g., IL-1, TNF, lipopolysaccharides, infectious agents). A **potent chemotactic activating factor for neutrophils,** IL-8 has a wide range of other proinflammatory effects. It causes degranulation of neutrophil specific granules in the presence of cytochalasin B and induces the expression of adhesion molecules by neutrophils. In addition to being chemotactic for neutrophils and enhancing neutrophil adherents, IL-8 has been reported to be chemotactic for T lymphocytes and eosinophils. In addition, it appears to have a significant degree of specificity for binding to neutrophils both *in vitro* and *in vivo.* It will also bind with much less avidity to eosinophils and erythrocytes. Virtually all cells that have receptors for IL-1 or TNF express IL-8 in response to these cytokines.

5. **Interleukin-9 (IL-9)** is synthesized and secreted by T helper cells and is encoded by a gene on chromosomes 5 (C5, q31). This factor **acts synergistically with IL-4 to potentiate antibody production by B cells.** It also stimulates erythroid colony formation and maturation of megakaryocytes *in vitro.* Synergism between IL-9 and Epo is apparent.

6. **Interleukin-10 (IL-10)** is **secreted by T cells and B cells** and is encoded by a gene on chromosome 1. This factor is a **potent immunosuppressant of macrophage function** because of its inhibitory effects on accessory function and antigen-presenting capacity of monocytes and macrophages. In addition, IL-10 can downregulate MHC class II antigen expression on macrophages, and it also inhibits numerous proinflammatory cytokines, including IL-1, TNF, and IL-6.

7. **Interleukin-11 (IL-11)** acts as an **inflammatory mediator** by stimulating the synthesis of hepatic acute phase reactants. This factor increases the number, size, and ploidy values of megakaryocyte colonies *in vitro*. IL-11 has been shown to have synergistic effects on the growth factor activity of IL-3 and IL-4 on early hematopoietic progenitors. It acts synergistically with thrombopoietin to induce megakaryocytic proliferation and maturation resulting in a substantial increase in platelets. Bioactivators of IL-11 are very similar to IL-6; these two cytokines have a common single transducer in their receptor, but they do not compete for receptor binding.

8. **Interleukin-12 (IL-12)** is produced by macrophages and B cells. This factor stimulates the production of interferon-gamma (IFN-γ) from T cells and NK cells and participates in the differentiation of helper T cells. In addition, it enhances the expansion of human helper T cells *in vitro* and augments cell-mediated response to infection by stimulating IL-2 and IFN-γ production (Table 3).

9. **Stem cell factor (SCF) and c-kit ligand** is synthesized and secreted by marrow stromal cells and fetal embryonic tissues. It synergizes with other hematopoietic growth factors that stimulate primitive or early hematopoietic progenitor cells and promotes mast cell proliferation and differentiation along with IL-3 and IL-4 and may have important therapeutic implications in bone marrow hypoplasia and marrow failure situations.

Other Interleukins and Cytokines
Other interleukins and cytokines that may be important contributors to the delicate balance and regulation of hematopoiesis include IL-1, TNF, transforming growth factor, and several of the interferons. IL-1, an important mediator of inflammation released by activated macrophages, is of particular importance because it suppresses erythroid production and leads to anemia in patients with infection or inflammatory disorders (see Chapter 2, section on **Anemia of Chronic Disease**). Its suppressive effect on the bone marrow can be potentiated by other cytokines such as TNF and IFN-γ.

Through recombinant DNA technology, many of these cytokines have become available in sufficient quantities to allow clinical studies to be performed. These studies will provide more information about the specificity, toxicity, and efficacy of various cytokines.

Some of these factors have even become commercially available for limited clinical use (Table 3). As additional information is compiled from clinical trials, it seems reasonable to predict that more of these specific agents will become available to the clinician and the indications for their use expanded.

Table 3. Commercially available hematopoietic
growth factors and approved clinical uses

Factor	Clinical uses
Recombinant human granulocyte-macrophage colony-stimulating factor (sargramostim [Leukine, Prokine])	Acceleration of myeloid recovery in patients with non-Hodgkin lymphoma, acute lymphoblastic leukemia, and Hodgkin disease who are undergoing autologous bone marrow transplantation
Recombinant human granulocyte colony-stimulating factor (filgrastim [Neupogen])	Neutropenia in nonmyeloid malignant disease in patients receiving myelosuppressive drugs or chemotherapy
Recombinant human erythropoietin (Epogen, Procrit)	Anemia of chronic renal disease (in predialysis and dialysis-dependent patients)
	Treatment of anemia in cancer patients on chemotherapy
	Anemia associated with HIV infection
Interleukin-2 (Proleukin)	Advanced renal cell carcinoma
Recombinant interleukin-11 (Neumega)	Treatment of severe thrombocytopenia due to myelosuppressive chemotherapy in patients with nonmyeloid malignancies

Suggested Readings
Hematopoiesis
Abbas AK, Lichtman AH, Pober JS, eds. *Cellular and molecular immunology.* Philadelphia: WB Saunders, 1991.
Andrew M, Paes B, Johnston M. Development of the hemostatic system in the neonate and young infant. *Am J Pediatr Hematol Oncol* 1990;12:95–104.
Brown BA, ed. Hematopoiesis. In: *Hematology: principles and procedures,* 5th ed. Philadelphia: Lea & Febiger, 1988:31–78.
Christensen RD. Hematopoiesis in the fetus and neonate. *Pediatr Res* 1989;26:531–535.
Dacie JV, White JC. Erythropoiesis with particular reference to its study by biopsy of human bone marrow; review. *J Clin Pathol* 1949;2:1–32.
Dessypris EN, Graber SE, Krantz SB, et al. Effects of recombinant erythropoietin on the concentration and cyling status of human marrow hematopoietic progenitor cells *in vivo. Blood* 1988;72:2060–2062.
Fauser AA, Messner HA. Granuloerythropoietic colonies in human bone marrow, peripheral blood and cord blood. *Blood* 1978;52:1243–1248.
Finne PH, Halvorsen S. Regulation of erythropoiesis in the fetus and newborn. *Arch Dis Child* 1972;47:683–687.
Gregory CJ, Eaves AC. Three stages of erythropoietic progenitor cell differentiation distinguished by a number of physical and biologic properties. *Blood* 1978;51:527–537.
Halvorsen K. Regulation of erythropoiesis in the fetus and neonate. In: Nakao K, Fisher JW, Takaku F, eds. *Proceedings of the Fourth International Conference on Erythropoiesis.* Baltimore: University Park Press, 1975.
Hesseldahl, H, Larsen FJ. Hemopoiesis and blood vessels in human yolk sac: an electron microscopic study. *Acta Anat (Basel)* 1971;78:274–294.
Kay NE, Douglas SD. Morphology and antigenic phenotypes of human blood lymphocytes. In: Williams WJ, Beutler E, Erslev AJ, et al., eds. *Hematology,* 4th ed. New York: McGraw-Hill, 1990: 905–918.
Kipps TJ, Meisenholder G, Robbins BA. New developments in flow cytometric analyses of lymphocyte markers. *Clin Lab Med* 1992;12:237–275.
Koury MJ, Bondurant MC, Atkinson JB. Erythropoietin control of terminal erythroid differentiation: maintenance of cell viability, production of hemoglobin, and development of the erythrocyte membrane. *Blood Cells* 1987;13:217–226.
Miale JB, ed. The reticuloendothelial system. I. Hemopoiesis. In: *Laboratory medicine hematology,* 6th ed. St Louis: Mosby, 1982:1–34.
Nakahata T, Gross AJ, Ogawa MA. A stochastic model of self-renewal and commitment to differentiation of the primitive hematopoietic stem cells in culture. *J Cell Physiol* 1982;113:455–458.
Nienhuis AW, Benz EJ Jr. Regulation of hemoglobin synthesis during the development of the red cell. *N Engl J Med* 1977;297:1318,1371,1430.
Paraskevas F, Foerster J. The lymphocytes. In: Lee GR, Wintrobe MM, eds. *Wintrobe's clinical hematology,* 9th ed. Philadelphia: Lea & Febiger, 1993:354–430.
Porter Pharr P, Ogawa M. Pluripotent stem cells. In: Golde DW, Takaku F, eds. *Hematopoietic stem cells.* New York: Marcel Dekker, 1985.
Prindull G. Maturation of cellular and humoral immunity during human embryonic development. *Acta Paediatr Scand* 1974;63:607–615.
Robinson WA, Mangalik A. The kinetics and regulation of granulopoiesis. *Semin Hematol* 1975;12:7–25.
Stohlman F. Kinetics of erythropoiesis. In: Gordon AS, ed. *Regulation of Hematopoiesis,* vol 1. New York: Appleton-Century-Crofts, 1970.
Weiss L, ed. *The blood cells and hematopoietic tissues,* 2nd ed. New York: Elsevier, 1984.
Wickramasinghe SN, ed. *Human bone marrow.* Philadelphia: Blackwell Scientific Publications, 1975.
Zanjani ED, Poster J, Burlington H, et al. Liver as the primary site of erythropoieting in the fetus. *J Lab Clin Med* 1977;89:640–644.

Hematopoietic Growth Factors
Alderson MR, Sassenfeld HM, Widmer MB. Interleukin 7 enhances cytolytic T lymphocyte generation and induces lymphokine-activated killer cells from human peripheral blood. *J Exp Med* 1990;172:577–587.

Bruno E, Hoffman R. Effect of interleukin-6 on *in vitro* human megakaryocytopoiesis: its interaction with other cytokines. *Exp Hematol* 1989;17:1038–1043.

Davis I, et al. Pharmacokinetic and clinical studies of interleukin-4 (IL-4) in patients with malignancy. *Proc Am Soc Clin Oncol* 1991;10:287(abst).

de Waal MR, Haanen J, Spits H, et al. Interleukin 10 (IL-10) and viral IL-10 strongly reduce antigen-specific human T cell proliferation by diminishing the antigen-presenting capacity of monocytes via downregulation of class II histocompatibility complex expression. *J Exp Med* 1991;174:915.

Dexter TM, Spooncer E. Growth and differentiation in the hematopoietic system. *Annu Rev Cell Biol* 1987;3:423–441.

Eschbach JW, Egrie JC, Downing MR, et al. Correction of the anemia of end-stage renal disease with recombinant human erythropoietin. *N Engl J Med* 1987;316:73–78.

Fiorentino DF, Zlutnik A, Vieira P, et al. IL-10 acts on the antigen-presenting cell to inhibit cytokine production by Th1 cells. *J Immunol* 1991;146:344–345.

Graber SE, Krantz SB. Erythropoietin and the control of red cell production. *Annu Rev Med* 1978;29:51–66.

Groopman JE, Molina JM, Scadden DT. Hematopoietic growth factors: biology and clinical applications. *N Engl J Med* 1989;321:14491459.

Hirano T, Akira S, Taga T, et al. Biological and clinical aspects of interleukin 6. *Immunol Today* 1990;11:443–449.

Howard M, O'Garra A, Ishida H, et al. Biological properties of interleukin 10. *J Clin Immunol* 1992;12:239–247.

Imai Y, Nara M, Tohda S, et al. Antiproliferative and differentiative effects of recombinant interleukin-4 on a granulocyte colony-stimulating factor-dependent myeloblastic leukemic cell line. *Blood* 1991;78:471–478.

Kitamura T, Sato N, Arai K, et al. Expression cloning of the human IL-3 receptor cDNA reveals a shared beta subunit for the human IL-3 and GM-CSF receptors. *Cell* 1991;66:1165–1174.

Lacombe C, Da Silva JL, Bruneval P, et al. Peritubular cells are the site of erythropoietin synthesis in the murine, hypoxic kidney. *J Clin Invest* 1988;81:620–623.

Manes KRT, et al. Treatment of the anemia of rheumatoid arthritis with recombinant human erythropoietin: clinical and *in vitro* results. *Blood* 1987;70(Suppl 1):139A.

Mazza JJ, Reding DJ, Plank GS. Hematopoietic growth factors. A promising future for use in bone marrow dysfunction. *Postgrad Med* 1992;91:299–302.

Moore MA. *In vivo* and *in vitro* action of hematopoietic colony stimulating factors. *Proc Am Assoc Cancer Res* 28:466, 1987.

Oster W, Schulz G. Interleukin 3: Biological and clinical effects. *Int J Cell Cloning* 1991;9:5–23.

Quesniaux VF. Interleukins 9, 10, 11 and 12 and kit ligand: a brief overview. *Res Immunol* 1992;43:385–400.

Paul SR, Schendel P. The cloning and biological characterization of recombinant human interleukin 11. *Int J Cell Cloning* 1992;10:135–143.

Paul WE. Interleukin-4: a prototypic immunoregulatory lymphokine. *Blood* 1991;77:1859–1870.

Renauld JC, et al. Cloning and expression of a cDNA for the human homolog of mouse T cell and mast cell growth factor P40. *Cytokine* 1990;2:9–12.

Robinson BE, Quesenberry PJ. Hematopoietic growth factors: overview and clinical applications. *Am J Med Sci* 1990;300:163–170.

Scott P. IL-12. Initiation cytokine for cell-mediated immunity. *Science* 1993;260:496–497.

Street NE, Mosmann TR. IL4 and IL5: the role of two multifunctional cytokines and their place in the network of cytokine interactions. *Biotherapy* 1990;2:347–362.

Takatsu K, Tominaga A, Harada N, et al. T cell-replacing factor (TRF)/interleukin 5 (IL-5): molecular and functional properties. *Immunol Rev* 1988;102:107–135.

Teshima H, Ishakawa J, Kitayama H, et al. Clinical effects of recombinant human granulocyte colony-stimulating factor leukemia patients: a phase II study. *Exp Hematol* 1989;17:853–858.

Tushinski RJ, McAllister IB, Williams DE, et al. The effects of interleukin 7 (IL-7) on human bone marrow *in vitro*. *Exp Hematol* 1991;19:749–754.

Wersall P, Masucci G, Mellstedt H. Interleukin-4 augments the cytotoxic capacity of lymphocytes and monocytes in antibody-dependent cellular cytotoxicity. *Cancer Immunol Immunother* 1991;33:45–49.

Williams DE, Straneva JE, Cooper S, et al. Interactions between purified murine colony-stimulating factors (natural CSF-1, recombinant GM-CSF, and recombinant IL-3) on the *in vitro* proliferation of purified murine granulocyte-macrophage progenitor cells. *Exp Hematol* 1987;15:1007–1012.

Winearls CG, Oliver DO, Pippard MJ, et al. Effect of human erythropoietin derived from recombinant DNA on the anemia of patients maintained by chronic haemodialysis. *Lancet* 1986;2:1175–1178.

2. THE ANEMIAS

Iron-deficiency Anemia

Virgil F. Fairbanks

The term *iron-deficiency anemia* is self-defining: It implies that anemia is due to a less than normal quantity of iron (Fe) in the body. The disorder has a long and interesting history, and many ambiguous terms have been considered synonymous. These include *hypochromic microcytic anemia, idiopathic hypochromic anemia, chlorosis, secondary anemia,* and *milk anemia.* All such imprecise terms should be avoided. *Iron-deficient erythropoiesis* is not synonymous with *iron-deficiency anemia* and should be avoided because it is easily misunderstood. Iron deficiency can often be demonstrated in the absence of anemia, especially in young women. *Iron depletion* denotes an earlier stage of iron deficiency, when iron stores have vanished but serum iron concentration and blood hemoglobin concentration are normal.

Iron Metabolism
Iron Compartments
Hemoglobin is normally the largest iron compartment of the body. It is 0.34% iron by weight. Thus, in an adult, the total iron content of the hemoglobin compartment is about 2 g, depending in part on sex and body size (Table 1).

Storage iron exists in two forms, either as ferritin or as hemosiderin. The storage compartment in men normally contains about 1,000 mg of iron. The storage iron is quite variable in women, ranging from 0 to about 500 mg. About one third of healthy young women have no significant amount of iron in the storage compartment. Most of the storage iron is in cells of the reticuloendothelial system of the liver, spleen, lymph nodes, and bone marrow, but nearly all nucleated cells of the body contain some storage iron.

1. **Ferritin** is a water-soluble iron storage protein. It consists of a spherical, hollow protein called **apoferritin** and a crystalline core that occupies the hollow interior of apoferritin. The crystal is a lattice of hundreds or thousands of ferrihydrite ($Fe_2O_3 \cdot 9H_2O$) molecules. The average ferritin molecule normally contains about 2,500 iron atoms in its interior crystal. Within the cytosol, ferritin acts as an iron buffer. When the cell has a surfeit of iron, Fe^{2+} readily enters pores in the apoferritin shell, is oxidized to Fe_2O_3, and is added to the interior $(Fe_2O_3 \cdot 9H_2O)_x$ crystal. Conversely, when the cell lacks sufficient iron for its metabolic needs, iron is readily released from the ferrihydrite crystal and passes out through apoferritin pores into the cytosol.

2. **Hemosiderin** is a water-insoluble derivative of ferritin. It is aggregated ferritin, partially stripped of the apoferritin component. Hemosiderin iron turnover is presumed to be less rapid than that of ferritin.

Transport iron is the iron bound to transferrin in plasma. This is the mechanism of iron exchange between storage iron or iron absorbed from the gastrointestinal tract and erythropoietic bone marrow. **Transferrin** is a protein of approximately 80,000 Da. Each molecule of apotransferrin can bind two atoms of trivalent iron. Normally, approximately one third of these Fe-binding sites are occupied at any time. Cell membranes contain **transferrin receptor,** which binds Fe^{3+}-transferrin. Transferrin receptor is particularly abundant on the surface of erythrocyte precursors. A small amount of soluble transferrin receptor is in blood plasma. Iron is taken into cells by internalization of the entire Fe^{3+}-transferrin–transferrin-receptor complex. The transport iron compartment is estimated by measurement of the serum iron concentration. The transferrin concentration in plasma usually is estimated by measurement of the total iron-binding capacity (TIBC). It also can be measured immunologically. Normally, the transport iron compartment contains approximately 3 mg of iron.

Table 1. Iron compartments in normal man[a]

Compartment	Iron content (mg)	Total body iron (%)
Hemoglobin iron	2,000	67
Storage iron (ferritin, hemosiderin)	1,000	27
Myoglobin iron	130	3.5
Labile pool	80	2.2
Other tissue iron	8	0.2
Transport iron	3	0.08

[a] These values represent estimates for an "average" person, that is, 70 kg weight, 177 cm (70 in.) height. They are derived from data in several sources.
From Fairbanks VF, Beutler E. Iron metabolism. In: Beutler E, Lichtman MA, Coller BS, et al., eds. *Williams' hematology,* 6th ed. New York: McGraw-Hill, 2001:195–304, with permission.

Myoglobin iron: Skeletal and cardiac muscle cells contain myoglobin, and the iron in this compartment normally amounts to about 130 mg.

Other tissue iron denotes iron that is part of enzymes, cytochromes, and myoglobin. Normally, a few milligrams of iron are bound to various enzymes and cytochromes. Ribonucleotide reductase is an iron-dependent enzyme that is required for synthesis of DNA. Approximately one half of the enzymes of the Krebs cycle contain iron or require it as a cofactor. Aconitase is an enzyme that catalyzes the interconversion of citric, iso-citric, and *cis*-aconitic acids at an early stage of the Krebs cycle. Each molecule of aconitase contains four iron atoms in an iron–sulfur cluster. When iron is in short supply, aconitase loses one of its four iron atoms. It then becomes the iron-regulatory protein, or IRP, that interacts with iron-responsive elements of messenger RNA to stimulate ribosomal synthesis of apotransferrin, transferrin receptor, delta amino levuelulinic acid synthase, and other proteins that are important in iron metabolism. Thus are iron metabolism and energy metabolism intricately intertwined. Many of the iron-dependent enzymes become iron depleted quite readily, and some of the clinical effects of iron deficiency are due to reduction in function of iron enzymes rather than to reduction in oxygen transport consequent to anemia.

The **labile iron pool** is not defined anatomically or functionally, but by analysis of data obtained in plasma iron clearance studies. The labia pool may represent either iron in the extravascular component of the intercellular fluid, such as lymph or iron that rapidly exchanges between plasma and cytosol, or both. Normally, the labile iron pool has approximately 80 mg of iron.

Absorption

Limited absorption of iron occurs at all levels of the intestinal tract, but absorption is most efficient in the duodenum. Inorganic iron must be in the divalent state for absorption to occur, although heme is absorbed together with its ferric component. The **amount** of iron absorbed increases with the dose of iron ingested, although the **percent** absorbed declines as the dose increases. Large doses of iron do not "block" iron absorption. In healthy persons, approximately 10% of the dietary iron is absorbed. In men, this amounts to about 1 mg daily. Ascorbic acid, gastric HCl, and mucin facilitate iron absorption. The proportion of iron absorbed is increased when there is anemia or accelerated erythropoiesis and decreased when there is bone marrow hypoplasia. The effect of alcohol ingestion on iron absorption is controversial; studies have yielded conflicting results. The physiologic mechanisms that regulate iron absorption are poorly understood.

Utilization and Catabolism

Major pathways of iron metabolism are shown in Fig. 1. Normal erythrocytes remain in circulation for about 4 months. By the end of that time, they are old and worn out (senescent) and must be removed, destroyed, and replaced. The signal for their removal and destruction is the appearance on the erythrocyte membrane of a protein called *erythro-*

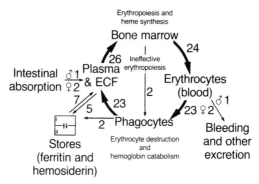

FIG. 1. The major pathways of iron metabolism. Numerals indicate milligrams of iron that normally enter or leave each compartment daily. Differences are also shown for male (♂) and female (♀) subjects. The milligrams of iron shown are only approximate; normal persons differ according to body size, sex, and other variables. Iron stores are represented as consisting of two distinct pools, designated I and II. The iron in pool I exchanges readily with plasma iron, but that of pool II exchanges very slowly. ECF, extracellular fluid.

cyte senescent antigen. Normally, about 25 mL of senescent erythrocytes are destroyed daily by phagocytic macrophages of the reticuloendothelial system. In these cells, hemoglobin is digested. The globin is digested, and the amino acids are reutilized. The heme is further degraded to bilirubin and excreted by the liver, but the iron is salvaged and recycled. Because 25 mL of erythrocytes contains approximately 25 mg of iron, the destruction of senescent erythrocytes releases about 25 mg of iron daily. About 80% of the iron released each day by hemoglobin catabolism is promptly reincorporated into newly formed hemoglobin. A portion of the rest is incorporated into other iron compounds in other tissues, but most is retained in the reticuloendothelial system as storage iron. To make up for the daily loss of about 25 mL of erythrocytes, approximately 25 mg of iron must be incorporated into newly synthesized hemoglobin, and 25 mL of newly formed erythrocytes must be released each day from the bone marrow into the circulating blood. About 20 mg of the needed iron comes from hemoglobin catabolism. The rest comes from iron stores or iron absorption. Effective utilization of iron requires the following:

1. Iron transport by transferrin
2. Binding of the transferrin–Fe^{+3} complex by transferrin receptor on the cell membrane of erythrocyte precursors in bone marrow
3. Internalization of the transferrin–Fe^{+3}–transferrin receptor complex into the cytosol
4. Release of Fe^{+3} from transferrin within the cytosol
5. Reduction of Fe^{+3}
6. Intracellular transport of Fe^{+2} to mitochondrial membranes
7. Internalization of iron by mitochondria
8. Formation of heme from protoporphyrin and iron within the mitochondria
9. Release of heme from mitochondria to cytosol
10. Incorporation of heme into hemoglobin. When sufficient hemoglobin has been formed, the cell extrudes its nucleus and is then released into the circulating blood.

Excretion

Very little iron is excreted by normal persons. Healthy adult males lose about 1 mg each day, mostly as hemoglobin, storage iron in desquamated intestinal epithelial cells, and erythrocytes in feces. Negligible amounts of iron are excreted in sweat and urine.

Sources of Iron

Although our physical environment exposes us all to vast quantities of iron, our food is generally iron poor, and our bodies conserve iron as if it were a trace element. Before the era of abundant aluminum, stainless steel, and plastic, much dietary iron came from cooking utensils. This is no longer true. There is virtually no release of iron into food, even from stainless steel. Foods that are relatively rich in iron include liver, oysters, and legumes. Beef, lamb, pork, poultry, and fish are only fair sources of iron. Cereals and flour, even though iron fortified, provide little absorbable iron because the iron is added at the mill as a finely powdered metal that cannot be absorbed until it has been converted first to Fe^{+3}, then to Fe^{+2}, and most of the ionic iron so formed is chelated by phytates in the cereal or flour. Most fruits and dairy products have negligible iron. Contrary to folk wisdom, spinach and raisins are poor sources of iron. In the United States, there has been, over the past several decades, a marked increase in the consumption of dairy products, cereal, and snack foods, poor sources of dietary iron, and a decrease in the consumption of iron-adequate food.

Prevalence of Iron Deficiency

Approximately two billion people, a third of the world's population, are believed to be iron deficient. In North America as well, iron deficiency is one of the most common organic disorders of humans; it is unquestionably the most frequent hematologic disorder. It occurs most commonly in children, poor people, and women of all ages. Surveys by the National Center for Health Statistics, of the U.S. Public Health Service, have shown significant declines in hemoglobin concentration, hematocrit, and red blood cell count (RBC) for U.S. adults since 1960, declines especially pronounced in African-American males and women, irrespective of ethnic origin. These trends, as yet unexplained, may reflect declines in the quality of iron nutrition in the U.S. population.

Children

Iron deficiency is common in children because their iron needs often exceed the amount of iron they can absorb from food during their rapid growth. This is particularly true of children who remain on a diet entirely of milk beyond the first few months of age.

Women

Iron deficiency is common in young women because many lose iron at twice the rate or more than do men as a consequence of menstruation and loss of blood at childbirth, and yet their iron intake is less than that of men. Among healthy young white women, at least one third have no demonstrable iron stores. Iron deficiency is common in older women who may not have compensated for the loss of iron earlier in life.

Lower Socioeconomic Groups

Iron deficiency is common among lower socioeconomic groups because their dietary sources of iron are poor (carbohydrates compose most of their diets). Furthermore, a large proportion of the world's poor people are living in tropical areas, where hookworm infestation is common. In many areas of Latin America, Africa, and India, iron-deficiency is nearly universal and iron deficiency anemia is prevalent.

African-Americans

Until a decade ago, iron deficiency was thought to be very prevalent among African-Americans because their mean hemoglobin concentration is below that for whites and also because erythrocyte microcytosis is common in African-Americans. The median value of blood hemoglobin concentration is about 1 g per deciliter lower in African-American persons who are not iron deficient than it is in whites. Twenty-eight percent of African-Americans have a mild form of α-thalassemia that is not associated with microcytosis, but about 3% of African-Americans are homozygous for this β-thalassemia and have microcytosis that is due not to iron deficiency but to thalassemia. Furthermore, about 1% of African-Americans have β-thalassemia trait and microcytosis due to this condition. If only because of the prevalence of thalassemias among African-Americans, at least 1 of every 25 may be expected to have microcytosis. Thus, in health surveys of African-Americans, hemoglobin concentration and mean corpuscular volume (MCV) cannot be relied on to indicate the prevalence of iron-deficiency anemia.

Southeast Asians
Because nearly half of southeast Asians have either α-or β-thalassemia or hemoglobin E in various combinations and these conditions cause microcytosis, MCV also cannot be used as an index of iron deficiency in southeast Asians.

Regular Blood Donors
Regular blood donors commonly are iron depleted unless they take iron supplements. (Most U.S. blood banks do not provide iron supplements.)

Elderly Persons
Iron-deficiency anemia is common in elderly persons as a result of chronic gastrointestinal bleeding.

Adverse Effects of Iron Deficiency
Many of the adverse effects of iron deficiency on cells of different tissues are not due to reduced oxygen transport.

Immunologic and Cellular Mechanisms
The immunologic and cellular mechanisms of defense against infection are impaired. Phagocytosis and killing of bacteria are impaired, but these impairments may be offset by reduced bacterial proliferation in an iron poor host. Bacteria depend on the iron of the host for their metabolic needs. The net effect is variable.

Brain and Motor Function
Rats that are iron depleted, but not anemic, have impaired exercise tolerance, which has been attributed to reduced activity of α-glycerophosphate dehydrogenase in skeletal muscle. Dysfunction of this enzyme has been disputed. Similar studies in humans have not yielded consistent results. Brain monoamine oxidase activity is reduced in iron-deficient animals. Iron deficiency in human infants is associated with disturbances in motor function and in attention span.

Epithelial Changes
The oral and buccal epithelium exhibits thinning and dyskeratotic changes in iron-deficient humans, and these changes may occur in the absence of anemia. The epithelial changes may cause fissuring at the corners of the mouth and glossitis, and web formation at the cricoid level of the hypopharynx.

Postcricoid Carcinoma
There is controversy about whether postcricoid carcinoma of the hypopharynx is a complication of chronic iron deficiency.

Koilonychia
Koilonychia, or spoon nails, a rare manifestation of chronic iron deficiency in North America. It also reflects a reduction of tissue iron rather than the effect of anemia. Other effects of iron deficiency include those that occur with anemias in general.

Causes of Iron Deficiency
Dietary
   1. **In infants and young children,** iron deficiency occurs when the body's net gain of iron is insufficient for growth. Often not enough iron is ingested. Loss of iron through bleeding also reduces the net gain of iron.
   2. **In adults,** dietary deficiency is very rarely the principal cause of iron deficiency, although it is a contributory cause in young women, especially with the marked decline in quality of iron nutrition in the United States during the past 20 to 40 years.

Blood Loss
Iron deficiency in adults must always be presumed to reflect bleeding (Table 2):

Table 2. Sources of blood loss

Respiratory tract
  Carcinoma
  Epistaxis
  Idiopathic pulmonary hemosiderosis
  Infections
  Telangiectases
Alimentary tract
  Esophagus
    Varices
  Stomach
    Angiodysplasia
    Antrial vascular ectasia
    Carcinoma
    Gastritis
    Helicobacter pylori
    Hemangioma
    Hiatus hernia
    Hypergastrinemia
    Leiomyoma
    Menetrier disease
    Mucosal hypertrophy
    Ulcer
    Varices
  Small bowel
    Aberrant pancreas
    Angiodysplasia
    Carcinoma
    Helminthiasis
    Hemangioma
    Intussusception
    Leiomyoma
    Meckle diverticulum
    Polyp
    Regional enteritis
    Telangiectasia
    Ulcer
    Vascular occlusion
    Volvulus

  Biliary tract
    Aberrant pancreas
    Carcinoma
    Cholelithiasis
    Intrahepatic bleeding
    Ruptured aneurysm
    Trauma
  Colon
    Amebiasis
    Angiodysplasia
    Carcinoma
    Diverticulum
    Hemangioma
    Polyp
    Telangiectasia
    Ulcerative colitis
  Rectum
    Angiodysplasia
    Carcinoma
    Hemorrhoids
    Ulceration

Genital tract
  Adenomyomas
  Carcinoma
  Inflammatory disease
  Menstruation/menorrhagia
Urinary tract
  Hematuria
  Carcinoma
  Goodpasture disease
  Hemoglobinuria
    March hemoglobinuria
    Paroxysmal cold hemoglobinuria
    Paroxysmal nocturnal hemoglobinuria
  Valvular hemolysis
Phlebotomy
  Blood donation
  Nosocomial
  Self-induced
  Therapeutic (e.g., in polycythemia vera)

From Fairbanks VF, Beutler E. Iron deficiency. In: Beutler E, Lichtman MA, Coller BS, et al., eds. *Williams' Hematology,* 6th ed. New York: McGraw-Hill, 2001:447–470, with permission.

1. **Menstruation** is the most common cause of blood loss in young women. Fibroid tumors of the uterus (adenomyomas) often exacerbate menstrual bleeding.

2. **Pregnancy** also imposes a drain on a woman's iron balance. The total iron cost of pregnancy is about 600 mg. This includes transfer of iron from mother to fetus during pregnancy and blood loss during labor, and it also takes into account the amount of iron saved as menses cease during pregnancy.

3. In men and postmenopausal women, iron deficiency most often reflects **chronic blood loss from the gastrointestinal tract.** Many different anatomic lesions can be responsible. The most common benign lesions are **hemorrhoids, peptic ulcer, large hiatus hernias,** and acquired **vascular anomalies,** such as **angiodysplasia.** The last of these is common in elderly patients and can occur at any level of the alimentary tract, although it is most common in the colon. Significant chronic blood loss may be due to this tiny vascular lesion, which cannot be visualized by barium enema radiography or sigmoidoscopy but may require endoscopy of the ascending colon. Gastrointestinal bleeding also may be due to **diverticula** or benign **polyps** of the colon or malignancy at any level of the alimentary tract. Blood loss that leads to iron deficiency also occurs in **ulcerative colitis** and **Crohn disease. Chronic aspirin use** can cause diffuse bleeding from the stomach. The blood loss is usually slight but can be copious. With the current popularity of long-distance running, a new cause of iron deficiency has become apparent. Many long-distance runners develop mild iron-deficiency anemia as a result of diffuse gastrointestinal bleeding. The amount of blood lost daily is only slight; no specific anatomic lesion has been identified. **Meckel's diverticulum** is a cause of chronic blood loss and iron deficiency, especially in infancy; it is notoriously difficult to diagnose. Scintigraphic studies with pertechnetate often help to demonstrate the diverticulum (Table 2). *Helicobacter pylori* causing chronic hemorrhagic gastritis may be a common cause of iron deficiency and appears to account for the high prevalence of iron deficiency among the Inuits of Alaska, Canada, and Greenland.

4. Bleeding from the respiratory tract can lead to iron deficiency. The blood loss is usually obvious, in the form of hemoptysis; however, small amounts of hemoptysis may be swallowed and thus detected in the feces. This has been observed in **idiopathic pulmonary hemosiderosis,** a condition characterized by chronic or recurrent hemoptysis, recurrent pneumonitis, and iron-deficiency anemia.

5. **Bleeding in the urinary tract** may point to a chronic inflammatory or neoplastic disorder of the bladder or to renal tumor. These conditions are characterized by **hematuria,** that is, increased numbers of erythrocytes in the urine. When there is hematuria, an orthotolidine (e.g., Hemastix, Bayer Corp., Diagnostic Division, Elkhart, IN USA) test for hemoglobin is positive, *and* microscopic examination of urinary sediment shows many erythrocytes:

- Neoplasm of the bladder or kidney can result in persistent significant hematuria that may be gross or microscopic.
- Chronic inflammation of the bladder mucosa can result in significant bleeding.
- Iron-deficiency anemia is also characteristic of paroxysmal nocturnal hemoglobinuria, in which hematuria is not demonstrable (the urine sediment is normal), but the orthotolidine test is often positive.
- Hemoglobinuria that leads to iron deficiency also may result from intravascular hemolysis resulting from faulty aortic valve prosthesis or interventricular septum patch (rarely from other intracardiac or valvular abnormalities).

Impaired Iron Absorption

Iron-deficiency anemia is a frequent aftermath of subtotal gastric resection. In most patients, the cause is impaired absorption of food iron, although medicinal iron is readily absorbed. A small portion of patients have chronic bleeding from recurrent peptic ulcer at the anastomosis site. The rate of blood loss may be only a few milliliters daily and thus difficult to detect. Iron malabsorption may accompany malabsorption of other nutrients, as in the sprue syndrome. Except following gastrectomy, **isolated malabsorption of iron is extremely rare.**

Phlebotomy

Therapeutic phlebotomy or that done for diagnosis when large-volume or repetitive blood sampling is undertaken, may lead to iron deficiency. **Blood donors** are commonly iron deficient (75% of female and 25% of male donors in the Mayo Clinic experience), and some donate repeatedly until they become anemic. Blood bank regulations in the United States permit acceptance of male donors even if they have mild anemia (hemoglobin concentration not <12.5 g/dL). **Autophlebotomy** is a rare cause of iron-deficiency anemia. Most cases are in women. It is extremely difficult to prove and equally difficult to treat.

Clinical Features
Symptoms and signs of iron deficiency include fatigue, palpitations, tinnitus, headache, sore tongue, pallor, glossitis, tachycardia, and "innocent" systolic cardiac murmur. The spleen tip is palpable in about 10% of patients. Koilonychia is apparently common in the United Kingdom but rare in the United States. Whereas some of these symptoms and signs are common to other anemias, koilonychia is not. **Pica** is a symptom that appears to be unique to iron deficiency and may be present before anemia develops. It may be manifested as compulsive ingestion of laundry starch, clay, earth, or ice. Often pica ceases within a few days of inception of treatment. Although many patients with iron deficiency are asymptomatic, they may admit to feeling better after treatment has been started. The lack of symptoms may reflect the very slow development of iron deficiency and the ability of the body to adapt to lower iron reserves and anemia.

Laboratory Features
Of the common laboratory tests, the serum ferritin (SF) concentration is the first to reflect iron deficiency, often when the blood hemoglobin concentration, erythrocyte count, erythrocyte indices, serum iron, TIBC, and erythrocyte morphology are all still normal. Examination of a Prussian blue–stained specimen of bone marrow also confirms iron depletion. As iron deficiency becomes progressively more severe, further abnormalities develop in approximately this sequence: anisocytosis, microcytosis, elliptocytosis, hypochromia, declining blood hemoglobin concentration, low serum iron concentration, and low transferrin saturation. Table 3 compares the costs of some of these tests.

Erythrocyte Morphology
Examination of a stained blood film is an insensitive and imprecise means for diagnosis of iron deficiency because morphologic changes are not early signs of iron deficiency

Table 3. Diagnosis of iron deficiency, comparison of fees (in $) of examinations[a]

Diagnostic test	Cost (U.S.$)
History and physical examination	150.00
CBC (excludes differential)	34.00
Serum iron and TIBC	24.50
Serum ferritin	48.00
Serum transferrin receptor	50.00
Erythrocyte zinc-protoporphyrin	24.00
Occult blood, feces (Hemoquant)	35.00
Review of blood film by physician	95.00
Chest radiograph, PA stereo	100.00
Marrow examination (with iron stain)	407.00
CT scan, abdomen	860.00
Colonoscopy	2,500.00

CBC, complete blood count; CT, computed tomography; PA, posteroanterior; TIBC, total iron-binding capacity.

[a] Approximate fees at a medical center in midwestern United States, July 1999. The fee for marrow examination includes costs of obtaining specimen, paraffin embedding, staining with Wright's stain and Perls' stain for iron, and physician examination. Charge for colonoscopy includes fee for physician service plus fee for administration of Versed and for postexamination recovery room. Costs vary between institutions and between laboratories.

Republished from Fairbanks VF, Beutler E. Iron deficiency. In: Beutler E, Lichtman MA, Coller BS, et al., eds. *Williams' Hematology*, 6th ed. New York: McGraw-Hill, 2001:447–470 with permission.

and because the classic findings of hypochromia and microcytosis are also characteristics of many other disorders.

Mild microcytosis often is not recognized when a blood film is examined microscopically. **Microcytosis** often is accompanied by **poikilocytosis** and **anisocytosis.** **Elliptocytosis** may be slight to marked. There may be elongated, cigar-shaped erythrocytes, inaptly called **pencil cells.** Microcytic erythrocytes are also thinner than normal erythrocytes (i.e., they are **leptocytes**). Thin erythrocytes transmit more light than do normal erythrocytes; hence, they appear hypochromic.

Anisocytosis may be evident on microscopic examination of the stained blood film or by measurement of the variability of erythrocyte size computed by an automated particle counter. Different instruments use various methods to calculate red cell distribution width (RDW) or a red cell morphology index (RCMI). These parameters are not the same, and results cannot be used reliably unless one understands how the calculations are made. A larger-than-normal value for RDW is found more often in iron deficiency than in thalassemia.

Erythrocyte Indices

Erythrocyte indices still are sometimes calculated from measured values of hemoglobin concentration, hematocrit, and RBC, as shown in Table 4. Today, however, in most laboratories, the measurements are made by automated instruments. Most automated instruments measure RBC hemoglobin, and MCV directly and, from these primary data, calculate "indices" as shown in Tables 4 and 5. The change in the methods of measurements and calculations has important practical consequences. With this shift in technology, the mean corpuscular hemoglobin concentration (MCHC) has become a poor indicator of iron-deficiency anemia because it is usually normal except when anemia is severe. Conversely, the MCV has become a much more sensitive indicator of iron-deficiency anemia. The MCV and the mean corpuscular hemoglobin (MCH) show concordant and proportional perturbations. The hematocrit, MCH, and MCHC have become redundant, except in calibration of instruments or monitoring measurements of Hb, RBC, and MCV. For example, when blood is lipemic or when erythrocytes are agglutinated, characteristic anomalies occur in the results of these measurements, and the anomalies can be recognized and analyzed by comparing the measured values (hemoglobin concentration, RBC, and MCV) with the calculated "indices" (Table 6).

Serum Ferritin

The concentration of SF normally reflects the size of the iron storage compartment, and a low value is the most reliable indicator of iron deficiency. Results are strongly influenced, however, by other conditions that commonly coexist with iron deficiency, thereby complicating interpretation of results. Values are increased with chronic inflammatory disease, malignancy, or hepatic injury. Gaucher disease is also characterized by high SF. Therefore, SF may be above normal when iron deficiency coexists with rheumatoid

Table 4. Definition of "erythrocyte indices"

$$MCV(fL) = \frac{Hct}{RBC} \times 10$$

$$MCH(pg) = \frac{Hb}{RBC} \times 10^6$$

$$MCHC\,(g/L) = \frac{Hb}{Hct} \times 0.1$$

$$Hct\,(\%)^a = MCV \times RBC \times 0.1$$

Hb, hemoglobin concentration (in g/d); Hct, hematocrit (in decimal notation); MCH, mean corpuscular hemoglobin; MCHC, mean corpuscular hemoglobin concentration; MCV, mean corpuscular volume; RBC, erythrocyte count/μL.

[a] When MCV is directly measured and Hct is calculated, by some automated instruments.

Table 5. Comparison of erythrocyte measurements and indices[a]

	Manual	Automated
Measured	Hb	Hb
	RBC	RBC
	Hct	*MCV*
Derived ("indices")	*MCV*	*Hct*
	MCH	MCH
	MCHC	MCHC

Hb, hemoglobin concentration; MCH, mean corpuscular hemoglobin; MCHC, mean corpuscular hemoglobin concentration; Hct, hematocrit; MCV, mean corpuscular volume; RBC, erythrocyte count.
[a] Italics emphasize differences. Some automated instruments measure Hct and calculate MCV, thus mimicking manual measurements.

arthritis, Gaucher disease, chronic lymphocytic leukemia, Hodgkin disease, or hepatitis, among many other disorders. Spuriously elevated values for SF also may occur for a few days following ingestion of medical iron or for many weeks after the parenteral administration of iron dextran. As a general rule, SF of 20 µg/L or less should be considered diagnostic of iron deficiency. Higher values are diagnostic of iron deficiency when accompanied by low MCV or anemia, or in the presence of chronic disease. Guyatt and colleagues examined the receiver-operator curve characteristics of SF, RDW, and erythrocyte zinc protoporphyrin (formerly called *free erythrocyte protoporphyrin*). They found that both sensitivity and specificity were quite poor for RDW, somewhat better for erythrocyte zinc protoporphyrin, and excellent for SF. Even at a SF of 40 µg/L, there was a high likelihood of iron deficiency, particularly in the elderly. Beck and associates proposed a bayesian approach to the diagnosis of iron deficiency, in which initial screening used MCV and SF. For various levels of MCV, they defined values of SF that were diagnostic of iron deficiency, values that excluded iron deficiency and values that were indeterminate. Table 7 is based on their data. For results in the intermediate range, additional studies were required, including serum iron, TIBC, and erythrocyte sedimentation rate. More recent studies showed that the serum ferritin assay is not a reliable test for iron deficiency in children.

Serum Iron, Total Iron-binding Capacity, and Transferrin Saturation
Measurement of serum iron concentration and serum TIBC and calculation of percent saturation of transferrin have been widely used for the diagnosis of iron deficiency. Results are often normal in patients with iron-deficiency anemia, however. Furthermore, results are strongly influenced by physiologic variations, concurrent inflammatory disease, and prior ingestion or injection of iron medicine. Thus, these tests have only limited diagnostic value.

Table 6. Spurious erythrocyte indices[a]

Causes	Hb	RBC	Effects: Hct	MCV	MCH	MCHC
Cold agglutinins	—	L	L	H	H	H
Lipemia	H	—	—	—	H	H

Hb, hemoglobin concentration; H, spuriously high; Hct, hematocrit; L, spuriously low; MCH, mean corpuscular hemoglobin; MCHC, mean corpuscular hemoglobin concentration; MCV, mean corpuscular volume; RBC, erythrocyte count; –, not affected.
[a] Pattern of spurious results typical for Coulter counters and some other automated instruments. The usual clue that results are spurious is an impossibly high MCHC, often much >36 g/dL. Thus, the MCHC has value in quality control in the laboratory.

Table 7. Serum ferritin and MCV as indicators of iron deficiency (>95% probability)[a]

MCV, fl	110	100	90	80	70	60	50
Serum ferritin, µg/L							
5	+	Ind	–	–	–	–	–
10	+	Ind	Ind	–	–	–	–
20	+	Ind	Ind	–	–	–	–
30	+	Ind	Ind	Ind	–	–	–
40	+	+	Ind	Ind	–	–	–
50	+	+	Ind	Ind	Ind	–	–
70	+	+	+	Ind	Ind	Ind	–
100	+	+	+	Ind	Ind	Ind	Ind
150	+	+	+	+	Ind	Ind	Ind
200	+	+	+	+	+	Ind	Ind
300	+	+	+	+	+	Ind	Ind
400	+	+	+	+	+	+	Ind

Ind, indeterminate (i.e., iron deficiency cannot be diagnosed or excluded; MCV, mean corpuscular) volume; +, no iron deficiency; –, iron deficiency.
[a] Readers must interpolate for intervening values of MCV and serum ferritin, or consult the original article.
From Beck JR, et al. The iron screen. *Hum Pathol* 1981;12:123–126, with permission.

Erythrocyte Ferritin
In both iron deficiency and chronic disease, erythrocyte ferritin is decreased, but it is normal or increased in thalassemias and hemolytic disorders. It is less sensitive than serum ferritin for the detection of iron deficiency.

Serum Transferrin Receptor
Usually serum transferrin receptor (sTfR) is increased in iron-deficiency anemia and in other conditions in which hematopoiesis is increased, such as hemolytic anemias, thalassemias, polycythemia vera, myeloid metaplasia, other myeloproliferative disorders, and in secondary polycythemias. sTfR is low in aplastic anemia and in anemia of chronic disease. In one small study, all patients with rheumatoid arthritis had elevated sTfR levels, although no patients were anemic and none had erythrocytic microcytosis. In another series of patients with proven uncomplicated iron deficiency, only 80% had low sTfR.

Bone Marrow Examination
Microscopic examination of a specimen of bone marrow, stained by the Perls' Prussian blue method, is still the most reliable test for iron deficiency. Inexperienced examiners are likely to err in reporting absence of stainable iron when iron is, in fact, abundant in marrow particles. Even experienced examiners do not always concur. Most of the iron that stains is in hemosiderin because ferritin, being soluble, is lost during fixation. The hemosiderin appears in irregular clumps, either in histiocytes or lying free as a consequence of rupture of histiocytes during preparation of the specimen. Globular or string-like structures that stain blue are artifacts. Besides the hemosiderin iron, tiny blue siderotic granules are seen in the cytoplasm of a fraction of normoblasts (normally about 20%). These siderotic granules are ferritin within cytoplasmic lysosomes, also called *siderosomes*. Normoblasts that contain siderotic granules are called *sideroblasts*. Normal sideroblasts contain one or a few such granules randomly distributed in the cytoplasm. In iron deficiency, both hemosiderin and sideroblasts are absent. When hemosiderin is present but sideroblasts are absent, one should suspect the presence of chronic disease, that is, chronic inflammation or malignancy, that impairs the uptake of iron by developing normoblasts. A patient may have iron-deficiency anemia and yet paradoxically have normal or increased stainable bone marrow iron. The usual explanation for this finding is that the patient has been treated by injections of iron dextran. Some patients utilize iron dextran very slowly. They may have persistent anemia, hypochromia,

microcytosis, low serum iron, low transferrin saturation, low serum ferritin concentration, and normal or increased stainable bone marrow iron. Such patients usually respond promptly to oral iron therapy.

Leukocytes and Platelets
Although leukocytes and platelets are usually normal, mild leukopenia is found in about 10% of patients with iron-deficiency anemia. The leukocyte count is usually not less than 3.0×10^9 per liter, and the 10^9 differential is normal. Rarely, hypersegmented neutrophils are seen, but this finding probably reflects concurrent deficiency of vitamin B_{12} or folate. Platelet counts often are increased in children who have iron deficiency. They are usually normal in adults but may either be increased or decreased.

Other Laboratory Tests
Measurement of the **erythrocyte zinc protoporphyrin** (EZP, formerly called *free erythrocyte protoporphyrin*) is a useful screening test for iron deficiency, especially in pediatrics. EZP concentration is increased in iron deficiency and lead poisoning; thus, the test screens for both conditions. Because EZP is normal in thalassemias, the results aid in the differential diagnosis of microcytic anemias. The method is simple and requires only a minute blood specimen.
Immunoassay of serum transferrin concentration, using an antibody as ligand, is an alternative to the TIBC, which uses iron as a ligand. Results are similar. Transferrin concentration may be calculated from TIBC by multiplying the latter by 0.7 and expressing the product in milligrams per deciliter (mg/dL). Transferrin concentration may be either normal or increased in patients with iron deficiency. The principal advantage of immunoassay of serum transferrin concentration is that the volume of sample required is much smaller than that required for measurement of TIBC.

Other Parameters
Several formulas, ratios, or other parameters, mostly using complete blood count (CBC) data, have been devised in the hope that they would have high sensitivity and specificity for the diagnosis of iron deficiency and the exclusion of the disorders discussed in the section entitled **Differential Diagnosis.** Most of these formulas have been abandoned or are little used. Only a few are mentioned here:

1. **Discriminant function (DF):**

$$(DF) = \left[MCV - (5 \times Hb\ Conc.) - RBC - K \right]$$

where $K = 3.4$ if the hematocrit is corrected for plasma trapping and 8.4 if it is not. The DF may be greater than 1.0 in iron-deficiency anemia and less than 1.0 in thalassemias. The validity of this formula depends on the relative proportions of patients with these two disorders in the population being examined, a qualification that severely limits the practical application of this formula.

2. **Red cell distribution width (RDW):** This parameter is determined in different ways by different instruments. In the past, it was sometimes designated *EVR 50,* and it was often determined by arbitrary upper and lower thresholds for erythrocyte volumes. At present, it is more frequently measured as the standard deviation or the coefficient of variation of the MCV. RDW is a quantitative measure of anisocytosis that helps distinguish uncomplicated iron deficiency from uncomplicated thalassemia. RDW values overlap greatly between groups of patients with these conditions. The sensitivity of RDW in many studies is at least 90% (i.e., it was elevated in at least 90% of patients who were proved by other means to have iron deficiency). In some studies, however, both the sensitivity and the specificity were poor, the latter being only about 50%. If the RDW is increased, one can be reasonably confident that there is a problem in erythropoiesis, but the probability that it is due to iron deficiency is only about 1:1. In nonanemic patients with early iron deficiency, as reflected in low serum ferritin concentration, the RDW is often normal.

3. **Serum ferritin concentration versus erythrocyte sedimentation rate (ESR):** By plotting these two variables on a graph, anemias can be classified as either due to iron deficiency or due to other etiology. This graphic method, based on gener-

ally available test results, merits consideration in anemic patients with chronic disease. It depends on the fact that inflammatory disease (e. g., rheumatoid arthritis) is associated with increases in both SF and in ESR but that the increase in SF levels is less if iron-deficiency anemia is concurrent. SF less than 12 µg per liter substantiates a diagnosis of iron deficiency anemia in all cases, and an SF greater than 80 µg per liter correctly excludes iron deficiency in nearly all cases. This method, which requires an ESR measured by the Westergren method, is not applicable for the detection of iron depletion before development of anemia (Witte et al., 1988). This graphic approach has two problems: First, the ESR must be measured using a dilution of EDTA-anticoagulated blood specimen with citrate solution in a ratio of 9:1 or by use of a Coulter Zetafuge (Beckman Coulter, Inc., Miami, FL USA), and results must be uncorrected for anemia. A conventional Westergren ESR does not suffice. A related method is to plot SF versus C-reactive protein (CRP) to help differentiate anemia of chronic disease from iron-deficiency anemia in the presence of the chronic disease (Fig. 2).

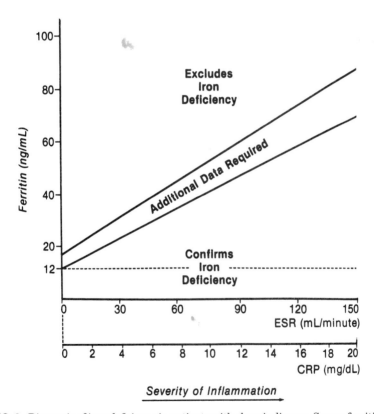

FIG. 2. Diagnosis of iron deficiency in patients with chronic disease. Serum ferritin is an acute phase reactant that increases in proportion to the severity of inflammatory disease. By determining either erythrocyte sedimentation rate or C-reactive protein, together with serum ferritin concentration, the latter may be interpreted in the presence of chronic disease. Results that are below the lower solid line are indicative of iron deficiency; results above the upper solid line exclude iron deficiency. Results that are between the lines neither confirm nor refute iron deficiency. (Modified and republished from Witte D. Laboratory tests to confirm or exclude iron deficiency. *Lab Med* 1985;16:671, with permission of the American Society of Clinical Pathologists).

4. **Serum soluble transferrin receptor (sTfR):** This analyte typically increases in iron deficiency, and it has been proposed as a test to differentiate iron deficiency from chronic disease. In my experience, however, all patients in a series of patients with uncomplicated rheumatoid arthritis had quite elevated values, thereby compromising use of this test in differentiating rheumatoid arthritis without iron deficiency from rheumatoid arthritis with iron deficiency. Others also found elevations of sTfR in patients with chronic disease or malignancy uncomplicated by iron deficiency. Further investigations are needed.

5. **Reticulocyte MCHC:** Flow cytometry permits this measurement that may be useful in identifying iron deficiency in patients who have been transfused. This method has been proposed particularly for chronic renal disease patients who are subjected to dialysis. It also appears to be more reliable than SF measurement ferritin for diagnosis of iron deficiency in children. Its general role as a diagnostic test for iron deficiency remains to be appraised. The **practical approach** for four common clinical situations follows:

- No anemia and normal indices: No action is indicated.
- Low MCV with normal hemoglobin concentration and normal or increased RBC: SF should be measured. If it is <20 µg per liter, the patient has iron deficiency; if SF is normal or increased, the patient may have thalassemia or chronic disease. Hemoglobin electrophoresis should be done, and hemoglobin A_2 and F should be measured. If these results are normal, the patient may have chronic disease or α-thalassemia. If the patient is African-American or Asian and there is no sign of chronic disease, these results are sufficient for a diagnosis of α-thalassemia, either homozygous α-thalassemia (if the patient is African-American) or α-thalassemia-1 trait (if the patient is Asian).
- Anemia and microcytosis: The diagnosis of iron deficiency is made if SF is <20 µg/L.
- Anemia, microcytosis, and SF > 20 µg/L: The patient may have anemia of chronic disease, thalassemia, or iron deficiency and anemia of chronic disease. If SF is greater than 80 µg per liter, iron deficiency is unlikely. The patient may have anemia of chronic disease, thalassemia, or sideroblastic anemia. Clinical information is needed. Does the patient have a chronic disease such as rheumatoid arthritis? If so, a bone marrow examination with iron stain may be required to exclude iron deficiency with confidence. Hemoglobin electrophoresis and measurement of hemoglobin A_2 and F may be needed if the patient does not have chronic disease or if the patient is of an ethnic group with a significant frequency of thalassemia. These considerations also apply if the patient has a chronic disease, such as rheumatoid arthritis, and SF between 15 and 80 µg per liter because concomitant iron deficiency is likely and cannot be excluded with confidence in such cases without bone marrow examination and iron stain. **Note:** In these suggested approaches to diagnosis, no mention is made of MCHC, serum iron, TIBC, blood smear, or examination. These omissions are not inadvertent but recognize the low sensitivity, low specificity, or high cost of each of these traditional methods. Both hematologists and pathologists prefer to examine blood smears; however, microscopic examination of such smears is not cost effective in the evaluation of microcytic anemias. (In other circumstances, however, examination of blood smears may be extremely useful for diagnosis.)

Differential Diagnosis
Anemia of Chronic Disease

The anemia of chronic disease that often accompanies chronic inflammatory disorders, such as rheumatoid arthritis and malignancies, is typically a microcytic anemia with changes in erythrocyte morphology that are indistinguishable from those of iron-deficiency anemia because iron uptake and utilization by normoblasts are impaired whenever there is an inflammatory process or malignancy. Usually, the presence of chronic disease is known, but sometimes it is occult, as in renal carcinoma. Typically, in both disorders, serum iron concentration is low, but usually, the TIBC is also reduced in patients with chronic disease, whereas it is usually increased in those with iron deficiency. As a corollary, percent transferrin saturation typically is normal in the former and low in iron-deficiency anemia. Exceptions are so common, however, that measurement of serum iron concentration and TIBC often leads to erroneous interpretations. Chronic disease typically causes elevation in serum ferritin concentration. When chronic disease and iron-deficiency anemia coexist, serum ferritin concentration may be normal. An increase in erythrocyte sedimentation rate, or in CRP, that is disproportionate to anemia is useful in distinguishing anemia of chronic disease from iron deficiency anemia complicating chronic disease (Fig. 2). Differentiation of these two disorders may require examination of the iron content of a bone marrow specimen.

Thalassemias

The thalassemias share many morphologic features with iron-deficiency anemia, and often these disorders cannot be distinguished morphologically. Both exhibit hypochromia and microcytosis. Target cells are more common in thalassemias but may be present in blood films from patients with iron-deficiency anemia and may be absent in specimens from patients with thalassemias. Coarse basophilic stippling and polychromasia favor a diagnosis of thalassemia, but these features are absent in half the cases of thalassemia trait. An important clue is that in the thalassemia traits, the RBC is usually normal or increased in blood specimens that have significant microcytosis, whereas in iron deficiency anemia, microcytosis usually is accompanied by a reduction in RBC. Further, in thalassemia traits, there is often microcytosis without anemia, a rare combination in iron deficiency. Measurement of hemoglobin A_2 usually permits the correct diagnosis of β-thalassemia trait when the proportion of hemoglobin A_2 is increased. When iron deficiency complicates β-thalassemia minor, however, hemoglobin A_2 is usually normal, and the diagnosis of β-thalassemia trait cannot be made until after adequate treatment of iron deficiency. Because α-thalassemia is very prevalent in African-Americans and in Asians, microcytosis of erythrocytes in persons in these ethnic groups often poses a problem for which there may be no simple, practical, inexpensive diagnostic test. Single α-chain gene deletion or α-thalassemia-2 trait, which occurs in 28% of African-Americans, usually, is not associated with microcytosis. Two–gene-deleted α-thalassemia typically causes microcytosis without anemia, although in some cases there may be mild anemia. The RBC is elevated. This occurs in about 20% of Southeast Asians, in whom it is usually α-thalassemia-1 trait, and in about 3% of African-Americans, in whom it is the expression of homozygous α-thalassemia-2. Both conditions are harmless. At present, the practical approach is to make these presumptive diagnoses by exclusion of other possible causes of microcytosis, such as iron deficiency, β-thalassemia, hemoglobin E or Lepore, and chronic disease. Current methods for the definitive diagnosis of α-thalassemia include globin gene DNA probe analysis using restriction endonucleases and Southern blot. These procedures are tedious and expensive (about $300 per specimen) and are not warranted in most cases. They may be justified for purposes of genetic counseling, however, if an Asian husband and wife both have unexplained microcytosis that may be due to α-thalassemia-1 trait because they would be at risk of having a pregnancy that results in lethal hemoglobin Bart hydrops fetalis. This is not a consideration for African-American couples, however, because if both are African-American, neither individual is likely to have α-thalassemia-1 trait (this condition is virtually unknown in African-Americans). As gene amplification (i.e., polymerase chain reaction, or PCR) technology becomes generally available at reasonable cost, more specific diagnosis of α-thalassemia may become justifiable for all cases.

Hemoglobinopathies

Hemoglobinopathies such as hemoglobin E and Lepore are characterized by microcytosis and hypochromic erythrocytes. Basophilic stippling and polychromasia are usually not present in blood films from patients with these hemoglobinopathies, and target cells may not be numerous. Diagnosis of these conditions requires hemoglobin electrophoresis, which usually is performed when tests for iron deficiency are negative. Unstable hemoglobins, such as hemoglobin Köln, also typically cause erythrocytic hypochromia that is accompanied by macrocytosis, polychromasia, and reticulocytosis.

Hemoglobin H is an unstable hemoglobin that results from α-thalassemia. Hemoglobin H disease also exhibits hypochromia, microcytosis, polychromasia, reticulocytosis, and basophilic stippling of erythrocytes.

Chronic Liver Disease
Chronic liver disease, such as Laennec cirrhosis, usually is characterized by the presence of round macrocytes and target cells in the blood film. Thin (hypochromic) macrocytes or microcytes also may predominate in the blood film, however, thereby sometimes leading to an erroneous diagnosis of iron deficiency. Because the serum ferritin concentration is normal or increased in patients with chronic liver disease, this test usually differentiates the anemia of *uncomplicated* chronic liver disease from that of *uncomplicated* iron deficiency. Often, however, iron-deficiency anemia complicates chronic liver disease because of bleeding from esophageal varices or from gastritis. In such cases, the serum ferritin concentration may be spuriously normal or elevated because of the release of ferritin from injured hepatocytes. Evaluation of iron stores may require examination of a bone marrow specimen with iron stain.

Chronic Renal Disease
Chronic renal disease is commonly accompanied by burr cells or fragmented erythrocytes (schistocytes) in the blood film. The presence of numerous schistocytes implies abnormalities of small blood vessels (microangiopathy), often the result of intravascular fibrin deposition. Hypochromic microcytosis may be present because of chronic inflammatory disease of the kidneys or because of iron deficiency. Furthermore, iron deficiency often accompanies chronic renal disease because of chronic blood loss, particularly as a consequence of repeated extracorporeal hemodialysis. Examination of blood film and measurement of serum iron concentration and TIBC are rarely helpful in differentiating these disorders. Further, the SF concentration is often spuriously normal. Confirmation of iron deficiency often requires examination of bone marrow iron content.

Myelodysplastic Disorders
Myelodysplastic disorders often are accompanied by hypochromia and microcytosis of erythrocytes. This is particularly true of the disorder called *refractory anemia with ringed sideroblasts,* or RARS *(formerly called idiopathic acquired sideroblastic anemia)*, in which the morphologic abnormalities of the peripheral blood are quite like those of iron-deficiency anemia. RARS may be suspected when the blood picture is strikingly **dimorphic,** that is, when there appears to be a mixture of normal erythrocytes with a hypochromic microcytosis. A dimorphic blood picture also may be seen in iron deficiency, however, particularly if the patient has undergone transfusion. Measurement of SF differentiates RARS from iron deficiency because the former commonly leads to iron overloading and the SF usually is elevated, often markedly. Bone marrow examination with iron stain is required for confirmation.

Myeloproliferative Disorders
Myeloproliferative disorders also may simulate iron-deficiency anemia. This is true particularly of **polycythemia vera** (PV), **essential thrombocythemia** (ET), and **agnogenic myeloid metaplasia.** PV and ET often exhibit microcytosis and hypochromia of erythrocytes, together with low serum iron concentration and absent stainable iron in bone marrow. Iron deficiency commonly accompanies these disorders as a consequence of spontaneous bleeding and, in PV, therapeutic phlebotomy. In addition, in PV, the enormous expansion of total red cell mass diverts iron from stores into circulating blood. In some cases of PV, chronic gastrointestinal bleeding is the dominant manifestation. Then the presence of splenomegaly, neutrophilia, thrombocytosis, and an elevated erythrocyte count should lead one to suspect that the correct diagnosis is PV masked by secondary iron-deficiency anemia. Similarly, if the platelet count exceeds $1,000 \times 10^9$ per liter in a patient with iron-deficiency anemia, ET should be suspected as the primary disorder. Bone marrow iron stores are also commonly depleted in chronic granulocytic leukemia and agnogenic myeloid metaplasia, although in these disorders, the mechanism is unclear.

Hereditary Sideroblastic Anemia

Also called *hereditary sex-linked anemia, hereditary hypochromic anemia,* and *hereditary sex-linked ovalocytosis,* hereditary sideroblastic anemia is a rare X chromosome–linked disorder that is often mistaken for iron deficiency or thalassemia because it is associated with hypochromic, microcytic anemia. The blood smear exhibits a dimorphic picture, a mixture of normal erythrocytes with cells that are hypochromic, microcytic, and elliptocytic. The serum iron and ferritin concentrations are normal or increased, and hemoglobin studies (electrophoresis and quantitation of Hb A_2 and HbF) are normal. Confirmation of diagnosis requires bone marrow examination and family studies. The former reveals normal or increased stainable iron and many ringed sideroblasts. Family studies demonstrate the typical pattern of X chromosome–linked transmission.

Congenital Dyserythropoietic Anemia

Congenital dyserythropoietic anemia is a term applied to several disorders that are characterized by lifelong anemia, poikilocytosis of erythrocytes in blood films, and abnormalities of maturation of erythrocyte precursors. These rare conditions cause morphologic changes in erythrocytes that may be mistaken for thalassemia or iron deficiency. The SF concentration is normal or increased. Confirmation requires bone marrow examination.

Myxedema

Often myxedema is accompanied by a mild normocytic, normochromic anemia. The serum iron concentration is usually reduced, which may lead to an erroneous diagnosis of iron deficiency. Furthermore, women with myxedema often have excessive menstrual bleeding that may lead to iron-deficiency anemia.

Congenital Atransferrinemia

Congenital atransferrinemia is an extremely rare hereditary disorder characterized by hypochromic, microcytic anemia, low serum iron concentration, low TIBC (<85 µg/dL), and absent serum transferrin by immunologic assay. There is marked progressive iron overloading of tissues because iron absorption is increased, but transport of iron to erythropoietic cells is impaired. In the few reported cases, no mention was made of marrow iron stores. To date, only nine cases of congenital atransferrinemia have been reported: three from Europe, two each from Japan and Mexico, and one each from Samoa and the United States. The mode of genetic transmission is autosomal recessive. Thus, within a family, only siblings are affected.

Therapeutic Trial

The ultimate proof of iron deficiency is the response to therapy. Physicians who provisionally diagnose iron deficiency by examining the blood film rely on a trial of iron therapy to prove the diagnosis. In such a therapeutic trial, it is important that the patient does not have a disorder that impairs iron absorption or utilization, that the iron is given in a form that is readily absorbed, that the patient takes the iron as instructed, and that the physician monitors the response to treatment. Treatment is stopped and other investigations made if the patient does not respond as expected. The expected response is that the anemia should be half corrected within 3 weeks and completely corrected within 2 months. In view of the potential hazard of iron administration to a person who already has or may develop iron overload and the relatively low cost of SF assay, a test that is universally available in North America, it is no longer justifiable to give iron therapy without adequate diagnostic tests. Table 3 compares the cost of diagnostic tests, including SF assay. Note that the SF assay is less expensive, and less ambiguous, than review of a blood film by a physician. Thus, provisional diagnosis of iron deficiency by examination of the blood film and therapeutic trial is no longer appropriate.

Treatment

Principles

The physician has four obligations:

1. To determine the cause of the iron deficiency, and if there is blood loss, the site and nature of the anatomic lesion

2. To eliminate that cause if feasible, for example, by changing the diet in a milk-fed child, or by surgical excision of a bleeding neoplasm of the colon
3. To administer effective replacement therapy for a sufficient time
4. To follow the response to treatment

Determining the Source of Blood Loss

Common sources of blood loss are shown in Table 2. Sometimes the source of blood loss is obvious, but often it is not. Whereas excessive menstrual bleeding is a common cause of iron deficiency in young women, patients' perceptions of what is excessive are often unreliable. A history of melena clearly indicates gastrointestinal bleeding. More often, however, the amount of blood is too small to discolor the stools; hence, it is occult, and it must be detected by chemical tests. Tests based on the benzidine reaction are too sensitive and yield too many false-positive results. On the other hand, tests based on the guaiac test yield too many false-negative results. A Hemoquant test, which measures products of heme catabolism, may resolve this problem.

Whereas bleeding from higher levels of the alimentary tract may cause melena or may be occult, bleeding from rectal lesions or hemorrhoids cause **hematochezia,** the presence of bright red blood on the surface of feces. The medical history often provides clues as to the site of bleeding.

Demonstration of occult fecal blood does not prove that bleeding is from the alimentary tract because hemoptysis also may result in positive test results. Investigations to determine the site of bleeding commonly include radiographic studies (upper gastrointestinal, colon, small bowel) and endoscopy (sigmoidoscopy, colonoscopy). To be demonstrable radiographically, a lesion must be at least several millimeters in diameter. Thus, many bleeding lesions are missed by radiographic studies. This is especially true of the tiny arteriovenous anomalies (angiodysplasia) that are a common cause of blood loss in elderly patients. Their identification requires endoscopy.

Surgery

Bleeding lesions, such as polyps or hemorrhoids, should be surgically excised. For many other lesions, however, surgery is often neither desirable nor feasible. This is true of the lesions of hereditary hemorrhagic telangiectasia and multiple angiodysplasia. Menorrhagia may be helped by curettage or by administration of progesterone derivatives. Rarely should hysterectomy be contemplated. These troublesome but benign conditions are best managed by long-term administration of iron in dosage sufficient to replace iron lost by bleeding.

Oral Iron Therapy

Iron can be administered either orally or parenterally. As shown in Table 8, the oral administration of simple ferrous salts is by far the least costly and safest form of therapy. Furthermore, such therapy is usually well tolerated and effective.

The iron compounds administered should be **plain ferrous salts,** not in combination with other substances or other hematinics. Enteric-coated or prolonged-release preparations should be avoided because they release iron where it is not efficiently absorbed. Indeed, sometimes they do not release iron at all! Generic prescribing of iron medications often results in the pharmacist dispensing an enteric-coated iron pill; the physician may discover this only when, after weeks of treatment, the patient's anemia is unaltered or worse. Contrary to much medical opinion and folk wisdom, generic medications may cost more and may be less effective than proprietary forms of iron. Generic prescribing simply leaves the choice to the pharmacist. Therefore, experienced physicians either prescribe by brand name or specify "nonenteric" in their prescriptions.

The optimal **dosage** is about 65 mg of elemental iron (equivalent to 0.2 g of ferrous sulfate exsiccated) three times daily between meals. Some examples of appropriate and undesirable iron preparations are shown in Table 8. Treatment should be started as soon as the diagnosis is made, without waiting for completion of ancillary studies. Such treatment should be continued for at least 6 months following correction of the anemia to replete the storage iron compartment. Thus, the total duration of treatment is usually about 8 months. If bleeding continues, treatment may be continued indefinitely.

Table 8. Comparison of different methods of iron therapy[a]

Form of iron	Iron content (mg/g)	Cost to patient (U.S.$/g Fe)	Palatability	Efficacy	Toxicity
Oral					
FeSO$_4$	66 mg/tablet	1.65	Mediocre	Excellent	Occasional abdominal discomfort
Beefsteak	1 mg/oz	500.00	Excellent	Mediocre	Weight gain, bloating
Parenteral					
Transfusion (packed RBC)	1 mg/mL	1,240.00	N/A	Good	Fever, jaundice, AIDS, anemia, shock, death
Iron dextran	50 mg/mL	2,078.00	N/A	Good	Fever, rash, arthralgia, lymphadenopathy, splenomegaly, death

AIDS, acquired immunodeficiency syndrome; N/A, not applicable; RBC, red blood cell count.
[a] Based on August 1999 charges for drawing, processing, and transfusing 4 U of packed red cells at a major midwestern medical center.

Some iron preparations contain other hematinics or substances believed to enhance iron absorption. These "combination hematinics" are unjustified and should not be prescribed.

A small proportion of patients experience **adverse effects,** such as heartburn, abdominal cramps, constipation, or diarrhea when taking iron orally in the recommended dosage. In such cases, it is often helpful to reduce the iron dosage to one pill daily for a few days, with subsequent gradual increase in dosage tolerated. Sometimes switching to a pill with a different color is sufficient to alleviate symptoms. Some patients respond well to iron pills with lower iron content and without these symptoms. Very rarely, patients are psychologically incapable of swallowing any kind of pill. Such patients can be treated successfully with 2 teaspoons of ferrous sulfate syrup USP thrice daily. This preparation contains 32 mg of iron per 4mL. Patients should be advised that while they take iron medications their stools will be black and that this should not alarm them. Those who must take ferrous sulfate syrup should be warned that their teeth may become discolored, a problem that can be avoided by using a straw and rinsing out the mouth after each dose of iron.

Parenteral Iron Therapy
Iron can be administered parenterally, either in the form of blood transfusions or as iron dextran. The following are indicators for parenteral therapy:

1. The inability or unwillingness of a patient to take oral iron medications in adequate dosage
2. Intestinal malabsorption, as in sprue, or following extensive intestinal
3. Continued bleeding from a lesion that cannot or should not be surgically treated, at such a rate that ingested iron in optimal dosage is insufficient
4. Prompt response may be an objective of transfusion, but accelerated response is not a rational purpose for parenteral administration of iron dextran.

Transfusion may be needed in severely anemic persons who may be in danger of ischemic injury to brain, heart, kidneys, or other vital organs. Such treatment, when urgently needed, should be given with caution. Packed erythrocytes should be transfused slowly to avoid cardiac decompensation and pulmonary edema. Several considerations argue against indiscriminate transfusion of anemic patients:

1. Physiologic mechanisms such as increased erythrocyte 2,3-diphosphoglycerate (2,3-DPG) and increased cardiac output usually compensate quite well for a moderate hemoglobin deficit.
2. Erythrocytes prepared from stored blood may not promptly improve the oxygen transport capacity of blood, because the low concentration of 2,3-DPG in stored blood results in high oxygen affinity and thus poor oxygen delivery. This impairment in oxygen transport of stored erythrocytes gradually improves over the course of several hours following transfusion. Modern blood-banking anticoagulant solutions have helped to alleviate the adverse effect of blood storage on oxygen transport.
3. Transfusion is the most expensive form of treatment. For example, if 1 g of medicinal iron costs about $1.65, the cost of 1 g that is absorbed by the gut would be about $10. By comparison, the total cost of transfusing each unit of packed erythrocytes derived from 480 mL of blood, containing 14 g of hemoglobin per deciliter, or 230 mg of iron, is about $310, or about $1,348/g of iron.
4. Transfusion carries greater risks than any other form of iron therapy. The risks include transmission of serious and sometimes lethal diseases, such as hepatitis, acquired immunodeficiency syndrome (AIDS), and cytomegalovirus infection. Furthermore, despite meticulous care, human errors can result in transfusion of mismatched, contaminated, or hemolyzed blood, with consequences of shock, renal shutdown, and death. Fortunately, such accidents are rare. Nevertheless, they do occur. Prudence dictates that transfusion not be administered casually or for the convenience of physicians or surgeons.

Iron dextran (InFeD, Schein, 100 Campus Drive, Florham Park, NJ, USA) is one of a few forms of medicinal iron presently available in the United States for parenteral administration. It contains 50 mg of iron per milliliter in the ferric form. It is usually administered by intramuscular injection into the buttocks, using a "Z-track" technique in which the skin is pulled sideways before injection to reduce brown staining of the skin.

The manufacturer recommends that 2 mL (100 mg) be given daily until the full dose has been administered. A simple and easily remembered formula for calculation of the total dose required is mg of Fe needed = Hb deficit (g/dL) × lean body weight (lb) + 1,000. The hemoglobin deficit may be estimated for men as 14–blood hemoglobin concentration; for women as 12–blood hemoglobin concentration. "Body weight in pounds" seems illogical but is a simplification that results from conversion factors that cancel each other. The addition of 1,000 mg is to ensure that not only is the hemoglobin deficit repaired but also that the iron storage compartment is adequately repleted. **Example:** A 60-year-old man who weighs 160 pounds has iron-deficiency anemia with a blood hemoglobin concentration of 8 g per deciliter. The number of milligrams of iron needed =160 (14 − 8) + 1,000

= 960 + 1,000 = 1,960 mg

Then the volume of iron dextran required = 1,960 ÷ 50 = 39.2 mL. Because the iron dextran comes in 2-mL ampules, this estimate of dose required may be rounded either to 38 or to 40 mL. (See Table 8 for 1994 cost estimate: $1,131 for 40 mL of iron dextran, exclusive of physician's office charges.)

Before a course of iron dextran therapy is begun, a test for **hypersensitivity** should be made by injection of 0.5 mL. The patient should be under medical observation by a physician who is prepared to treat anaphylactic shock. If no adverse reaction occurs, the planned course of treatment may be started after a few hours or on the following day.

Total dose intravenous infusion of iron dextran is not presently approved by the U.S. Food and Drug Administration. **The toxicity of iron dextran** is often troublesome. **The most common adverse effects** are pain and swelling at the injection site, arthralgias, and fever, which may begin several hours to a few days following administration of the drug. These effects are often accompanied by leukocytosis (neutrophilia). Rheumatoid arthritis may be exacerbated following administration of iron dextran. A generalized urticarial eruption may appear. There may be generalized lymphadenopathy, splenomegaly, or aseptic meningitis. Examination of cerebrospinal fluid may disclose pleocytosis. These benign but unpleasant side effects subside after a few days or a few weeks.

A more serious problem is **anaphylactic shock.** This may occur during or immediately following injection, and it must be treated promptly with epinephrine and other supportive measures. Otherwise, the anaphylactic shock may be fatal.

A few cases have been reported of **sarcomas** at sites of injection of iron dextran both in experimental animals and in humans. Because such cases have been very rare, one is tempted to discount sarcoma as a possible adverse effect from iron dextran; but the rare association of sarcoma with prior iron dextran injection should encourage physicians not to administer iron dextran casually.

Injudicious administration of iron dextran to a patient who has a microcytic anemia that is not due to iron deficiency (e.g., thalassemia or sideroblastic anemia) may exacerbate iron overload and lead to **hemochromatosis.** In such cases, removal of iron is particularly difficult and costly.

Response to Therapy

The rate of response to medicinal iron therapy (i.e., other than transfusion) depends not on the route of administration but on the adequacy of dose and the responsiveness of the bone marrow. Thus, oral iron therapy, in optimal amount, results in a response as rapid as that to parenteral administration of iron dextran. The blood hemoglobin deficit should be half corrected within 3 weeks and fully corrected in 8 weeks. Young people may respond more promptly and elderly patients more slowly.

Sometimes patients fail to respond as expected. Such cases require reevaluation, not more of the same iron pills. One must ask the following questions:

1. Is the bleeding controlled?
2. Did the pharmacist dispense a proper iron pill, or is it enteric-coated or slow-release? Ask the pharmacist.

3. Is the dose adequate?
4. Is the patient taking the pills as prescribed?
5. Is there intestinal malabsorption (a rare explanation)?
6. Is there a complicating problem, inflammatory or neoplastic, that might retard the response to iron?
7. Is the diagnosis of iron deficiency correct?

Some patients respond poorly to iron dextran administration either because they mobilize it very slowly from injection sites or because their bone marrow macrophages catabolize iron dextran very slowly, thus providing iron at an insufficient rate to developing normoblasts. Often such patients have ample bone marrow iron but have low serum ferritin concentration and microcytic erythrocytes. Usually, most of these patients will respond promptly to oral iron therapy.

Acute Iron Poisoning

Physicians who prescribe iron medications must be aware that severe, and sometimes lethal, iron poisoning occurs in young children who swallow their parents' iron pills. A child's hand can easily hold enough sugar-coated iron pills to cause severe iron poisoning. **Always warn parents to keep iron medications out of reach of little children.**

Suggested Readings

Annibale B, Marignani M, Monarca B, et al. Reversal of iron deficiency anemia after *Helicobacter pylori* eradication in patients with asymptomatic gastritis. *Ann Intern Med* 1999;131:668–678.

Bainton DF, Finch CA. The diagnosis of iron deficiency anemia. *Am J Med* 1964;37:62–70.

Beck JR, Cornwall GG, French EEA, et al. The iron screen. *Hum. Pathol* 1981; 12:118–126.

Bessman JD, Feinstein DI. Quantitative anisocytosis as a discriminant between iron deficiency and thalassemia minor. *Blood* 1979;53:288–293.

Beutler E, Fairbanks VF. The effects of iron deficiency. In: Jacobs A, Worwood M, eds. *Iron in biochemistry and medicine,* 2nd ed. New York: Academic Press, 1980:393–425.

Brittenham GM, Danish EH, Harris JW. Assessment of bone marrow and body iron stores: Old techniques and new technologies. *Semin Hematol* 1981;18:194–221.

Brugnara C, Zurakowski D, DiCanzio J, et al. Reticulocyte hemoglobin content to diagnose iron deficiency in children. *JAMA* 1999;281:2225–2230.

Cesana BM, Maiolo AT, Gidiuili R, et al. Relevance of red cell distribution width (RDW) in the differential diagnosis of microcytic anaemias. *Clin Lab Haematol* 1991;13:141–151.

Charache S, Gittlesohn AM, Allen H, et al. Noninvasive assessment of tissue iron stores. *Am J Clin Pathol* 1987;88:333–337.

Coenen JL, van Diejien-Visser MP, van Pelt J, et al. Measurements of serum ferritin used to predict concentrations of iron in bone marrow in anemia of chronic disease. *Clin Chem* 1991;37:560–563.

Dallman PR. Manifestations of iron deficiency. *Semin Hematol* 1982;19:19–30.

Doube A, Davis M, Smith JG, et al. Structured approach to the investigation of anaemia in patients with rheumatoid arthritis. *Ann Rheum Dis* 1992;51:469–472.

England JM, Fraser PM. Differentiation of iron deficiency from thalassemia trait by routine blood count. *Lancet* 1974;1:449–452.

Fairbanks VF, Beutler E. Iron metabolism. In: Beutler E, Lichtman MA, Coller BS, et al., eds. *Williams' hematology,* 6th ed., 2001:295–304.

Fairbanks VF, Beutler E. Iron deficiency. In: Beutler E, Lichtman MA, Coller BS, et al., eds. *Williams' hematology,* 6th ed., 2001:447–470.

Guyatt GH, Oxman AD, Ali M, et al. Laboratory diagnosis of iron deficiency: an overview. *J Gen Intern Med* 1992;7:145–153.

Guyatt GH, Patterson C, Ali M, et al. Diagnosis of iron-deficiency anemia in the elderly. *Am J Med* 1990;88:205–209.

Hines JD, Hoffbrand AV, Mollin DL. The hematologic complications following partial gastrectomy: a study of 292 patients. *Am J Med* 1967;43:555–569.

Johnson CS, Tegos C, Beutler E. Thalassemia minor: routine erythrocyte measurements and differentiation from iron deficiency. *Am J Clin Pathol* 1983;80:31–36.

Lin CK, Lin JS, Chen SY, et al. Comparison of hemoglobin and red blood cell distribution width in the differential diagnosis of microcytic anemia. *Arch Pathol Lab Med* 1992;116:1030–1032.

Meloni T, Gallisai D, Demontis M, et al. Free erythrocyte porphyrin (FEP) in the diagnosis of beta-thalassaemia trait and iron deficiency anaemia. *Haematologica (Pavia)* 1982;67:341–348.

Meyer CT, Troncale FJ, Galloway S, et al. Arteriovenous malformation of the bowel: an analysis of 22 cases and a review of the literature. *Medicine* 1981;60:36–48.

Pollitt E, Leibel RL. *Iron seficiency: brain biochemistry and behavior.* New York: Raven Press, 1982.

Punnonen K, et al. Serum transferrin receptor and its ratio to serum ferritin in the diagnosis of iron deficiency. *Blood* 1997;89:1052–1057.

Schwartz S, Ahlquist D, McGill D. Hemoquant, a new quantitative assay for fecal hemoglobin: comparison with hemoccult. *Ann Int Med* 1984;101:297–302.

Shek CC, Swaminathan R. A cost-effective approach to the biochemical diagnosis of iron deficiency. *J Med* 1990;21:313–322.

Stewart JG, et al. Gastrointestinal blood loss and anemia in runners. *Ann Intern. Med* 1984;100:843–845.

van Zeben D, et al. Evaluation of microcytosis using serum ferritin and red blood cell distribution width. *Eur J Haematol* 1990;44:106–109.

Vreugdenhil G, Baltus CA, van Eijk HG, et al. Anaemia of chronic disease: diagnostic significance of erythrocyte and serological parameters in iron-deficient rheumatoid arthritis patients. *Br J Rheumatol* 1990;29:105–110.

Witte DL. Laboratory tests to confirm or exclude iron deficiency. *Lab Med* 1985;16:671.

Witte DL, Angstadt DS, Davis SH, et al. Predicting bone marrow iron stores in anemic patients in a community hospital using ferritin and erythrocyte sedimentation rate. *Am J Clin Pathol* 1988;90:85–87.

Witte DL, Kraemer DF, Johnson GF, et al. Prediction of bone marrow iron findings from tests performed on peripheral blood. *Am J Clin Pathol* 1986;85:202–206.

Yip R, Limburg PJ, Ahlquist DA, et al. Pervasive occult gastrointestinal bleeding in an Alaska native population with prevalent iron deficiency: role of *Helicobacter pylori* gastritis. *JAMA* 1997;277:1135–1139.

Megaloblastic Anemia

John D. Hines

Megaloblastic anemia is a descriptive morphologic term that refers to abnormal hematomyelopoiesis characterized by dyssynchronous nuclear and cytoplasmic maturation in all myeloid and erythroid cell lines. Arrest in the S phase of DNA synthesis of developing cell lines is common. This is the direct result of aberrant DNA synthesis provoked by a single or combined deficiency of either cobalamin (Cbl) (vitamin B_{12}) or folate. This also occurs in patients who are receiving a variety of antineoplastic agents and is less commonly observed in a number of rare inborn errors of pyrimidine or purine metabolism. Macrocytic red cell indices also occur in patients with aplastic anemia, myelodysplastic syndrome, and hemolytic anemias associated with an elevated reticulocyte count. Significantly earlier detection of megaloblastic anemia was afforded the medical community with the advent of the Coulter Counter (Beckman Coulter, Inc., Miami, FL, USA) Model S type of cell counter. Macrocytic red cell alterations occur prior to the onset of anemia in nearly all subjects with Cbl and folate deficiency and not infrequently when the patients are asymptomatic. Mean corpuscular volume (MCV) values greater than 95 fL should prompt the physician to institute further diagnostic investigation. A normal MCV may, however, be encountered in patients with Cbl or folate deficiency when complicated by a coexistent iron deficiency or by one of the thalassemia traits. Microscopically, the earliest morphologic sign of folate or Cbl deficiency is the detection of hypersegmented ([35] lobed) neutrophils. Detection of this finding should mandate further diagnostic studies.

The bone marrow morphologic abnormalities produced by deficiency of Cbl and folate are identical. In all marrow cell lineages, there is a disparity between the nuclear and cytoplasmic maturation, which is most graphically displayed in the intermediate and more mature erythroblasts. Within the bone marrow, erythropoiesis and myelopoiesis are ineffective, and relatively few of the developing erythroblasts survive to the reticulocyte stage. Cytogenetic analysis of marrow from patients with megaloblastic anemia often reveals extensive chromosomal disruption, particularly breakage and elongation. All these marrow disfigurements are rapidly reversed after therapy with the appropriate vitamin.

It is also worth emphasizing that these same types of nuclear-cytoplasmic anomalies occur in other body cells with a relatively brisk cell cycle. Cells derived from the aerodigestive tract or uterine cervix become grossly enlarged and distorted, and this appearance may lead to an erroneous diagnosis of dysplasia or even neoplasia when viewed on cytologic smears. Treatment with Cbl or folate for the appropriate deficiency promptly restores normal cellular morphology.

Megaloblastic Anemia: Cobalamin Deficiency
Structure and Function

The **structural formula** of the Cbl molecule is depicted in Fig. 3. Its composition includes a corrin nucleus (planar group), which is linked to a ribonucleotide by d-1-amino-2-propanol. The nucleotide is composed of a base, 5,6-dimethybenzimidazole, which is attached to ribos-3-phosphate by an α-glycoside linkage. Two bonds exist between the major sections of the molecule. One connects the central cobalt atom within the corrin ring to the four reduced pyrrol rings and to an anionic ligand (-R group). The second connects the cobalt atom to one of the nitrogen atoms of the nucleotide base. The vitamin B_{12} molecule without the anionic ligand has been termed *cobalamin*. Two commercially available therapeutic forms of the vitamin are cyanocobalamin and hydroxycobalamin, the former being the most widely used for treatment. The two coenzyme forms of the vitamin are methylcobalamin and 5-deoxyadenosylcobalamin. Both are extremely unstable in light and photolyase to aquacobalamin and, in the presence cyanide, convert to cyanocobalamin.

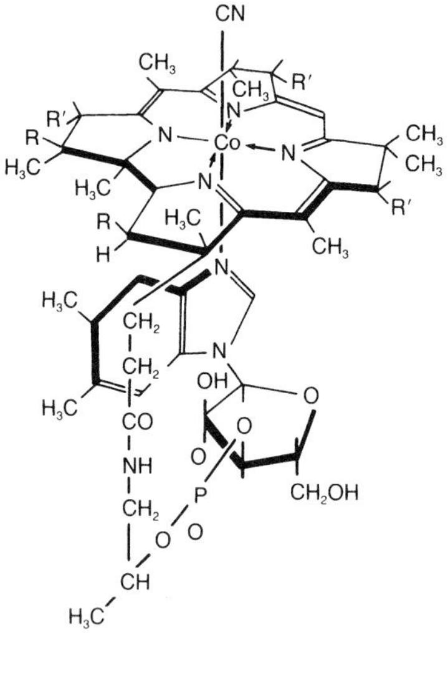

$$R = CH_2CONH_2, \quad R' = CH_2CH_2CONH_2$$

FIG. 3. Structural formula for cyanocobalamin.

Only two known **enzymatic functions** exist in humans. The first is methyl-malonate–succinate isomerization, and the second is methylation of homocysteine to methionine. We still do not have a precise molecular understanding of how deficiency of Cbl leads to perturbed DNA synthesis and megaloblastic anemia. Figure 4 schematically depicts the intracellular interrelationship of Cbl and folate. Most evidence to date points to deficiency of Cbl leading to intracellular methionine deficiency, which theoretically would block the availability of reduced folate within the cell. This then would perturb DNA synthesis by reducing the quantity of thymidylate precursor. This model has been termed the methyl folate trap hypothesis because Cbl deficiency causes a "pile up" of 5-methltetrahydrofolate. Prolonged deficiency of Cbl in humans ultimately results in defective conversion of propionate to succinyl-CoA, which in some patients (and other mammals) results in defective myelin synthesis within the central nervous system. It has now been demonstrated that elevated levels of serum methylmalonic acid (MMA) and total homocysteine (tHCYS) are positively correlated with Cbl-dependent neurologic dysfunction in humans. This suggests that perturbed metabolism of these enzymes may be etiologically related to neurologic disease. Certain hereditary defects in methionine synthase reactions are associated with similar neurologic dysfunctions, whereas methylmalonyl CoA deficiency is not. These and other recent findings have promoted the importance of methionine synthase as potentially protecting the integrity of myelin in humans. This "demyelination" results in subacute diseases of the spinal cord and subsequent neurologic disability. Thus, the two known enzymatic functions of Cbl correlate with the clinical findings in deficiency of the vitamer.

Cobalamin Absorption, Transport, and Cellular Uptake
   1. **Absorption:** Cbl is found in bacteria and animal tissue but not in fruits and vegetables. Cbl in food is usually coenzyme form methyl-Cbl (methyl Cbl) or (5′-deoxyadenosyl Cbl (Ado-Cbl) bound to proteins. Gastric peptic digestion at low pH is a prerequisite for Cbl release from protein. This can be clinically relevant in patients over the age of 70 years, in whom the incidence of hypohydria or achlorhydria ranges from 20% to 25%, potentially resulting in inadequate pepsin activation and decrease in free Cbl.

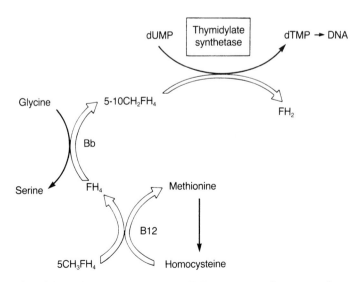

FIG. 4. Simplified schema showing intracellular coenzyme function and interrelationship between vitamin B_{12} (cobalamin) and folate in thymidylate synthesis. dUMP, deoxyuridine monophosphate; dTMP, deoxythymidine monophosphate; FH4, tetrahydrofolate; 5CH3FH4, 5-methyltetrahydrofolate.

Once released by proteolysis Cbl preferentially binds to R protein, so named because it migrates more rapidly than the gastric Cbl-binding protein, intrinsic factor (IF). Both gastric juice and salivary R protein have higher affinity for Cbl than IF at acidic and neutral pH, respectively. Once the Cbl-R protein and IF pass into the second portion of the duodenum, pancreatic proteases degrade R proteins but not IF. This results in transfer of Cbl to IF within 10 to 15 minutes. Failure to degrade proteolytically R proteins may result in marked decrease of Cbl-IF and impede adequate Cbl absorption. In fact, 30% of patients with pancreatic insufficiency malabsorb Cbl. R proteins bind with high affinity both Cbl and Cbl analogs, whereas IF binds only Cbl. IF is generated in the rough endoplasmic reticulum of parietal cells in the fundus and cardia of the stomach. IF has two binding sites, one for Cbl and one for the ileal IF-Cbl receptor. IF is produced in great excess of physiologic need; only 2 to 4 mL of normal gastric juice is necessary to restore normal Cbl in deficient adults. IF secretion is inhibited by long-term intake of H_2 blockers but not by the "proton pump" inhibitors unless they are administered over many months. IF efficiently binds the biliary Cbl but not Cbl analogs. The Cbl–IF dimers and oligomers pass through the jejunum to the distal ileum, where the receptors for Cbl–IF complex reside in the microvilli. The Cbl–IF complex is absorbed, and "free" Cbl binds to transcobolamin II, the major plasma Cbl transport protein.

2. **Transport:** Greater than 90% of absorbed (or injected) Cbl is bound to TC II, the specific transport protein for deliver of Cbl to tissues. TC II also will bind a variety of Cbl analogs, but it is immunologically distinct from the other two Cbl binding R-proteins, TC I and TC II. All plasma Cbl is protein bound, approximately 15% to 30% to TC II, and most remaining Cbl binds to TC I. The latter appears to act as a storage protein with no known physiologic significant. TC I is secreted by secondary granules of polymorphonuclear granulocytes. TC III is derived from the primary granules and has no primary transport role.

3. **Cellular uptake:** Cbl is released into lysosomes after TC II–mediated endocytosis. The Cbl is released after lysosomal degradation of TC II. Most Cbl (>95%) is bound to two intracellular enzymes, methionine synthase and methylmalonyl-CoA mutase. The oxidized form of Cbl is reduced, and in mitochondria it is converted to its coenzyme form Ado–Cbl, which participates in the conversion of methylmalonyl CoA to succinyl CoA, allowing for conversion of products or proportionate metabolites into easily metabolized products. Cbl, as Methyl-Cbl functions intracytoplasmically acts as a coenzyme for methionine synthase allowing transfer to methyl groups to homocystine (Hcys) to form methionine. The methyl group of 5-methyltetrahydrofolate (5-methyl FH4) is donated to Cbl, thus regenerating methyl-Cbl. Folates and Cbl are therefore both required for one carbon (transfer) metabolism.

Adult Cobalamin-deficiency States
   1. **Pernicious anemia**
   • Etiology: The prototype adult deficiency state is pernicious anemia (PA), which arises as a consequence of long-standing gastritis leading to eventual atrophy of all the secretory cellular components of the stomach. This disease produces an almost complete malabsorption of ingested Cbl and leads to megaloblastic anemia. In some severely depleted patients, subacute disease of the spinal cord arises. The precise etiology of PA remains unknown. Some indirect evidence points toward a possible "immune disturbance" whereby autoantibodies are directed against gastric IF. Such antibodies can be detected in the serum of nearly two thirds of patients with PA. The atrophic gastritis in these patients precedes the onset of megaloblastic anemia by many years. The clinical manifestations of megaloblastic anemia in PA usually occur after the age of 40. The red cell MCV increases many months before the patient exhibits anemia or other clinical symptoms. Additional diagnostic features of PA and of the other Cbl deficiency states include glossitis, elevated serum lactic dehydrogenase (LDH) levels, and, in prolonged deficiency, neurologic abnormalities (demyelination of dorsal columns).
   • **Diagnosis:** All PA patients will exhibit a very low serum Cbl level, usually less than 100 pg per milliliter. Serum folate levels are either normal or increased. Correct diagnosis of PA can be made by several methods: (a) Detection of a circulat-

ing IF ("blocking") antibody in the patient's serum is found in more than two thirds of PA patients. (b) Direct measurement of gastric IF after pentagastrin stimulation can be performed using radioimmune techniques. Patients with PA will have virtually no detectable gastric IF. (c) Radiolabeled B_{12} absorption tests (the Schilling test) are more cumbersome but can be used to establish a correct diagnosis. This test reveals a very reduced absorption of the Cbl isotope, which is corrected to normal only when coadministered with a source (usually human) of gastric IF (see Appendix D).

- **Treatment:**

  Transfusion therapy. There exists a significant mortality among severely anemic elderly patients with hemoglobin levels below 5 g per deciliter. These patients often have incipient cardiac failure with a greatly expanded plasma volume. Generally, patients older than 50 years of age with severe anemia should receive 1 U of packed red cells given over 10 to 12 hours with appropriate diuretic measures. In subjects with hemoglobin levels below g per deciliter, it may be prudent to remove judiciously 250 to 300 mL of anemic blood while administering packed red cells.

  Treatment of concurrent infections. Urinary tract and pulmonary infections are common in elderly PA patients. Close culture surveillance is required, and appropriate antimicrobial therapy should be given at the earliest sign of active infection.

  Specific replacement therapy. As soon as blood has been obtained for serum B_{12} and folate assay, treatment with parenteral vitamin B_{12} and folic acid should be instituted. The daily requirement for Cbl is 1 µg daily, and an initial "loading" dose of 1,000 µg is customary. Oral folic acid is administered as 1 mg each day until serum assay results are available to establish the specific deficiency causing the megaloblastic anemia. PA patients are subsequently administered monthly doses of 1,000 mcg of cyanocobalamin for life. Many PA patients present with subnormal serum K+ levels. On institution of replacement therapy with parenteral Cbl, most patients require careful monitoring, and supplemental K+ therapy is often necessary.

2. **Other cobalamin deficiency states**

- **Nutritional deficiency** is quite rare in the Western Hemisphere, but it is common in India, where a substantial percentage of the population adheres to a strict vegetarian diet. Because Cbl is derived only from microorganisms, such a diet may lead to deficiency, particularly in multiparous women and their offspring.

- **Gastrectomy syndromes:** Cbl deficiency is an inevitable complication after total gastrectomy if the patient survives more than 4 years without Cbl supplementation. This delay is accounted for by the slow exhaustion of the liver storage pool. All patients should receive monthly or bimonthly parenteral vitamin B_{12} replacement following total gastrectomy. Cbl deficiency is an uncommon, but still significant, complication following partial gastrectomy, occurring in some series in as many as 10% of patients more than 5 years after surgery. Annual assay of serum Cbl levels should provide adequate monitoring of these patients to allow institution of parenteral replacement with Cbl before anemia occurs.

- **Small-intestinal syndromes:** The following intestinal disorders predispose a patient to Cbl deficiency:

  Surgical resection of the distal ileum

  Regional ileitis

  Tropical sprue

  Chronic pancreatic insufficiency

  Chronic ingestion of p-aminosalicylic acid or colchicine

  Cobalamin malabsorption associated with hypothyroidism

  These disorders are not infrequently associated with Cbl deficiency in clinical practice.

  - **Small-intestinal parasitic syndromes:** There are two well-known intestinal parasitic causes of Cbl deficiency: Infestation with the cestode *Diphyllobothrium* *latum,* is indigenous to areas surrounding the Baltic Sea and, to a lesser extent, the Great Lakes. This parasite is transmitted to humans through the ingestion of raw fish or fish roe. Only about 5% of patients harboring the tapeworm become vitamin B_{12} deficient through the worm's ability to parasitize the ingested vitamin within the small bowel as has been amply demonstrated. Correct diagnosis resides in the demonstration of the tapeworm ova in feces, and treatment usually involves administration of quinacrine (Atabrine) or niclosamide for eradication.

In blind-loop syndrome, either because of prior surgery, stricture, or diverticula, a loop of small intestine fails to empty normally, allowing for parasitization by various strains of *Escherichia coli* and other gram-negative bacteria. These can effectively parasitize the ingested vitamin attached to IF and ultimately cause significant Cbl deficiency. Abnormal radiolabeled Cbl absorption tests are not corrected by addition of exogenous IF, but after a therapeutic trial of tetracycline for 2 weeks, the radiolabeled Cbl absorption often normalizes. Severely deficient Cbl subjects with this syndrome usually require parenteral Cbl maintenance therapy or require surgical intervention to ablate the blind loop.

Childhood Cobalamin Deficiency

Table 9 outlines the four major subtypes of childhood Cbl deficiency, sometimes referred to as *juvenile pernicious anemia:*

Adult-type pernicious anemia is an exceedingly rare entity wherein the child is born with gastric atrophy and nearly total lack of gastric IF production analogous to pernicious anemia seen in adults. Many of these children possess associated endocrine organ dysfunction, which also may occur in their siblings. Hypoadrenalism and hypoparathyroidism are the most common of the endocrinopathies. Circulating antibodies to gastric IF are universally found, but detection of parietal cell antibodies occurs in only half of these patients. Cbl malabsorption is corrected by adding exogenous IF in all these infants.

Children who develop **congenital absence of intrinsic factor** usually present with megaloblastic anemia after 1 to 1.5 years of life, after exhausting maternally supplied Cbl. The gastric mucosa in these children is histologically normal and exhibits normal acid production. Their Cbl malabsorption is completely corrected with exoge-

Table 9. Classification of cobalamin (Cbl) deficiency

A. Nutritional Cbl deficiency
   Absolute vegetarians, vegans, breast-fed infants of mothers with Cbl deficiency
B. Gastric
   1. Pernicious anemia–total gastric atrophy
   2. Atrophic gastritis, H_2 blockers, proton-pump inhibitors
   3. Total gastrectomy, chemical injury
C. Small bowel malabsorption
   1. Pancreatic insufficiency or Zollinger–Ellison syndrome
   2. Blind loop syndrome–bacterial overgrowth
   3. *Diphyllobothrium latum* (fish tapeworm)
D. Abnormal ileal mucosa
   1. Decreased or absent IF-Cbl receptors
   2. Abnormal mucosal surface: tropical–nontropical sprue, Crohn disease, granulomatous ileitis amyloid
   3. TC II deficiency
   4. Drug inhibition: Slo-K, biguanides, cholestyramine, colchicine, neomycin
E. Metabolic disorders
   1. Inborn metabolic errors (rare)
   2. Acquired: oxidation by N_2O exposure

IF, intrinsic factor; Slo-K, slow-release potassium; TC II, transcobalamin II.

nous gastric IF, and these patients do not have demonstrable circulating antibodies to gastric IF or parietal cells. These children require parenteral Cbl therapy for life and do not exhibit other associated endocrine deficiencies.

Imerslund-Gräsbeck syndrome is a rare autosomal recessive condition wherein the afflicted children are unable to absorb the Cbl that attaches to normal gastric IF. The defect appears to involve the microvilli of the terminal ileum, which are histologically normal. Additional defects found in all these patients are proteinuria and renal tubular dysfunction. The gastric IF is normal in these subjects, as is the gastric function. There are no other associated endocrine defects, and these children respond appropriately to parenteral Cbl therapy.

Production of biologically inert gastric IF is an exceedingly rare entity in which secretion by the stomach or a biologically inert IF molecule that is immunologically indistinguishable from normal gastric IF occurs. No other associated deficiencies have been noted, and no detectable IF or parietal cell antibodies are found.

Drug-induced malabsorption can occur as a result of long-term use of H_2 antagonists, which inhibit IF secretion. Omeprazole does not appear to alter IF secretion, but several cases of Cbl malabsorption in chronic long-term omeprazole users have been reported. Metformin analogs inhibit acid and IF secretion in healthy volunteers and may inhibit intestinal absorption in approximately 7% of users. Other drugs capable of interference with Cbl absorption include Slo-K, cholestyramine, colchicine, and neomycin and may be rarely associated with mild to negligible Cbl deficiency.

Transcobalamin II deficiency is a rare condition that usually manifests by megaloblastic anemia of infancy associated with normal serum Cbl levels (due to Cbl bound to TC I, a storage protein). Because TC II is essential to intestinal transport and absorption, malabsorption of Cbl occurs. Treatment with parenteral cyanocobalamin or hydroxycobalamin is effective in restoring hematologic homeostasis.

Defective intracellular utilization: There now exist seven very rare congenital disorders of Cbl metabolism. The combination of megaloblastic anemia with increased MMA or t-Hcys in serum/urine with normal serum Cbl levels should direct investigation into inborn errors of Cbl metabolism. It also reemphasizes the paradigm that any patient with cerebral, myelopathic, or neuropathic disorders should be screened with serum MMA or t-Hcys levels, which might diagnose a disorder of Cbl metabolism.

Acquired disorder of Cbl utilization—nitrous oxide (N_2O) exposure: N_2O efficiently oxidizes reduced Cbl and inactivates the Cbl coenzymes. Either long-term intermittent or intensive short-term exposure to N_2O can lead to cellular Cbl deficiency and may eventuate in megaloblastosis or myeloneuropathy. Elevated serum levels of t-Hcy invariably occur in these situations.

Laboratory Features: Cobalamin Deficiency
Numerous investigations help to assess the Cbl status, and a precise diagnosis requires their consideration. The serum Cbl level is now performed with radioimmune assay "kits" that use some type of R-binder. Most laboratories report "normal" serum levels between 200 and 600 pg per milliliter. Although virtually all patients with megaloblastic anemia resulting from Cbl deficiency exhibit low serum Cbl levels (<170 pg/mL), a low Cbl serum level does not correlate with Cbl deficiency in many instances. Notable examples include normal pregnancy, atrophic gastritis, and a vegetarian diet. In a few cases, a low serum Cbl level is seen accompanying folate deficiency; this is normalized by replacement therapy with folate. The observation that a significant number of elderly patients have Cbl deficiency despite serum Cbl levels between 150 and 200 pg per milliliter is of clinical relevance. Another valuable test in assessing for Cbl deficiency is the quantitation of plasma or urine methylmalonic acid. It is relatively specific for Cbl deficiency; however, if levels are increased in plasma or urine either with or without serum t-Hcy, levels are elevated in cellular cobalamin deficiency and are particularly valuable in assessment of patients with normal serum Cbl levels and megaloblastic anemia with or without neurologic deficits.

Megaloblastic Anemia: Folate Deficiency
Table 10 outlines the etiologic classification of folate deficiency in humans. The major basic factors leading to ensuing folate deficiency include nutritional deficiency,

Table 10.   Causes of folate deficiency

Reduced intake
  Nutritional
    Alcoholism
    Infancy and prematurity
    Elderly "tea and toasters"
    Hemodialysis
    Chronic debilitating disease states
    Anorexia nervosa
  Malabsorption
    Alcoholism
    Celiac and tropical sprue
    Partial gastrectomy
    Small-bowel resection or shunting
    Crohn disease
    Dermatitis herpetiformis
    Scleroderma
    Drugs: anticonvulsants, oral contraceptives
    Intestinal lymphoma
    Hypothyroidism
Increased requirements
  Pregnancy
  Hemolytic anemias
  Neoplastic diseases
  Hyperthyroidism
  Exfoliative dermatitis
  Ineffective erythropoiesis (pernicious anemia, sideroblast anemia)
Defective utilization
  Alcoholism
  Folate antagonists: methotrexate, primethamine, trimethoprim
  Enzyme deficiency states
Reduced hepatic stores
  Alcoholism
  Nonalcoholic cirrhosis
  Hepatoma

---

malabsorption of ingested food folate, increased cellular requirements for folate, and impaired intracellular utilization of available folate.

Folates: Structure and Function
Figure 5 illustrates the biochemical structure of folic acid (pteroylglutamic acid). This structure is a monoglutamate and does not exist as such in natural food products. Polyglutamic forms or folic acid (usually heptaglutamates) compose the so-called *naturally* occurring folates in nature. These are larger molecules that require enzymatic digestion by the small-bowel microvilli of the mucosa for subsequent absorption (*vida infra*). In humans, only the reduced forms of folic acid are active coenzymes and are termed tetrahydrofolates (FH 4). Figure 4 illustrates the coenzyme pathway and demonstrates the mechanism by which a deficiency of folate produces perturbed DNA synthesis and ensuing megaloblastic anemia. It should be emphasized here, however, that numerous other folate coenzymes catalyze other enzymatic steps in single carbon–unit transfer reactions. Thus, folate deficiency of any cause leads to decreased intracellular FH 4, which, in turn, causes perturbed thymidylate synthesis, leading to the morphologic expression of retarded DNA synthesis, megaloblastic cellular maturation.

Nutritional Requirements and Absorption
• **Folate and nutrition:** Nutritional requirements of folate for the average adult approximate 75 to 100 µg per day. Most dietary folate exists in the form of complex

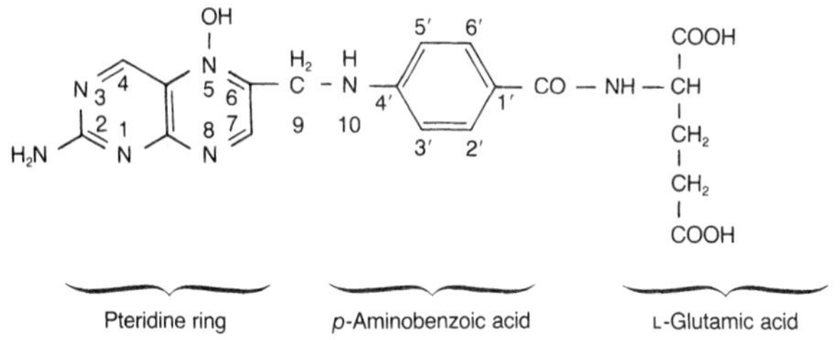

FIG. 5. Structural formula for folic acid (pteroylglutamic acid).

pteroyl-polyglutamates, which require deconjugation by the mucosal microvilli enzymes of the small intestine prior to absorption. Green vegetables are an excellent source of polyglutamate folate, in particular asparagus, broccoli, spinach, lettuce, and green beans. Cooking, however, destroys the nonprotein-bound folates found in these vegetables. Yeast and liver contain protein-bound folates that are not destroyed by cooking. It is estimated that the so-called nutritionally normal or standard diet in this country contains 200 to 300 µg of available folate daily, which is obviously in excess of the usual daily requirement. Noteworthy is the fact that the body is capable of storing up to 5 mg of folate, which is approximately a 3- to 4-month supply. This contrasts with the 3- to 5-year hepatic storage supply of Cbl. Despite the published "adequacy" of the hypothetical standard American diet, folate status in most adults is fragile. Some notable nutritional surveys have determined that fully 10% of the American public is deficient in folate stores. The incidence of overt folate deficiency is especially high in most large metropolitan teaching hospitals. Folate deficiency is particularly common among more affluent subjects who are engaged in diet fads.

- **Folate absorption and transport:** As previously noted, most food folate exists in complex polyglutamate forms, usually pentaglutamates and heptaglutamates. Recent studies with purified radiolabeled synthetic heptaglutamate demonstrated an efficiency of absorption between 70% and 90% of that for folic acid. These studies dispelled previous doubts concerning the bioavailability of food folates when ingested in physiologic dietary guidelines.

  A process of polyglutamate hydrolyzation occurs in the microvilli of the small intestine by hydrolase, an enzyme that efficiently converts the complex polyglutamate molecule to a tri-, di-, or monoglutamate form, which is then absorbed into the cell. Reduced folate carriers (RFCs) probably mediate most of the folates absorbed in the jejunum. At physiologic folate concentrations, a substantial amount of the monoglutamate folate is reduced and methylated intracellularly prior to its emergence in the mesenteric circulation. Higher "nonphysiologic" concentrations of intestinal human monoglutamic folate can be absorbed by diffusion without methylation or reduction. The proximally jejunum is generally acknowledged to be the primary site of absorption. Folate transport is thought to be a saturable process or physiologic concentrations of the vitamin. With higher concentrations, absorption may occur by diffusion. 5-Methyl-FH 4 is the only physiologic form of circulating folate and is loosely bound to albumin.

- **Folate receptors (FR):** Three isoforms exist: FRα, FR$_b$, and FRγ. Much *in vitro* work has accumulated on the various roles of these FR in many cellular systems. FR transfers folate intracellularly where polyglutamination occurs, thus allowing for intracellular retention. The FR is expressed in normal and malignant epithelial cells. The precise *in vivo* role for these FRs remains to be elucidated. A second mechanism for folate uptake occurs via reduced folate carriers (RFCs). Most studies have been carried out in malignant cells and appear to be carried and mediated by a pH- and energy-dependent process that transports reduced folates (FH 4) efficiently. The RFCs probably mediate most intestinal "physiologic" absorption. This form of the vitamin is coenzymatically inactive and is converted within the cell to FH 4, which then may be converted to various other coenzyme forms. In most laboratories, the normal range of

serum folate concentrations falls between 5 and 20 ng per milliliter. All cellular folate coenzymes are polyglutamate forms of the vitamin. Most cells, especially hematopoietic ones, contain an adenosine triphosphate (ATP)-dependent synthetase for
converting FH 4 to the polyglutamate storage form. The lysosomal hydrolases cleave
tissue polyglutamates to FH 4, which is ultimately converted to 5, 10-methylene FH 4,
the cofactor of thymidylate synthetase. This balance between the hydrolase and
polyglutamate synthetase activities appears necessary for regulation of the rate of
DNA synthesis. The pteroylpolyglutamates are the nature substitutes for various
enzymes involved in one-carbon metabolism.

Causes of Folate Deficiency
1. **Nutritional deficiency**
Nonalcoholic causes of folate deficiency include the following:
* Premature infants
* "Tea and toast" diets in the elderly
* Hyperalimentation
* Renal dialysis patients
* Prolonged cooking of vegetables
* Synthetic diets
* Pregnancy

Alcoholism is probably the leading cause of folate deficiency encountered in most
large urban health care centers. Additional causes of folate deficiency in these subjects
include the following:
* Dietary malabsorption
* Decreased hepatic storage
* Decreased intracellular folate utilization
* Depression of serum folate levels

Prolonged excessive ingestion of alcohol often produces abnormal bone marrow sideroblasts and vacuolization of myeloid cells in addition to the megaloblastic changes
secondary to folate deficiency.

2. **Malabsorption of folate in disease:** Table 10 outlines a list of disease conditions in which folate malabsorption has been documented. Malabsorption can occur in
diseases where there is a loss of normal mucosa (celiac and tropical sprue), infiltration
of the submucosa (lymphoma, amyloid), or loss of intestinal surface by surgical resection, shunting, or granulomatous changes in the intestinal wall.

Tropical sprue is a well-recognized clinical entity that occurs in patients who have
spent days or years in tropical areas such as Southeast Asia, Puerto Rico, and other
Caribbean sites. The clinical manifestations are diverse and range from no symptoms
to classic sprue (with steatorrhea) with attendant megaloblastic anemia due to folate
deficiency. The most precise characteristic of this disorder is the rapid correction of
malabsorption following institution of folic acid therapy. Most patients exhibit a low
serum folate whether or not they are anemic. Excessive fecal fat can be demonstrated
in nearly all subjects when placed on a 70-g fat diet for several days preceding the
analysis. When performed, a jejunal biopsy invariably demonstrates subtotal or total
villous atrophy. Patients with long-standing tropical sprue frequently manifest coexisting Cbl deficiency. This requires supplemental vitamin B_{12} therapy. The precise
etiology of tropical sprue has not been well elucidated. Most investigators agree that
there is a pertubation of transport of monoglutamate folate and possibly a reduction
in hyrdolase-mediated polyglutamate folate absorption, which is corrected by daily
oral administration of pharmacologic (1–5 mg) doses of folic acid. There has been a
great deal of speculation that in some patients the underlying pathogenesis may be
due to pathogenic microorganisms within the small intestine.

Nontropical sprue (celiac disease, gluten-induced enteropathy) is a disease that
results from generalized small-intestinal malabsorption and appears to be caused or
induced by wheat gluten (or glutamine-rich peptides). The diagnosis usually is made
when a child or adult manifests recurring bouts of folate deficiency, often accompanied
by a coexisting iron deficiency. Small-bowel biopsy in these patients reveals subtotal
villous atrophy, which reverts to normal after institution of a gluten-free diet. As in

tropical sprue, most patients exhibit steatorrhea when challenged with a 70-g fat intake. The excretion of D-xylose provides and inexpensive and accurate means to confirm malabsorption in these patients. Urinary excretion of less than 1.5 g of xylose within 5 hours of ingestion of a 5-g loading dose is presumptive evidence of malabsorption. Following the institution of a gluten-free diet, the folate malabsorption gradually corrects itself. Adequate treatment of the associated folate deficiency is achieved by oral administration of between 1 and 5 mg of folic acid daily. In contrast, patients with tropical sprue, Cbl deficiency rarely occurs in patients with this disorder. Of interest is the inexplicable higher-than-expected occurrence of non-Hodgkin lymphomas in patients with adult celiac disease.

Other miscellaneous intestinal disorders: Folate malabsorption also commonly occurs in association with a variety of other diseases afflicting the small bowel. These include the following:

- Regional ileitis
- Extensive small-bowel resection
- Excessive alcohol ingestion
- Amyloid
- Whipple disease
- Systemic bacterial infection
- Scleroderma
- Dermatitis herpetiformis
- Small-bowel lymphoma
- Diabetic enteropathy
- Protracted cardiac failure

Anticonvulsant drugs: Many published studies have documented a strong association between the ingestion of all classes of anticonvulsants and the finding of low serum folate levels. Overt megaloblastic anemia, however, occurs infrequently, most likely in subjects on a subnormal dietary folate intake. Clinical studies to date have not provided a precise explanation for this association, but most investigators concede that malabsorption of dietary folate is the most likely cause. Whether this is due to reduced intestinal conjugase or not remains speculative. Treatment with oral folic acid, 1 mg daily, is adequate for patients exhibiting megaloblastic anemia, and this regimen does not place the patient in jeopardy for increased seizure activity.

3. **Increased folate requirements:**

- In **pregnancy,** prior to folate supplementation by prenatal vitamin preparations, folate deficiency was commonly encountered in pregnant women. The folate requirements for pregnant women increase fivefold to tenfold by the third trimester. The fetus is remarkably efficient in its ability to accumulate folate, even when the mother is severely deficient. The association of multiple fetuses, infection, coexisting hemolytic anemia, or the ingestion of anticonvulsants further serves to increase folate requirements. Because Cbl deficiency is extremely rare in pregnancy, it is now recommended that all pregnant women take a prenatal vitamin–iron preparation containing 1 mg of folic acid daily during gestation.

- **Increased hemopoietic demands.** Folate requirements are sharply increased in all the hemolytic anemias and are particularly increased in sickle cell anemia, thalassemia syndromes, hereditary spherocytosis, and paroxysmal nocturnal hemoglobinuria. Continuous folate supplementation is recommended for these patients at a dosage of 1 mg daily of folic acid. Patients with myeloproliferative disorder and myeloma also have increased folate requirement and should receive folate supplementation.

- **Exfoliative cutaneous disorders.** Folate deficiency is commonly associated with a number of exfoliative dermatitis disorders. These patients may lose up to one-fourth of their dietary folate requirements in exfoliated skin. The prototype of these exfoliative disorders is psoriasis. Many medical centers are using methotrexate, a folate antagonist, to treat these patients. It has been suggested that this subgroup of patients should receive folate supplementation prior to methotrexate institution to minimize the development of folate deficiency. This does not appear to affect the therapeutic effects of the methotrexate adversely.

- **Neoplastic disorders.** Folate deficiency and megaloblastic anemia are frequently encountered in patients with metastatic carcinoma and acute leukemia. The presumed mechanism for the development of folate deficiency in these patients is the preferential utilization of folate by the tumor cells over the host tissues. Other important contributing factors include poor nutritional intake of the vitamin, cachexia, decreased hepatic stores, and malabsorption.

4. **Impaired folate utilization:** Two major classes of drugs impair cellular utilization of folate: alcohol and specific folate antagonists.

- When ingested in excessive amounts, **alcohol** appears to influence the cellular utilization of folate. Clinical studies confirmed the fact that a patient ingesting excessive amounts of alcohol, with an adequate dietary intake of folate, frequently develops morphologic signs of deficiency in the face of a normal serum folate level. The precise mechanism by which this phenomenon occurs remains obscure.

Folate antagonists compose a group of drugs that specifically inhibit dihydrofolate reductase (DHFR), the enzyme necessary for replenishment of reduced intracellular folates. Chief among these agents is methotrexate, which is the most potent inhibitor of DHFR. This drug is widely used in the treatment of acute lymphatic leukemia, lymphomas, and a variety of solid tumors (e.g., breast carcinoma, sarcoma). This drug is rapidly excreted by the kidneys, and any reduction in glomerular filtration rate (GFR) enhances toxicity. It also readily diffuses into extravascular spaces, and it must be administered with extreme caution in patients with effusions. Citrovorum factors (leucovorin, 5-formyl-FH 4) rapidly reverse the toxicity of this agent by "bypassing" the effects of the drug on DHFR. Many therapeutic regimens now use high doses of methotrexate with "leucovorin rescue." Other less potent inhibitors of DHFR include pyrimethamine, an antimalarial agent, and trimethoprim, an agent that is combined with sulfamethoxazole (Bactrim, Septra). This combination is widely used in the treatment of urinary tract infections and in immunocompromised patients for prophylaxis against *Pneumocystis carinii* infection. Of interest is the observation that coadministration of leucovorin with this combination does protect the patient but does not protect the parasite against the effects of the drugs.

Clinical Features

It is important to reemphasize here that the initial clinical presentations in either folate or Cbl deficiency may be indistinguishable from each other. Depending on the severity of the deficiency, patients may present with minimal symptoms or with anorexia, glossitis, fatigue, and other symptoms of anemia. The only clinical feature that occurs in some patients with Cbl deficiency, but not with folate deficiency, is neurologic evidence of either neuropathy or dorsal spinal column disease. This is seen exclusively in Cbl-deficient patients with megaloblastic anemia. Physical signs may include pallor, a "lemon color" reflecting mild icterus, a smooth tongue, and a cardiac "hemic" systolic murmur. With more severe degrees of anemia, the liver may become readily palpable, but clinically detectable splenomegaly is uncommon. The neurologic picture in Cbl-deficient patients ranges from subtle signs of mental inattentiveness to severe mental confusion with or without dorsal column spinal tract signs. Fortunately, for most patients with neurologic sequelae, Cbl therapy results in significant objective reversal of these neurologic abnormalities.

Laboratory Features

Like the serum Cbl level, the serum folate level is not a precise indicator of depleted body stores of the vitamin. The serum folate level, however, is the single most useful laboratory test in the diagnosis of folate deficiency. There is an indeterminate range in serum folate values wherein the patient may or may not have actual cellular deficiency of the vitamin. In most hospital laboratories, the normal range for serum folate extends from 5 to 15 ng per milliliter. Values from 3 to 5 ng per milliliter often are considered indeterminate in interpretation. Red cell folate usually is not used in diagnosing folate deficiency because it has lacked the precision formerly ascribed to its diagnostic importance. When the red cell folate concentration becomes subnormal, however, it is always associated with cellular folate deficiency of the vitamin. Red cell folate concentrations do not fall into the subnormal range until all of the body stores have become depleted. A subnormal red cell folate level usually accompanies Cbl deficiency despite an increased serum folate level. As with Cbl deficiency, megaloblastic anemia patients with folate deficiency frequently exhibit elevated serum LDH levels. The use of the so-called FiGlu (formiminoglutamic acid) excretion after oral histidine loading is no longer used in the diagnosis of folate deficiency. Occasionally, the so-called DU (deoxyuridine) suppression test is used when inborn errors of Cbl metabolism are suspected.

Treatment of Folate Deficiency

Irrespective of the etiology of folate deficiency, adequate therapy is provided with the institution of 1 mg daily of folic acid. It should be reemphasized here that initial therapy of any patient presenting with megaloblastic anemia should consist of parenteral B_{12} and oral folic acid therapy until the serum vitamin concentrations are known with certainty. The rationale of this treatment strategy is that Cbl-deficient patients can exhibit a hematologic response to 100 µg of folic acid. Once the serum assay results are available, the clinician's responsibility is to direct investigations into the specific cause of the deficiency.

Megaloblastic Anemias Not Responsive to Cobalamin or Folate

Three categories of patients exhibit megaloblastic bone marrow morphology and yet do not respond hematologically to therapy with Cbl or folate. The first and most commonly observed category is that associated with the administration of antineoplastic drugs. The second category is the megaloblastic hematopoiesis that results from rarely encountered inborn errors of metabolism. The final category of patients who exhibit megaloblastic and dysplastic hematopoiesis not responsive to vitamin therapy comprises the myelodysplastic syndromes (MDSs).

Antineoplastic Agents

Most antineoplastic agents that can produce megaloblastic hematopoiesis are antimetabolites that either block DNA synthesis solely or in concert with similar effects on RNA and protein synthesis. Each year, this list expands nearly exponentially. Only the major classes of these agents are considered here.

1. **Purine inhibitors:** The most commonly used of these are 6-mercaptopurine, 6-thioguanine, and azathioprine (Imuran). Prior to producing bone marrow hypoplasia, these agents produce a mild megaloblastic anemia that is unresponsive to vitamin therapy. This condition resolves with cessation of drug use.

2. **Pyrimidine inhibitors** include 5-fluorouracil, 5-fluoro-2-deoxyuridine, bromodeoxyuridine, 5-azauridine, and 5-azauracil. These agents likewise produce a mild megaloblastic anemia that is responsive only to drug cessation.

3. **Deoxyribonucleotide inhibitors** include cytosine arabinoside, which is widely used in treatment of acute leukemia and hydroxyurea and also is used in chronic myelocytic leukemia regimens. These agents produce a most pronounced megaloblastic marrow soon after administration.

4. **Intercalating agents** include doxorubicin, daunorubicin, and idarubicin as well as amsacrine and mitoxantrone. All are used in treatment of leukemia and lymphoma and can produce rather pronounced megaloblastic hematopoiesis and other dysplastic cellular perturbation before producing profound myelosuppression.

Inborn Errors of Metabolism

1. Hereditary orotic aciduria is very rare and produces megaloblastic anemia in childhood as a result of disordered pyrimidine metabolism and renal excretion of large quantities of orotic acid.

2. Inborn errors of folate metabolism: There are numerous exceptionally rare examples of abnormal folate coenzyme deficiencies, and most are unresponsive to folic

acid. In some instances, hematologic responses were elicited following very high doses of folic acid or leucovorin.

Myelodysplastic Syndromes
The diverse group of patients is the subject of another chapter (see Chapter 10) and consists of the following syndromes:

1. Refractory anemia with ring-sideroblasts
2. Refractory anemia with excess blasts
3. Refractory anemia without sideroblasts
4. Chronic myelomonocytic leukemia

In addition to megaloblastic-appearing erythroid cells, all these patients display varying degrees of other dysplastic features in erythroid and often in all myeloid cell lines. A significant number of these patients will also demonstrate abnormal marrow cytogenetics and develop acute leukemia (see Chapter 11).

Suggested Readings

General
Allen RH. Megaloblastic anemia. In: Wyngaarden JB, Smith LH Jr, Bennett JC, eds. *Cecil textbook of medicine,* 19th ed. Philadelphia: WB Saunders, 1992:846.
Beck WF. Diagnosis of megaloblastic anemia. *Annu Rev Med* 1991;42:311.
Castle WB. The conquest of pernicious anemia. In: Wintrobe MM, ed. *Blood, pure and eloquent.* New York: McGraw-Hill, 1980:283.
Chanarin I. *The megaloblastic anemias,* 3rd. ed. Oxford: Blackwell Scientific Publications, 1990.
Chanarin I, Deacon R, Lumb M, et al. Cobalamin and folate: recent developments. *J Clin Pathol* 1992;45:277–283.
Heath CW Jr. Cytogenetic observations in vitamin B_{12} and folate deficiency. *Blood* 1996;27:800–815.
Herbert V. Biology of disease: megaloblastic anemias. *Lab Invest* 1985;52:3–19.

Vitamin B_{12} Deficiency
Babior BM. In:Williams WJ, et al., eds. *Hematology,* 4th ed. New York: McGraw-Hill, 1990.
Babior BM, Strossel TP. *Hematology: a pathophysiologic approach,* 2nd ed. New York: Churchill Livingstone, 1990.
Carmel R. Pernicious anemia: the expected findings of very low serum cobalamin levels, anemia, and macrocytosis are often lacking. *Arch Intern Med* 1988;148:1712–1714.
Carmel R. Prevalence of undiagnosed pernicious anemia in the elderly. *Arch Intern Med* 1996;56:1097–1100.
Carmel R, Karnaze DS. The deoxyuridine suppression test identifies subtle cobalamin deficiency in patients without typical megaloblastic anemia. *JAMA* 1985;253: 1284–1287.
Carmel R, Watkins D, Goodman SI, et al. Hereditary defect of cobalamin metabolism (cblG mutation) presenting as a neurologic disorder in adulthood. *N Engl J Med* 1988; 318:1738–1741.
Chanarin I, Deacon R, Lumb M, et al. Cobalamin and folate: recent developments. *J Clin Pathol* 1992;45:277–283.
Chanarin I, Deacon R, Lumb M, et al. Cobalamin-folate interrelations. *Blood Rev* 1989;3:211–215.
Dawson DW, Fish DI, Frew ID, et al. Laboratory diagnosis of megaloblastic anemia: current methods assessed by external quality assurance trials. *J Clin Pathol* 1987; 40:393–397.
Donaldson RM Jr. Mechanisms of malabsorption of cobalamin. In: Babior BM, ed. *Cobalamin, biochemistry, and pathophysiology.* New York: John Wiley and Sons, 1975:335–368.
Giannela RA, Broitman SA, Zamcheck N. Vitamin B_{12} uptake by intestinal microorganisms: mechanisms and relevance to syndromes of bacterial overgrowth. *J Clin Invest* 1971;50:1100.

Hines JD, Hoffbrand AV, Millin DL. Hematologic complications following partial gastrectomy. *Am J Med.* 1967;43:555–569.

Imerslund O, Bjornstad P. Familial vitamin B_{12} malabsorption. *Acta Haematol (Basel)* 1963;30:1.

Irvine WJ. Immunologic aspects of pernicious anemia. *N Engl J Med* 1975;273:432.

Koblin DD, Tomerson BW, Waldman FM, et al. Effects of nitrous oxide on folate and vitamin B_{12} metabolism in patients. *Anesth Analg* 1990;71:610–617.

Lindenbaum J, Healton EB, Savage DG, et al. Neurophsychiatric disorders caused by cobalamin deficiency in the absence of anemia or macrocytosis. *N Engl J Med* 1988;318:1720–1728.

Lindenbaum J, Rosenberg IH, Wilson, PW, et al. Prevalence of cobalamin deficiency in the Framingham elderly population. *Am J Clin Nutr* 1994;60:2–11.

Lindenbaum J, Savage DG, Stabler SP, et al. Diagnosis of cobalamin deficiency: II. Relative sensitivities of serum cobalamin, methylmalonic acid, and total homocysteine concentrations. *Am J Hematol* 1990;34:99–107.

Minot GR, Murphy WP. Landmark article (*JAMA* 1926). Treatment of pernicious anemia by a special diet. *JAMA* 1983;250:3328–3335.

Rosenblatt DS, Cooper BA. Inherited disorders of vitamin B_{12} utilization. *Bioessays* 1990;12:331–334.

Schade S, Abels J, Schilling RF. Studies on antibody to intrinsic factor. *J Clin Invest* 1967;46:615–620.

Schulman R. Psychiatric aspects of pernicious anemia. *BMJ* 1967;3:266.

Scudmore HH, Thompson JH, Owen CA. Absorption of 58 co-labeled vitamin B_{12} in man and uptake by parasites including **Diphyllobothrium latum.** *J Lab Clin Med* 1961;57:240.

Shields RW, Harris JW. Subacute combined degeneration of the spinal cord and brain. In: Johnson, RT, ed. *Current therapy in neurologic disease—2.* Philadelphia: BC Decker, 1987.

Folate Deficiency

Antony AC. The biological chemistry of folate receptors. *Blood* 1992;79:2807–2820.

Bertino JR. Folate antagonists: toward improving the therapeutic index and development of new analogs. *J Clin Pharmacol* 1990;30:291–295.

Chabner BA, Myers CE, Coleman CN, et al. The clinical pharmacology of antineoplastic agents. *N Engl J Med* 1975;292:1107–1113.

Chabner BA, Allegra CJ, Curt GA, et al. Polyglutamation of methotrexate—is methotrexate a prodrug? *J Clin Invest* 1985;76:907–912.

Cook GC, Morgan JO, Joffbrand AV. Impairment of folate absorption by systemic bacterial infection. *Lancet* 1974;2:1416–1417.

Chanarin I, Deacon R, Lumb M, et al. Cobalamin and folate: recent developments. *Clin Pathol* 1992;45:277–283.

Folate deficiency and pregnancy outcome. *Nutr Rev* 1991;49:314.

Frenken EP, Arthur C. Induced riboside reductive conversion and its relationship to megaloblastosis. *Cancer Res* 1967;27:1016.

Halsted CH, Reisenauer AM, Shane B, et al. Availability of monoglutamyl and polyglutamyl folates in normal subjects and patients with coeliac sprue. *Gut* 1978;19:886–891.

Herbert V. Minimal daily adult folate requirement. *Arch Intern Med* 1962;110:649.

Hines JD. Hematologic abnormalities involving vitamin B_6 and folate metabolism in alcoholic subjects. *Ann NY Acad Sci* 1975;252:316–327.

Hines JD, Cowan DH. Anemia and alcoholism. In: Dimitrov NV, ed. Drugs and hematologic reactions, 29th ed. Hahnemann International Symposium. New York: Grune & Stratton, 1973.

Hoffbrand AV, Peltit JE. In: *Clinical hematology illustrated: an integrated text and color atlas.* London: Gower Medical Publishing, 1987.

Hoffbrand AV, Jackson BF. Correction of the DNA synthesis defect in vitamin B_{12} deficiency by tetrahydrofolate: evidence in favor of the methyl-folate trap hypothesis as the cause of megaloblastic anemia in vitamin B_{12} deficiency. *Br J Haematol* 1993;83:643–647.

Jeffries GH, Wesser E, Sleisinger MH. Malabsorption. *Gastroenterology* 1969;56: 777–797.

Johns DG, Bertino JR. Folates and megaloblastic anemia. *Clin Pharmacol Ther* 1965; 6:372.

Kane MA, Wakman S. Biology of disease: role of folate binding proteins in folate metabolism. *Lab Invest* 1989;60:737–746.

Kim JH, Eidinhoff ML. Action of 1-b-arabinofuranosylcytosine on the nucleic acid metabolism and viability of HeLa cells. *Cancer Res* 1965;25:698.

Klipstein FA. Tropical sprue in New York City. *Gastroenterology* 1964;47:457.

Lawrence C, Klipstein FA. Megaloblastic anemia of pregnancy in New York City. *Ann Intern Med* 1967;66:25–34.

Lieber C. Metabolism and metabolic effects of alcohol. *Semin Hematol* 1980;17:85–99.

Lindenbaum J. Folate and vitamin B_{12} deficiency in alcoholism. *Semin Hematol* 1980; 17:119–129.

Lindenbaum J, Lieber CS. Hematologic effects of alcohol in man in the absence of nutritional deficiency. *N Engl J Med* 1969;281:333–338.

Moscow JA, Gong M, He R, et al. Isolation of a gene encoding a human reduced folate carrier (RFC1) and analysis of its expression in transport-deficient, methotrexate-resistant human breast cancer cells. *Cancer Res* 1995;55:3790–3794.

Nunn JF, Chanarin I, Tanner AG, et al. Megaloblastic bone marrow changes after repeated nitrous oxide anesthesia. *Br J Anaesth* 1986;58:1469–1470.

O'Brien W, England NW. Military tropical sprue from Southeast Asia. *BMJ* 1966;2:1157.

Rosenberg IH, Mason JB. Folate, dysplasia, and cancer. *Gastroenterology* 1989;97: 502–503.

Shanahan F, Weinstein WM. Extending the scope in celiac disease. *N Engl J Med* 1988;319:782–783.

Skipper HT, Schabel FM. In: Holland JF, Frei E, eds. *Cancer medicine*. Philadelphia: Lea & Febiger, 1973.

Sullivan LW, Herbert V. Suppression of hemopoiesis by alcohol. *J Clin Invest* 1964; 43:2048.

Anemia of Chronic Disease

Joseph J. Mazza

The anemia of chronic disease (ACD) is a common and often clinically important malady. Unfortunately, however, it is commonly underdiagnosed by the clinician and frequently misunderstood and treated inappropriately. ACD most often is associated with chronic infection, inflammatory diseases, trauma, and neoplastic diseases.

Characteristic Features and Abnormalities of Iron Metabolism

Disturbed iron metabolism, characterized as this type of anemia and hypoferremia, is the rule despite normal body iron stores. This anemia goes under the guise of different synonyms, all having the same characteristic features and abnormalities of iron metabolism.

Synonyms for the Anemia of Chronic Disease
1. Sideropenic anemia
2. Simple anemia
3. The anemia of chronic disorders

Renal, Hepatic, and Endocrinologic Diseases
These diseases are not consistently associated with the characteristic abnormalities of iron metabolism seen in ACD. Hypoferremia does not usually accompany the anemia of hypothyroidism or Addison disease.

Renal Insufficiency and Cirrhosis
These conditions are also not associated with the characteristic disturbance in iron and metabolism unless inflammation or infection is present.

Common Clinical Features
Most often, the signs and symptoms seen in patients with ACD are referable to the underlying disease. Common symptoms elicited from the history include weight loss, anorexia, fever, chills, myalgias, and arthralgias. Sometimes the symptoms are unimpressive and vague and often antedate the anemia by weeks or even months. The anemia is usually mild and nonprogressive. The hemoglobin rarely is less than 9 g unless other factors are present to contribute to the anemia. The anemia usually occurs insidiously over a period of approximately 3 to 4 weeks and thereafter remains stable or unchanged.

Laboratory Features
Hypoferremia is the hallmark of ACD with specific characteristic abnormalities in iron metabolism as reflected in the plasma, storage sites, and erythrocytes.

1. The anemia is most often normochromic and normocytic.
2. Not infrequently, it is hypochromic and microcytic, as reflected by the red blood cell count (RBC) indices (approximately 30% of patients) and therefore may be confused with β-thalassemia minor.
3. The serum iron is almost always decreased.
4. Transferrin levels or iron-binding capacity is low.
5. Saturation index is decreased and is often less than 15%.
6. Iron stores are usually normal or increased in the bone marrow.
7. Serum ferritin (SF) is usually normal or increased.
8. There is a reduced bone marrow sideroblastic iron because of the reduced supply of iron going to the marrow erythrocytes.
9. Free erythrocyte protoporphyrin is increased.

Plasma Proteins
Acute-phase Response
There is usually an acute-phase response characterized by an increase in a variety of plasma proteins with a significant decline in plasma albumin.

1. C-reactive protein
2. Amyloid A-protein
3. Fibrinogen
4. Ceruloplasmin
5. Haptoglobin
6. Components of the complement system, β-1-C or C′3 in particular

Synthesis
These proteins are synthesized at an increased rate and persist as long as the cause for the anemia is present. They are synthesized at the expense of albumin and transferrin by the hepatocytes. The levels of these proteins can be used to measure the activity of the underlying disease and the effectiveness of treatment (Fig. 6).

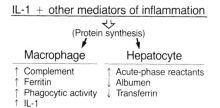

FIG. 6. Alterations in plasma protein levels induced by inflammatory mediators seen in anemia of chronic disease (ACD). IL-1, interleukin-1.

Interleukin-1
It is thought that interleukin-1 (IL-1), an inflammatory mediator synthesized and secreted by leukocytes, plays a major role in the pathophysiology of ACD and ties together the various diseases associated with ACD. The disturbance in iron metabolism with the resulting anemia is thought to be linked to IL-1 and other mediators of inflammation.

The effects and properties of IL-1 can be found in a recent review of this low-molecular-weight mediator substance, but its effects on macrophages and hepatocytes may induce the acute-phase response that occurs with the alterations in plasma proteins seen with infections and inflammatory diseases.

Iron Metabolism
Disturbance in iron kinetics is the hallmark of ACD. Hypoferremia with normal to increased body stores of iron is the common presenting picture. Impaired flow of iron from the tissues to the plasma appears to be the major explanation for the decreased serum iron. Multiple factors seem to contribute to this problem, but its kinetics are not completely understood.

It appears that iron is not released from the intracellular sites when infection or inflammation is present. Macrophages responsible for normal hemolysis of senescent RBCs in the reticuloendothelial system seem to sequester the iron and are mainly responsible for the hypoferremia. Hepatocytes and the epithelial cells of the gastrointestinal mucosa also sequester iron and fail to release it to the plasma at a normal rate and to other storage compartments such as the bone marrow.

The macrophages of the reticuloendothelial system are the major cells controlling iron dynamics and metabolism. The iron extracted from the RBCs is held and stored and not released promptly into the plasma for transport as an iron-deficiency anemia. Thus, these macrophages contain an increased amount of iron. The factors leading to this restricted or impaired iron release in ACD are poorly understood.

Lactoferrin
Lactoferrin is an iron-binding protein found in milk and virtually all body secretions in fairly high concentrations. Its concentration in plasma, however, is relatively low. It is synthesized and stored in specific granules in neutrophils and is released during phagocytosis. It is found in high concentrations at the site of inflammation (Fig. 7).

The release of lactoferrin from granulocytes appears to be stimulated by IL-1, which is synthesized and secreted by monocytes and macrophages. Interestingly, lactoferrin is similar to transferrin, the major iron transporting protein in the plasma, with respect to its size, shape, and affinity for binding iron. Immunologically and structurally, however, it is different from transferrin and has an even greater affinity for binding iron.

Other properties of lactoferrin include the following:

1. It does not transfer its bound iron to erythroid precursors.
2. It is taken up actively and rapidly by macrophages.
3. It can compete with and remove iron from transferrin.
4. It returns iron to macrophages of the reticuloendothelial system, where it becomes incorporated into the intracellular storage form.
5. It does not cause decrease in iron absorption from the gastrointestinal tract.

Thus, if the fundamental processes in iron metabolism are active in ACD, the expected results would be hypoferremia as a result of diversion of iron from the dynamic pool to the intracellular storage pool and an insufficient supply of iron for erythropoiesis in the bone marrow.

Ferritin Kinetics
The hypoferremia of inflammation stimulates ferritin synthesis. This surplus of apoferritin binds a larger than normal proportion of the iron entering the cell and prevents it from rapid release. Apoferritin essentially behaves like an acute-phase reactant and increases before there is increase in intracellular iron.

The SF levels reflect the amount of storage ferritin (intracellular ferritin). An increase in SF with inflammation occurs within 24 hours and lasts several weeks. Augmented synthesis of this binding protein continues as long as the inflammatory response persists.

ACD

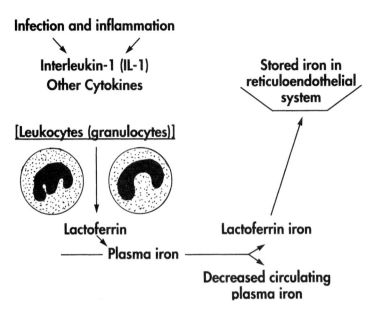

FIG. 7. The role of lactoferrin in causing hypoferremia and ultimately anemia. Potent binding of plasma iron leads to increased storage and decreased circulating iron.

It is clear that storage iron is less available to the plasma iron transport system than iron recently derived from destroyed RBCs. The fundamental process of ACD seems to divert the intracellular iron into storage iron, resulting in hypoferremia.

The reasons for the alterations in ferrokinetics and iron metabolism in the clinical setting of inflammation and infection are at best speculative at this point. There is a convincing body of literature supporting host defense mechanisms aimed at denying iron to invading microorganisms, however, thus providing a less than optimum environment for the propagation and progression of infection.

It is well known that most microorganisms require a specific iron concentration for optimal growth. When infection occurs, there is competition for the iron made available between the iron-binding proteins in the plasma and the microorganisms. Thus, transferrin and lactoferrin have an indirect antibacterial effect by binding to available iron and transporting it to intracellular compartments, where it is unavailable for utilization by microorganisms. The high concentration of lactoferrin in human breast milk is thought to have significant antibacterial effects through this mechanism.

Of additional interest is the increased susceptibility to infection noted in a variety of conditions associated with hyperferremia or iron overload syndromes such as hemochromatosis, Bantu siderosis, and thalassemia.

It has been shown that hypoferremia induced by endotoxin or IL-1 administration increases resistance to infection. Administration of parenteral iron to circumvent the hypoferremia response increases the incidence of infection and death in experimental animals. Thus, it would appear that the mechanisms to sequester iron have evolved as part of the host response to infection and, if chronic, could lead to anemia.

Generally, ACD is regarded as refractory to iron therapy, but when iron is given parenterally in saccharated iron oxide form, a reticulocytosis can be elicited with mild increase in hemoglobin levels. Such therapy and response are neither required nor desirable and may be dangerous to the patient.

Erythrokinetics
There is believed to be a hemolytic component that contributes to the anemia in ACD. The RBC survival is mildly decreased (80–90 days). Cross-transfusion studies seem to indicate that the hemolysis factor is outside the erythrocyte. Hyperactivity of the reticuloendothelial system with increased phagocyte capacity of the macrophages is believed to be responsible for increased RBC uptake and their shortened survival. Activated macrophages have an increased number of membrane receptor sites. Intracellular changes indicating increased metabolic activity are also noted. These postulated events contributing to ACD may be directly or indirectly attributable to the release of inflammatory mediators as part of the underlying systemic disease (Fig. 8).

Erythropoiesis
The decrease in erythropoiesis is due to limited iron stores made available in these conditions:

1. Hypoxemic stimulation of erythropoietin secretion is decreased with respect to the degree of anemia present, and thus the bone marrow response is less than expected (Fig. 9).
2. Erythroid iron turnover is decreased, and this decrease correlates with the decreased serum iron levels.
3. Measured serum erythropoietin levels are normal.

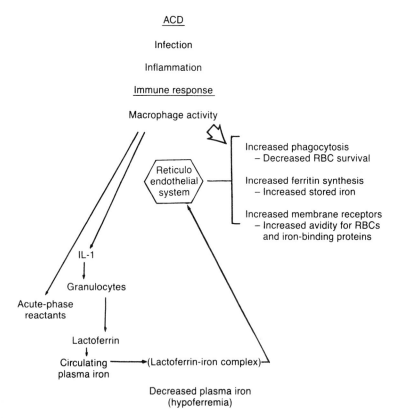

FIG. 8. Proposed interaction of the host immune response with the reticuloendothelial system, resulting in decreased circulating iron and anemia.

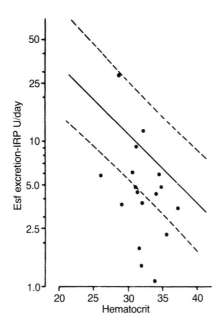

FIG. 9. Relation between hematocrit and erythropoietin (Esf) excretion in 17 patients with the anemia of chronic disorders. Values in normal subjects are shown as mean (*solid line*) and 95% limits (*dashed line*). IRP, international reference preparation. (From Douglas SW, Adamson JW. The anemia of chronic disorders: studies of marrow regulation and iron metabolism. *Blood* 1975;45:55–65, with permission.)

Decreased availability of iron explains the limitations on the erythroid elements of the bone marrow to proliferate. Ineffective erythropoiesis is not confirmed, however, and the erythroid-granulocyte ratio is usually normal. Thus, no erythroid hyperplasia to compensate for the degree of anemia present is apparent.

Other Unique Factors
The reason for the inappropriate lack of response of erythropoietin levels for the degree of anemia is unclear. Under these conditions, where ACD is present, however, the correlation between erythropoietin levels and the degree of anemia is lost. Even when septic laboratory animals are exposed to hypoxemia, their serum erythropoietin increase is much less than that seen in uninfected control animals. Similar results have been obtained when turpentine abscesses are induced in iron-deficient rats:

1. RBC 2,3-diphosphoglycerate (2,3-DPG) levels are increased.
2. Erythropoietin is not increased as would be expected with the degree of anemia.
3. Hemoglobin oxygen affinity is reduced or shifted to the right, indicating appropriate intraerythrocyte response to the anemia and hypoxemia.

Erythropoiesis increases if erythropoietin is given or if hypoxemia is present; but a greater degree of hypoxemia appears necessary for a given level of erythropoietin secretion under the circumstances associated with ACD.

It is possible that IL-1 inhibits erythropoietin synthesis or a precursor of erythropoietin. IL-1 can cause a decrease in the synthesis of a variety of proteins by the liver and other tissues while stimulating or increasing the synthesis of other proteins and mediators associated with inflammation.

Recent studies have shown that IL-1 can suppress bone marrow activity when systemic inflammatory or infectious processes are active. This may be the main factor responsible for the lack of compensatory marrow changes (e.g., hyperplasia) during these clinical situations.

Other cytokines have been implicated in the inhibition of erythropoiesis. In fact, it appears that multiple factors synthesized by a variety of cells that participate in the host response to infection or in the inflammatory milieu act synergistically to inhibit bone marrow function.

Elegant *in vitro* studies have shown direct inhibitory effects on erythropoiesis by IL-1, tumor necrosis factor (TNF), interferon-γ, and interferon-β. Other studies have shown that a variety of cytokines may indirectly play an adjuvant role in inhibiting erythropoiesis resulting in ACD.

Malignancy

The anemia associated with malignant diseases is far less clear than that associated with inflammatory and infectious diseases. It has been well established that suppression of erythropoietin by certain malignancies can occur and can lead to sufficient deficiency to result in anemia. Other studies showed that there may be a defect in the bone marrow's ability to respond to the erythropoietin in malignancy. Thus, the factors contributing to ACD may not be completely operational or, in some instances, may be altered when a malignant disease is present.

Treatment

To reiterate, iron therapy and other hematinic agents are unnecessary in the treatment of ACD. The anemia will resolve when the underlying inflammatory or infectious process is successfully treated, and frequently, the anemia will improve with effective chemotherapy for malignant disease.

Suggested Readings

Birgegard G. The source of serum ferritin during infection: studies with concanavalin A-sepharose absorption. *Clin Sci* 1980;59:385–387.

Blick M, Sherwin SA, Rosenblum M, et al. Phase I study of recombinant tumor necrosis factor in cancer patients. *Cancer Res* 1987;47:2986–2989.

Bornstein DL. Leukocytic pyrogen: a major mediator of the acute phase reaction. *Ann NY Acad Sci* 1982;389:323–337.

Brock JH, Esparza I. Failure of reticulocytes to take up iron from lactoferrin saturated by various methods. *Br J Haematol* 1979;42:481–483.

Cartwright GE. The anemia of chronic disorders. *Semin. Hematol* 1966;3:351–375.

Cartwright GE, Lee GR. The anaemia of chronic disorders. *Br J Haematol* 1971;21:147–152.

Cavill I, Bently DP. Erythropoiesis in the anaemia of rheumatoid arthritis. *Br J Haematol* 1982;50:583–590.

Chernow B, Wallner SF. Is the anemia of chronic disorders normocyticnor-mochromic? *Milit Med* 1978;43:345–346.

Dinarello CA. Interleuken-1 and the pathogenesis of the acute-phase response. *N Engl J Med* 1984;311:1413–1418.

Douglas SW, Adamson JW. The anemia of chronic disorders: studies of marrow regulation and iron metabolism. *Blood* 1975;45:55–65.

Eastgate JA, Symons JA, Wood NC, et al. Correlation of plasma interleukin 1 levels with disease activity in rheumatoid arthritis. *Lancet* 1988;2:706–709.

Fillet G, Cook JD, Finch CA. Storage iron kinetics: VII. A biologic model for reticuloendothelial iron transport. *J Clin Invest* 1974;53:1527–1533.

Hershko C, Cook JD, Finch CA. Storage iron kinetics: VI. The effect of inflammation on iron exchange in the rat. *Br J Haematol* 1974;28:67–75.

Kampschmidt RF, Upchurch HF, Johnson HL. Iron transport after injection of endotoxin in rats. *Am J Physiol* 1965;208:68.

Kauchansky K, Lin N, Adamson JW. Interleuken-1 stimulates fibroblasts to synthesize granulocyte-macrophage and granulocyte colony-stimulating factors: mechanism for the hematopoietic response to inflammation. *J Clin Invest* 1988;81:92.

Konijn AM, Hershko C. Ferritin synthesis in inflammation: I. Pathogenesis of impaired iron release. *Br J Haematol* 1977;37:7–16.

Kushner I. The phenomenon of the acute phase response. *Ann NY Acad Sci* 1982;389:39–48.

Lipschitz DA, Cook JD, Finch CA. A clinical evaluation of serum ferritin as an index of iron stores. *N Engl J Med* 1974;290:1213.

Lynch SR, et al. Iron and the reticuloendothelial system. In: Jacobs A, Worwood M, eds. *Iron in biochemistry and medicine.* New York: Academic Press, 1974:563–587.

Mackaness GB. The monocyte in cellular immunity. *Semin Hematol* 1970;7:172–184.

Mahmood T, Robinson WA, Vautrin R. Granulopoietic and erythropoietic activity in patients with anemias of iron deficiency and chronic disease. *Blood* 1977;50:449–455.

Maury CP, Salo E, Pelkonen P. Mechanism of the anaemia in rheumatoid arthritis: demonstration of raised interleukin 1b concentrations in anaemic patients and of interleukin 1 mediated suppression of normal erythropoiesis and proliferation of human erythroleukemia (HEL) cells *in vitro. Ann Rheum Dis* 1988;47:972–978.

Means RT, Dessypris EN, Krantz SB. Inhibition of human erythroid colony-forming units by interleukin-1 is mediated by gamma interferon. *J Cell Physiol* 1992;50:59–64.

Means RT, Krantz SB. Progress in understanding the pathogenesis of the anemia of chronic disease. *Blood* 1992;80:1639–1647.

Schade SG, Fried W. Suppressive effect of endotoxin on erythropoietin-responsive cells in mice. *Am J Physiol* 1976;231:73–76.

Van Snick JL, Markowetz B, Masson PL. The ingestion and digestion of human lactoferrin by mouse peritoneal macrophages and the transfer of its iron into ferritin. *J Exp Med* 1977;46:817–827.

Van Snick JL, Masson PL, Heremans JF. The involvement of lactoferrin in the hyposideremia of acute inflammation. *J Exp Med* 1974;140:1068–1084.

Zaroulis CG, Kourides IA, Valeri CR. Red cell 2,3-diphosphoglycerate and oxygen affinity of hemoglobin in patients with thyroid disorders. *Blood* 1978;52:181–185.

Zarrabi MH, Lysik R, Zucker S. The anemia of chronic disorders: studies of iron reutilization of the anaemia of experimental malignancy and chronic inflammation. *Br J Haematol* 1977;35:647–658.

Zucker S, Friedman S, Lysik RM. Bone marrow erythropoiesis in the anemia of infection, inflammation and malignancy. *J Clin Invest* 1974;53:1132–1138.

Zucker S, Lysik RM, DiStefano M. Cancer cell inhibition of erythropoiesis. *Lab Clin Med* 1980;96:770–782.

Aplastic Anemia

William G. Hocking

Aplastic anemia is characterized by peripheral blood pancytopenia in association with bone marrow hypocellularity involving granulocytic, erythroid, and megakaryocytic cell lines. Aplastic anemia is a relatively uncommon disease with an annual mortality in the United States of approximately 0.5 per 100,000. The disease is infrequent during the first year of life, with a progressively rising incidence until the age of 20 years and a plateau between ages 20 and 60 years, followed by an increase after the age of 60 years. There may be a genetic predisposition in some families.

Etiology
The causes of aplastic anemia are diverse (Table 11).

Idiopathic Aplastic Anemia
Idiopathic aplastic anemia accounts for approximately one half of all cases and is a diagnosis of exclusion.

Drugs and Toxins
Drug-induced aplastic anemia is the second leading cause. A large number of agents have been associated with the development of aplastic anemia (Table 12). Chloramphenicol is by far the most frequently implicated drug. Phenylbutazone, sulfonamides,

Table 11. Etiology of aplastic anemia

Idiopathic

Drug-induced
  Dose-dependent
  Idiosyncratic

Chemical or toxin

Radiation

Infection
  Hepatitis
  Parvovirus
  Tuberculosis
  Human immunodeficiency virus (HIV)

Pregnancy

Thymoma

Associated with myelodysplasia

Paroxysmal nocturnal hemoglobinuria (PNH)

Constitutional
  Fanconi anemia
  Familial aplastic anemia
  Dyskeratosis congenita

---

and the anticonvulsants are associated relatively often. Drug-induced bone marrow aplasia may occur by either a dose-dependent or an idiosyncratic mechanism, and a single drug may act in both ways under appropriate circumstances. A host of chemicals, including benzene, carbon tetrachloride, and several insecticides, has been associated with the development of aplastic anemia. Radiation exposure may produce bone marrow aplasia in a dose-related fashion.

Infections

1. **Viral hepatitis** is the infection most often associated with aplastic anemia, most commonly in males, occurring from a few weeks to 8 months after the onset of hepatitis. The incidence appears to be less than 1%. The hepatitis is usually non-A, non-B, non-C, and non-G type (1), but occurrence in association with hepatitis C has been reported (2). Approximately one third of patients undergoing liver transplantation for posthepatic liver failure develop aplastic anemia (3). Aplastic anemia associated with hepatitis is particularly severe, with long-term survival less than 10% for patients who receive only supportive care, but it generally responds to immunosuppressive therapy.

2. **Cytomegalovirus**

3. **Infectious mononucleosis**

4. **Parvovirus** may cause aplastic crises in patients with sickle cell disease or other chronic hemolytic anemias (4) and appears to be directly toxic to erythroid progenitors, but it is not associated with other causes of aplastic anemia.

5. **Human immunodeficiency virus (HIV)** has been associated with aplastic anemia (5).

6. **Nonviral infections:** Tuberculosis can be associated with pancytopenia, but the bone marrow is not usually aplastic.

Pregnancy

Aplastic anemia associated with pregnancy remits following delivery in some patients, although the mechanism for aplasia in pregnancy is not understood.

Thymoma

The most frequent hematologic disorder associated with thymoma is pure red cell aplasia; however, rare cases of aplastic anemia associated with thymoma have been described.

Table 12. Drugs associated with aplastic anemia[a]

Class	Frequent reports	Few reports
Antimicrobials	Chloramphenicol	Streptomycin
		Penicillins
	Quinacrine	Tetracyclines
		Sulfonamides
		Amphotericin B
Anticonvulsants	Methylphenylhydantoin	Methyophenylhydantoin
	Trimethadione	Diphenylhydantoin
		Ethosuximide
		Carbamazepine
Antithyroid agents		Carbethoxythiomethylgly-oxaline (carbimazole)
		Methylenemercaptoimida-zole (tapazole)
		Potassium perchlorate
		Prophylthiouracil
Antidiabetic agents		Tolbutamide
		Chlorpropamide
		Carbutamide
Antihistamines		Tripelennamine
Analgesics	Phenylbutazone	Acetylsalicylic acid
		Indomethacin
Sedative/tranquilizer		Meprobamate
		Chlordiazepoxide
		Phenothiazines
		Methyprylon
Miscellaneous	Gold compounds	Acetazolamide
		D-Penicillamine
		Cimetidine
		Methazolamide
		Thiocyanate
		Bismuth
		Metolazone
		Ticlopidine

[a] Drugs listed are those that produce idiosyncratic reactions; agents causing dose-dependent aplasia (e.g., cancer chemotherapeutic agents) are not included.
Adapted from Wintrobe MM. *Clinical hematology,* 8th ed. Philadelphia: Lea & Febiger, 1981:702.

Clonal Stem Cell Disorders
A relationship between paroxysmal nocturnal hemoglobinuria (PNH), myelodysplasia, and aplastic anemia has been recognized for many years.

1. **PNH** is a clonal disorder characterized by a mutation in the phosphatidylinositol glycan (PIG-A) gene, resulting in deficiency of phosphatidylinositol glycan-anchored cell proteins (e.g., CD55, CD59) that protect cells from complement-mediated lysis (6). This same defect can be identified from 15% up to 50% of newly diagnosed patients with aplastic anemia (7,8). Progenitor or stem cells with this defect may have a survival advantage over normal cells, possibly as a result of resistance to apoptosis (9). Overt PNH may evolve into aplastic anemia, particularly after immunosuppressive treatment.

2. **Myelodysplasia** is the second clonal disorder seen in patients with aplastic anemia; it occurs in 15% to 25% of long-term survivors after immunosuppressive therapy

(10,11). The risk of myelodysplasia appears to be higher for patients who receive multiple courses of immunosuppressive therapy. Acute leukemia also may occur as a late complication.

Constitutional Aplastic Anemia
This category includes patients with a congenital or genetically transmitted predisposition to aplastic anemia.

   1. **Fanconi's anemia:** These patients have familial bone marrow failure that usually develops within the first 10 years of life and often is associated with other phenotypic abnormalities, such as skin pigmentation, renal or splenic hypoplasia, hypoplastic thumbs or radii, microcephaly, and mental retardation. Fibroblasts and lymphocytes from these patients have a high incidence of gaps, breaks, chromatid exchanges, and endoreduplication. These patients have an increased incidence of acute myelogenous leukemia.
   2. **Familial aplastic anemia:** Rare families have been described in whom aplastic anemia occurs without the other stigmata of Fanconi's anemia.
   3. **Dyskeratosis congenita:** This rare X-linked recessive disorder has an approximately 50% incidence of aplastic anemia.

Pathophysiology
Several mechanisms appear to be responsible for aplastic anemia (12). Clonal hematopoiesis can be detected in some patients and may result from a neoplastic transformation that causes an intrinsic abnormality in stem cells, but it also may occur because of an immunologically mediated decrease in the size of the stem cell compartment (13,14). Defective hematopoietic microenvironment or cytokine production may contribute to aplastic anemia in some patients, but it does not appear to play a primary role in most patients.

Clinical Features
The presenting manifestations and clinical features of aplastic anemia usually are related to pancytopenia.

Initial Manifestations
   1. **Bleeding** is a direct result of thrombocytopenia and is the most frequent presenting manifestation. It may occur as ecchymoses, petechiae, epistaxis, or other more serious hemorrhagic events. The frequency and severity of bleeding depends on the severity of thrombocytopenia, with spontaneous hemorrhage likely when the platelet count is less than 20,000 per microliter. Infection may aggravate the thrombocytopenia and bleeding diathesis.
   2. **Weakness, fatigue,** and other manifestations of impaired tissue oxygenation (e.g., angina pectoris) resulting from anemia.
   3. **Infection,** most frequently upper respiratory, cellulitis, or perirectal infection: Bacterial pathogens are predominant initially. In hospitalized patients, particularly those receiving antibiotics, fungal infections may occur.

Physical Examination
1. Pallor
2. Purpura: ecchymoses or petechiae
3. Noncutaneous hemorrhage: retinal or oral mucosal
4. Gingivitis, stomatitis, pharyngitis, or proctitis
5. Splenomegaly, although uncommon at presentation, may develop later in the course of the disease.
6. Hepatomegaly is infrequent unless related to an underlying associated disease process (e.g., hepatitis).
7. Generalized lymphadenopathy is infrequent.
8. Presence of splenomegaly, hepatomegaly, or lymphadenopathy at the presentation of aplastic anemia should prompt a search for an associated disease process.

Laboratory Features
Peripheral Blood
1. **Anemia** is always present and is usually normocytic and normochromic, although mild macrocytosis may occur. The reticulocyte count is less than 5%. The corrected reticulocyte count (reticulocyte % × actual hematocrit ÷ normal hematocrit) is low and may more accurately reflect the suppression of erythropoiesis.

2. **Neutropenia** (absolute neutrophil count < 1,500/μL) is invariably present and often accompanied by monocytopenia.

3. **Lymphocytes:** (a) quantitatively normal; (b) abnormalities in lymphocyte subsets and function have been described in some patients (15–18). These changes may play a role in the pathogenesis of aplasia through suppression of hematopoiesis through direct cytotoxicity or release of inhibitory cytokines.

4. **Thrombocytopenia:** Platelet count is less than 150,000 per microliter, but severity is variable.

5. **Peripheral blood smear:** Red cell morphology is usually normal except for mild macrocytosis. Granulocytes and platelets are reduced in number. The presence of nucleated red cells or a leukoerythroblastic picture is not typical of aplastic anemia and should raise the suspicion of another disease process. The blood smear should be examined for large granular lymphocytes, which sometimes is associated with erythroid hypoplasia.

6. **Serum iron** is elevated with increased saturation of iron-binding capacity.

Bone Marrow
Bone marrow aspiration often yields a small amount of material with few spicules. Smears reveal a predominance of lymphocytes, plasma cells, and occasional residual granulocytic, erythroid, or megakaryocytic elements. Bone marrow biopsy shows hypocellularity with a predominance of fat cells, and iron stores usually are increased. Occasionally, small foci of hypercellular bone marrow may be identified, and repeated bone marrow aspiration and biopsy may be required to clarify the diagnosis.

Cytogenetics
Cytogenetic abnormalities are present in a few patients at diagnosis (19,20). Some markers, such as monosomy 7, may predict a higher risk of myelodysplasia and acute leukemia.

Flow Cytometry
Abnormalities in the peripheral blood lymphocyte markers and the PNH abnormalities in CD56 and CD59 may be present and indicate the presence of associated disorders.

Magnetic Resonance Imaging
Magnetic resonance imaging (MRI) may demonstrate areas of bone marrow cellularity in patients with otherwise typical aplastic anemia (21). Some of these patients subsequently develop myelodysplasia or acute leukemia.

Differential Diagnosis
The differential diagnosis for aplastic anemia is that of pancytopenia with a hypocellular bone marrow. This includes primarily hypoplastic myelodysplasia. Generally, the bone marrow aspirate and biopsy distinguish aplastic anemia from other diseases associated with pancytopenia.

Prognosis
Patterns of Survival
Survival is biphasic, with high early mortality and then a slower decline. Twenty-five percent of patients survive 4 months or less, 25% survive for approximately 4 to 12 months, 35% survive for more than 1 year, and 10% to 20% spontaneously recover partially or completely. Overall mortality is approximately 70%, and the median survival is about 12 months (22).

Prognostic Features

The etiology of aplastic anemia may have prognostic importance. Constitutional aplastic anemia is usually a fatal illness. Two months after diagnosis, aplastic anemia associated with hepatitis has a mortality rate in excess of 60%. In contrast, aplastic anemia secondary to a known drug or toxin may have a more favorable prognosis.

There is no clear correlation of the prognosis with age or sex. Several attempts at multivariate analysis produced complex formulas for prediction of outcome. With these formulas, it is possible to predict with reasonable accuracy which patients will clearly have severe disease and early death and which will have mild disease and more prolonged survival, but an indeterminate group that is difficult to classify remains (23). The International Aplastic Anemia study group has established criteria for severe aplastic anemia (Table 13). Patients who meet these criteria have a very poor prognosis with a median survival of 6 months and a 20% one-year survival (24). Patients with a white blood cell count of less than 200 per microliter appear to have an even worse prognosis (25). Patients with deterioration in blood counts during the initial phase of observation also have a poor prognosis.

Complications

Long-term complications of aplastic anemia are in part determined by the therapy selected (10,26). Patients treated for aplastic anemia have an increased risk of malignancy, with a relative risk of 5.5.

Risk of myelodysplasia and acute leukemia is greatest for patients who receive immunosuppressive treatment compared with those who undergo bone marrow transplantation. Both groups have an increased risk of solid tumors (10). Patients treated with only androgens appear to have a lower rate of subsequent neoplasia (26).

Treatment

Patients who meet the criteria for severe aplastic anemia under the age of 50 years should be evaluated immediately for the possibility of bone marrow transplantation. Transfusion of blood products should be minimized in any potential bone marrow transplantation candidate, and if blood product transfusion is needed, family members should not be used as donors.

General Measures

1. When the granulocyte count is less than 500 per microliter, patients should avoid crowd exposure and contact with persons known to have infections. Anyone who is in contact with the patient should wash his or her hands thoroughly using a bacteriostatic soap. In hospitalized patients, protective isolation measures, including regular hand washing with antiseptic soap, should be instituted. It is not clear whether the regular use of face masks, gowns, or gloves is of additional benefit. Prophylactic use of oral nonabsorbable antibiotics may reduce the incidence of bacteremias of bowel origin. Alternatively, cotrimoxazole (one double-strength tablet twice daily) or a quinolone (Ciprofloxacin) are also effective.

2. Regular use of antiseptic soaps on the skin may reduce the risk of skin infection.
3. Electric razors should be used in place of blades to avoid bleeding.
4. A soft toothbrush should be used for dental care to avoid gingival bleeding.
5. A stool softener should be taken to avoid constipation and rectal bleeding.
6. Intramuscular injections should be avoided.

Table 13. Criteria for severe aplastic anemia[a]

Blood	Neutrophils <500 μL
	Platelets <20,000/μL
	Reticulocytes <1% (corrected)
Bone marrow	Severe hypocellularity
	Moderate hypocellularity with <30% of residual cells being hematopoietic

[a] Any two blood criteria and either marrow criterion.

7. Menstrual bleeding may be prevented by using an anovulatory agent (e.g., Ovral, 1–2 tablets daily). Breakthrough bleeding may occur, and withdrawal bleeding occurs when the medication is stopped. Excessive menstrual flow may be interrupted with Premarin, 25 mg administered intravenously, every 6 to 12 hours until bleeding stops; then oral anovulatory agents should be started.

Blood Product Replacement
Patients who are potential bone marrow transplant candidates should not receive blood product support unless this is unavoidable. Blood products should be leukocyte depleted and irradiated. Patients without evidence of cytomegalovirus immunity should receive cytomegalovirus-negative products.

1. **Packed red blood cell transfusions:** Red cell transfusions may become necessary with a hemoglobin below 8 g per deciliter. Patients who are not acutely ill and with no cardiac, pulmonary, or peripheral vascular disease may tolerate a hemoglobin of 6 g per deciliter for some time.
2. **Platelet transfusions:** Pooled random-donor platelets or single-donor platelets obtained by apheresis should be administered prophylactically in patients with a platelet count less than 10,000 per microliter. In the face of bleeding, infection, fever, or an associated coagulation abnormality, platelet transfusions are necessary at higher platelet counts. Patients often become refractory after repeated platelet transfusions and may benefit from use of family donors or unrelated human leukocyte antigen (HLA)-compatible patients. Family donors should be avoided, however, for patients who are candidates for a transplant from a family member. Refractory patients may respond to ABO blood type–specific pooled random platelets (see Chapter 17).
3. **Granulocyte transfusion** is not helpful prophylactically, but it may be efficacious during an episode of documented bacterial infection that has not responded to antibiotic therapy. Daily administration of 1×10^{10} neutrophils for 4 to 7 days should be considered (27).

Antibiotic Therapy
1. **Fever** or any sign of infection is an indication for empiric broad-spectrum antibiotic therapy.
2. **Pretreatment evaluation:** History and physical examination; cultures (blood, urine, throat, skin lesions, or any site of apparent infection). When a venous access device is present, blood cultures are drawn from the catheter and culturing the exit site should be considered.
3. **Choice of antibiotics:** A regimen containing a semisynthetic penicillin (e.g., piperacillin) plus an aminoglycoside (e.g., tobramycin or gentamicin) is a reasonable initial empiric choice. In penicillin-allergic patients, a third-generation cephalosporin, such as ceftazidime with or without the aminoglycoside, can be substituted. If gram-positive infection is suspected, vancomycin should be included. Antibiotic choice also depends on institutional infection experience and should be adjusted after sensitivities have been determined.
4. **Evaluate for opportunistic infections** requiring specific therapies: fungal, *Nocardia, Listeria, Pneumocystis carinii*.
5. Patients with persistent fevers while receiving broad-spectrum antibacterial therapy should empirically receive antifungal therapy.

Hematopoietic Growth Factors
1. **Aplastic anemia** is not characterized by deficiencies of the known hematopoietic growth factors, with the possible exception of stem cell factor (SCF) (28).
2. Both **granulocyte colony stimulating factor (G-CSF) and granulocyte-macrophage colony stimulating factor (GM-CSF)** can improve neutrophil counts, with the best responses more likely in less severe aplastic anemia.
3. G-CSF has a better toxicity profile than GM-CSF, and there is no apparent advantage in efficacy for GM-CSF in aplastic anemia.
4. **Erythropoietin (EPO)** alone has no role in the treatment of aplastic anemia. EPO (400 IU/kg three times weekly) combined with G-CSF (400µg/m² daily) has improves erythropoiesis in nonsevere aplastic anemia (29), but the role of this treatment

is limited to a small group of patients and probably has little value for patients with severe aplasia.

5. G-CSF has been used in combination with immunosuppression to reduce the severity and duration of neutropenia. Although this may result in improved early neutrophil counts and reduce the incidence of infections, there is no evidence for improved response rate or survival (30).

6. There is some evidence, primarily from Japan, that patients treated with both immunosuppression and G-CSF may have a higher incidence of evolving into myelodysplasia (31).

7. G-CSF can shorten the duration of neutropenia following bone marrow transplantation.

8. The role of SCF and thrombopoietin in managing aplastic anemia has not been determined, but it is not likely these growth factors will become primary treatment.

9. Hematopoietic growth factors should not be used as the primary treatment for aplastic anemia. This can result in dangerous and potentially fatal delays in definitive management with bone marrow transplantation or immunosuppressive therapy.

Androgens

1. **Mechanism:** Androgens increase erythropoietin production and stimulate proliferation of erythroid and granulocytic progenitors.

2. **Androgens** have not been shown to improve survival, but occasionally patients may benefit.

3. **Androgens should be** considered for use in patients not eligible for bone marrow transplantation after failure of immunosuppressive therapy. Oxymetholone, 3 to 5 mg per kilogram of weight daily orally for 3 to 6 months, may be used to assess response.

Bone Marrow Transplantation

1. Allogeneic bone marrow transplantation is the treatment of choice for patients younger than 40 years of age with severe aplastic anemia and an HLA-identical sibling donor. About 25% to 30% of patients will have an acceptable donor. Referral should be made to a transplant center as soon as possible after diagnosis.

2. Patients over 40 to 50 years of age with an HLA-identical sibling donor also may be considered for bone marrow transplantation, but they are at increased risk for graft-versus-host disease (GVHD) and have higher mortality.

3. Patients over 50 years are generally not considered for allogeneic bone marrow transplantation because of the associated toxicity with the procedure.

4. Patients with an identical twin donor should receive a bone marrow transplantation regardless of age and without immunosuppressive conditioning. If the syngeneic bone marrow transplantation is unsuccessful, a second one with immunosuppressive conditioning should be attempted.

5. Transfusion of blood products should be minimized before transplantation in all bone marrow transplant candidates.

6. Unrelated, HLA-compatible donor bone marrow transplantation can be considered for patients without a sibling donor who fail to achieve sustained response to immunosuppressive therapy (32). Current results show about 36% with a 3-year survival (33). High-resolution DNA based HLA typing will improve the accuracy of compatibility testing and should improve the outcomes of nonsibling donor transplantation. In patients younger than 20 years of age with a molecularly matched unrelated donor, transplantation should be considered after failure of one course of immunosuppression. Based on current results, patients over the age of 20 should receive a second course of immunosuppression before undergoing unrelated donor transplant.

7. Successful bone marrow transplantation is curative for aplastic anemia.

8. Complications of bone marrow transplantation (34) include the following: (a) graft rejection; (b) GVHD [Note: The addition of antithymocyte globulin (ATG) to cyclophosphamide in conditioning regimens and the use of cyclosporine have reduced the incidence of both graft rejection and GVHD]; (c) interstitial pneumonia; (d) infection; (e) organ toxicities [e.g., skin problems (scleroderma-like), cataracts, chronic lung dis-

ease, hypothyroidism, chronic bone and joint problems, gonadal dysfunction]; and (f) neoplasia, most commonly, squamous carcinomas.

9. **Long-term results:** Five-year survival rates for HLA-identical sibling transplants have progressively improved over the past three decades and in most recent studies are about 66%. Survival is best in young patients (<20 years), patients who have not undergone transfusion, patients who have undergone transplantation early in their disease, and patients in good overall condition without infection at the time of transplant. For patients who live 6 years after transplantation for aplastic anemia, mortality rates become indistinguishable from the general population (35). Long-term functional status for transplant patients is excellent.

Immunosuppressive Therapy

Immunosuppression is the initial choice of treatment for patients over the age of 40 and those without an HLA-matched sibling donor. ATG is the most effective single agent, with response rates of 40% to 70% (36). The addition of cyclosporin A to ATG results in better early response rate and can reduce the need for repeated courses of immunosuppression. The combination of ATG and cyclosporine is currently the standard immunosuppressive regimen for severe aplastic anemia (37). Prednisone is given during the ATG treatment to prevent serum sickness (immune complex) reactions. ATG is contraindicated for patients with horse serum allergy, but desensitization may be considered.

The role of **growth factors,** specifically G-CSF, is uncertain. G-CSF appears to improve neutrophil counts early in treatment and may reduce infectious complications, but the impact of growth factors on survival has not been determined. At present, routine growth factor administration during immunosuppressive therapy is not recommended.

In terms of **dosage,** ATG protocols vary but have ranged from 10 to 20 mg per kilogram of body weight daily for 8 to 14 days to 40 mg per kilogram of body weight daily for 4 days. ATG is given as an infusion over 4 to 8 hours. An intradermal test dose is given before the first infusion. Cyclosporine is given in a total daily dose of 12 mg per kilogram daily administered orally in two divided doses for 14 days and then adjusted weekly to maintain a level of 200 to 400 ng per milliliter by radioimmunoassay. Treatment is continued for 6 months and then tapered or discontinued.

Responses are gradual, with initial improvement requiring about 4 weeks of therapy. Median time to response is about 2 months, and almost all responses have occurred by 4 months. Most responses are incomplete in that residual abnormalities of the hemoglobin, neutrophil, or platelet count may persist. For patients who do not respond to an initial course of ATG, a second course is effective in 40% of cases.

Relapse occurs in about 35% of patients treated with immunosuppression and is often in association with tapering or discontinuation of cyclosporine. Patients who have a relapse have an excellent chance of responding to another course of ATG (38).

Long-term results were studied retrospectively by researchers in Seattle who studied patients treated from 1978 through 1991. They compared the results of bone marrow transplantation with those of immunosuppression in acquired aplastic anemia. Actuarial survival at 15 years was 69% for transplant patients and 38% for those who received immunosuppressive therapy. Only one of the 227 patients who underwent immunosuppression received cyclosporine (39). Five-year survival for the patients treated with immunosuppressive therapy since 1990 was 73%. Older age is associated with worse survival (40). There is continuing risk for relapse and development of clonal hematologic disorders, PNH, or myelodysplasia (36).

Toxicities from ATG include lymphopenia, neutropenia, thrombocytopenia, fever, arthralgias, rash, infection, anaphylaxis (<3%), and serum sickness (>90%). From high-dose **cyclosporine,** the toxicities include mild, reversible azotemia, hepatic injury, hypertension, gum hypertrophy, neuropsychiatric syndrome, and infection.

Other Approaches

1. **High-dose cyclophosphamide:** After high-dose cyclophosphamide given as preparative regimen for bone marrow transplantation, some patients recover autologous hematopoiesis. In a small series, high-dose cyclophosphamide induced a complete

response in seven of ten 10 patients. None of the responders relapsed or developed clonal hematologic disorders with a median follow-up of 10.8 years (41). This therapy requires more intensive initial supportive care than ATG–cyclosporine therapy because of the severe pancytopenia that ensues. A randomized trial of high-dose cyclophosphamide with cyclosporine versus ATG with cyclosporine is in progress (42). The ultimate place of this therapy in treating aplastic anemia may become evident as the results of this trial become available.

2. The role of **splenectomy** in aplastic anemia is limited. Splenectomy can be performed safely and results in more rapid improvement in blood counts for patients who receive immunosuppressive therapy (43). It may be helpful to patients refractory to platelet transfusions.

Overview of Treatment
1. All patients under the age of 40 years with an HLA-identical sibling donor should be offered an allogeneic bone marrow transplant.
2. Patients aged 40 to 50 years can be considered for bone marrow transplant or immunosuppressive therapy.
3. Patients of any age with an identical twin donor should receive a bone marrow transplant.
4. Patients who are not candidates for HLA-matched sibling transplant should receive primary immunosuppressive therapy with ATG and cyclosporine.
5. For patients who do not respond to immunosuppressive therapy after two courses, (a) if younger than 40 years of age, consider HLA-matched unrelated donor bone marrow transplant; and (b) if over 40 years of age or otherwise unable to receive unrelated bone marrow transplant, consider high-dose cyclophosphamide, androgens, or experimental approaches via clinical trials.

References
1. Brown KE, Tisdale J, Barrett AJ, et al. Hepatitis-associated aplastic anemia. *N Engl J Med* 1997;336:1059–1064.
2. Hibbs JR, Frickhofen N, Rosenfeld SJ, et al. Aplastic anemia and viral hepatitis: non-A, non-B, non-C? *JAMA* 1992;267:2051–2054.
3. Tzakis AG, Arditi M, Whitington PF, et al. Aplastic anemia complicating orthotopic liver transplantation for non-A, non-B hepatitis. *N Engl J Med* 1988;319: 393–396.
4. Young NS, Mortimer PP, Moore JG, et al. Characterization of a virus that causes transient aplastic crisis. *J Clin Invest* 1984;73:224–230.
5. Spivak JL, Bender BS, Quinn TC. Hematologic abnormalities in the acquired immune deficiency syndrome. *Am J Med* 1984;77:224–228.
6. Rosse WF. Paroxysmal nocturnal hemoglobinuria as a molecular disease. *Medicine* 1997;76:63–93.
7. De Lord C, Tooze JA, Saso R, et al. Deficiency of glycosylphosphatidyl inositol-anchored proteins in patients with aplastic anaemia does not affect response to immunosuppressive therapy. *Br J Haematol* 1998;101:90–93.
8. Schrezenmeier H, Hertenstein B, Wagner B, et al. A pathogenetic link between aplastic anemia and paroxysmal nocturnal hemoglobinuria is suggested by a high frequency of aplastic anemia patients with a deficiency of phosphatidylinositol glycan anchored proteins. *Exp Hematol* 1995;23:81–87.
9. Luzzatto L, Bessler M, Rotoli B. Somatic mutations in paroxysmal nocturnal hemoglobinuria: a blessing in disguise? *Cell* 1997;88:1–4.
10. Socie G, Henry-Amar M, Bacigalupo A, et al. Malignant tumors occurring after treatment of aplastic anemia: European Bone Marrow Transplantation-Severe Aplastic Anaemia Working Party. *N Engl J Med* 1993;329:1152–1157.
11. Tichelli A, Gratwohl A, Wursch A, et al. Late haematological complications in severe aplastic anaemia. *Br J Haematol* 1988;69:413–418.
12. Castro-Malaspina H. Aplastic anemia: current concepts on pathogenesis and therapy. *Nouv Rev Fr Hematol* 1993;35:183–186.
13. Young NS. The problem of clonality in aplastic anemia: Dr Dameshek's riddle, restated. *Blood* 1992;79:1385–1392.

14. Young NS, Maciejewski J. The pathophysiology of acquired aplastic anemia. *N Engl J Med* 1997;336:1365–1372.
15. Mentzel U, Vogt H, Rossol R, et al. Analysis of lymphocyte subsets in patients with aplastic anemia before and during immunosuppressive therapy. *Ann Hematol* 1993;66:127–129.
16. Moebius U, Herrmann F, Hercend T, et al. Clonal analysis of CD4$^+$/CD^8 T cells in a patient with aplastic anemia. *J Clin Invest* 1991;87:1567–1574.
17. Viale M, Merli A, Bacigalupo A. Analysis at the clonal level of T-cell phenotype and functions in severe aplastic anemia patients. *Blood* 1991;78:1268–1274.
18. Zoumbos NC, Ferris WO, Hsu SM, et al. Analysis of lymphocyte subsets in patients with aplastic anaemia. *Br J Haematol* 1984;58:95–105.
19. Appelbaum FR, Barrall J, Storb R, et al. Clonal cytogenetic abnormalities in patients with otherwise typical aplastic anemia. *Exp Hematol* 1987;15:1134–1139.
20. Geary CG, Harrison CJ, Philpott NJ, et al. Abnormal cytogenetic clones in patients with aplastic anaemia: response to immunosuppressive therapy. *Br J Haematol* 1999;104:271–274.
21. Negendank W, Weissman D, Bey TM, et al. Evidence for clonal disease by magnetic resonance imaging in patients with hypoplastic marrow disorders. *Blood* 1991;78:2872–2879.
22. Cartwright GE, Williams DM, Lynch RE. Natural history, cause and prognosis of aplastic anemia. In *Proceedings of the Conference on Aplastic Anemia: A Stem Cell Disease.* NIH Publication 81–1008, 1981.
23. Najean Y, Pecking A. Prognostic factors in acquired aplastic anemia: a study of 352 cases.*Am J Med* 1979;67:564–571.
24. Gewirtz AM, Hoffman R. Current considerations of the etiology of aplastic anemia. *Crit Rev Oncol Hematol* 1985;4:1–30.
25. Marsh JC, Hows JM, Bryett KA, et al. Survival after antilymphocyte globulin therapy for aplastic anemia depends on disease severity. *Blood* 1987;70:1046–1052.
26. Najean Y, Haguenauer O. Long-term (5 to 20 years) evolution of nongrafted aplastic anemias. The Cooperative Group for the Study of Aplastic and Refractory Anemias. *Blood* 1990;76:2222–2228.
27. Wright DG. Symposium on infectious complications of neoplastic disease (part II): leukocyte transfusions: thinking twice. *Am J Med* 1984;76:637–644.
28. Kumar M, Alter BP. Hematopoietic growth factors for the treatment of aplastic anemia. *Curr Opin Hematol* 1998;5:226–234.
29. Bessho M, Hirashima K, Asano S, et al. Treatment of the anemia of aplastic anemia patients with recombinant human erythropoietin in combination with granulocyte colony-stimulating factor: a multicenter randomized controlled study. Multicenter Study Group. *Eur J Haematol* 1997;58:265–272.
30. Marsh JC. Hematopoietic growth factors in the pathogenesis and for the treatment of aplastic anemia. *Semin Hematol* 2000;37:81–90.
31. Kaito K, Otsubo H, Sekita T, et al. Long-term administration of G-CSF for aplastic anemia may be a risk factor to develop myelodysplastic syndrome with monosomy 7 in adults. *Blood* 1997;90(Suppl 1):582a.
32. Margolis DA, Casper JT. Alternative-donor hematopoietic stem-cell transplantation for severe aplastic anemia. *Semin Hematol* 2000;37:43–55.
33. Deeg HJ, Seidel K, Casper J, et al. Marrow transplantation from unrelated donors for patients with severe aplastic anemia who have failed immunosuppressive therapy. *Biol Blood and Marrow Transplantation* 1999;5:243–252.
34. Horowitz MM. Current status of allogeneic bone marrow transplantation in acquired aplastic anemia. *Semin Hematol* 2000;37:30–42.
35. Socie G, Stone JV, Wingard JR, et al. Long-term survival and late deaths after allogeneic bone marrow transplantation: Late Effects Working Committee of the International Bone Marrow Transplant Registry. *N Engl J Med* 1999;341:14–21.
36. Frickhofen N, Rosenfeld SJ. Immunosuppressive treatment of aplastic anemia with antithymocyte globulin and cyclosporine. *Semin Hematol* 2000;37:56–68.
37. Frickhofen N, Kaltwasser JP, Schrezenmeier H, et al. Treatment of aplastic anemia with antilymphocyte globulin and methylprednisolone with or without cyclosporine: the German Aplastic Anemia Study Group. *N Engl J Med* 1991;324: 1297–1304.

38. Rosenfeld SJ, Kimball J, Vining D, et al. Intensive immunosuppression with anti-thymocyte globulin and cyclosporine as treatment for severe acquired aplastic anemia. *Blood* 1995;85:3058–3065.
39. Doney K, Leisenring W, Storb R, et al. Primary treatment of acquired aplastic anemia: outcomes with bone marrow transplantation and immunosuppressive therapy: Seattle Bone Marrow Transplant Team. *Ann Intern Med* 1997;126:107–115.
40. Tichelli A, Socie G, Henry-Amar M, et al. Effectiveness of immunosuppressive therapy in older patients with aplastic anemia: European Group for Blood and Marrow Transplantation Severe Aplastic Anaemia Working Party. *Ann Intern Med* 1999;130:193–201.
41. Brodsky RA, Sensenbrenner LL, Jones RJ. Complete remission in severe aplastic anemia after high-dose cyclophosphamide without bone marrow transplantation. *Blood* 1996;87:491–494.
42. Tisdale JF, Dunn DE, Rosenfeld SE, et al. Report on a randomized trial comparing cyclophosphamide and cyclosporine versus antithymocyte globulin and cyclosporine as initial treatment for severe aplastic anemia. *Blood* 1999;94(Suppl 1):407a.
43. Speck B, Tichelli A, Widmer E, et al. Splenectomy as an adjuvant measure in the treatment of severe aplastic anaemia. *Br J Haematol* 1996;92:818–824.

Suggested Reading

Vincent PC. Drug-induced aplastic anemia and agranulocytosis. Incidence and mechanisms. *Drugs* 1986;31:52–63.

3. PRIMARY AND SECONDARY ERYTHROCYTOSIS

William G. Hocking

Erythrocytosis is characterized by pathologic elevation of the red blood cell mass. At sea level, the normal red cell mass for a woman is 23 to 29 mL per kilogram of body weight and for men 26 to 32 mL per kilogram of body weight. *Erythrocytosis* can be defined as any increase in the red cell mass above these limits. *Polycythemia* is often used synonymously with erythrocytosis but more correctly refers to an increase in two or more hematopoietic cell lines.

Classification

Erythrocytosis can be classified by the underlying pathophysiologic mechanisms (Table 1).

Primary Erythrocytosis
Primary erythrocytosis represents autonomous proliferation of erythroid progenitors as a result of an intrinsic cellular defect or infrequently to altered regulation of erythropoiesis.

Polycythemia vera (PV) is a neoplastic clonal proliferation, probably arising in a pluripotent hematopoietic progenitor cell with clinical manifestations involving erythroid, granulocytic, and megakaryocytic cell lines.

Primary "pure" erythrocytosis (erythremia) is a heterogeneous syndrome characterized by isolated elevation of the red cell mass without the other stigmata of PV and no apparent cause of secondary erythrocytosis. Both sporadic and familial syndromes have been described (1). Erythropoietin levels are normal or low (2). In some families, erythrocytosis may result from a mutation in the erythropoietin receptor gene, which increases the sensitivity of erythroid progenitors to erythropoietin (3). These mutations result in truncation of the erythropoietin receptor with loss of a negative regulatory mechanism (4). Some patients develop overt PV during the course of observation (5).

Secondary Erythrocytosis
This heterogeneous group of disorders is associated with erythrocytosis because of either a physiologically appropriate response to decreased tissue oxygenation or the physiologically inappropriate production of erythropoietin or other factors that stimulate erythropoiesis. **Physiologically appropriate conditions** cause erythrocytosis by virtue of physiologic mechanisms triggered by a decrease in tissue oxygenation.

1. **High altitude:** People who ascend to altitudes above 2,000 m (6,500 feet) undergo a sequence of adaptive changes. During the first 24 hours, the plasma volume decreases, resulting in a relative erythrocytosis. Erythropoietin levels rise, and enhanced erythropoietic activity ultimately leads to a rise in the red cell mass. Initial hyperventilation alkalosis causes a leftward shift of the oxyhemoglobin dissociation curve, but subsequent increase in synthesis of red cell 2,3-diphosphoglycerate (2,3-DPG) causes the curve to shift back to the right. The principal long-term human adaptation to high altitude is an increase in red cell mass.

2. **Chronic lung disease** with arterial hypoxemia is often associated with an elevation of the red cell mass, which correlates with the degree of arterial desaturation. Whereas the mechanism of erythrocytosis in these patients is believed to be related to stimulation of erythropoietin release by hypoxia, activation of the renin–angiotensin system also appears to play a role (6).

3. **Alveolar hypoventilation** can produce secondary erythrocytosis as a result of arterial hypoxemia.

4. **Cardiovascular right-to-left shunt:** These patients often have pronounced arterial hypoxemia and extreme secondary erythrocytosis with hematocrits in excess of 70%.

Table 1. Classification of erythrocytosis

I. Primary (autonomous)
  A. Polycythemia vera
  B. "Pure" erythrocytosis ("erythremia")
    1. Familial
    2. Sporadic
II. Secondary
  A. Physiologically appropriate (decreased tissue oxygenation)
    1. High altitude
    2. Chronic lung disease
    3. Alveolar hypoventilation
    4. Cardiovascular right-to-left shunt
    5. High-oxygen-affinity hemoglobinopathy
    6. Carboxyhemoglobinemia ("smoker's erythrocytosis")
    7. Congenitally decreased erythrocyte 2,3-DPG
  B. Physiologically inappropriate erythropoietin or other erythropoietic substances
    1. Tumors producing erythropoietin or other erythropoietic substances
      a. Renal cell carcinoma
      b. Hepatocellular carcinoma
      c. Cerebellar hemangioblastoma
      d. Uterine leiomyoma
      e. Ovarian carcinoma
      f. Pheochromocytoma
      g. Other tumors
    2. Renal diseases
      a. Cysts
      b. Hydronephrosis
      c. Diffuse parenchymal disease
      d. Bartter syndrome
      e. Renal transplantation
      f. Long-term hemodialysis
    3. Andrenal cortical hypersection
    4. Exogenous androgens
    5. Unexplained ("essential")
III. Apparent polycythemia (Gaisböck syndrome, relative, spurious, or stress
    erythrocytosis)

2,3-DPG, 2,3-diphosphoglycerate.

5. **High-oxygen-affinity hemoglobinopathies:** These disorders result from genetic point mutations leading to single amino acid substitutions, which produce a hemoglobin with increased oxygen affinity. Erythrocytosis results from impaired release of oxygen to the tissues.

6. **Carboxyhemoglobinemia (smoker's erythrocytosis):** Erythrocytosis results from a functional anemia and left shift of the oxyhemoglobin dissociation curve caused by binding of carbon monoxide to hemoglobin (7).

7. **Congenitally decreased erythrocyte 2,3-DPG:** Mild erythrocytosis has been reported in association with hereditary reduction in 2,3-DPG. The erythrocytosis is probably due to leftward shift of the oxyhemoglobin dissociation curve.

In patients with **physiologically inappropriate conditions,** erythrocytosis does not represent a physiologic compensatory mechanism. Most of these patients have inappropriately elevated erythropoietin production from a benign or malignant tumor or as a result of regional renal hypoxia. Occasionally, erythrocytosis is mediated by other substances that are stimulating erythropoiesis:

1. **Tumors producing erythropoietin or other erythropoietic substances** (8): Praneoplastic erythrocytosis occurs in 1% to 5% of renal cell carcinomas, 5% to 10% of hepatocellular carcinomas, and 15% to 20% of cerebellar hemangioblastomas. Because renal cell carcinoma is the most common of these tumors in the United States, it represents the most frequent cause of paraneoplastic erythrocytosis. A wide variety of other neoplasms may be associated with erythrocytosis. Unexplained erythrocytosis may be an early indication of an otherwise occult neoplasm.

2. **Renal disease:** These disorders lead to regional renal hypoxia, presumably affecting the tissue oxygen sensor and resulting in increased erythropoietin production. In addition, activation of the renin–angiotensin system plays a role in stimulating erythropoiesis in some forms of renal disease. This effect is mediated both by stimulation of erythropoietin production (9) or by the direct stimulation of erythroid progenitors by angiotensin II (10).

3. **Adrenal cortical hypersecretion:** Erythrocytosis may result from the production of adrenal androgens, thus stimulating erythropoiesis.

4. **Exogenous androgens:** Androgens lead to increased erythropoiesis by increasing erythropoietin production and having a direct stimulatory effect on erythroid progenitor cells.

5. **Unexplained or "essential" erythrocytosis** (2): Patients with this disorder have elevated erythropoietin levels but no obvious cause or abnormality in tissue oxygenation to explain the enhanced erythropoietin production. Some patients appear to have a recessive familial form of erythrocytosis. Human immunodeficiency virus (HIV) infection and the use of zidovudine have recently been associated with erythrocytosis, but the causal relationship and mechanism are not clear (11).

Apparent Polycythemia
This heterogeneous syndrome is known by a variety of designations, including Gaisböck syndrome and spurious, or stress, or relative erythrocytosis. These patients have a high normal red cell mass and low normal or reduced plasma volume (5,12).

Hereditary or Familial Erythrocytosis
Hereditary or familial forms of erythrocytosis are rare, but different pathophysiologic mechanisms exist (Table 2). These entities are discussed in the appropriate classification.

Physiologic Effects of Erythrocytosis
Increased Oxygen-carrying Capacity
Effects on Viscosity
1. In normovolemic subjects, a hematocrit in excess of 45% may lead to hyperviscosity.
2. In hypervolemic subjects, the optimal hematocrit for tissue oxygen delivery is higher, approximately 55% to 60%; hematocrits in excess of 60% are likely to impair tissue oxygen delivery.

Physiologic Benefits
1. Patients with primary autonomous erythropoiesis or physiologically inappropriate secondary erythrocytosis derive no physiologic benefit from their elevated hematocrit.

Table 2. Hereditary erythrocytosis

High-affinity hemoglobinopathies (autosomal dominant)
Decreased erythrocyte 2,3-diphosphoglycerate (DPG)
DPG mutase deficiency (autosomal recessive)
Hereditary high-erythrocyte adenosine triphosphate
Increased erythropoietin production—essential erythrocytosis (autosomal recessive)
Erythropoietin-receptor mutations (autosomal dominant)
Unknown mechanisms
Hereditary polycythemia vera (polygenic)

2. Cerebral blood flow is significantly reduced in patients with hematocrits over 45% and improves after phlebotomy (13). Thus, for patients with no physiologic need for increased oxygen-carrying capacity, the optimal hematocrit is 42% to 46%.

3. Patients with physiologically appropriate secondary erythrocytosis develop an elevated red cell mass as a compensatory process, which may eliminate a deficit in tissue oxygenation and establish a new equilibrium at a higher-than-normal red cell mass. In some patients, a new equilibrium is not established and the red cell mass rises progressively, leading to hyperviscosity and impairment of oxygen delivery. This overcompensation is observed most frequently in patients with cyanotic congenital heart disease or hypoxemia due to chronic pulmonary disease.

The mechanism for overcompensation may be development of hyperviscosity, worsening tissue oxygenation, stimulus to erythropoietin production, and further expansion of the red cell mass. Other factors, such as activation of the renin–angiotensin system in chronic obstructive pulmonary disease (COPD), also may play a role (8).

Physiologic Control of Erythropoiesis

Erythropoietin (Fig. 1) is a 34,000-Da glycoprotein, encoded for by a gene located on the long arm of chromosome 7 (C7q), that is the principal regulator of red cell production (Fig. 1). It is produced predominantly by kidney in adults. The cellular site of production is not clearly established but is most likely a tubular or peritubular cell. The liver is the major extrarenal site of production and accounts for about 10% of erythropoietin in adults. Secretion is regulated by a putative renal tissue oxygen sensor and occurs in response to a reduction of tissue oxygen delivery. It stimulates proliferation and maturation of erythroid progenitors.

Tissue oxygen delivery is determined by a variety of factors:

1. Cardiac output
2. Arterial oxygen saturation
3. Red cell mass
4. Hemoglobin oxygen affinity:
   - Oxyhemoglobin dissociation curve (see Appendix E) reflects the affinity of hemoglobin for oxygen.
   - Increasing oxygen affinity occurs with increasing hemoglobin saturation (heme–heme or cooperative interaction).
   - Hemoglobin oxygen affinity can be expressed as the oxygen tension at which hemoglobin becomes 50% saturated or P_{50}: normal P_{50} is 27.5 mm Hg; decreased P_{50} reflects increased oxygen affinity; increased P_{50} reflects decreased oxygen affinity. Factors affecting P_{50} are illustrated in Table 3.

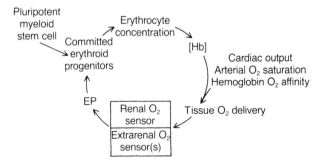

FIG. 1. Regulation of erythropoiesis by erythropoietin (EP). Hb, hemoglobin concentration.

Table 3. Factors that affect hemoglobin oxygen affinity (P_{50})

Increased oxygen affinity ($\downarrow P_{50}$, leftward shift)
   Alkalosis (Bohr effect)
   Decreased erythrocyte 2,3-diphosphoglycerate (DPG)
   Decreased temperature
   Carboxyhemoglobinemia
   High-affinity hemoglobinopathies
Decreased oxygen affinity ($\uparrow P_{50}$, rightward shift)
   Acidosis (Bohr effect)
   Increased erythrocyte, 2,3-DPG
   Increased temperature
   Hemoglobinopathies

Diagnosis and Differential Diagnosis
Establishing the Diagnosis
Erythrocytosis is considered initially on the basis of an elevated hematocrit. A hematocrit above 60% reliably predicts an elevated red cell mass, but an elevated hematocrit below 60% may be associated with a normal, or even low, red cell mass. In patients with borderline elevation of the hematocrit, other clinical or hematologic findings (e.g., splenomegaly, leukocytosis) may lead to a diagnosis of PV. In other patients, the association with an underlying disease process (e.g., obstructive lung disease with hypoxia) may explain mild erythrocytosis. In some patients, mild erythrocytosis occurs in the absence of other findings or disease. In these situations, a definitive diagnosis may not be possible at initial presentation. These patients require longer-term monitoring for development of findings consistent with a myeloproliferative disorder.

Differential Diagnosis
In some patients, [51]chromium red cell mass and [125]iodine plasma volume measurements may be helpful, but interpretation of these studies can be difficult in some patients, particularly in the presence of obesity.

Full-blown PV usually can be recognized easily by its clinical manifestations:

1. **Pruritus** occurs in about 40% of patients and is uncommon in other forms of erythrocytosis.
2. **Splenomegaly** occurs in 75% of PV patients and is an uncommon finding in other forms of erythrocytosis. Hepatomegaly may be present in about one third of patients.
3. **Panmyelosis:**
   * **Leukocytosis and granulocytosis** occur in about 60% of patients, often with a left shift and basophilia.
   * **Thrombocytosis,** usually of modest degree (400,000–800,000/mL), is present in approximately 50% of patients.
   * **Peripheral blood smear abnormalities** are uncommon early in the course of disease; however, mild anisocytosis and poikilocytosis, and rarely a nucleated red blood cell, may be present on the smear. Macrothrombocytes and hypogranular thrombocytes may be present.
4. **Bone marrow hyperplasia** involving erythroid, myeloid, and megakaryocytic lines is invariably present, and mild myelofibrosis also may be detected.
5. The Polycythemia Vera Study Group (PVSG) established criteria for inclusion of patients into their studies (Table 4). These criteria may serve as useful guidelines for diagnosis of PV, but they are relatively stringent and undoubtedly exclude patients with early PV or mild manifestations of the disease.

In patients without definitive evidence for PV, the differential diagnosis includes **early or mild PV, pure erythrocytosis, or secondary erythrocytosis. History** of cardiac or pulmonary disease, tobacco smoking, hematuria, or other symptoms of renal disease or a family history of erythrocytosis should be sought.

Table 4. Criteria for diagnosis of polycythemia vera (PV)[a]

Category A
1. Total red cell mass
   Male ≥36 mL/kg
   Female ≥32 mL/kg
2. Arterial oxygen saturation ≥92%
3. Splenomegaly

Category B
1. Thrombocytosis (platelets >400 × 10^3/μL)
2. Leukocytosis (white blood cells >12 × 10^3/μL)
3. Increased leukocyte alkaline phosphates (LAP) score
4. Serum B_{12} >900 pg/mL or B_{12}-binding capacity >2,200 pg/mL

From Berk PD, Goldberg JD, Donovan PB, et al. Therapeutic recommendations in polycythemia vera based on Polycythemia Vera Study Group protocols. *Semin Hematol* 1986;23:132.
[a] PV is diagnosed when A1 + A2 + A3 or A1 + A2 and any two from category B are present.

Physical examination may provide clues to the etiology:

- Obesity suggests alveolar hypoventilation.
- Cyanosis indicates arterial desaturation.
- Palpable splenomegaly suggests PV.

The **initial laboratory evaluation** (Table 5) includes a **complete blood count (CBC), including platelet count.** This test can distinguish isolated erythrocytosis from polycythemia.

Bone marrow aspiration and biopsy, although not indicated in all patients, are indicated in patients with neither clear evidence for PV nor secondary erythrocytosis. The finding of hypercellularity with trilinear hyperplasia and decreased or absent stainable iron supports a diagnosis of PV. Furthermore, although uncommon in early PV, the presence of myelofibrosis also supports this diagnosis. Cytogenetic analysis should be performed for patients in whom a myeloproliferative disorder is suspected because specific nonrandom cytogenetic markers, such as deletion of a portion of the long arm of chromosome 20 (20q-), occurs in about 30% of PV patients at diagnosis (14).

Arterial blood gases: In PV, the arterial oxygen saturation is greater than 92% unless there is an associated abnormality in gas exchange, and values less than this suggest that hypoxemia may be the cause for erythrocytosis. Arterial desaturation in carboxyhemoglobinemia is not apparent when saturation is determined from the PO_2 and a standard oxyhemoglobin dissociation curve but will be detected by direct measurement of saturation by oximetry. In some patients, desaturation may not be detected unless arterial blood is obtained while the patient is supine or sleeping. This is particularly important for patients with obesity hypoventilation or sleep apnea syndromes.

Table 5. Erythrocytosis—diagnostic tests

Complete blood count and platelet count
Bone marrow aspiration and biopsy
Arterial blood gases (consider supine)
Leukocyte alkaline phosphatase
P_{50}
Intravenous pyelogram or renal ultrasound
Liver ultrasound or CT scan
Erythropoietin level
Erythroid progenitor assays
Sleep apnea evaluation

CT, computed tomography; P_{50}, oxygen half-saturation pressure of hemoglobin.

Leukocyte alkaline phosphatase (LAP): This enzyme of neutrophil secondary granules is increased in approximately 70% of patients with PV. LAP also may be elevated by a variety of nonspecific stimuli, however, and thus is of limited value in differential diagnosis.

Oxygen half-saturation pressure of hemogrlobin (P_{50}): In patients with high-oxygen-affinity hemoglobinopathies, the P_{50} is decreased. Usually, it is less than 20 mm Hg, in contrast to the normal value of 27.5 mm Hg. P_{50} is also reduced in carboxy-hemoglobinemia, but it is normal in PV.

Intravenous pyelogram, renal ultrasound, or abdominal computed tomographic (CT) scan: One of these studies is indicated in all patients with unexplained erythrocytosis to exclude a benign or malignant renal abnormality.

Liver ultrasound or CT scan: In selected patients, hepatic imaging may be indicated to exclude a hepatic tumor.

Brain CT scan: In selected patients, this evaluation for cerebral hemangioblastoma is warranted.

Erythropoietin level: In primary erythrocytosis, erythropoietin levels are, by definition, suppressed. In secondary erythrocytosis, erythropoietin levels are generally normal or increased unless the erythrocytosis is mediated through an erythropoietin-independent mechanism.

Plasma or serum erythropoietin levels can be measured by radioimmunoassay or enzyme immunoassay. Erythropoietin levels can help discriminate between primary and secondary erythrocytosis (15,16). In some cases, however, erythropoietin levels may not distinguish these two groups (17). The degree of erythropoietin elevation in secondary erythrocytosis may depend on the underlying disorder. Abnormalities in erythropoietin levels may be intermittent, making a single normal level unreliable for exclusion of secondary erythrocytosis. In general, an elevated erythropoietin level is indicative of secondary erythrocytosis, a subnormal level suggests PV, and a normal level may be seen in either condition. The greatest use for erythropoietin levels may be in patients without clear-cut PV and with no obvious cause for secondary erythrocytosis.

Culture of erythroid progenitors *in vitro*: Growth of erythroid progenitors [burst-forming unit erythroid (BFU-E)] *in vitro* normally requires the addition of erythropoietin. In PV, BFU-E shows "endogenous" colony formation in the absence of added erythropoietin. Patients with secondary erythrocytosis do not exhibit endogenous colony formation. This may be a useful diagnostic test in difficult cases (18). These assays are available only at specialized centers.

Sleep apnea evaluation may be warranted in patients with erythrocytosis with no clearly established etiology (19).

Erythrocytosis-specific Syndromes
Polycythemia Vera

1. **Incidence:** PV is an uncommon disease with a peak age of onset of 50 to 60 years. Rare cases are diagnosed in adolescence.

2. **Pathophysiology:** PV is due to autonomous proliferation of erythroid progenitor cells. This autonomous proliferation is due to a clonal abnormality of the pluripotent stem cell, giving rise to erythrocytes, granulocytes, platelets, and probably lymphocytes. Normal hematopoietic stem cells are present but are suppressed by unknown mechanisms.

3. **Clinical features:** PV is often of insidious onset and usually is discovered incidentally on a routine blood count. Five stages have been proposed for the evolution of PV from (a) pure erythrocytosis, (b) erythrocytosis and thrombocytosis, (c) myeloid metaplasia/fibrosis, (d) spent phase with osteomyelosclerosis, and (e) acute leukemia (20). Stage I patients may be difficult to distinguish from patients with pure erythrocytosis.

Symptoms are often nonspecific. Symptoms related to impaired oxygen delivery include headache dizziness, vertigo, tinnitus, visual disturbances, angina pectoris, or intermittent claudication. Venous thrombosis or thromboembolism may occur. Hemorrhage may involve epistaxis, gingival bleeding, ecchymoses, or gastrointestinal bleeding. Abdominal pain secondary to peptic ulcer disease may be seen. Early satiety due to splenomegaly is characteristic. Pruritus, often exacerbated by a warm bath, occurs in about 40% of patients and may be due to increased granulocyte histamine release. A peripheral sensory neuropathy associated with axonal degeneration has been described in patients with PV (21).

The **physical examination** may reveal any of the following findings:

- Splenomegaly is present in 75% of patients at the time of diagnosis.
- Hepatomegaly is present in approximately 30% of patients at the time of diagnosis.
- Hypertension is commonly found in PV.
- Facial plethora.

4. **Laboratory features:**
- An **elevated red cell mass** is an essential feature of PV. The plasma volume is usually normal or mildly elevated. If the hematocrit is greater than 0.60, the red cell mass does not need to be measured by radionuclide techniques. Likewise, patients with hematocrit of 0.55 to 0.60 and other manifestations of PV do not require red cell mass measurement.
- **Red cell morphology** is usually normal early in the disease unless iron deficiency exists. Later, as myeloid metaplasia develops, marked anisocytosis, poikilocytosis, and increasing numbers of nucleated red cells often occur.
- **Leukocytosis** (white blood count > 12,000/mL) occurs in about 60% of patients. Neutrophilia with a left shift and the appearance of immature granulocytes may be present.
- **Mild basophilia** is observed in about 60% of patients.
- **Mild to moderate thrombocytosis** (platelet count 400,000–800,000/mL) is seen in about 50% of patients. Morphologic abnormalities of the platelets, including macrothrombocytes and deficient platelet granules, may be observed.
- **Abnormal platelet aggregation** with adenosine diphosphate (ADP), epinephrine, and collagen may be demonstrated, but the bleeding time is usually normal.
- **Routine coagulation tests** are normal, but fibrinogen turnover is accelerated. In patients with marked erythrocytosis, the amount of anticoagulant present in the blood collection tube increases relative to the amount of plasma and may result in artifactual prolongation of coagulation tests.
- **Bone marrow** hypercellularity and hyperplasia of erythroid, granulocytic, and megakaryocytic cell lines are typically present. Iron stores are decreased or absent. Fibrosis may be present and is detected early by the use of reticulin silver stains.
- The **LAP score** is elevated in about 70% of patients.
- A **vitamin B_{12}** level greater than 900 pg per milliliter is present in about 30% of patients and elevation of the unbound vitamin B_{12}-binding capacity greater than 2,200 pg per milliliter occurs in about 75% of patients. The binding capacity is elevated predominantly due to an increase in transcobalamin III.

Cytogenetic abnormalities with clonal karyotypic abnormalities are detected in about 30% of previously untreated patients and approximately 50% of patients who have received myelosuppressive therapies. Karyotypic abnormalities may develop during the course of the disease. The presence of clonal markers does not convey a poor prognosis. The most common karyotypic abnormalities are a deletion of the long arm of C5 (5q-), deletion of the long arm of C20 (20q-), trisomy-8, or trisomy-9 (14). The development of acute myelogenous leukemia almost always is associated with complex karyotypic abnormalities detected at the time of leukemic evolution.

- **Hyperuricemia** occurs in about 40% of patients.
- **Pseudohyperkalemia** related to release of potassium from platelets during *in vitro* coagulation may occur in patients with thrombocytosis. Plasma potassium concentration is normal.

5. **Complications:**
Thromboembolism occurs in 15% to 60% of patients and is the cause of death in 10% to 40%. Thromboses may be either venous or arterial. Intraabdominal venous thrombosis and arterial thromboembolism also occur. The pathophysiology of thromboembolism in PV is probably related to erythrocytosis in combination with thrombo-

cytosis and abnormalities of platelet function, but the precise mechanisms have not been clarified. Erythromelalgia is a unique clinical syndrome seen in patients with PV and essential thrombocythemia. It is characterized by red, painful, burning toes, feet, or fingers (22). Erythromelalgia responds dramatically to aspirin.

Hemorrhage occurs in 15% to 35% and is a cause of death in 6% to 30% of patients with PV. The risk of bleeding does not correlate well with the degree of thrombocytosis, platelet function abnormalities, or bleeding time. Treatment with antiplatelet agents may increase the risk of hemorrhage (23), but recent studies demonstrated the safety of low-dose aspirin in patients who have no risk factors for bleeding (24). A randomized placebo-controlled clinical trial of low-dose aspirin (100 mg daily) in PV is now being conducted in Europe to determine the efficacy in reducing thrombotic events and safety of this treatment (25).

Peptic ulcer disease occurs with three to five times greater frequency than in the normal population.

Postpolycythemic myeloid metaplasia ("spent" polycythemia) is reported to occur in 3% to 0% of patients with PV in most series, although in patients not dying from other causes, the incidence may approach 100%. These patients develop progressive hepatosplenomegaly, anemia, leukocytosis, and increasing numbers of immature granulocytes, including myeloblasts in the peripheral blood. Median survival in this phase of PV is approximately 2 years (26).

The incidence of **acute leukemia** incidence was studied prospectively by the PVSG (27) and subsequently updated (28). Patients treated with phlebotomy alone have an approximate 1.5% incidence of acute leukemia. Patients treated with chlorambucil have a 17% incidence, and patients treated with radioactive phosphorus (^{32}P) have a 10.9% incidence. About 50% of the chlorambucil-associated cases occur within 5 years of diagnosis, whereas most of the ^{32}P-associated cases occur 6 to 10 years after diagnosis. The incidence of leukemia in hydroxyurea-treated patients is 5.9% after a median of 8.6 years of follow-up (28). Although this value is not statistically greater than historical controls treated with phlebotomy, it raises concern that hydroxyurea carries some leukemogenic risk. There is also the suggestion that exposure to multiple myelosuppressive agents further increases this risk. The vast majority of leukemias in PV are nonlymphoblastic in type.

Nonhematologic malignancies: Patients treated with chlorambucil or ^{32}P have a higher incidence of skin and gastrointestinal tumors than those treated by phlebotomy alone.

6. **Treatment:** Guidelines for management of PV are summarized in Table 6.

Diagnosis: Establishing a definite diagnosis, particularly prior to administration of myelosuppressive therapy, is of particular importance, since no other form of erythrocytosis is treated with myelosuppression.

Table 6. Guidelines for management of polycythemia vera

Establish correct diagnosis.
Individualize therapy:
    Patients >70 yr: ^{32}P or hydroxyurea plus phlebotomy.
    Patients 50–70 yr: Phlebotomy with or without hydroxyurea. Consider interferon-α.
    Patients <50 yr: Phlebotomy alone when possible. Consider interferon-α.
    Anagrelide in selected patients.
Initially reduce hematocrit by phlebotomy.
Maintain hematocrit <46.
Administer myelosuppressive therapy in patients who have thrombosis risk factors.
When possible, avoid myelosuppressive therapy in patients <50 yr of age.
Postpone elective surgery until the disease is controlled for >2 mo.
Treat complications.
Administer symptomatic care.
Avoid severe iron deficiency.

Therapy must be individualized. Factors such as the age and sex of the patient, presenting clinical manifestations, and hematologic picture influence the treatment plan.

Phlebotomy: In all patients, the hematocrit initially should be normalized by phlebotomy. In younger patients with normal cardiovascular function, a 450-mL phlebotomy can be performed every other day until the hematocrit is less than 46%. Older patients or those with underlying cardiovascular disease should undergo smaller phlebotomies (20)–300 mL) twice weekly until the hematocrit is less than 46%. Subsequently, the hematocrit should be maintained between 42% and 46%.

Myelosuppressive therapy: Patients who are managed with phlebotomy alone have a substantially higher risk of thrombotic complications during the initial 5 to 7 years after diagnosis. Patients treated with chlorambucil or ^{32}P have a lower incidence of thrombosis but a substantially increased risk of acute leukemia and other malignancies. The latent interval for the development of leukemia is relatively short for chlorambucil and longer for ^{32}P treated-patients. Risk factors for thrombosis for patients treated by phlebotomy alone are a history of prior thrombosis and advanced age. Other factors, including increased hematocrit and platelet count, do not correlate well with this complication. Therefore, for patients younger than 50 years of age with no history of prior thrombosis, phlebotomy alone may be appropriate unless there is other reason to suspect an increased risk of thrombosis. For patients over 70 years of age, ^{32}P or hydroxyurea plus phlebotomy is recommended. Patients between the ages of 50 and 70 present a difficult problem in choosing optimal therapy; in general, when myelosuppression is required, hydroxyurea should be considered the agent of choice.

- **Hydroxyurea** (Hydrea) is an inhibitor of ribonucleoside reductase and has been shown to be effective in controlling PV in dosages of 15 to 30 mg per kilogram of body weight daily. In a PVSG protocol, hydroxyurea was not associated with an increased risk of acute leukemia. The use of hydroxyurea requires frequent monitoring of blood counts and continuous therapy because unmaintained remissions generally last less than 2 weeks.
- ^{32}P in a dosage of 2.3 millicuries per m^2 of body surface area, administered intravenously, has the advantage of longer duration of effect, often 6 to 24 months. It may be useful in treatment of noncompliant patients in patients for whom follow-up is difficult, or in elderly patients in whom leukemogenic potential is of less concern.
- **Busulfan** (Myleran) is a bifunctional alkylating agent that may be used for myelosuppression in PV. Patients are initially treated with 4 to 6 mg daily, and maximal response occurs in 2 to 4 months. Patients may achieve unmaintained remissions lasting for several years. In a European study, the leukemogenic potential of busulfan was less than ^{32}P (29). Prolonged myelosuppression, particularly thrombocytopenia, however, and nonhematologic toxicities, such as pulmonary fibrosis and cutaneous hyperpigmentation, make busulfan a less desirable agent for control of PV.
- **Interferon-α** was shown to be effective in (a) controlling the myeloproliferation of PV and (b) reducing thromboembolic events in a small uncontrolled study (30,31), and in some patients with a cytogenetic marker, suppression of the PV clone in the bone marrow has been observed (32). One of the advantages of interferon-α is that it has not been associated with induction of second malignant neoplasms. It also was suggested that interferon-α, because of the effects on suppression of fibroblast-stimulatory cytokines in the bone marrow, may reduce the incidence of evolution to postpolycythemic myeloid metaplasia and myelofibrosis. This has not been demonstrated in any prospective trial, however. The ultimate role of interferon-α in PV treatment will require prospective randomized trials to compare with hydroxyurea (33). The other drawback to interferon-α treatment is the side effects, which have resulted in discontinuation of this agent in about 20% of patients. It is reasonable to offer interferon-α to patients requiring myelosuppression who are willing to accept the inconvenience of subcutaneous administration and the potential for greater side effects.
- **Anagrelide** is a drug that specifically reduces platelet counts without affecting white or red blood cells numbers. This agent is generally well tolerated and does not appear to be associated with carcinogenesis (34). Anagrelide may be useful, partic-

ularly in younger patients, when trying to avoid long-term toxicities of myelosuppressive agents.
- **Elective surgery** should be postponed until the disease has been under control for
approximately 2 months.

Treatment of complications:

- **Hyperuricemia** should be treated with allopurinol in conventional doses because
the elevation in uric acid usually reflects increased cellular turnover. Acute gout
should be managed in the conventional manner, but particular caution should be
used in administering nonsteroidal antiinflammatory agents, which may predispose
to bleeding or gastric irritation.
- **Peptic ulcer disease** patients should be treated in a conventional manner using
antacids, H_2 histamine antagonists, proton-pump inhibitors, and other measures as
needed.
- **Postpolycythemic myeloid metaplasia** usually requires supportive blood product therapy. It is important to exclude iron, folic acid, or vitamin B_{12} deficiencies in
the anemic patient, and replacement of these substances should be given when appropriate. The anemia may respond to androgen therapy. Some patients have evidence of decreased red cell survival and may benefit from prednisone therapy (26).
Patients with severe cytopenias that are not responsive to other treatment or massive splenomegaly with pressure symptoms may require splenectomy. Splenomegaly
also may respond to myelosuppressive therapy. Radiation therapy may be useful in
producing temporary reduction in splenic size, but these responses are generally of
short duration. In carefully selected, young patients with this complication, allogeneic bone marrow transplantation may be effective (35).
- **Acute leukemia** in PV patients usually responds poorly to antileukemic therapy
and has a very poor prognosis. In these patients, who are often elderly and in poor
medical condition, a decision must be made whether to treat in a palliative and supportive fashion only, or to attempt aggressive induction therapy.
- **Thromboembolic risk** is not diminished by the prophylactic use of antiplatelet
agents (aspirin and dipyridamole), but these agents do increase the risk of hemorrhagic complications (23). Recently lower doses of aspirin (40 mg daily) have been
shown to be safe in selected patients (24). The efficacy of low-dose aspirin in prophylaxis of thromboembolism in PV patients requires further study in controlled
clinical trials (25). Patients with transient ischemic attacks or peripheral arterial
ischemic lesions may benefit from the use of antiplatelet agents until the PV is controlled by myelosuppression. Established thromboembolic complications should be
treated in a conventional manner.
- **Hemorrhagic complications** should be managed in the usual manner with blood
transfusion and correction of any existing coagulation abnormalities. Platelet transfusion may be justified in patients with dysfunctional platelets, even with a normal
platelet count.

Symptomatic care: Pruritus may respond to the administration H_1 or H_2 histamine antagonists, either alone or in combination.

Iron deficiency: Avoid severe iron deficiency. It has been previously reported that
microcytic red blood cells have a higher intrinsic viscosity, and in the presence of
microcytosis, whole blood viscosity is higher at any given hematocrit. Although there
is some conflicting evidence in this regard, it is advisable to avoid severe microcytosis
induced by repeated phlebotomy. When the mean corpuscular hemoglobin concentration is less than 22 pg, consideration should be given to cautious iron supplementation
with careful monitoring of the hemoglobin and hematocrit to avoid rapid or excessive rise.

7. **Prognosis:** Survival of untreated patients with PV historically ranges from 1.5 to
3.0 years (36). In recent results from the PVSG, median survival of patients treated with
^{32}P or phlebotomy alone is approximately 10 years, whereas survival of chlorambucil-
treated patients is significantly shorter. The major causes of death in PV are thrombotic events, acute leukemia, secondary neoplasms other than leukemia, bleeding, and

complications of myelofibrosis, which together account for approximately 75% of mortality in PV.

Secondary Erythrocytosis

1. **Smoker's erythrocytosis (carboxyhemoglobinemia):** Carboxyhemoglobin is formed when carbon monoxide binds to the ferrous iron of hemoglobin with an affinity 200 times that of oxygen. Carboxyhemoglobin has a biologic half-life of 4 hours and appears to be an important cause of erythrocytosis in tobacco smokers. The elevated red cell mass results both from the functional reduction in oxygen-carrying capacity and from the left shift of the oxyhemoglobin dissociation curve, which impairs oxygen unloading to the tissues (24). Diagnosis is established by history and measurement of carboxyhemoglobin levels, although the levels may return to normal if the patient has abstained from smoking for several hours before obtaining the blood sample. Arterial oxygen saturation is normal if calculated from the partial pressure of oxygen (PO_2) and a standard oxyhemoglobin dissociation curve, but directly measured saturation is reduced.

2. **High-oxygen-affinity hemoglobinopathies:** More than 20 known high-oxygen-affinity hemoglobinopathies, which result from genetic point mutations causing single amino acid substitutions, stabilize oxyhemoglobin, destabilize deoxyhemoglobin, or lead to altered binding of 2,3-DPG to hemoglobin and result in a left shift in the oxyhemoglobin dissociation curve. These are autosomal dominant traits in which homozygosity is incompatible with life. Diagnosis is made by measurement of oxygen half-saturation pressure of hemoglobin (P), which is usually less than 20 mm Hg. Standard hemoglobin electrophoresis discloses an abnormal band in approximately 50% of these hemoglobinopathies and cannot be relied on to exclude this cause of erythrocytosis.

3. **Chronic obstructive pulmonary disease (COPD):** Hypoxemia from chronic lung disease often is associated with erythrocytosis. The elevation of red cell mass correlates with the degree of arterial desaturation. Plasma volume often is increased so that the hematocrit and hemoglobin concentrations often underestimate the severity of erythrocytosis. Activation of the renin–angiotensin system also may play a role in stimulation of erythropoiesis in COPD patients (6). The degree of erythrocytosis may be related in part to continued exposure to tobacco smoking (carboxyhemoglobinemia). Phlebotomy probably is indicated for patients whose hematocrits are above 60%. Phlebotomy results in a reduction in arteriovenous oxygen content difference, pulmonary artery resistance, improved hemodynamic response to exercise, and mental alertness. Patients with an element of congestive heart failure are most likely to benefit. The ideal hematocrit for these patients is unknown and may vary among patients but is probably around 50% (37).

4. **Cyanotic congenital heart disease:** These patients have severe arterial hypoxemia secondary to right-to-left shunting. Some patients achieve an elevated but stable (compensated) hematocrit, whereas others have a continued tendency for a rising hematocrit, which is detrimental because hyperviscosity counteracts the benefit of increased oxygen-carrying capacity (38). The optimal hematocrit range in most of these patients is 55% to 60%.

5. **Alveolar hypoventilation:** The syndrome of hypoventilation associated with obesity (pickwickian) or upper-airway obstruction may be associated with erythrocytosis. The hypoxemia may not be apparent on arterial blood gases obtained with the patient awake and upright during the daytime, and it may be necessary to obtain supine or sleeping blood gases to confirm this diagnosis. Sleep apnea syndrome in the absence of obesity may explain some cases of secondary erythrocytosis. Patients may not have elevated erythropoietin levels (19).

6. **High-altitude erythrocytosis:** With ascent to altitudes above 2,000 m (approximately 6,500 ft), the plasma volume decreases by about 20% during the first 24 hours, causing a relative erythrocytosis. Erythropoietin levels rise and enhanced erythropoiesis results, leading to an increase in red cell mass. Initially, as a result of respiratory alkalosis, the oxyhemoglobin dissociation shifts to the left, but because of higher erythrocyte 2,3-DPG, the curve subsequently returns to a normal position. No treatment is specifically required for high-altitude erythrocytosis in most circumstances.

7. **Tumor-associated erythrocytosis:** Ectopic erythropoietin secretion occurs in a variety of tumors (8). In some tumors, there is circumstantial evidence that indicates the production of other erythropoietic stimulatory substances. The red cell mass may be more than twice normal in these patients. This syndrome is important because paraneoplastic erythrocytosis may provide an early clue to the presence of an otherwise occult tumor at a potentially curable stage. This is most likely to be true of renal cell carcinoma, and the erythrocytosis usually responds to successful treatment of the tumor.

8. **Renal disease:** Erythrocytosis has been associated with renal cysts, hydronephrosis, the nephrotic syndrome, diffuse parenchymal renal disease, and Bartter syndrome. Between 4% and 17% of renal transplant recipients develop erythrocytosis that appears to be mediated by increased erythropoietin production by the native kidneys (39). Activation of the renin–angiotensin system is also important and has implications for treatment (9,39). Recently, two patients on long-term hemodialysis were reported to develop erythrocytosis. Both these patients developed acquired renal cystic disease, and it was suggested that the renal cysts may have been responsible for elevation of erythropoietin secretion and the erythrocytosis. The alternative is that dialysis simply unmasked a preexisting propensity to erythrocytosis by correcting some of the metabolic consequences of renal failure.

9. **Adrenal cortical hypersecretion:** Erythrocytosis in these patients is mild and presumed to be secondary to stimulatory effect of adrenal cortical hormones. In some cases, androgen secretion may be involved.

10. **Exogenous androgens:** Androgens with the 5-α configuration stimulate erythropoietin production in both renal and extrarenal sites. 5-β androgens directly stimulate erythroid progenitor cells. Both mechanisms may be involved in the development of erythrocytosis in patients who are receiving therapeutic androgens.

11. **Unexplained ("essential") secondary erythrocytosis:** This group of patients is characterized by high erythropoietin titers and erythrocytosis with no evidence of another underlying cause of erythrocytosis (2).

Treatment of Secondary Erythrocytosis (Table 7)
The specific etiology of erythrocytosis should be determined whenever possible by appropriate diagnostic evaluation. **Factors that may aggravate or cause erythrocytosis** should be eliminated when possible:

1. **Smokers** should be encouraged to discontinue tobacco use.
2. **Diuretics** may aggravate hyperviscosity caused by erythrocytosis by reduction of plasma volume and should be avoided if feasible.
3. **Androgen** administration should be discontinued or dosage reduced if possible.

Avoid severe **iron deficiency** because it may have an adverse effect on intrinsic red cell viscosity. The reduction of hemoglobin concentration per red blood cell (mean corpuscular hemoglobin) may further impair oxygen transport. This effect may be of particular concern for patients with erythrocytosis secondary to arterial hypoxemia.

In some types of secondary erythrocytosis, **specific interventions** may improve or reverse the process:

Table 7. Guidelines for management of secondary erythrocytosis

---

Determine specific etiology if possible.
Eliminate aggravating factors.
Avoid severe iron deficiency.
Apply specific measures when applicable (see text).
Consider phlebotomy after asking:
    1. Does the elevated hematocrit provide a physiologically important adaptation for this patient?
    2. Is the degree of erythrocytosis detrimental?
Avoid myelosuppressive therapy.

---

1. **Smoking cessation** reverses the erythrocytosis associated with carboxyhemo-globinemia and may improve erythrocytosis in patients with chronic pulmonary disease (7).
2. **Supplemental oxygen therapy:** Low-flow continuous oxygen therapy may result in a reduction of the hematocrit and improved functional status in patients with hypoxemia due to chronic lung disease (40).
3. **Weight reduction:** In patients with the obesity–hypoventilation syndrome, weight reduction may improve nocturnal desaturation and decrease the level of erythro-cytosis.
4. **Removal of erythropoietin-producing tumors:** Successful surgical excision of an erythropoietin-producing tumor is associated with resolution of erythrocytosis.
5. **Correction of underlying renal disease:** Surgical repair of benign renal lesions results in reversal of erythrocytosis.
6. **Posttransplant erythrocytosis may respond to removal of the native kidneys:** (41). Theophylline reduces erythropoietin production in this condition and results in a decrease in hematocrit (42). Angiotensin-converting enzyme inhibitors were shown to be highly effective in controlling posttransplant erythrocytosis (43).

Before performing a **phlebotomy** in a patient with secondary erythrocytosis, it is important to determine whether the patient has physiologically appropriate or inappropriate erythrocytosis:

1. **Physiologically appropriate erythrocytosis:** The elevated red cell mass serves as the principal physiologic compensatory mechanism for decreased tissue oxygenation. In some instances, there may be "excessive" compensation, leading to hyperviscosity and a net detrimental effect on the patient; phlebotomy may be beneficial in these circumstances. It is inappropriate to reduce the red cell mass or hematocrit to normal levels in these patients, who depend on some increase in oxygen-carrying capacity to compensate for arterial hypoxemia or impairment in oxygen transport. The optimal red cell mass or hematocrit in these patients varies with the underlying disorder and may vary among patients with the same disease. The optimal hematocrit in these patients is a compromise between maximizing oxygen-carrying capacity and minimizing the effects of hyperviscosity on cardiovascular function of cerebral blood flow.

2. **Physiologically inappropriate erythrocytosis:** Patients in this category do not benefit physiologically from the elevated red cell mass, and phlebotomy can be done safely to a hematocrit of 42% to 46%. Before elective surgery, phlebotomy should be performed, following the same guidelines for PV.

Myelosuppressive therapy is contraindicated in secondary erythrocytosis.

Apparent Polycythemia

These patients have an elevated hematocrit; when measured directly, however, the red blood cell mass is normal. The elevation of hematocrit results from either a high normal red cell mass in combination with low normal plasma volume or a normal red cell mass associated with reduced plasma volume (5,12). Some patients with high normal red cell mass may be in the early phase of true erythrocytosis, and on follow-up, this possibility should be considered in all patients whose diagnosis is apparent polycythemia.

Pathophysiology

The underlying mechanism for the elevated hematocrit in patients with the high normal red cell mass and low normal plasma volume may explained be explained by carboxyhemoglobinemia in many patients. For patients with normal red cell mass and contracted plasma volume, the mechanism of plasma volume reduction remains uncertain. Hypertension with resultant volume contraction may play a role in many patients (44). Chronic alcohol consumption has been implicated in some patients, and elevated venous tone also may be a factor.

Clinical Features

1. **Males** are predominantly affected, and they are often anxious and mildly obese.
2. **Smoking** is common among patients with relative polycythemia. True erythrocytosis attributable to carboxyhemoglobinemia must be distinguished.

3. **Symptoms** are generally nonspecific and similar to those seen in PV: (a) headache, paresthesias, and dizziness; (b) weakness and fatigue; (c) dyspnea and epigastric pain; (d) angina pectoris; and (e) pruritus (uncommon).
4. **Physical findings:** (a) plethora and conjunctival injection; (b) hepatomegaly in about 20% of patients; (c) splenomegaly, which is uncommon, occasionally has been observed; and (d) hypertension is common, particularly in patients with plasma volume contraction.

Laboratory Features
1. The hematocrit is mildly elevated.
2. White blood cell count, platelet count, and reticulocyte count are normal.
3. Hypercholesterolemia is frequent.
4. LAP is normal to mildly elevated.
5. Bone marrow cellularity and megakaryocyte numbers are normal, but iron stores may be absent. There is no evidence of myelofibrosis.

Complications
1. Hypertension is a frequent finding.
2. Thromboembolism occurs in about 30% of patients and is most frequent in those with a contracted plasma volume (45).

Prognosis
Patients with relative polycythemia have a survival rate that is lower than age-matched controls. These patients suffer from a high incidence of cardiovascular and cerebrovascular complications.

Treatment
   1. An **initial period of observation** is warranted in these patients unless symptoms of ischemia or thrombotic events are present. In some patients, the hematocrit normalizes spontaneously.
   2. **Smoking cessation or reduction in alcohol consumption** may be helpful in some patients.
   3. **Control of hypertension** has been shown to reverse relative polycythemia in many patients and is probably the single most important intervention in hypertensive patients with this syndrome. No formal studies have determined optimal antihypertensive therapy in these patients. Based on our understanding of the pathophysiology, however, it is recommended that diuretics be avoided and agents with antirenin or vasodilatory properties be selected to control the hypertension.
   4. **Phlebotomy:** In the past, phlebotomy has not been generally recommended in patients with relative polycythemia. Studies have revealed, however, that cerebral blood flow is reduced in these patients and can be normalized by phlebotomy to a hematocrit less than 46%. Phlebotomies should be considered in patients with (a) persistent hematocrit elevation after other measures have been used and (b) symptoms attributed to hyperviscosity.

References
   1. Emanuel PD, Eaves CJ, Broudy VC, et al. Familial and congenital polycythemia in three unrelated families. *Blood* 1992;79:3019–3030.
   2. Erslev AJ, Caro J. Pure erythrocytosis classified according to erythropoietin titers. *Am J Med* 1984;76:57–61.
   3. de la Chapelle A, Sistonen P, Lehvaslaiho H, et al. Familial erythrocytosis genetically linked to erythropoietin receptor gene. *Lancet* 1993;341:82–84.
   4. Kralovics R, Indrak K, Stopka T, et al. Two new EPO receptor mutations: truncated EPO receptors are most frequently associated with primary familial and congenital polycythemias. *Blood* 1997;90:2057–2061.
   5. Pearson TC, Wetherley-Mein G. The course and complications of idiopathic erythrocytosis. *Clin Lab Haematol* 1979;1:189–196.
   6. Vlahakos DV, Kosmas EN, Dimopoulou I, et al. Association between activation of the renin-angiotensin system and secondary erythrocytosis in patients with chronic obstructive pulmonary disease. *Am J Med* 1999;106:158–164.

7. Smith JR, Landaw SA. Smokers' polycythemia. *N Engl J Med* 1978;298:6–10.
8. Thorling EB. Paraneoplastic erythrocytosis and inappropriate erythropoietin production: a review. *Scand J Haematol Suppl* 1972;17:1–166.
9. Vlahokos DV, Balodinios C, Papachristopoulous V, et al. Renin-angiotensin system stimulates erythropoietin secretion in chronic hemodialysis patients. *Clin Nephrol* 1994;43:53–59.
10. Mrug M, Stopka T, Julian BA, et al. Angiotensin II stimulates proliferation of normal early erythroid progenitors. *J Clin Invest* 1997;100:2310–2314.
11. Kennedy GA, Griffin HS. Erythrocytosis after zidovudine for AIDS. *Ann Intern Med* 1991;114:250–251.
12. Pearson TC. Apparent polycythemia. *Blood Rev* 1991;5:205–213.
13. Thomas DJ, du Boulay GH, Marshall J, et al. Cerebral blood-flow in polycythaemia. *Lancet* 1977; 2:161–163.
14. Testa JR, Kanofsky JR, Rowley JD, et al. Karyotypic patterns and their clinical significance in polycythemia vera. *Am J Hematol* 1981;11:29–45.
15. Birgegard G, Wide L. Serum erythropoietin in the diagnosis of polycythaemia and after phlebotomy treatment. *Br J Haematol* 1992;81:603–606.
16. Koeffler HP, Goldwasser E. Erythropoietin radioimmunoassay in evaluating patients with polycythemia. *Ann Intern Med* 1981;94:44–47.
17. Cotes PM, Dore CJ, Yin JA, et al. Determination of serum immunoreactive erythropoietin in the investigation of erythrocytosis. *N Engl J Med* 1986;315: 283–287.
18. Weinberg RS. *In vitro* erythropoiesis in polycythemia vera and other myeloproliferative disorders. *Semin Hematol* 1997;34:64–69.
19. Carlson JT, Hedner J, Fagerberg B, et al. Secondary polycythaemia associated with nocturnal apnoea—a relationship not mediated by erythropoietin. *J Intern Med* 1992;231:381–387.
20. Michiels JJ, Barbui T, Finazzi G, et al. Diagnosis and treatment of polycythemia vera and possible future study designs of the PVSG. *Leuk Lymph* 2000;36: 239–253.
21. Yiannikas C, McLeod JG, Walsh JC. Peripheral neuropathy associated with polycythemia vera. *Neurology* 1983;33:139–143.
22. Van Genderen PJ, Michiels JJ. Erythromelalgia: a pathognomonic microvascular thrombotic complication in essential thrombocythemia and polycythemia vera. *Semin Thromb Hemostasis* 1997;13:357–363.
23. Tartaglia AP, Goldberg JD, Berk PD, et al. Adverse effects of antiaggregating platelet therapy in the treatment of polycythemia vera. *Semin Hematol* 1986;23: 172–176.
24. Low-dose aspirin in polycythaemia vera: a pilot study. Gruppo Italiano Studio Policitemia (GISP). *Br J Haematol* 1997;97:453–456.
25. Landolfi R, Marchioli R. European Collaboration on Low-dose Aspirin in Polycythemia Vera (ECLAP): a randomized trial. *Semin Thromb Hemost* 1997;23: 473–478.
26. Silverstein MN. The evolution into and the treatment of late stage polycythemia vera. *Semin Hematol* 1976;13:79–84.
27. Landaw SA. Acute leukemia in polycythemia vera. *Semin Hematol* 1986;23: 156–165.
28. Fruchtman SM, Mack K, Kaplan ME, et al. From efficacy to safety: a Polycythemia Vera Study group report on hydroxyurea in patients with polycythemia vera. *Semin Hematol* 1997;34:17–23.
29. Treatment of polycythaemia vera by radiophosphorus or busulphan: a randomized trial. "Leukemia and Hematosarcoma" Cooperative Group, European Organization for Research on Treatment of Cancer (EORTC). *Br J Cancer* 1981;44:75–80.
30. Silver RT. Interferon-alpha 2b: a new treatment for polycythemia vera. *Ann Intern Med* 1993;119:1091–1092.
31. Silver RT. Interferon alfa: effects of long-term treatment for polycythemia vera. *Semin Hematol* 1997;34:40–50.
32. Sacchi S, Leoni P, Liberati M, et al. A prospective comparison between treatment with phlebotomy alone and with interferon-alpha in patients with polycythemia vera. *Ann Hematol* 1994;68:247–250.

33. Lengfelder E, Berger U, Hehlmann R. Interferon alpha in the treatment of polycythemia vera. *Ann Hematol* 2000;79:103–109.
34. Petitt RM, Silverstein MN, Petrone ME. Anagrelide for control of thrombocythemia in polycythemia and other myeloproliferative disorders. *Semin Hematol* 1997;34:51–54.
35. Anderson JE, Sale G, Appelbaum FR, et al. Allogeneic marrow transplantation for primary myelofibrosis and myelofibrosis secondary to polycythemia vera or essential thrombocytosis. *Br J Haematol* 1997;98:1010–1016.
36. Chievitz E, Thiede T. Complications and causes of death in polycythemia vera. *Acta Med Scand* 1962;172:513–523.
37. Chetty KG, Light RW, Stansbury DW, et al. Exercise performance of polycythemic chronic obstructive pulmonary disease patients. Effect of phlebotomies. *Chest* 1990;98:1073–1077.
38. Rosove MH, Perloff JK, Hocking WG, et al. Chronic hypoxaemia and decompensated erythrocytosis in cyanotic congenital heart disease. *Lancet* 1986;2:313–315.
39. Sumrani NB, Daskalakis P, Miles AM, et al. Erythrocytosis after renal transplantation. A prospective analysis. *ASAIO J* 1993;39:51–55.
40. Nocturnal Oxygen Therapy Trial Group. Continuous or nocturnal oxygen therapy in hypoxemic chronic obstructive lung disease: a clinical trial. *Ann Intern Med* 1980;93:391–398.
41. Friman S, Nyberg G, Blohme I. Erythrocytosis after renal transplantation: treatment by removal of the native kidneys. *Nephrol Dial Transplant* 1990;5:969–973.
42. Bakris GL, Sauter ER, Hussey JL, et al. Effects of theophylline on erythropoietin production in normal subjects and in patients with erythrocytosis after renal transplantation. *N Engl J Med* 1990;323:86–90.
43. Gaston RS, Julian BA, Barker CV, et al. Enalapril: safe and effective therapy for posttransplant erythrocytosis. *Transplant Proc* 1993;25:1029–1031.
44. Emery AC Jr, Whitcomb WH, Frohlich ED. "Stress" polycythemia and hypertension. *JAMA* 1974;229:159–162.
45. Weinreb NJ, Shih CF. Spurious polycythemia. *Semin Hematol* 1975;12:397–407.

Suggested Readings

Berk PD, Goldberg JD, Donovan PB, et al. Therapeutic recommendations in polycythemia vera based on Polycythemia Vera Study Group protocols. *Semin Hematol* 1986;23:132–143.
Golde DW, Hocking WG, Koeffler HP, et al. Polycythemia: mechanisms and management. *Ann Intern Med* 1981;95:71–87.
Rao AK, Walsh PN. Acquired qualitative platelet disorders. *Clin Haematol* 1983; 12:201–238.

4. HEMOLYTIC ANEMIA: HEREDITARY AND ACQUIRED

Stephan D. Thomé and Lawrence D. Petz

Normal Red Cell Kinetics

An average adult weighing 70 kg with a red blood cell mass of roughly 30 mL per kilogram of body weight has a total red blood cell (RBC) volume of 2,100 mL (24×10^{12} RBC). To maintain a constant red cell mass, this adult produces and destroys about 21 mL of RBC (2×10^{11} RBC) every day containing 6 to 7 g of hemoglobin. RBCs leave the bone marrow as reticulocytes and normally survive in the circulation for approximately 100 to 120 days. Erythrocyte reticulin is degraded within 1 day of entering the circulation unless there is severe anemia with accelerated erythropoiesis, when the degradation time can be prolonged up to 2 to 3 days. On a blood smear, we therefore normally find one reticulocyte per 100 erythrocytes (1% of 5 million RBC/μL = 50,000/μL absolute reticulocyte count). Given sufficient micronutrients (folate, cobalamin, iron) and hormonal stimulation (erythropoietin), the rate of RBC production can be increased fivefold to tenfold, with resultant reticulocytosis. At the other extreme in the life of a RBC is the senescent spherocyte, transformed from a biconcave and pliable disk to a fragile sphere, awaiting phagocytosis by sinusoidal macrophages in the spleen, liver, or bone marrow. If, for some reason, the bone marrow ceases to produce reticulocytes (e.g., Parvovirus B19 infection, chemotherapy, radiation, pure red cell aplasia), we would see a daily decrease of 1% in the RBC count, in parallel with hemoglobin and hematocrit. This is the rate of normal senescent hemolysis. **Accelerated hemolysis (>1% decrease in hemoglobin per day) is defined as shortened red blood cell survival (<100–120 days) and is the topic of this chapter.**

The signal that triggers disappearance of normal senescent red cells from the circulating blood is still unresolved. The mature red cell, lacking a nucleus and unable to synthesize protein, must survive while utilizing its enzymatic legacy. The activities of many red cell enzymes decrease as the cells age. Initially, there is rapid loss of reticulocyte remodeling enzymes such as pyrimidine 5′-nucleotidase. Thereafter, a slow, rather modest decline in the activities of various housekeeping enzymes occurs, suggesting that enzymatic failure alone probably does not trigger the destruction of senescent red cells. Normal human immunoglobulin G (IgG) has been reported to bind selectively to autologous erythrocytes, thereby opsonizing them and promoting their phagocytosis by reticuloendothelial cells. Senescent red cells assume the shape of spherocytes, and no longer can pass through narrow sinusoids, thus also promoting phagocytosis. Indeed, examination of spleens from patients with hereditary spherocytosis (HS) has shown red pulp trapping and phagocytosis of senescent spherocytes in the splenic cords of Billroth, consistent with the latter mechanism. In HS, splenectomy clearly prolongs the shortened red cell survival. Still the relative physiologic importance of the proposed clearance mechanisms remains unclear, especially because nonhemolyzing patients with agammaglobulinemia, as well as asplenic patients exhibit normal, not prolonged, red cell survival.

Overview of Red Cell Physiology and Pathophysiology

The mean diameter of a red cell is about 8 μm. Yet, on its travels through the circulation of 100 to 200 miles, it must repetitively traverse the much narrower tissue capillaries, where oxygen and carbon dioxide exchange occurs, and then pass through the 2- to 3-mm, slit-like orifices that separate the splenic cords from the splenic sinusoids. To accomplish this, the cells must remain exquisitely deformable. This requires a biconcave resting shape, a constant intracellular environment maintaining hemoglobin in a reduced and soluble state, and a high degree of membrane elasticity. Because a sphere packs the largest volume possible in the smallest surface area and the lipid bilayer is not elastic, spherocytes are poorly deformable and thus easily trapped in capillaries and sinusoids. The excess surface area of a normal biconcave erythrocyte is thus one prerequisite for a normal life span. Hemolytic disorders occur either because the red cells produced are inherently defective or as a result of injurious factors within the extracellular environment. Intrinsic abnormalities that predispose to hemolysis may be present in the red cell membrane, in the contained hemoglobin, or in the enzymes required for metabolic homeostasis.

Red Cell Membrane
The human red cell membrane (Fig. 1) contains three major parts: a lipid bilayer, integral or transmembrane proteins within the bilayer, and a membrane cytoskeleton providing structural support.

1. **Lipid bilayer:** Phospholipids are arranged in a bilayer with their negatively charged phosphate groups oriented externally and their aliphatic fatty acid chains internally. On the red cell surface, the phosphate groups interact with the aqueous plasma environment and, in conjunction with sialic acid residues, contribute to the negative charge (the zeta potential) of the erythrocyte, which serves mutually to repel these cells. Cholesterol is inserted into the internal hydrophobic core of the phospholipid bilayer. Red cell cholesterol readily exchanges with free plasma cholesterol. A membrane protein (flipase) polarizes phospholipids and contributes to the biconcave shape. Hereditary abnormalities of lipid metabolism are rare causes of altered red cell shape and hemolysis (abetalipoproteinemia, sitosterolemia). Acquired lipid changes occur in severe liver and renal disease (spur cells, acanthocytes, echinocytes) and also may cause hemolysis.

2. **Intrinsic membrane proteins** traverse the lipid bilayer and mediate forces perpendicular or vertical to the membrane. They contain external (environmental) and internal (cytoplasmic) domains. Red cell membrane proteins are enumerated according to their relative electrophoretic mobility in sodium dodecyl sulfate (SDS)-polyacrylamide gels. The principal intrinsic protein, **band 3,** represents the anion transport channel through which rapid exchange of chloride and bicarbonate occurs. In its cytoplasmic domain, band 3 contains an attachment site for **ankyrin,** a protein (band 2.1) that anchors the membrane cytoskeleton to spectrin. Another intrinsic membrane protein, **glycophorin C** (GP) serves as an attachment site for the cytoskeleton (Fig. 1). Abnormal membrane protein interactions (spectrin–ankyrin interaction, glycophorin, ankyrin, band 3 protein) result in loss of "vertical" forces, forces perpendicular or at right angle to the membrane. This type of structural deficiency is believed to be at the root of the clinical picture of hereditary spherocytosis.

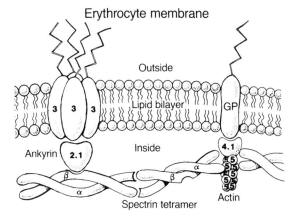

FIG. 1. Erythrocyte membrane structure. Membrane proteins have been numbered, by convention, in a sequence corresponding to decreasing molecular weight. GP, glycophorin; α and β refer to the respective chains of spectrin.

3. The major constituent of the **cytoskeletal proteins** is **spectrin,** a high-molecular-weight protein dimer composed of entwined α (240 kDa) and β (220 kDa) chains. α and β chain interactions cause spectrin dimers to associate into tetramers and higher oligomers. The β chains serve to attach oligomeric spectrin to ankyrin. Spectrin tetramers are bound to **F-actin** (band 5), an interaction enhanced by **band 4.1.** This cytoskeletal network confers a remarkable degree of resilient elasticity to the erythrocyte membrane and mediates "horizontal" forces parallel to the membrane. The loss of horizontal force as a result of abnormal cytoskeletal protein interactions (actin, band 4.1 protein, spectrin dimer–dimer interaction) results in hereditary elliptocytosis or ovalocytosis and red cell fragmentation.

Hemoglobin
The red cell must maintain its highly concentrated hemoglobin [30 g/dL mean corpuscular hemoglobin concentration (MCHC), or 2.5 mmol/L $\alpha_2\beta_2$ tetramer] reduced and functional in solution at 37°C for 4 months, a feat that protein chemists would find difficult to duplicate. The viscosity of red cell stroma rises rapidly between 30 to 40 g per deciliter of MCHC, leading to decreased deformability. Mutations in the hemoglobin molecule may alter its solubility, stability, and ability to resist oxidation to methemoglobin. These mutations also adversely affect the survival of the cell that transports it and therefore cause hereditary hemolysis (see Chapter 6). Hereditary methemoglobinemia, whether due to abnormal hemoglobin or due to methemoglobin reductase deficiency, presents with a lifelong history of cyanosis. Acquired methemoglobinemia usually results from toxic or drug injury and is present in glucose-6-phosphate dehydrogenase (G6PD) deficiency.

Red Cell Enzymes (Fig. 2)
Red cells contain two classes of enzymes:

1. **Remodeling enzymes,** such as those responsible for the degradation and disposal of reticulocyte organelles (mitochondria and ribosomes). An example is pyrimidine 5′-nucleotidase, which facilitates the removal of residual ribonucleotides from maturing reticulocytes. A hemolytic syndrome attributable to hereditary nucleotidase deficiency can be diagnosed easily by the specific finding of prominent basophilic stippling on a peripheral blood smear. Acquired nucleotidase deficiency occurs in lead poisoning and can manifest with identical basophilic stippling.
2. **Housekeeping enzymes** maintain iron in its divalent form; the electrolyte gradients for sodium, potassium and calcium; the sulfhydryl groups of red cell enzymes, hemoglobin and membrane proteins in the reduced, active form; and the biconcave shape of the red cell. Enzymes of the housekeeping group are frequently responsible for hereditary hemolytic disorders. The normal red cell is equipped with several enzymes that protect against oxidative damage (e.g., catalase, glutathione peroxidase, superoxide dismutase) and various repair enzymes that functionally preserve its hemoglobin and other cellular constituents (e.g., methemoglobin reductase, glutathione reductase). In addition, red cell nucleotide salvage enzymes conserve nucleotide coenzymes, such as adenosine triphosphate (ATP), that cannot be synthesized from precursors.

- **Direct glycolytic pathway:** The Embden-Meyerhof (E-M) anaerobic glycolytic pathway generates 2 M of ATP per mole of glucose catabolized to pyruvate or lactate. Another role of the E-M pathway is to reduce nicotinamide-adenine dinucleotide (NAD) to NADH, the latter being required to reduce trivalent methemoglobin (Fe^{3+}) to the functional divalent Fe^{2+} form. A shunt (Rapoport-Luebering) in the E-M pathway allows the production of 2,3 diphosphoglycerate (2,3 DPG), an important regulator of the oxygen affinity of hemoglobin.
- **Direct oxidative pathway:** The pentose phosphate shunt (PPS) yields 2 M of NADPH per mole of glucose shunted and a triose and hexose, which are normal intermediary metabolites of the direct glycolytic pathway. G6PD is the key enzyme in this pathway directly oxidizing G6P at position 1 yielding 2 NADPH, carbon dioxide, and a pentose. NADPH is required for reduction of oxidized glutathione (GSSG) by glutathione reductase. Reduced glutathione (GSH) acts with glutathione peroxidase to destroy hydrogen peroxide, protecting the red cell against this ubiquitous

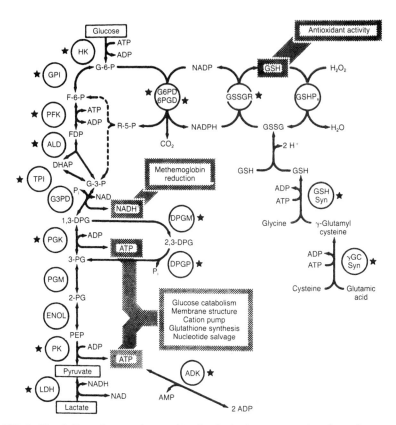

FIG. 2. Metabolic pathways of anaerobic glycolysis, the pentose–phosphate shunt, and glutathione metabolism available to the human erythrocyte. Clearly documented inherited deficiencies of enzymes, marked with a star, have been reported in erythrocytes from one or more patients. Enzymes of anaerobic glycolysis Embden–Meyerhof pathway). HK, hexokinase; GPI, glucosephosphate isomerase; PFK, phosphofructokinase; ALD, aldolase; TPI, triosephosphate isomerase; G3PD, glyceraldehyde 3-phosphate dehydrocgenase; PGK, phosphoglycerate kinase; PGM, monophosphoglycerate mutase; ENOL, enolase; PK, pyruvate kinase; LDH, lactate dehydrogenase; ADK, adenylate kinase. Enzymes of the Rapoport–Luebering shunt; BPGM, bisphosphoglycerate mutase; BPGP, dephosphoglycerate phosphatase (both activities reside in the same enzyme protein). Enzymes of the aerobic pentosephosphate pathway and glutathione metabolism; G6PD and 6PGD, glucose-6-phosphate and glucose-6-phosphogluconate dehydrogenases; GSSGR, glutathione reductase; GSHP, glutathione peroxidase; GSH Syn and g GC Syn, glutathione and glutamylcysteine synthetases. Glycolytic intermediates and cofactors; G-6-P, F-6-P, and R-5-P, glucose-6-, fructose-6, and ribose-5-phosphates; FDP, fructose-1,6-bisphosphate; DHAP, dihydroxyacetone phosphate; 1,3-DPG and 2,3-DPG, 1,3- and 2,3-diphosphoglycerate; PI, inorganic phosphate; 3-PG and 2-PG, 3- and 2-phosphoglycerate; PEP, phosphoenolpyruvate; AMP, ADP, and ATP, adenosine monophosphate, diphosphate, and triphosphates; NAD and NADH, oxidized and reduced nicotinamide adenine dinucleotide; NADP and NADPH, oxidized and reduced nicotinamide adenine dinucleotide phosphate; GSH and GSSG, reduced and oxidized glutathione. (Modified from Valentine WN, moderator. Hemolytic anemias and erythrocyte enzymopathies. *Ann Intern Med* 1985;103:245–257, with permission.)

oxidant. Moreover, GSH is required to maintain the integrity of sulfhydryl groups present in hemoglobin, in various red cell enzymes, and within the membrane itself. The antidote methylene blue used for the acute treatment of methemoglobinemia is dependent on the presence of NADPH and thus at best unhelpful and potentially fatal in G6PD deficiency.

Extrinsic Abnormalities
These abnormalities are rare causes of hereditary hemolysis (arteriovenous malformations, such as cavernous hemangiomas in Kasabach-Merritt syndrome, and copper toxicity in Wilson disease). Acquired extrinsic abnormalities such as microangiopathic hemolytic anemia [hemolytic uremic syndrome (HUS); thrombotic thrombocytopenic purpura (TTP); hemolysis, elevated liver enzymes, and low platelet count (HELLP)], burns, intravascular coagulation, and fibrinolysis (or disseminated intravascular coagulation), mechanical heart valves, chemical and infectious injuries are more common. Of note is the intraerythrocytic infectious agent most notorious worldwide for causing life-threatening hemolysis: malaria. In the United States, infectious agents such as Babesia, *Ehrlichia, Rickettsia, Bartonella* species, and clostridia can present with hemolysis resulting from intraerythrocytic infection or lipolytic toxins. Finally, because of its unique vascular architecture, an enlarged spleen can entrap and randomly destroy normal red cells in excess of normal senescence. In malignant or secondary histiophagocytic syndrome, a picture of hemolysis results from activated macrophages and histiocytes in bone marrow, liver, and spleen; clues are fevers, high lactate dehydrogenase (LDH), and very high ferritin in a sick patient.

Clinical and Laboratory Recognition of Accelerated Hemolysis
Most important is to determine the presence of accelerated hemolysis. Unfortunately, no single laboratory test or physical or historical finding is sufficiently sensitive and specific, and a high index of suspicion coupled with considerable clinical acumen is required.

History in a Patient with Hemolysis
Symptoms of anemia and decreased tissue oxygen delivery, such as weakness, fatigue, light-headedness, palpitations, angina, and central nervous system ischemia, as well as symptoms of compensatory increased cardiac output leading to congestive heart failure and tachycardia, may be present. Mild hemolysis may not result in significant symptoms; however, other historical features more specifically may suggest a hemolytic process.
    The history of a hereditary hemolytic disorder is frequently characterized by recognition of an anemia refractory to conventional medical treatment early in infancy or childhood. Obtaining all prior hemoglobin results can be helpful; often a family history of anemia, jaundice, unexplained splenomegaly or splenectomy, and cholecystectomies at an early age is present. Intermittent jaundice after infections and drug exposures can be another clue to red cell enzyme abnormalities. Mild hereditary hemolytic disease may be asymptomatic and may present in older patients with aplastic crisis, iron overload, nutritional deficiency, and hemolytic crisis.
    An acquired hemolytic process is strongly suggested by the rapid onset of anemia in a patient with no evidence of blood loss. The presence of a collagen vascular disease or neoplasm (particularly a lymphoproliferative disorder) suggests an acquired hemolytic process, probably of an immune etiology. The patient's use of drugs, which should be comprehensively explored, may suggest a possible etiology for the hemolysis.

Physical Findings
The physical findings are determined largely by the suddenness of onset, the rate, and the presence of associated or underlying disease processes (e.g., leukemia, lymphoma, lupus erythematosus). Severe anemia of any cause may result in pallor, tachycardia, and signs of congestive heart failure. Findings more characteristic of a hemolytic disorder include jaundice without bilirubinuria, splenomegaly, and ankle ulcers (occur in severe hereditary anemias). Significant hemolysis dating from early childhood may be associated with characteristic skeletal abnormalities (e.g., hypertrophied maxillae resulting in "chipmunk" facies) secondary to chronic marrow hyperplasia.

Laboratory Testing

Laboratory findings should document increased red cell production (reticulocyte count), increased red cell destruction (indirect bilirubin), and always include a personal or expert hematopathologist review of the peripheral blood smear. If all three tests are normal, hemolysis is going to be mild or nonexistent at examination.

1. **Reticulocytosis** can be determined with automated counters or by manual review. Reticulocytosis may be present because of recent blood loss, recent correction of nutritional deficiencies, hemoglobins with low oxygen affinity, unstable hemoglobins and increased erythropoietin levels (hypoxia, kidney cancer). The absolute reticulocyte count is more informative in a patient with severe anemia than an uncorrected relative reticulocyte percentage because of the low RBC count. Morphologic examination of the normal bone marrow discloses approximately three myeloid (M) cells for every erythroid (E) progenitor. Bone marrows of hemolyzing patients characteristically exhibit erythroid hyperplasia with a significant decrease, or inversion, of the normal M : E ratio. This morphologic picture is so predictable that diagnostic bone marrow studies are generally not indicated unless an underlying malignancy, such as leukemia or lymphoma, is suspected. Reticulocytosis may be absent when bone marrow function is suppressed by infection, nutritional deficiency (folate, cobalamin, iron), and myelotoxins.

2. **Indirect bilirubin** is elevated only in increased hemoglobin catabolism or in Gilbert syndrome. Thus, it is a specific marker for hemolysis in the absence of a history of Gilbert syndrome. Mild cases of hemolysis may not result in elevated levels of indirect bilirubin. Total bilirubin may not be elevated and is not helpful as a single test.

3. **Peripheral Blood Smear:** The single most helpful laboratory test in the recognition of a hemolytic disorder is the careful examination of the patient's peripheral blood film. In addition to polychromasia (increased reticulocytes), this may reveal morphologic abnormalities of red cells characteristic of a specific hemolytic process (e.g., schistocytes or helmet cells of microangiopathy, spherocytes of hereditary spherocytosis or immune hemolysis, agglutination, sickle cells, target cells, acanthocytes and spur cells of liver disease, elliptocytes, basophilic stippling of pyrimidine 5'-nucleotidase deficiency) (Table 1).

4. **Haptoglobin** binds to hemoglobin released by intravascular hemolysis or during incomplete phagocytosis ("messy macrophages"). Unbound haptoglobin has a half-life of 5 days, whereas the haptoglobin–hemoglobin complex is cleared from the bloodstream within 10 minutes. This rapid clearance explains the value of measuring haptoglobin in suspected cases of acute intravascular hemolysis (e.g., major transfusion reaction). The haptoglobin contained in 100 mL of plasma can bind about 100 to 140 mg hemoglobin. Thus, acute hemolysis of about 8 to 10 mL of RBC would deplete the total plasma haptoglobin and result in an unmeasurable haptoglobin concentration. Haptoglobin is an acute phase reactant and may be measurable in cases of mild hemolysis and inflammation. It is a glycoprotein produced in the liver and may be decreased in severe liver disease in the absence of hemolysis. When the hemoglobin-binding capacity of haptoglobin is exceeded, plasma hemoglobin may enter the glomerular filtrate because free hemoglobin disassociates rapidly into $\alpha\beta$-chain dimers (34 kDa) small enough to pass the glomerular basement membrane.

5. **Coombs' testing** is important to rule out immune mediated hemolytic anemias. In more than 95% of patients with immune hemolysis, the direct antiglobulin (Coombs') test is positive. This test detects the presence of immunoproteins (immunoglobulin or fragments of activated complement) that have adhered to the patient's red cells. A polyspecific Coombs' antiserum containing antibodies to human immunoglobulins and complement components is added to a washed suspension of the patient's red cells. The appearance of agglutination indicates membrane-bound immunoprotein and is presumptive evidence of an immune hemolytic disorder. The nature of the cell-bound immunoprotein can be defined better by using specific antiglobulin agents (i.e., anti-IgG, anti-C3, anti-C4). In fewer than 5% of patients with immune hemolytic anemia, the direct antiglobulin test is negative. More sensitive immunologic techniques available in some research laboratories are able to detect quantities of cell-bound immunoprotein too small to be recognized by conventional direct Coombs' testing. The indirect antiglobulin test is designed to detect antibodies present in patient's serum that are capable of

Table 1. Recognition and diagnosis of common hemolytic disorders: helpful morphologic findings

Red cell abnormality	Major diagnostic possibilities
Permanently sickled cells	Sickle disease (SS, SC, S-thal)
Target cells	Hemoglobin C disease (CC)
Liver disease	
Spherocytes	Hereditary spherocytosis
Immune hemolytic anemia (IgG antibody)	
Hypersplenism	
Elliptocytes	If >25%, hereditary elliptocytosis
Acanthocytes	Spur-cell anemia
Fragmented red cells (schistocytes) prostheses	Valvular disease (heart/aorta), malfunctioning
Microangiopathic disorders (disseminated intravascular coagulation, hemolytic-uremic syndrome, thrombotic thrombocytopenic purpura)	
Agglutination	Immune hemolytic anemia (IgM cold agglutinin)
Basophilic stippling	Pyrimidine 5'-nucleotidase, lead poisoning, thalassemia
Parasitic inclusions	Malaria, babesiosis, Carrion disease
Cookie-bite cells	Heinz body hemolytic anemia (especially drug-induced)

IgG, immunoglobulin G; IgM, immunoglobulin M; SC, sickle cell disease; SS, sickle cell Hgb and HgbC; S-thal, sickle cell thalassemia.

attaching to normal red cells of the same ABO and Rh type. A positive indirect Coombs' test may be due to alloantibody as well as autoantibody; consequently, only the direct Coombs' test yields unequivocal evidence of an immune hemolytic disorder. A Donath–Landsteiner antibody test occasionally is required for cases of suspected paroxysmal cold hemoglobinuria.

6. **Lactic dehydrogenase** is an insensitive marker for mild hemolysis and can be elevated in other disorders unrelated to hemolysis.

7. **Hemosiderinuria** results when free hemoglobin in the form of $\alpha\beta$-chain dimers (34 kDa) is filtered through the glomerular membrane and enters the tubular system. The renal tubular cells try to break down hemoglobin to amino acids, heme, hemosiderin, and ferritin but are unable to return the iron to the body stores in an efficient manner. Within a few days, hemosiderin granules in sloughed tubular cells are detectable in the urinary sediment using the Prussian blue iron stain. This test is helpful in screening for chronic intravascular hemolysis such as PNH or several days after a suspected acute hemolytic crisis.

8. **Serial determination of hemoglobin, hematocrit, or RBC count:** A sustained decrease of more than 1% per day is consistent with accelerated blood loss. It is important not to neglect the possibility of occult bleeding (e.g., renal cell carcinoma, gastrointestinal tract). A slow decrease of 1% per day may be due to a bone marrow production problem.

9. **Laboratory findings in intravascular and extravascular hemolysis:** The primary site(s) of destruction of normal red cells is unclear. In some hemolytic disorders, red cells may be destroyed within the circulation (intravascular hemolysis). Intravascular hemolysis is heralded by the release of hemoglobin into the plasma, where it is bound by haptoglobin. A low haptoglobin is thus a hallmark of significant intravascular hemolysis. Because red cells contain much LDH, elevated serum LDH levels are also present in patients with significant intravascular hemolysis. Most hemolytic disorders are characterized by extravascular red cell destruction; the erythro-

cytes are initially culled from the blood principally by macrophages lining the sinusoids in spleen, liver, and bone marrow. Although little of their contained hemoglobin escapes into the plasma, plasma haptoglobin levels may fall nevertheless, especially if the hemolytic process is chronic ("messy macrophages"). No hemoglobin is detectable in the plasma or urine, nor is hemosiderinuria present. Serum LDH levels may be modestly elevated. Heme derived from hemolyzed erythrocytes is normally catabolized within reticuloendothelial cells to biliverdin and iron. Biliverdin is further broken down into unconjugated (indirect-reacting) bilirubin. The unconjugated bilirubin is bound by albumin, transported to the liver, and there converted into the "direct-reacting," water-soluble conjugate. Serum concentrations of unconjugated bilirubin reflect the quantity of heme catabolized as well as its rate of conjugation. When no hepatic or biliary pathology is present, hemolyzing patients usually have normal conjugated bilirubin levels and bilirubinuria does not occur. Bacteria reduce bilirubin to water-soluble urobilinogen in the gastrointestinal tract, where a small part is reabsorbed and renally excreted causing urobilinogenuria. Therefore, laboratory features suggesting hemolysis include **anemia** (the severity being determined by the degree of bone marrow compensation), **reticulocytosis, unconjugated hyperbilirubinemia without bilirubinuria,** and **decreased serum haptoglobin** and increased LDH levels. To document the presence of a hemolytic process, it is rarely necessary to measure a patient's red cell survival using a radioisotope such as ^{51}Cr. This test occasionally is used to detect the primary site of *in vivo* red cell destruction by external gamma scintillation scanning.

10. **Defining the etiology of hereditary hemolysis in the laboratory:** A reasonably comprehensive screening strategy incorporates the review of all known clinical data and examination of the blood smear with testing for osmotic fragility, erythrocyte G6PD, pyruvate kinase, and glucose phosphate isomerase and tests for abnormal hemoglobins. Despite this battery of tests and referral of unsolved problem samples to national central laboratories, the overall success rate of making the laboratory diagnosis is only about 20% to 30%.

Hereditary Hemolytic Disorders
Caused by Membranopathies

Hereditary spherocytosis (HS) of autosomal dominant inheritance is the most common hemolytic disorder in patients of Northern European descent, occurring in at least 0.02% of this population. About 1% of normal blood donors exhibit increased osmotic fragility on screening consistent with the possibility of a higher prevalence of asymptomatic, subclinical RBC membrane defects. HS appears also to be prevalent among Japanese and blacks from South Africa. The molecular defects defined all appear to decrease vertical forces between skeleton and lipid bilayer and result in membrane loss and destabilization so that the cell becomes spherocytic.

1. **Etiology and pathobiology:** Two major factors lead to the premature destruction of erythrocytes in HS:
   - A quantitative or qualitative abnormality in the vertical interactions between vital skeletal and transmembrane proteins shaping the erythrocyte membrane. Several pathognomic red cell membrane defects have been elucidadated at a molecular level, all of which lead to deficiency of forces vertical to the membrane: (a) isolated partial spectrin deficiency (β-spectrin autosomal dominant, most common in whites, α-spectrin autosomal recessive), (b) ankyrin deficiency leading to combined ankyrin and spectrin deficiency, (c) partial deficiency of band 3 protein, (d) decreased band 4.2 protein (Japanese), and (e) other various causes. This results in the loss of lipids from the membrane in the form of microvesicles, leading to a significant loss of surface area and altered erythrocyte morphology. That is, the red blood cells lose their normal biconcave morphology and become spherocytic.
   - Splenic enlargement that impedes the sojourn of these abnormal erythrocytes through microcirculation of the spleen and increases phagocytosis of poorly deformable spherocytic RBC leading to premature destruction (Fig. 3).

2. **Clinical features** of HS may vary within families and from family to family, even with the same primary molecular defect. A strong family history of anemia, jaundice, splenomegaly, and cholelithiasis may be present. Twenty-five percent of HS patients

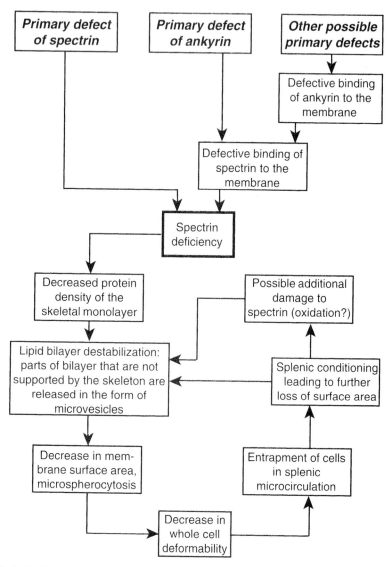

FIG. 3. Pathobiology of the red cell lesion in hereditary spherocytosis. Partial deficiency of spectrin, resulting from either a primary defect of spectrin of a spectrin-binding protein ankyrin (and possibly, other primary defects) leads to a reduced density of the skeletal monolayer. As a result, the membrane lipid bilayer is destabilized, and the bilayer lipids are released from the membrane in the form of microvesicles. The ensuing loss of cell surface area and a decrease in surface-to-volume ratio lead to a decrease in red cell deformability that predisposes cells to splenic trapping. Subsequent splenic conditioning inflicts additional damage on the cells. (Adapted from Palek J. Hereditary elliptocytosis, spherocytosis and related disorders: Consequences of a deficiency or a mutation of membrane skeletal protein. *Blood Rev* 1987;1:147–168, with permission.)

have mild, compensated hemolysis and may present late in life with asymptomatic isolated splenomegaly. A review of the blood smear and osmotic fragility screen can help prevent an invasive and costly workup for splenomegaly. Two thirds present with moderate anemia, intermittent jaundice, and splenomegaly. Occasionally, patients have severe, transfusion-dependent anemia. Where severe hemolysis occurs in childhood, growth retardation, as well as bone changes secondary to marrow hypertrophy, may be seen. Aplastic, megaloblastic, and hemolytic crises may lead to acute presentations.

3. **Laboratory features:** The laboratory finding most suggestive of HS is an abnormal peripheral blood smear containing numerous microspherocytes as well as polychromatophilic reticulocytes. Typically, the MCHC is elevated as a result of the loss of membrane microvesicles. The diagnosis of HS requires a negative direct antiglobulin test because spherocytosis commonly occurs in immune hemolytic disorders. The diagnosis is strengthened by a positive osmotic fragility test (see Appendix F): Red cells, when exposed to a series of hypotonic saline solutions, hemolyze at higher salt concentrations in HS than do normal cells. This increased sensitivity to osmotically induced swelling reflects an inability of the spherocytic red cells to increase their volume without rupturing due to lack of excess membrane. If the patient's sterile anticoagulated blood is incubated for 24 hours at 37°C before the osmotic fragility test is performed, the glucose-deprived red cells exhibit an even more strikingly increased osmotic fragility compared with normal as a result of excessive sodium influx during the incubation period. If sterile incubation is simply prolonged to 48 hours (no osmotic challenge), the patient's red cells undergo more spontaneous hemolysis (autohemolysis) than normal. The excessive autohemolysis is largely prevented by the prior addition of glucose because glycolysis and active cation transport in HS red cells are normal.

4. **Hemolytic crises** in HS patients usually are precipitated by infection. They are characterized by worsening jaundice, increased splenomegaly, and more profound anemia despite persistent reticulocytosis. Supportive care includes hydration and attention to the underlying precipitating disorder.

5. **Aplastic crises** may occur as well; they appear to be caused primarily by parvovirus infections. The typical picture is one of fever, abdominal pain, vomiting, and worsening anemia with reticulocytopenia. Iron stores need to be assessed carefully before any replacement therapy is initiated because hemolyzing patients may be more likely to suffer from iron overload. Aplastic crisis needs to be differentiated from megaloblastic crisis.

6. **Megaloblastic crises** may occur most commonly because of increased folate requirements, especially during pregnancy. This particular issue underscores the importance of making the diagnosis and recommending family screening of incident cases: Folate deficiency of pregnancy is associated with increased risk of neural tube defects. Vitamin B_{12} deficiency also can cause megaloblastic changes and needs to be considered if clinical neurologic symptoms or hematologic findings are present. Acutely, cobalamin deficiency resulting from the inhibitory effects of the anesthetic nitrous oxide (N_2O) on cobalamin-dependent enzymes may present days to weeks after inhalational anesthesia in depleted patients (reportedly as short as 65 minutes) and after heavy N_2O abuse, even in B_{12}-replete patients (dental and paramedical professionals with access to N_2O).

7. **Treatment:** In HS, the spleen is the principal site of red cell destruction, the splenic cords being engorged with spherocytic red cells. Here the decreased pH and glucose levels, as well as the low oxygen tension, appear to potentiate the sphering and entrapment of HS red cells. Splenectomy is the treatment of choice for HS. Although this does not correct the underlying cellular defect, removal of the spleen usually slows the rate of hemolysis dramatically. Splenectomy should precede or it should be performed concurrently with cholecystectomy when the latter procedure is required. If cholecystectomy alone is performed, persistent intrasplenic hemolysis may result in deposition of bilirubin stones within the smaller biliary radicals. Splenectomy removes an important organ in the body's defense against infection, particularly by encapsulated bacteria, such as the pneumococcus, meningococcus, or *Haemophilus* species. The excess risk of sudden death as a result of sepsis from encapsulated organisms is on the order of 1 per 1,000 patient years. Therefore, in young children, splenectomy should be postponed until age 6 years or older, if possible. All patients scheduled for splenectomy should receive pneumococcal, meningococcal, and *Haemophilus influenzae* type B

vaccinations 1 to 2 months before surgery. Postoperatively, prophylaxis with oral penicillin or other suitable antibiotic should be instituted and continued throughout the life of the patient.

Hereditary elliptocytosis (HE) consists of a clinically and molecularly heterogeneous group of diseases that share a common morphologic feature: At least 25% of red cells present in the peripheral smear are elliptocytic with the classic discoidal shape. Ovalocytosis is a HE variant that occurs in as many as 30% of Southeast Asians and Melanesians; it is the only HE type with increased membrane rigidity and is characterized by a longitudinal or transverse slit in spoon-shaped RBC (stomatocytosis). Occasional patients present with spherocytic (ovalocytic) HE, a hybrid between HS and HE. The severity of HE ranges from an asymptomatic carrier state recognizable by a defect in spectrin to severe hemolytic disease associated with abnormalities either in band 4.1 or in that portion of the spectrin chain involved in spectrin polymerization. To date, at least ten HE variants have been described in which a specific membrane protein abnormality has been identified. In all forms of HE, defects in horizontal forces weaken the lattice of proteins in the cytoskeleton supporting the membrane; this destabilizes the whole red cell and leads to fragmentation and poikilocytosis. Electron microscopy easily demonstrates the absence of the regular hexagonal lattice in the various forms of HE. Most HE types are inherited as a dominant or codominant trait leading to variable presentations within a kindred.

1. The **diagnosis** of HE is complicated by the fact that, in some apparently normal persons, as many as 10% of red cells may be elliptocytic. Indeed, small percentages of elliptocytes are commonly seen in a wide variety of disorders including iron deficiency, thalassemia, sickle disease, and myelodysplastic syndromes. To be confident of the diagnosis of HE, these more common disorders first must be ruled out and the presence of a hereditary hemolytic process characterized by marked elliptocytosis must be documented.

2. **Treatment:** Patients with HE who present with severe, chronic hemolysis are improved by splenectomy. Southeast Asian or Melanesian ovalocytosis is associated with increased resistance to malarial infection and little, if any, hemolysis. Such patients require no treatment.

Hereditary pyropoikilocytosis (HPP) is closely related to HE and indeed is indistinguishable from HE with severe homozygous spectrin deficiency. HPP occurs predominantly in black patients and is associated with severe hemolysis. This disorder exhibits double heterozygous, autosomal recessive inheritance. Frequently, one parent has apparent elliptocytosis, whereas the other parent has a clinically inapparent red cell membrane defect. The patient's peripheral blood film discloses striking micropoikilocytosis with apparent red cell budding. The morphologic picture strongly resembles that of heat-injured normal red cells. Indeed, HPP erythrocytes fragment at temperatures lower than normal (46°C versus 49°C) and have been found to contain heat-unstable spectrin. This is thought to explain the tendency of HPP red cells to undergo fragmentation even at physiologic temperatures. Splenectomy has been reported to improve the anemia of HPP patients.

Hereditary Hemolytic Disorders Caused by Hemoglobinopathies
See Chapter 6 for a discussion of sickling disorders, unstable hemoglobins, M hemoglobins, and hemoglobins with altered oxygen affinity.

Hereditary Hemolytic Disorders Caused by Enzymopathies (Fig. 2)
Abnormalities of the pentose phosphate shunt: Any impediment to this pathway, which is responsible for generating NADPH, the coenzyme required for reduction of GSSG to GSH, greatly increases the risk of oxidant damage to the red cell. Red cells synthesize the tripeptide GSH from constituent amino acids utilizing the enzymes glutamylcysteine synthetase and GSH synthetase. A mutation involving either enzyme causes GSH deficiency and a moderately severe hemolytic disorder exacerbated by oxidant drugs. GSH deficiency is rarely caused by a biosynthetic defect, however. A much more

common problem is an abnormality in G6PD, the first enzyme of the pentose phosphate pathway.

Oxidant damage to red cells, whatever its cause, initiates a characteristic sequence of events:

1. Hemoglobin is oxidized, initially to methemoglobin (reversible) and then irreversibly to sulfhemoglobin and Heinz bodies.
2. Heinz bodies, composed of denatured, precipitated globin, are "pitted" from red cells by the spleen, resulting in a characteristic "cookie-bite" morphology.
3. Disulfide-linked membrane protein aggregates are formed.
4. Rigid red cell membranes result, predisposing to hemolysis.

Potentially injurious oxidant drugs are usually aromatic compounds capable of accepting and donating electrons to molecular oxygen.

G6PD deficiency: To date, more than 400 G6PD mutants have been described at a biochemical level and more than 70 at a molecular level. These have been associated with a broad spectrum of global familial hemolytic disease (increased G6PD incidence in Kurdish Jews, West African American, African American, Chinese, Southeast Asian, and Mediterranean). The gene for G6PD is contained within the X chromosome; therefore, clinical G6PD deficiency occurs almost exclusively in males. In female heterozygotes, variable percentages of red cells have low G6PD activity, depending on the proportion of normal and affected X chromosomes inactivated during embryogenesis. One classic proof of the Lyon–Beutler hypothesis of selective X-chromosomal inactivation came from examination of individual red blood cells for G6PD deficiency in heterozygous in females. G6PD mutants have been classified in the past by the World Health Organization (WHO) into five classes based on the severity of the associated hemolysis. Because of the imprecision of biochemistry in this particular area, however, the WHO classification is likely to be superseded by a molecular classification based on specific genetic mutations (at catalytic site, at NADPH binding site, at C or N terminus, at promoter region).

The **five WHO classes of G6PD deficiencies** are the following:

1. **Class I mutations** result in very low residual activity of G6PD (<5%) and occur primarily in white patients with chronic, hereditary nonspherocytic hemolytic anemia. Oxidant drugs (Table 2) may greatly accelerate the rate of hemolysis, however. These patients derive only limited benefit from splenectomy. They should avoid oxidant drugs and discouraged from using any medication not prescribed by a responsible and knowledgeable physician.

2. **Class II G6PD mutants** exhibit only episodic hemolysis due to oxidants despite severe G6PD deficiency (from 1% to 10% of normal). A small percentage of patients with class II mutations, who are usually of Mediterranean extraction, exhibit a peculiar sen-

Table 2. Glucose-6-phosphate dehydrogenase (G6PD) deficiency: potentially oxidant drugs and chemicals

Drugs	
Acetanilid	Pentaquine
Amyl nitrite	Phenazopyridine (Pyridium)
Doxorubicin (Adriamycin)	Primaquine
Isosorbide dinitrate	Sulfacetamide
Methylene blue	Sulfamethoxazole (Gantanol)
Nalidixic acid (NegGram)	Sulfanilamide
Niridazole (Ambilhar)	Sulfapyridine
Nitrofurantoin (Furadantin)	Sulfasalazine (Azulfidine)
Pamaquine	Thiazolsulfone
Chemicals	
Naphthalene (mothballs)	Toluidine blue
Nitrates and nitrites	Trinitrotoluene
Phenylhydrazine	

sitivity to the **fava** bean. When such patients ingest fava beans, severe intravascular hemolysis ensues within hours to days, characterized by headache, dizziness, fever, chills, jaundice, hemoglobinuria, and Heinz bodies on peripheral smear. Compounds present in *Vica fava* seeds may play an important role in the pathophysiology of **favism.**

3. **Patients with class III G6PD deficiency** appear hematologically normal until they are stressed by severe infection of exposure to oxidant drugs (10%–60% activity). The class III molecular variant, G6PD A⁻, is the most frequently encountered of all the erythrocyte enzymopathies, being present in 10% of African Americans. Within 2 to 3 days of administration of an oxidant drug such as primaquine, a transient hemolytic episode occurs, which subsides even if the patient continues to take the drug. G6PD A— is inherently unstable so that with progressive aging of red cells *in vivo*, their G6PD activities decline, and they become increasingly susceptible to oxidative stress. G6PD activity, being normal in younger red cells, protects them from oxidative destruction so that hemolysis subsides after the older red cell population has been destroyed.

4. **Class 4 G6PD deficiency** is asymptomatic (activity 60%–150%).

5. **Class 5 G6PD deficiency** has increased activity (>100%) and abnormal electrophoretic mobility.

Diagnostic tests for G6PD: Numerous simple diagnostic screening tests for G6PD deficiency are available. These estimate red cell susceptibility to oxidant stress by measuring the magnitude of Heinz body formation or glutathione loss when patient red cells are exposed to acetylphenyl-hydrazine or by quantitating the amount of methemoglobin induced by ascorbate after red cell catalase has been inactivated by cyanide. Unfortunately, these tests are relatively nonspecific. An enzymatic test that quantifies red cell NADPH generation specifically identifies the G6PD-deficient male. To make the diagnosis of G6PD deficiency resulting from the A—variant, it is best to measure the patient's red cell G6PD activity during a hematologically quiescent period. If quantified immediately after an acute hemolytic episode, red cell G6PD levels may be normal because the older cells have been destroyed and younger, G6PD-replete cells have been spared. The same principle, that is, avoiding enzyme tests during acute hemolytic episodes, holds true for a number of other enzymopathies. Of course, genetic screening, although costly, uses DNA in white cells and can be performed anytime. Routine G6PD screening of black populations has been advocated in an effort to prevent drug-induced hemolysis and, in newborns, kernicterus.

G6PD treatment: Patients with class III G6PD mutations should avoid drugs and chemicals that have oxidant properties. Because methylene blue is used for the treatment of life-threatening methemoglobinemia, it is important to realize that the dye requires NADPH for the reduction of methemoglobin. In the absence of NADPH, the dye has oxidant properties. Thus, giving methylene blue for methemoglobinemia in a patient with G6PD deficiency, who cannot produce sufficient NADPH, is contraindicated and potentially fatal. Indeed, methylene blue has caused acute hemolysis in persons with G6PD deficiency. A rapid screen for G6PD deficiency and a look at the patient's ancestry as well as a prior history of drug-induced hemolytic episodes can help with the acute differential diagnosis and management of severe methemoglobinemia. In severe cases that are acutely symptomatic due to functional anemia, immediate red blood cell transfusion may be required to correct the oxygen carrying defect.

Abnormalities of the Embden-Meyerhof (E-M) glycolytic pathway: Enzymopathies that interfere with normal functioning of the E-M pathway result in ATP deficiency. How a deficiency of this energy-transferring coenzyme results in premature red cell destruction is not known. An important by-product of the glycolytic pathway is 2,3-BPG (old name: 2,3-DPG). This compound, which modulates the oxygen affinity of hemoglobin, may be either increased or decreased in enzymopathies affecting the E-M pathway, depending on the level of the enzymatic block.

Pyruvate kinase (PK) deficiency is the most common enzymopathy of the E-M pathway, its incidence approximating that of class I G6PD deficiency. Except where there is consanguinity, PK-deficient patients are usually mixed heterozygotes, inheriting different mutant PK genes from each parent. The severity of hemolysis is quite variable, ranging from transfusion-dependent anemia occurring primarily in newborns to well-compensated hemolysis in asymptomatic adults. Although patients in the latter group usually present with moderately severe anemia (hemoglobins 7–10 g/dL), they generally tolerate this well because their oxyhemoglobin dissociation curves are right-shifted as a result of the increased red cell 2,3 DPG levels. The diagnosis of PK deficiency is usually difficult to make.

As in most enzymopathies there are no characteristic morphologic changes in the peripheral blood film. An elevated P 50 secondary to supranormal 2,3 DPG levels strongly suggests the presence of PK deficiency. However, the diagnosis can be made with certainty only by specifically assaying red cell PK activity. Treatment of the PK-deficient patient who presents with significant hemolysis consists of splenectomy and red cell transfusions as required. Splenectomy usually improves the anemia, probably by enhancing the ability of reticulocytes to survive. Splenectomy is not as efficacious in this disease as it is in HS, however, because significant extrasplenic destruction of PK-deficient red cells appears to occur. To avoid iron overload, judicious use of red cell transfusions and chelation therapy with desferrioxamine has been advocated.

Miscellaneous enzyme deficiencies of the E-M pathway: Other enzymopathies involving the E-M glycolytic cycle are exceedingly rare. Hexokinase deficiency results in the diminution of all metabolic intermediates of glucose as well as 2,3 DPG, which causes increased hemoglobin oxygen affinity. The resultant tissue hypoxia accentuates the symptoms of anemia so that these patients are more incapacitated clinically, at the same levels of hemoglobin, than those suffering from PK deficiency.

Enzymopathies involving nucleotide salvage pathway: A deficiency in pyrimidine 5′-nucleotidase, an enzyme that converts pyrimidine monophosphate to diffusible nucleosides, causes premature red cell destruction. As a consequence of this deficiency, intracellular pyrimidine nucleotide concentrations increase dramatically, interfering with erythrocyte metabolism. Because ribosomal nucleoproteins present in reticulocytes are poorly degraded, striking basophilic stippling of the red cells is present in the peripheral smear and is pathognomic. Lead poisoning represents an acquired form of pyrimidine 5′-nucleotidase deficiency, the enzyme being inactivated by heavy metals.

Environmentally Induced Hemolytic Disorders
Hypersplenism

A portion of the arterial blood supply to the spleen enters the splenic cords, nonendothelialized channels filled with tissue macrophages. To escape the cords into the venous circulation, red cells must squeeze through 3-μm fenestrations between epithelial cells that line the splenic sinusoids. This vascular filter efficiently retains poorly deformable red cells, which are then destroyed by the macrophages. The survival of normal red cells is not significantly jeopardized by the physiologic splenic filtration process; however, if for any reason the spleen enlarges and hypertrophies, it may begin to sequester and destroy normal erythrocytes (as well as neutrophils or platelets) randomly. Hemolysis associated with this hypersplenic state is generally mild; moreover, the rate of hemolysis correlates poorly with overall spleen size.

The **diagnosis** of hypersplenism usually is made by exclusion. It requires demonstrable splenomegaly (on physical examination or radiographically) and some understanding of the pathophysiology of the underlying disease process (e.g., portal hypertension, infectious processes, lymphoma/leukemia, collagen vascular disorders such as systemic lupus or Felty syndrome, lipid storage disease). Small numbers of spherocytes are commonly present in the peripheral blood film. The direct antiglobulin test is characteristically negative.

Treatment of hypersplenism should be directed at correction or management of the underlying disorder. Splenectomy is rarely indicated.

Hemolysis from Physical Trauma

1. **March hemoglobinuria:** Mechanical trauma to red cells associated with prolonged intense physical exertion (e.g., marching, running) may cause transient intravascular hemolysis with hemoglobinemia and hemoglobinuria. Paradoxically, the peripheral blood film discloses no red cell morphologic abnormalities. Usually, no treatment is required.

2. **Fragmentational hemolysis caused by abnormalities of the heart or large vessels:** Red cell fragmentation may result from excessive shear stress associated

with turbulent blood flow. This may originate in the heart, primarily with left-sided lesions, where pressures are high. Mild fragmentational hemolysis has been observed most frequently in patients with tight aortic stenosis or regurgitation, a ruptured sinus of Valsalva, traumatic arteriovenous fistulas, and aortofemoral bypass procedures. More rapid intravascular hemolysis may occur in patients with prosthetic heart valves, particularly when they malfunction.

- **Diagnosis:** Patients usually present with mild to moderate anemia, a reticulocytosis, and numerous schistocytes (fragmented red cells) in the peripheral blood smear. Typical laboratory findings include low haptoglobin and increased serum LDH levels and hemosiderinuria. Frank hemoglobinemia and hemoglobinuria occur much less commonly. Iron deficiency resulting from chronic urinary loss of iron is frequently present. The direct Coombs' test is usually negative.
- **Treatment:** Oral iron should be administered to correct the iron deficiency. If the anemia cannot be controlled without transfusion, surgical correction of the cardiovascular abnormality should be strongly considered.

3. **Microangiopathic hemolytic disorders:** Fragmentational hemolysis may result when blood flow through small vessels is impeded by the presence of microthrombi or by intrinsic disease of the vessel wall. Schistocytes or helmet cells on the peripheral blood smear are the hallmarks of these disorders.

- **Disseminated intravascular coagulation (DIC):** The clinical picture of DIC results from the introduction of procoagulant(s) into the systemic circulation. The procoagulant may result from the interaction of an infectious agent (particularly a gram-negative bacterium) with the host's immune system, or it may be elaborated by disseminated neoplasms such as acute promyelocytic leukemia or adenocarcinomas. A particularly explosive form of DIC is initiated by amniotic fluid embolism. Systemic triggering of coagulation is attended by consumption of platelets and coagulation factors with widespread formation of microthrombi and activation of fibrinolysis.

  Laboratory features suggesting the diagnosis of severe DIC include thrombocytopenia; prolongation of the prothrombin, activated partial thromboplastin, and thrombin times; reduced concentrations of plasma coagulation factors V, VIII, and fibrinogen; and elevated levels of fibrin degradation products ("split products"). The peripheral blood film typically discloses a decrease in platelets and variable numbers of schistocytes and polychromatophilic cells (reticulocytes). Hemolysis is usually mild; when more severe, low haptoglobin and elevated LDH serum levels may be present. DIC rarely causes rapid intravascular hemolysis with hemoglobinemia and hemoglobinuria.

  Treatment of DIC should be directed at correcting or ameliorating the underlying disease process and supporting the patient with transfusions of platelets, coagulation factors, and red cells as required. Rarely, systemic anticoagulation with heparin may be indicated. Treatment of patients with life-threatening DIC must be highly individualized and requires integrated efforts by clinical and laboratory personnel.
- **Localized or diffuse microvascular disease.** Red cell fragmentation may be seen in patients with cavernous hemangiomas (Kasabach-Merritt syndrome); vasculitis associated with infection, hypersensitivity states, malignant hypertension, and eclampsia; and widely metastatic neoplasms. Hemolysis may be slow and well compensated or very rapid, resulting in severe anemia. Prominent red cell fragmentation is usually present, and laboratory evidence suggesting significant intravascular hemolysis occurs commonly. Coagulation abnormalities that are prominent in DIC are usually minimal or absent. Again, treatment should be directed at the underlying disease process.
- **Microocclusive syndromes associated with hemolysis, thrombocytopenia, and renal failure:** Three clinical entities that closely resemble one another are idiopathic TTP; HUS, which occurs primarily in children due to *Escherichia coli* O157 (raw hamburger syndrome, antibiotics contraindicated); and a drug-induced TTP syndromes (mitomycin C, ticlopidine, cyclosporine, post-bone marrow transplantation). Infections, drug hypersensitivity, systemic lupus erythematosus, and pregnancy have been proposed as possible precipitating factors for the first two. The

pathophysiology of TTP was illuminated by the finding of abnormally large von Willebrand factor (vWf) multimers in some patients. The abnormally large multimers cause platelet thrombi and are due to an IgG antibody inhibiting the vWf cleaving protease in acquired TTP. Patients commonly have fever, jaundice, a bleeding diathesis, neurologic abnormalities, and renal failure. There is evidence of rapid fragmentational hemolysis, thrombocytopenia, and deteriorating renal function accompanied by hematuria or otherwise abnormal urinary sediment. Although biopsy (and autopsy) specimens characteristically reveal hyaline microthrombi composed of platelet detritus and fibrin, there is usually very little laboratory evidence of a DIC-like coagulopathy. In a high percentage of patients with TTP, aggressive plasmapheresis followed by replacement with normal or cryo-poor plasma (plasma exchange) totally suppresses the disease process; however, 10-year relapse rates are greater than 30%. A similar therapeutic approach has been less effective in HUS and in the drug-induced process. Glucocorticoids and platelet inhibitory drugs have been used frequently in all three disorders with unconvincing efficacy.

Hemolysis Accompanying Systemic Metabolic Derangements
Serious malnutrition or liver dysfunction associated with profound disturbances of the plasma environment of the erythrocyte may lead to accelerated red cell destruction.

1. **Spur-cell hemolytic anemia:** Patients with severe hepatic disease are usually anemic. Blood loss, folate deficiency, marrow suppression due to alcohol, and portal hypertension with hypersplenism may contribute to this; however, some patients with end-stage liver disease present with brisk hemolysis characterized by the presence of misshapen erythrocytes exhibiting irregular, spur-shaped projections (acanthocytes) on peripheral smear. Red cell membranes from these patients contain excessive cholesterol without a concomitant increase in phospholipids. The red cells are pathologically rigid and are rapidly destroyed within the enlarged spleen. The etiology of this abnormality is unknown. The diagnosis of spur cell hemolytic anemia is usually apparent from the clinical picture, that is, severe liver disease with jaundice, ascites, and encephalopathy in conjunction with a characteristic spiculated appearance of the peripheral red blood cells (acanthocytes). These patients have an exceedingly poor prognosis and splenectomy has been associated with significant mortality.

2. **Hypophosphatemia:** Profound hypophosphatemia (serum phosphorus levels 1 mg/dL) may predispose to hemolysis. Phosphate depletion of this severity has been seen primarily in profoundly malnourished patients after treatment with oral phosphate-binding antacids, intravenous glucose, or hyperalimentation regimens lacking phosphate. The patient's red cells become ATP depleted, lose deformability, and are destroyed primarily within the spleen. Phosphate supplementation promptly corrects the hemolytic process.

Immune Hemolytic Disorders
Immune hemolytic anemias are a diverse group of disorders characterized by the presence of red cell antibodies that result in a shortened red cell life span. This is the major mechanism of the etiology of the anemia.
Pathophysiology of immune hemolysis: Antibody-mediated red blood cell destruction can occur as a result of activation of the complement system and resultant intravascular hemolysis, cellular mechanisms leading to extravascular hemolysis, or a combination of both mechanisms.
Complement activation: Activation of the entire complement system leads to disruption of the red cell membrane and "intravascular hemolysis" that is characterized by the presence of hemoglobinemia and hemoglobinuria. The complement system may be activated by two pathways: the *classic* pathway and the *alternative* pathway. The predominant mechanism of complement-mediated cytolysis is through activation of the classic pathway. Antibodies that are capable of activating the classic complement cascade are the immunoglobulins IgM, IgG1, IgG2, or IgG3. IgG4 and IgA antibodies do not activate the complement cascade.
The classic pathway of complement activation: Complement consists of a complex of at least 14 components with four fluid-phase inhibitors and an unknown

number of membrane-bound inhibitors. These react in a given set of sequences such that a series of complexes are generated on the membrane surface of the target cell (Fig. 4).

The initiation reaction: The initiation reaction of the classic pathway lies in the activation of C1, the protein that has been referred to as the *recognition unit*. C1 circulates in a precursor state, and after activation by antigen-antibody immune complexes or certain nonimmune substances, it acquires the ability to initiate the classic complement pathway. The resultant activation provides a supply of enzymatically active fragments of C1, which catalyze the reactions required by the next unit of the classic complement pathway, the activation unit.

The activation unit: C4, C2, and C3: In succession, C4 and C2 are activated by fragments of C1 and form a bimolecular complex, C4b-2a. This complex, also known as C3 convertase, has only one substrate, the next component of complement to be activated, C3. Activation of C3 gives rise to a number of distinct fragments (Fig. 5), many of which can interact with one or more of the cellular receptors for activated C3. The native molecule is cleaved and two fragments, C3a and C3b, are produced. The C3b fragment undergoes a rapid conformational change that allows for its covalent. Binding with the complement-activating particle (e.g., an antibody-coated red blood cell) C3 is further cleaved into fragments called C3d, g, and C3c. The C3d, g fragment remains associated with the red cell, whereas C3c is eluted. C3d, g appears to be the final product of *in vivo* C3 activation in plasma and on red cells. Red blood cells of patients with immune hemolytic anemias may be coated with C3d, g. In the immunohematology laboratory, complement sensitization of red blood cells is demonstrated by their agglutination by an antiglobulin serum (Coombs' serum) that has antibodies against C3d.

The formation of C5 convertase: The C3b fragment that is produced during the activation of C3 has a dual function in the complement sequence. First, it associates with its own activating C3 convertase to form a trimolecular complex consisting of C4b, 2a, 3b, which is termed *C5 convertase*. This complex causes cleavage of C5 in much the same way as C3. C5a is produced, which exits from the complement sequence to function as an anaphylatoxin. A larger fragment, C5b, becomes the focal point for the membrane attack complex. Second, and very important, C3b is involved in the generation of numerous monomeric C3b sites on the surface of the target cell. A C3b-coated erythrocyte presents specific receptors for lymphocytes, polymorphonuclear leukocytes, monocytes, macrophages, and various other effector cells.

The membrane attack complex: The "killer molecule" of complement is the membrane attack complex, which contains one molecule of C5b, C6, C7, C8, and multiple molecules of C9. The complex functions by inserting itself into membranes, thus impairing the normal permeability barrier by formation of a transmembrane channel and weakening the lipid bilayer structure. Water and ions enter the cell causing the cell to swell and rupture, releasing hemoglobin into the plasma.

The alternative pathway: In comparison, not much is known about the role of the alternative pathway of complement activation in cell destruction (Fig. 4). Few data implicate the alternative pathway in the destruction of circulating blood cells, but it is highly probable that it can play a role.

Extravascular hemolysis: If red cells become sensitized with noncomplement-fixing IgG antibodies, or if cells are sensitized with components of complement but do not proceed through the cascade completely to lysis, they may be destroyed or damaged by the cells of the reticuloendothelial system, resulting in "extravascular hemolysis," which is manifested by hyperbilirubinemia, elevated lactic dehydrogenase, and low serum haptoglobin but not hemoglobinemia or hemoglobinuria. The process of immune adherence is fundamental to such cell-mediated destruction of erythrocytes.

Immune adherence is the process by which the phagocytic or destructive cell attaches to the target cell. Bifunctional immunoproteins, which can adhere to the target cell (e.g., erythrocyte) as well as to specific components on the destructive cell (e.g., mononuclear phagocyte), are essential. The two major types of such immunoproteins that possess such bifunctional properties are antibodies (especially IgG) and components of complement (e.g., C4b, C3b).

The following are **consequences** of immune adherence:

1. IgG molecules bound to erythrocytes interact with Fc receptors on polymorphonuclear leukocytes, monocytes, and destructive lymphocytes. This results in binding of the

Reaction Sequence	Comments (A = Activation, I = Inhibition)

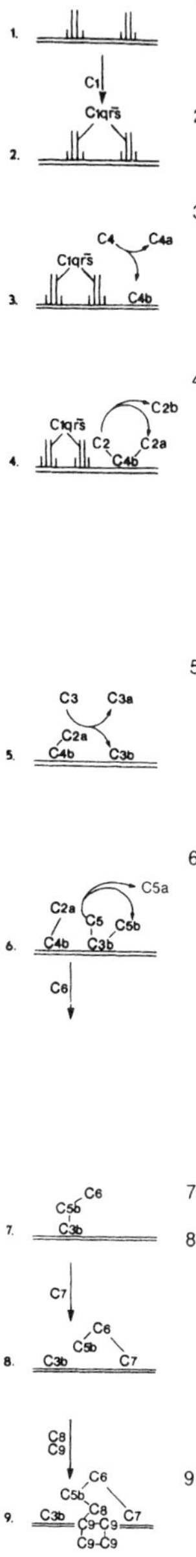

1. Complement-fixing antibody (≡) binds to an antigen present in RBC membrane (═).

2. A:C1 binds to Fc portion of antibody and develops protease activity.

3. A:C1ŝ cleaves C4. Nascent C4b may covalently bind to the RBC membrane. I:C1-inhibitor inactivates C1qr̄s̄ by dissociating C1rs from C1q.

4. A:C4b binds C2, which is then cleaved by C1ŝ. C2a, a serine protease, remains bound to C4b. I:(a) C4b is degraded to iC4b by I (the plasma C3b/C4b inactivator) (see Fig. 3-4). (b) Decay accelerating factor (DAF) inhibits c2a binding by C4b.

5. A:C2a cleaves C3. Nascent C3b may bind covalently to the RBC membrane. I:DAF inhibits C3 cleavage by accelerating the dissociation of C2a from C4b.

6. A:C3b binds C5, which is then cleaved by C2a. C5b remains bound to C3b. (Note that C3b may bind factor B, instead of C5, thereby activating the alternative pathway—see reaction 2 of the alternative pathway sequence.) I:C3b is degraded by I to iC3b, then to C3dg (see Fig. 3-4).

7. A:C5b binds C6.

8. A:C7, after binding to C5b6, inserts into the RBC membrane, simultaneously translocating the C5b-7 complex from C3b. I:S-protein in plasma competitively inhibits C5b67 binding to the RBC membrane.

9. A:Assembled C5b-9 complex (containing polymerized C9), when inserted into the RBC membrane, results in loss of osmotic integrity.

A

Reaction Sequence	Comments

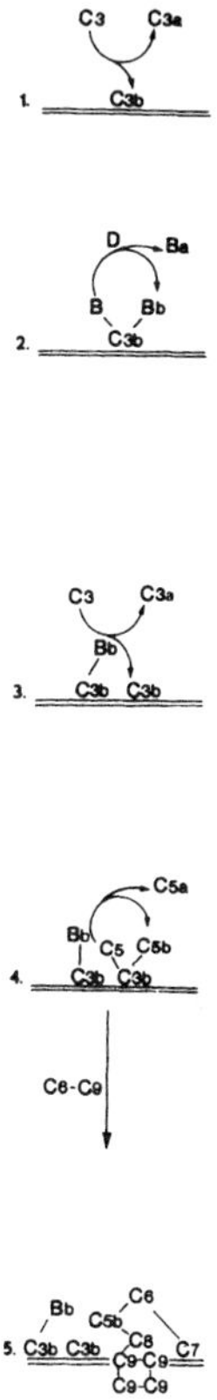

1. A:C3 activation may occur spontaneously or via alternative pathway activators. Nascent C3b may covalently bind to RBC membranes.

2. A:Factor B binds to C3b and is cleaved by D into Ba and Bb. Bb, a serine protease, remains bound to C3b; this association is stabilized by properdin. I:(a) C3b is degraded by I (see Fig. 3-4). (b) DAF inhibits C3 binding by C3bBb.

3. A:C3bBb cleaves C3 to generate additional nascent C3b, which may bind to RBC membranes. I:DAF inhibits C3 cleavage by accelerating the dissociation of Bb from C3b.

4. A:C5 binds to C3b and is then cleaved by Bb. C5b remains bound to C3b. (Note that C3b may bind B instead of C5 (reaction 2 above) augmenting alternative pathway activation.) I:DAF inhibits C5 cleavage by accelerating the dissociation of Bb from C3b.

5. A:See classical pathways reaction sequences 7–9. Loss of membrane osmotic integrity leads to red cell swelling and subsequent hemoglobinemia. I:S-protein inhibits assembly and insertion of C5b-9 complex into the RBC membrane (see classical pathway reaction sequence 8).

B

FIG. 4. A: Activation of the classic complement pathway by red cell antibodies. **B:** Activation of the alternative complement pathway on the red cell membrane.

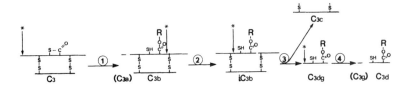

1. Activation occurs when C3 is cleaved into C3a and C3b by the C3 convertase of the classical (C4b2a) or alternative (C3bBb) complement pathway. Nascent C3b binds covalently either to an adjacent membrane site or to a soluble immune complex.

2. CR1 binds C3b, facilitating cleavage of the latter by I. First, iC3b is formed.

3. iC3b is further degraded by I (utilizing CR1 as a cofactor) to C3dg.

4. Degradation of C3dg to C3d may not occur in vivo to any significant degree, since this proteolytic step requires plasmin or a tryptic enzyme.

*Site of enzymatic cleavage.

FIG. 5. Sequential activation and degradation of C3 at the red cell membrane.

erythrocyte to the destructive cell, which may result in phagocytosis. The entire red cell or only a portion of it may be internalized. In the latter case, the membrane of the red blood cell left on the outside of the phagocyte is often able to reseal and escape from the phagocyte. Because more membrane has been lost than contents, the red blood cell must assume a more nearly spherical shape; it is recognized on blood films as a spherocyte.

2. Alternatively, antibody-dependent cellular destruction can occur without phagocytosis. If an antibody-coated red cell is adherent to a phagocytic cell but is not ingested, lysis may occur by a process known as *antibody-dependent cell-mediated cytotoxicity.* Cytoplasmic granules are apparently able to spill their contents onto the adherent cell with resulting red cell lysis.

3. Circulating cells coated with IgG or complement components are destroyed primarily in the liver and spleen because these organs possess effector cells within the channels through which the blood flows. The Kupffer cells, which line the hepatic sinusoids, are the effector cells in the liver, and the effector cells that lie in the cords of Billroth or the red pulp are the effector cells in the spleen.

Clinical and laboratory features: Immune hemolytic anemias may be classified as in Table 3. It is essential that a precise diagnosis be made in each case because prognosis and management of the various hemolytic anemias differ significantly. Characteristic serologic features of the various kinds of autoimmune hemolytic anemia (AIHA) are summarized in Table 4.

Warm-antibody AIHA: About 70% of cases of AIHA are associated with warm autoantibodies, that is, antibodies optimally reactive at 37°C. About 50% of patients with warm-antibody AIHA have an associated disease. Although the pathogenetic mechanisms are poorly understood, a relationship is defined either on the basis of a higher incidence in patients with AIHA than in the general population (e.g., chronic lymphocytic leukemia and systemic lupus erythematosus) or because reversal of the AIHA occurs with correction of the associated disease (e.g., surgical removal of certain ovarian tumors or colectomy for ulcerative colitis). Another, less definitive reason for suspecting a relationship consists of evidence of immunologic aberration as part of the underlying disorder, especially if the associated disease is thought to have an autoimmune pathogenesis.

1. **Symptoms and signs:** In some patients, the onset is insidious, with the gradual emergence of symptoms of anemia, and often is associated with fever and jaundice. In

Table 3. Classification of immune hemolytic anemias

I. Autoimmune hemolytic anemias (AIHAs)
  A. Warm-antibody AIHA
    1. Idiopathic
    2. Secondary (e.g., chronic lymphocytic leukemia, lymphomas, systemic lupus erythematosus)
  B. Cold agglutinin syndrome
    1. Idiopathic
    2. Secondary
      a. *Mycoplasma pneumoniae* infection, infectious mononucleosis, virus infections
      b. Lymphoreticular malignancies
  C. Paroxysmal cold hemoglobinuria
    1. Idiopathic
    2. Secondary
      a. Viral syndromes
      b. Syphilis
  D. Atypical AIHA
    1. Antiglobulin test-negative AIHA
    2. Combined cold and warm AIHA
II. Drug-induced immune hemolytic anemia
III. Alloantibody-induced immune hemolytic anemia
  A. Hemolytic transfusion reactions
  B. Hemolytic disease of the newborn

---

others, the onset is sudden, with pain in the abdomen and back, malaise, and manifestations of rapidly increasing anemia. A history of dark urine is common as a result of the presence of bile pigments or hemoglobinuria. This is a prominent finding in the most seriously ill patients. Jaundice evident on physical examination is present in about 40% of patients. In idiopathic AIHA, splenomegaly occurs in 50% to 60% of patients, hepatomegaly in 30%, and lymphadenopathy in about 25%. Only about 25% of patients have no enlargement of spleen, liver, or lymph nodes.

2. **Hematologic findings:** The anemia is frequently severe, with an initial hemoglobin level of 7 g per deciliter or less. Progression of the anemia frequently occurs before therapy becomes effective. Although platelet counts and white blood cell counts are usually normal, they are elevated in a minority of patients, often with the presence of occasional metamyelocytes and myelocytes. In other instances, however, platelet antibodies and leukocyte antibodies have been documented, resulting in thrombocytopenia or leukopenia. As in other types of hemolytic anemias, a persistently raised reticulocyte count is a characteristic, although not invariable finding. The peripheral blood film often reveals spherocytosis and mild to moderate poikilocytosis. Polychromatophilia is present except in patients with reticulocytopenia. In AIHA, erythroid hyperplasia in the bone marrow is characteristic; hyperplasia of all marrow elements is found less frequently.

3. **Immunohematologic findings:** The cardinal feature of immune hemolytic anemia is a positive direct antiglobulin test (DAT), often referred to as the direct Coombs' test. Monospecific antiglobulin sera (Coombs' sera) that contain antibodies only to IgG or C3d are manufactured; polyspecific antisera contain antibodies to both IgG and C3d. These monospecific sera cause agglutination when reacted with RBCs coated with the appropriate globulin. In warm-antibody AIHA, the patient's red cells, almost all warm autoantibodies, which are typically found in the serum, can be eluted from the patient's red blood cells. They are usually in the IgG immunoglobulin class and react with all normal red blood cells. Occasionally, investigators have shown that they react preferentially with antigens on the patient's own RBCs, most frequently antigens of the Rh blood group system.

4. **Prognosis and survival:** The prognosis for a given patient with warm-antibody AIHA is unpredictable. A minority of patients will have complete resolution of their

Table 4. Characteristic serologic findings in autoimmune hemolytic anemias

Type of anemia	Result of DAT	Eluate	Tests for serum antibody	Antibody specificity
Warm-antibody autoimmune hemolytic anemia (most common type)	IgG or complement (C3) or both	IgG antibody	Indirect antiglobulin test or agglutination or hemolysis of enzyme-premodified cells	Usually within Rh system; other specificities include LW, U, I^t, K, Kp^b, K13, Ge, Jk^a, En^a, and Wr^b
Cold agglutinin syndrome	Complement (C3) alone	Negative	Agglutinating activity up to 30°C; high titer at 4°C (usually >500)	Usually anti-I; other specificities include I, Pr, Gd, and Sd^x
Paroxysmal cold hemoglobinuria	Complement (C3) alone	Negative	Biphasic hemolysin (i.e., sensitizing erythrocytes in the cold and then hemolyzing them when moved to 37°C)	Anti-P (reacts with all erythrocytes except the very rare p or P^k cells)

DAT, direct antiglobulin test; IgG, immunoglobulin G.

disease, and others have a chronic but manageable course. The estimated mortality rate of patients followed up for 5 to 10 years is 15% to 25%.

Cold agglutinin syndrome (CAS): About 15% of patients with AIHA have CAS. Patients with CAS are typically middle-aged or elderly; the peak age of onset ranges from 51 to 60 years.

1. **Symptoms and signs:** Symptoms are frequently those of a chronic anemia. Some patients may experience hemoglobinuria, particularly in cold weather, and may complain of acrocyanosis of the ears, nose tip, fingers, and toes in cold temperatures. This condition vanishes quickly on warming. Physical findings may include pallor and jaundice and, in most cases, splenomegaly. Hepatomegaly and lymphadenopathy are not prominent.

2. **Hematologic findings:** In classic cases, the degree of anemia varies with the degree of cold exposure. A fairly stable anemia that is mild or moderate in severity, however, is much more common. Autoagglutination of blood specimens is characteristic; this reaction creates problems in making satisfactory blood films and in performing blood counts. Erythrocyte morphology is less abnormal than in warm antibody AIHA, with lesser degrees of spherocytosis, anisocytosis, and poikilocytosis. Reticulocytopenia is rare, as are abnormalities of white blood cells and platelets.

3. **Immunohematologic findings:** Patients with CAS have a positive DAT because of the presence of C3d on their red blood cells. The IgM antibody responsible for the fixation of complement to the red cells usually is not demonstrated by the DAT because antiglobulin serum does not readily detect IgM antibodies. The autoantibody in the patient's serum causes agglutination of normal red cells to a higher titer than normal at 4°C (i.e., >50) and reacts to a lesser titer up to a temperature of at least 30°C. In classic cases, the cold agglutinin titer at 4°C is greater than 1,000, and it may be as high as 256,000. In about 40% of cases, however, the cold agglutinin titer is less than 1,000. The antibody usually has specificity within the Ii blood group system, most commonly anti-I.

4. **Associated diseases:** Usually CAS is idiopathic, but it may be associated with a number of infectious diseases, particularly *Mycoplasma pneumoniae* infections and infectious mononucleosis. Some patients develop CAS in association with hematologic malignancies, especially chronic lymphocytic leukemia, Hodgkin disease, and the lymphocytic lymphomas, although this is unusual.

5. **Prognosis:** The prognosis of patients with idiopathic CAS is significantly better than in patients with warm-antibody AIHA. Many patients have a chronic course and can tolerate their mild or moderate anemia quite well. In most patients, the response to therapy is poor, however, so that when more severe hemolysis is present, death may ensue from complications of slowly progressive anemia or chronic blood transfusion therapy. In patients with secondary CAS associated with *M. pneumoniae* infections or infectious mononucleosis, spontaneous resolution of the hemolysis usually occurs within several weeks.

Paroxysmal cold hemoglobinuria (PCH) is a rare disorder, making up fewer than 1% of cases of AIHA. Historically, PCH has occurred after cold exposure in patients who had hereditary syphilis or who were in the quiescent stage of late syphilis. Presently, the disorder is most common in children, and most patients have a history of a recent viral infection or flu-like illness. Almost all recent reports of PCH describe an acute, transient, nonrecurring hemolytic anemia that is not related to cold exposure.

Hemolysis is acute in onset and causes severe and rapidly progressive anemia. Patients may have chills, fever, malaise, abdominal distress, aching in the back or legs, and nausea. Hemoglobinemia and hemoglobinuria are frequently present. The blood film may reveal spherocytosis, anisocytosis, poikilocytosis, erythrophagocytosis, and nucleated erythrocytes.

The causative antibody is an IgG antibody that readily elutes from the patient's red cells and therefore is usually not detected with the DAT. This test is often only weakly positive as a result of complement sensitization. PCH is diagnosed by the presence of a red cell autoantibody that fixes to normal red cells at cold temperatures (0–4°C) and subsequently causes hemolysis of the cells when they are warmed to 37°C in the presence of complement (the Donath–Landsteiner test). The autoantibody almost always has anti-P specificity. The acute illness characteristically resolves spontaneously after several weeks and usually does not recur.

Combined cold-antibody and warm-antibody AIHA: About 8% of patients with AIHA have serologic findings that satisfy the criteria for both warm-antibody AIHA and CAS. The cold antibody in such cases may be elevated only in titer at 4°C but reacts up to at least 30°C. An association between combined cold-antibody and warm-antibody AIHA and systemic lupus erythematosus appears to exist; systemic lupus has been found in more than 25% of these patients. Most patients have severe hemolysis and, although the initial response to therapy is generally excellent, many have a chronic course.

AIHA with a negative DAT: Some patients who ultimately are diagnosed as having AIHA have a negative DAT. These patients have findings suggestive of AIHA, that is, an acquired hemolytic anemia, spherocytes on the peripheral blood film, no other apparent diagnosis after exhaustive evaluation, and a response to therapy similar to that in patients with AIHA who have characteristic immunohematologic findings. Small concentrations of autoantibodies are usually demonstrated on the patient's red cells or in an eluate from the red cells using techniques that are more sensitive than the routine DAT (e.g., tests using radiolabeled antiglobulin sera or agglutinating potentiators).

Drug-induced immune hemolytic anemia: About 15% of acquired immune hemolytic anemias are related to drug administration. Some drugs lead to true autoimmune hemolytic anemia by causing the development of antibodies with specificity for red cell antigens. Other drugs cause development of drug-dependent antibodies that react with red cells only in the presence of the drug. These antibodies may be reacting at least in part with drug absorbed onto the red cell membrane. Some drugs are very loosely bound to the erythrocyte, however, and in this instance, it seems possible that the antibody forms a complex with the drug in the plasma. This complex then attaches to the red cell resulting in hemolysis; this reaction frequently is augmented by complement activation. It is convenient to categorize the drugs that cause immune hemolytic anemia according to the proposed mechanism by which they lead to the development of red cell antibodies. Clinical and laboratory correlations are presented in Table 5. The mechanisms by which various drugs lead to the development of immune hemolysis, however, may be less dissimilar than has been suggested in the past. A unifying hypothesis suggests that all drugs that result in the development of antibodies that react with red cells first bind to the cell. Even if the binding is quite loose, it leads to an alteration of red cell membrane proteins. Resultant antibodies can be directed against drug–cell com-

Table 5. Drug-induced immune hemolysis

Type of serologic reaction	Severity of hemolysis	Detection of drug-induced antibody	Prototype drugs
Drug-dependent antibody	Severe, often with intravascular hemolysis and renal failure	Serum + drug + RBCs	Quinidine, quinine
Passive agglutination	Moderate severity usually without intravascular hemolysis	Serum + drug-coated RBCs	Penicillins, cephalosporins
Autoantibody	Moderate severity, usually without intravascular hemolysis	Serum + RBCs	Methyldopa, procainamide

RBC, red blood cells.

plexes (drug-dependent antibodies) or against cell antigens alone (autoantibodies), or both types of antibodies may develop in the same patient.

Drugs that are firmly bound to the erythrocyte: Several drugs are firmly bound to the erythrocyte, in which case the optimal means of detection of the drug-dependent antibody in the laboratory involves the use of drug-coated red blood cells. Available data suggest that the drug becomes coupled to the red blood cell surface as a primary event, and circulating anti-drug antibody binds to the cell-bound drug secondarily. This mechanism of cell sensitization leading to hemolysis has been called the *drug-absorption mechanism:*

1. Prototype drugs are the penicillins and cephalosporins; other drugs are cisplatin, erythromycin, tetracycline, and tolbutamide.
2. The antibody, which is usually of the IgG immunoglobulin class, reacts with the drug-coated cells *in vitro* to produce a positive indirect antiglobulin test. Clinically, the hemolysis is usually, but not always, moderate in severity with no signs of intravascular hemolysis.

Drugs that are loosely bound to the erythrocyte: Drugs that are loosely bound to the red cell *in vitro* lead to the development of a drug-dependent antibody, that is, an antibody that can be detected only in the presence of the drug *in vitro*. The optimal means of detection involves adding a solution of the drug to the patient's serum; adding red cells to the incubation mixture; and observing for agglutination, sensitization to antiglobulin serum, or lysis. The drugs frequently cause severe hemolytic anemia with manifestations of acute intravascular hemolysis, such as hemoglobinemia and hemoglobinuria. Renal insufficiency is a common occurrence.

Antibody formation has generally been thought to occur as a consequence of the drug's reacting with cell membrane constituents to act as a hapten (hapten mechanism). The resultant antibody has specificity for the drug–cell complex. Alternatively, it has been proposed that the drug-dependent antibody has specificity for the drug and that immune complexes develop as a result of interaction of the antibody with drug in the plasma. These complexes, which then are absorbed onto the red cell membrane, result in complement activation and hemolysis (immune complex mechanism). Such drugs include acetaminophen, cefotaxime, ceftriaxone, chlorpromazine, chlorpropamide, phenacetin, quinidine, and quinine.

Drug-induced AIHA is caused by methyldopa, procainamide, and a small number of other drugs, including chlorpromazine, L-dopa, mefenamic acid, phenacetin, and streptomycin. AIHA caused by methyldopa has been particularly well characterized. A remarkable feature is the fact that serologic findings are indistinguishable from idiopathic warm antibody AIHA. Indeed, no serologic evidence of a relationship between the antibodies and the drug has ever been demonstrated; proof that methyldopa causes AIHA has come from clinical observations. Cessation of the drug results in a prompt remission of the hemolytic anemia, and the DAT slowly reverts to negative. Readministration of the drug causes the AIHA to reappear. In about 15% of patients receiving methyldopa, the DAT becomes positive after 3 to 6 months of treatment. Fewer than 1% of the patients with a positive test develop hemolysis. The serologic findings in these cases are identical to those described above in patients with warm antibody AIHA.

Management of Immune Hemolytic Anemias
Corticosteroids are the initial therapy for patients with **warm antibody AIHA.** An appropriate regimen is prednisone, 1 to 1.5 mg per kilogram daily, administered orally. The increased effectiveness of higher doses or parenteral administration has not been documented.

A large majority of patients manifest a clinical response within 2 weeks of treatment initiation, and a complete lack of response at 21 days should be considered a steroid failure. A response is indicated by an increasing hematocrit, often with an increasing reticulocyte count, until the hematocrit nears normal levels. The DAT often remains positive (although weaker); the indirect antiglobulin test, which detects antibody in the patient's serum, usually becomes negative. For those patients who respond to corticosteroids, a normal or stable hematocrit and reticulocyte count are found in 30 to 90 days. At this time, the dose of prednisone should be reduced weekly by 0.5 mg per kilogram daily or by 10 to 20 mg daily. Alternate-day therapy may be used with doses less than 30 mg daily.

Some patients may be maintained on acceptably low doses of prednisone, but if more than 10 to 15 mg per day is required to keep the hematocrit at an acceptable level, the response should be considered inadequate and other treatments should be strongly considered. The decision regarding the use of other therapies should be made within several months of diagnosis to prevent the adverse effects of long-term corticosteroid administration, which can be devastating.

If the response to corticosteroids is inadequate, **splenectomy** should be performed unless surgery is strongly contraindicated.

About 50% to 75% of patients show marked improvement or have a complete hematologic remission after splenectomy. Remissions are not always permanent, however, and relapse may occur after months or years. If an incomplete remission or a relapse occurs following splenectomy, much lower corticosteroid doses may prove effective in controlling the disease activity.

After splenectomy, patients have a lifelong increased risk of fulminant bacteremia, with a particular susceptibility to encapsulated organisms such as pneumococcus. Although potentially fatal, postsplenectomy sepsis is unusual; this risk must be balanced with the more common adverse effects of prolonged high-dose corticosteroid administration. Pneumococcal vaccine is undoubtedly effective in raising antibody concentrations, particularly when administered before splenectomy, but also when given postoperatively. Revaccination may be necessary after 5 to 10 years. A strategy for antibiotic prophylaxis is less clear, but many investigators recommend that all patients receive penicillin prophylaxis for at least 2 years after the operation. Patients should be educated about this risk and told to contact their physicians at once when symptoms of an infection develop.

Patients whose hemolysis is inadequately controlled by steroids and splenectomy may benefit from **immunosuppressive drugs.** Oral azathioprine (Imuran), 50 to 200 mg per day, or cyclophosphamide (Cytoxan), 50 to 150 mg per day, is commonly used. Although therapeutic responses are generally not very dramatic, they may be sufficient to avoid transfusion therapy.

Other therapies: Anecdotal reports describe the beneficial effects of plasma exchange. Acute hemolytic episodes are reported to have stabilized after other therapies have been ineffective. In almost all cases, however, it has been difficult to separate the effects of the plasma exchange from the effects of other therapies given concomitantly.

Danazol, a modified androgen with reduced masculinizing effects, may be used in doses of 600 to 800 mg daily. Treatment with danazol usually has been used in conjunction with prednisone either as initial therapy or after inadequate response to corticosteroids alone. Limited experience suggests that danazol may lead to improvement, typically within 1 to 3 weeks. Thereafter, corticosteroids may be tapered to a low dose or discontinued. Once remission is sustained, the dose of danazol may be reduced to 200 to 400 mg daily.

Although some patients with AIHA have responded to high-dose intravenous immunoglobulin, there are numerous reports of its ineffectiveness. This treatment usually has been given in association with other therapies and, when effective, has produced only temporary benefit.

Transfusion therapy: *Transfusion therapy must never be considered contraindicated,* even though the crossmatch test may be strongly incompatible. When life-threatening manifesta of anemia are present, transfusion is mandatory. Even at hemoglobin levels of 5 to 8 g per deciliter, however, most patients tolerate the anemia well if treated with bed rest, oxygen, and institution of high doses of corticosteroids as described previously.

Recently, emphasis has been given to improved pretransfusion compatibility testing in AIHA. The patient's autoantibodies usually react with all red cells tested, making all crossmatch tests incompatible. Such broadly reactive autoantibodies make the detection of red cell alloantibodies, such as anti-D, anti-Kell, and anti-Kidd, more difficult, which can cause hemolytic transfusion reactions. Several methods are available by which autoantibodies can be absorbed from the serum, which then can be used to test for alloantibodies.

Despite *in vitro* incompatibility caused by red cell autoantibodies, acute hemolytic transfusion reactions are uncommon. The transfused erythrocytes survive about as well as the patient's own cells, thus affording temporary benefit while more definitive treatment is becoming administered.

Consideration of the optimal volume of blood to be transfused is particularly important. The kinetics of red cell destruction are such that the number of cells removed in a unit of time is a percentage of the number of cells present at the start of this time interval.

Thus, the more cells present at zero time, the greater the absolute number of cells that will be destroyed per unit time. Therefore, a rapid increase in red cell volume by transfusion of several units of red cells may result in the development of increased signs of hemolysis, such as hemoglobinemia and hemoglobinuria, even though the rate of hemolysis has not changed. This marked increase in the amount of hemolysis may potentially precipitate disseminated intravascular coagulation DIC, possibly as a result of procoagulant substances present in red cell lysates. This risk can best be minimized by transfusion of relatively small volumes of red blood cells with the aim of maintaining a tolerable level of hematocrit while other therapy is becoming effective.

Cold agglutinin syndrome is frequently not severe and often results in chronic mild hemolytic anemia with a hemoglobin of 9 to 12 g/dL. Patients with a hemoglobin in this range require no therapy other than avoidance of exposure to cold, which can precipitate more severe hemolytic episodes. Even with strict avoidance of cold, however, some hemolysis usually persists. For more severely anemic patients, immunosuppressive therapy may be tried. Prednisone may be used in doses similar to that used for warm-antibody AIHA, but a good response is much less likely. Other immune manipulations, such as cytotoxic chemotherapy with chlorambucil, 2 to 4 mg per day, with careful monitoring for leukopenia or thrombocytopenia, also may be useful. Plasmapheresis, although theoretically effective in removing IgM antibody, is difficult to accomplish because spontaneous agglutination usually occurs even if attempts are made to keep the blood from cooling. Furthermore, it is frequently not effective and is only temporarily beneficial.

Paroxysmal cold hemoglobinuria: Corticosteroid therapy has been disappointing, although it is still used empirically. Patients are best managed with avoidance of cold and, when necessary, with blood transfusion. Usually, treatment should last a period of days to several weeks, by which time spontaneous resolution of the disease occurs.

Drug-induced immune hemolytic anemia: Recognition of drug-induced immune hemolysis is important because the hemolysis can be life threatening if the drug therapy is continued. Usually, the only therapy necessary is cessation of the drug. Corticosteroids and blood transfusion also may be helpful when hemolysis is severe, however.

Paroxysmal nocturnal hemoglobinuria (PNH): Classic PNH involves hemolytic anemia accompanied by nocturnal hemoglobinuria. PNH is the only acquired hemolytic anemia characterized by an abnormality intrinsic to the erythrocyte. PNH is not just a red cell abnormality but is a clonal stem cell disorder associated with the formation of abnormal erythrocytes, platelets, and granulocytes. The following are the **clinical findings** in patients with PNH:

1. These patients manifest all the clinical and laboratory signs of chronic hemolytic anemia. Nocturnal hemoglobinuria occurs in a minority of patients. More commonly, hemoglobinuria is irregular in its occurrence and may be infrequent or even absent. Other symptoms are recurrent abdominal pain, vomiting, severe headaches, and pain in the eyes. Iron loss occurs in the urine and hemosiderinuria, frequently leading to iron deficiency, a constant feature of the disease.

2. One of the most serious manifestations of PNH is the formation of venous thromboses at several unusual sites. The Budd–Chiari syndrome, which results from hepatic vein thrombosis, is a particularly common development with an ominous prognosis. Clots in the cerebral veins, splenic vein, and dermal veins have occurred; dermal–vein clots can result in unusual necrotic skin lesions.

The following are the **hematologic findings** in patients with PNH:

1. The characteristic blood findings are anemia accompanied by reticulocytosis. If the patient is iron deficient, the red cells may be microcytic and hypochromic.

2. The bone marrow is usually hypercellular due to increased erythropoiesis, and the myeloid-to-erythroid ratio may be reversed. Hypoplasia of the marrow is not unusual, however. Indeed, PNH is frequently associated with aplastic anemia. Severe aplastic anemia may be the presenting disorder or, less commonly, may develop during the course of PHN. A decrease in red cell membrane acetylcholinesterase activity and a diminished leukocyte alkaline phosphatase activity are other associated findings.

Pathophysiology: An abnormality in the glycolipid-anchored proteins of the membranes of blood cells has been implicated in the pathogenesis of PNH. Research has shown that at least nine such proteins are missing from the membrane of the abnormal blood cells; the lack of these proteins appears to be the cause of the clinical syndrome. The absence of at least three complement-controlling proteins—decay accelerating factor (DAF), membrane inhibitor of reactive lysis (MIRL or CD59), and C8 binding protein—results in the intravascular lysis of the abnormal cells. How the abnormality of the PNH cells arises is not clear. It is probably a somatic mutation; the abnormal cells are clonal in origin, and the abnormality (a stem cell) is passed to its progeny.

Diagnostic tests: The most convenient screening test for PNH is the sucrose hemolysis test. If this test is positive, the diagnosis should be confirmed using the acidified serum lysis test (Ham test). These tests demonstrate the red blood cell defect, an unusual susceptibility to lysis by complement. A similar defect can be demonstrated in platelets and granulocytes. In addition, the urine should be examined for hemosiderin because it is invariably present. Some laboratories are able to document the characteristic red cell membrane protein abnormalities.

Course and prognosis: The course of PNH is highly variable; some patients die within months of onset of symptoms, whereas others survive for decades. Although the long-term outlook is good for many patients, the disease may be fatal, particularly because of the thrombotic manifestations or complications of pancytopenia.

Management of patients with PNH should be treatment with iron in addition to receiving folic acid because chronic hemosiderinuria and hemoglobinuria often result in iron deficiency. Iron administration may cause increased hemoglobinuria; however; this probably results from increased formation and destruction of complement-sensitive reticulocytes.

Treatment with androgens may improve the anemia. A 2-month trial of fluoxymesterone (5–40 mg per day administered orally), oxymetholone (1–5 mg/kg body weight daily administered orally), or nandrolone decanoate (25–200 mg once weekly administered intramuscularly) may produce a hematologic response. The side effects of these drugs include masculinization in women and prostatic enlargement in men.

Corticosteroids, 15 to 45 mg every other day, are reported to be beneficial in about 60% of patients. Bone marrow transplantation has been used in selected patients, especially for those with manifestations associated with severe defects in hematopoiesis. Blood transfusion is necessary in some patients. Rarely, hemolytic episodes with destruction of the patient's own red cells have been reported following transfusion. This has been attributed to activation of the complement system by alloantibodies against white cells or by the presence in the infused blood of compounds capable of activating complement in the patient's plasma. The problem can be avoided by the use of washed or frozen, reconstituted red blood cells.

Suggested Readings

Beutler E. Glucose-6-phosphate dehydrogenase deficiency and other enzyme abnormalities In: Beutler E, Lichtman MA, Kipp TJ, eds. *Williams' hematology*, 5th ed. New York: McGraw-Hill, 1995:564–581. (This is an excellent current summary of enzymopathies.)

Beutler E, Luzatto L. Hemolytic anemia: a century of hematology. *Semin Hematol* 1999;36(Suppl 7):38–47. (This is an excellent historical review.)

Dacie JV. The haemolytic anaemias. In: *The autoimmune haemolytic anaemias,* 3rd ed, vol 3. New York: Churchill Livingstone, 1992:1–452.

Engelfriet CP, Overbeeke MAM, von dem Borne AEGK. Autoimmune hemolytic anemia. *Semin Hematol* 1992;29:3–12.

Garratty G. Mechanisms of immune red cell destruction, and red cell compatibility testing. *Hum Pathol* 1983;14:204–212.

Garratty G, ed. Symposium on drug-induced immune cytopenia. *Transfus Med Rev* 1993;7:213–214.

Palek J, Jarolim P. Hereditary spherocytosis, elliptocytosis and related disorders. In: Beutler E, Lichtman MA, Kipp TJ, eds. *Williams' hematology,* 5th ed. New York: McGraw-Hill, 1995: 536–557.

Palek J, Sahr KE. Mutations of the red blood cell membrane proteins: from clinical evaluation to detection of the underlying genetic defect. *Blood* 1992;80:308–330.

Petz LD, Branch DR. Drug-induced immune hemolytic anemia. *Methods Hematol* 1985;18:47.

Petz LD, Swisher SN. Blood transfusion in acquired hemolytic anemias. In: *Clinical practice of transfusion medicine,* 2nd ed. New York: Churchill Livingstone, 1989: 549–582.

Rosse WF. Autoimmune hemolytic anemia. *Hosp Practice* 1985;20:105–111.

Rosse WF. *Clinical immunohematology: basic concepts and clinical applications.* Boston: Blackwell Scientific Publications, 1989.

Rosse WF, Parker CJ. Paroxysmal nocturnal haemoglobinuria. *Clin Haematol* 1985;14:105–125.

Sokol RJ, Hewitt, S. Autoimmune hemolysis: a critical review. *CRC Crit Rev Oncol Hematol* 1985;4:125–154.

Tanner MJA, Anstee DJ, eds. Red cell membrane disorders. *Baillieres Clin Haematol* 1999;12:605–762.

Valentine WN, moderator. Hemolytic anemias and erythrocyte enzymopathies. *Ann Intern Med* 1985;103:245–257.

Zanella A, ed. Inherited disorders of red cell metabolism. *Baillieres Clin Haematol* 2000;13:1–148.

5. HEREDITARY HEMOCHROMATOSIS AND OTHER IRON-OVERLOAD DISORDERS

Gordon D. McLaren

The term *iron overload* refers to any condition in which body iron stores greatly exceed the normal level, which is generally about 1 g in adult men and somewhat less in women, approximately 300 mg (see Chapter 2). Clinically relevant systemic iron overload occurs most often in **hereditary** *(idiopathic, primary)* **hemochromatosis,** an inherited disorder of iron metabolism characterized by abnormal regulation of dietary iron absorption, leading to gradual accumulation of markedly increased amounts of storage iron. In this condition, total body iron stores may reach 20 to 40 g or more. Several other disorders often produce a similar clinical picture. Examples include iron overload from multiple blood transfusions or as a result of increased iron absorption associated with increased ineffective erythropoiesis (Table 1). A type of iron overload seen among indigenous peoples of sub-Saharan Africa is associated with ingestion of a traditional home-brewed beer having a high iron content. The amount of excess body iron in this condition can reach levels comparable to those seen in hereditary hemochromatosis, with similar deleterious effects (see section entitled **African Iron Overload**).

It is possible to detect relatively minor degrees of iron overload in some patients with alcoholic liver disease and in patients with porphyria cutanea tarda. In the following sections, the pathogenesis of hereditary hemochromatosis and the causes of the various other types of iron overload are outlined, and the diagnostic and therapeutic implications of their differing etiologies are emphasized.

Hereditary Hemochromatosis

This disorder also has been called *idiopathic* hemochromatosis, *primary* hemochromatosis, *genetic* hemochromatosis, *human leukocyte antigen (HLA)-linked* hemochromatosis, and, most recently, hemachromatosis gene (HFE)-related hemochromatosis. For purposes of this chapter, the term *hereditary* hemochromatosis (or simply *hemochromatosis*) is used throughout.

Pathophysiology

Iron overload in hereditary hemochromatosis is attributable to excessive dietary iron absorption. Over the course of many years, increased absorption leads to accretion of toxic levels of iron in multiple organs, resulting in organ damage and dysfunction.

Most patients are homozygous for a mutation in the hemochromatosis gene (designated *HFE*), which was identified in 1996 (see section entitled **Genetics**). The condition is characterized early on by increased plasma iron and transferrin saturation levels, and, with the passage of time, by a progressive rise in the plasma ferritin concentration as well, reflecting the progressive increase in body iron stores.

The liver is the primary target organ and the major site of initial iron deposition. The resulting hepatocellular damage leads to fibrosis, cirrhosis, and hepatic failure. The cirrhosis can occur in affected homozygotes whether or not they consume alcohol (although alcohol abuse can accelerate the process); that is, iron overload alone is sufficient to produce the lesion. Primary hepatocellular carcinoma (hepatoma) often develops as a terminal event.

Hyperpigmentation is often seen in advanced disease and represents increased deposition of melanin, rather than iron, in the dermis. Another common complication is glucose intolerance, the result of iron deposition in the pancreatic islets. (Before the recognition of the role of iron in the disease, this combination of hyperpigmentation and glucose intolerance was referred to as *bronze diabetes*).

Other organs that may be involved include the heart, pituitary, joints, and central nervous system. Patients with advanced disease may present with hepatomegaly, as-

Table 1. Classification of iron overload disorders[a]

Primary iron overload
    Hereditary hemochromatosis (*HFE* related)
    Non-*HFE* related iron overload
        Juvenile hemochromatosis
        Transferrin receptor 2 related iron overload
    Autosomal dominant iron overload

Other disorders associated with severe iron overload
    African iron overload[b]
    Medicinal iron overload
    Transfusional hemosiderosis
    Ineffective erythropoiesis
    Hereditary atransferrinemia
    Neonatal iron overload
    Hereditary aceruloplasminemia[c]

Disorders associated with minor to moderate iron overload
    Alcoholic liver disease
    Porphyria cutanea tarda
    Dysmetabolic hepatosiderosis[d]

---

[a] Other disorders, not listed here, include pulmonary hemosiderosis (focal, rather than generalized, iron overload involving only the lungs) and the hereditary hyperferritinemia cataract syndrome, which is not associated with iron overload (see text).
[b] There is evidence that iron overload among indigenous peoples of sub-Saharan Africa has a genetic component (see text), suggesting that this disorder may be re-classified as a form of primary iron overload in the future, although the gene has not yet been identified.
[c] Whereas the underlying defect in this disorder is a lack of ceruloplasmin, a copper-containing protein, the major phenotypic manifestation is iron overload, possibly resulting from loss of ceruloplasmin's plasma ferroxidase activity, which may be required for release of iron from reticuloendothelial cells.
[d] Also called insulin-resistance-associated liver siderosis, this disorder is characterized by mild to moderate iron excess, often in association with hyperlipidemia, diabetes, and obesity. The etiology is unknown but appears not to be related to *HFE* gene mutations.

cites, congestive heart failure or cardiac arrhythmias, evidence of gonadal dysfunction (impotence, amenorrhea), loss of body hair, arthritis, or dementia, or any combination of these manifestations. Fortunately, through early diagnosis and removal of excess iron by serial phlebotomy (see section entitled **Therapy and Prognosis**), all such complications can be prevented entirely.

Genetics
Hereditary hemochromatosis is inherited in an autosomal recessive manner. The hemochromatosis gene, designated *HFE* (formerly called *HLA-H*), encodes a major histocompatibility complex (MHC) class I–like protein, the function of which is not fully understood (see section on **Etiology and Pathogenesis**). The gene is closely linked to the HLA locus on the short arm chromosome 6 (C6p).

Most patients with hemochromatosis are homozygous for a mutation that produces a single amino acid substitution of cysteine with tyrosine at amino acid 282 of the protein (Cys282Tyr; C282Y). Homozygous (C282Y/C282Y) affected persons typically develop clinically significant iron overload by the fifth or sixth decade of life, although there is considerable variability in the age of onset and extent of disease expression.

Heterozygotes generally do not have increased iron stores, although some may have slightly increased hepatic iron levels; however, iron overload to the extent seen in homozygotes does not occur except rarely in the presence of another coexisting condition that is also associated with a predisposition for excess iron accumulation (see section on **Interactions between the Hemochromatosis Gene and Other Disorders**).

A second common missense mutation in *HFE* results in substitution of aspartic acid for histidine at amino acid 63 (His63Asp; H63D). This mutation does not appear to confer an increased risk for the development of iron overload in most cases, even in homozygous (H63D/H63D) persons, although some compound heterozygotes (persons who are heterozygous for both C282Y and H63D; C282Y/H63D) have clinically relevant degrees of iron overload. A third relatively common mutation occurs at position 65, with substitution of cysteine for serine (Ser65Cys; S65C) and may be involved in causing iron storage disease.

Other, less common *HFE* mutations have been described, occasionally in patients with iron overload. Most of these mutations are still under investigation, and some are "private" (i.e., found in only one or two families). Thus, it is not the general practice to test for such mutations on a routine basis.

Inheritance Pattern
A diagnosis of hemochromatosis in one family member (the proband) means that the proband's siblings are also at risk for the disease (Fig. 1). Because hereditary hemochromatosis is an autosomal recessive disorder, both of the proband's parents must carry a copy of the mutant allele, and each of the proband's siblings will have a one in four

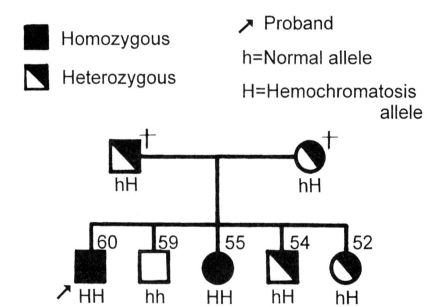

FIG. 1. Hypothetical family with several members affected by hereditary hemochromatosis, illustrating the autosomal recessive mode of inheritance. Squares and circles represent males and females, respectively, with ages shown to the upper right of each (†, deceased). Although the parents could not be tested, they are obligatorily heterozygous because they had children with homozygous disease. (*Note:* The probability that individual offspring will be homozygous is one in four, but in a given family, any combination of hemochromatosis homozygotes, heterozygotes, and normal homozygotes can occur.) The hemochromatosis allele identified in most hemochromatosis patients contains a single mutation in the hemochromatosis gene (*HFE*) resulting in substitution of tyrosine for cysteine at position 282 (C282Y) of the HFE protein (see **Genetics** in the **Hereditary Hemochromatosis** section).

chance of being homozygous (e.g., C282Y/C282Y). Each sibling also has a one in four chance of being homozygous for the *normal* allele and a 50:50 chance of being heterozygous. In contrast, all the proband's offspring will be heterozygous and therefore unlikely to develop iron overload unless the proband's partner also carries the defective gene.

In some families, homozygous affected persons are identified in successive generations. This "vertical" transmission can occur as the result of a mating between a homozygous, affected person and a heterozygous carrier, or, less often, a mating between two homozygotes.

Sometimes the disease can appear to "skip" a generation as the result of a mating between a hemochromatosis patient's heterozygous child and another heterozygous carrier. The occurrence of such matings is not surprising, given the high frequency of the gene (see the following section).

Disease Frequency and Origin

1. **Frequency in Europeans:** Among populations of European (particularly Northern European) origin, including those in the United States, Canada, Australia, and other countries that have large European populations, the frequency of hereditary hemochromatosis appears to be quite high, although estimates vary considerably from one study to another (Table 2). Some of this variability is attributable to geographic differences. In addition, several methods of ascertainment have been used (e.g., family studies, autopsies, population screening), and these may provide different estimates. Taking all these estimates together, the overall disease frequency appears to be approximately 3 to 5 per 1,000 persons, making hereditary hemochromatosis the most common autosomal recessive disorder in whites.

2. **Carrier frequency:** The frequency of heterozygous carriers of the gene is calculated to be approximately one in every eight persons (i.e., about 12% of the population), with most estimates ranging from 1 in 7 (14%) to 1 in 11 (9%). Similar estimates for U.S. whites have been derived by distribution analysis of transferrin saturation measurements in nutrition surveys.

Table 2. Hereditary hemochromatosis: prevalence gene frequency[a]

Geographic area or population group	Basis[b]	Disease prevalence (%)	C282Y frequency	Heterozygote prevalence (%)[c]
Australia (Queensland)	f,p,d	0.36	0.064	11.3
France (Brittany)	f,p,d	0.1–0.4	0.029	6.1–11.8
Italy (North)	p,d	0.20	0.045	8.5
United Kingdom	p,d	0.30	0.06	10.4
United States (Utah)	p,d	0.45	0.062	12.5

[a] Disease prevalence estimates for hemochromatosis are based on phenotypic manifestations, and C282Y frequencies are derived from results of genotyping for *HFE* mutations in the same geographic areas. Table represents a selective composite for illustrative purposes only; the different types of studies are not directly comparable. (For references, see *Suggested Readings*. Comprehensive summaries of most of the available studies may be found in Fairbanks VF. Hemochromatosis: population genetics. In: Barton JC, Edward CQ, eds. *Hemochromatosis genetics, pathophysiology, diagnosis and treatment*. Cambridge: Cambridge University Press, 2000:42–50; and Porto G, de Sousa M. Variation of hemochromatosis prevalence and genotype in national groups. *Ibid.*)
[b] Indicates basis of estimates: d, DNA analysis for *HFE* alleles; f, family; p, population.
[c] Heterozygote prevalence estimates are calculated according to the Hardy-Weinberg equilibrium equation on the basis of disease prevalence estimates, without reference to frequencies of the C282Y mutation.

3. **Frequency of *HFE* mutations in patients with hemochromatosis and in the general population:**
- In North America, about 85% to 90% of hemochromatosis patients are homozygous for the C282Y mutation (C282Y/C282Y). Most of the remainder are homozygous for the normal allele (wild type, wt). Some are heterozygotes (C282Y/wt), and others are doubly heterozygous for C282Y and another *HFE* mutation such as H63D (C282Y/H63D) or occasionally S65C (C282Y/S65C). Rare individuals having iron overload consistent with hemochromatosis are homozygous for H63D.
- The occurrence of clinically relevant iron overload in patients who are not C282Y homozygotes suggests the existence of other genes that are important in controlling iron metabolism and may modify the hemochromatosis phenotype (see discussion of **Genotypic/phenotypic correlation**).
- The proportion of hemochromatosis patients who are C282Y/C282Y varies widely among geographic areas across the world, from 60% in Southern Italy to greater than 95% in Brittany, France. Among patients in Australia, the proportion of C282Y homozygotes is essentially 100%.
- The C282Y mutation is very common among persons of European ancestry, such that in the United States, about 10% are heterozygous (C282Y/wt) and 0.5% are homozygous (C282Y/Y282Y). It is not known how many of these C282Y homozygotes are at risk for the development of iron overload, however, and this is the subject of current research (see section entitled **Factors that Affect the Severity of Disease in Hemochromatosis Homozygotes**).
- The frequency of the H63D mutation is even higher, with up to 25% of persons in European populations being heterozygous carriers. As noted earlier, however, the H63D allele usually is not causally related to iron overload, except in some compound heterozygotes (C282Y/H63D). The S65C mutation is less common, with a carrier frequency of 2% to 4%.

4. **Frequency in other populations:** Hemochromatosis is essentially unknown among Native Americans, and the frequency also is thought to be low in African Americans, Ashkenazic Jews, and Japanese. The probable frequency of hereditary hemochromatosis in African Americans is about three to six per 10,000, or about one tenth the frequency among whites. There is evidence, however, of a different iron-loading gene in Africans, and this gene may be common among African Americans as well (see discussion of **genetic studies** in section entitled **African Iron Overload**).

Factors that Affect the Severity of Disease in Hemochromatosis Homozygotes
Expressivity in hemochromatosis is quite variable. Some homozygotes manifest no clinical abnormalities, and others develop only moderate degrees of iron overload. About one third to one half of all homozygotic persons in the United States develop a full-blown picture of severe parenchymal iron overload and organ damage.

Individual factors that affect the extent of iron overload include the following:

1. **Age:** Typically, patients become symptomatic in the fifth or sixth decade of life, although symptoms may develop at an earlier age. Younger homozygous persons, who have not yet accumulated an appreciable amount of iron, often have a normal serum ferritin (SF) level, but transferrin saturation in affected persons usually is elevated even in earlier stages of the disease, despite the fact that iron stores may still be normal. (This is the time to make the diagnosis, however, before the patient begins to develop symptoms or signs, rather than years later when disease manifestations already have supervened).

2. **Sex:** Female homozygotes are partially protected by iron losses associated with menstrual blood loss and childbearing. As a result, only about one tenth to one fifth of patients with clinical manifestations of hemochromatosis are women. Iron stores increase more rapidly after cessation of menses, however, and the rate of accumulation subsequently may approach that of homozygous affected men. In some homozygous women, the rate of iron accumulation is much more rapid and can lead to the onset of clinical symptoms and signs during the third or fourth decade of life. In such patients, amenorrhea secondary to pituitary damage may be the first clinically apparent manifestation of the disease.

3. **Blood loss:** Iron accumulation may occur slowly or not at all in hemochromatosis patients who are frequent blood donors or who suffer chronic gastrointestinal blood loss from ulcers or other hemorrhagic disorders.

Genetic factors that affect disease expression: The foregoing discussion focused on factors that are unrelated to the genetic defect in hemochromatosis *per se* and yet can account for some of the variability in disease expression. In the following sections, evidence will be reviewed indicating that *genetic* factors also may affect phenotypic expression of the mutant *HFE* allele in hemochromatosis patients:

1. **Genotypic/phenotypic correlation:** Although most patients with hemochromatosis are homozygous for the C282Y mutation of the *HFE* gene (see section entitled **Disease Frequency and Origin**), not all C282Y homozygotes show full expression of the disease. The (mutant) gene for hemochromatosis is associated with a number of different HLA haplotypes, but the predominant (ancestral) haplotype carries HLA A3, which is found in three fourths of patients and is associated with more severe disease. Thus, it is possible that the greater severity of disease manifestations in hemochromatosis patients carrying the ancestral haplotype may be attributable to the presence of genetic modifiers in this region of 6p that influence *HFE* expression.

2. **Heterogeneity of phenotypic manifestations:** In addition to variation in overall expressivity in patients with hemochromatosis, there can be heterogeneity with regard to the pattern of biochemical expression. The reasons for this heterogeneity are unknown, although some of the reported cases may have represented variant forms of hemochromatosis (see section entitled **Non-*HFE* Hemochromatosis**) or other iron-overload disorders (see section entitled **Other Iron-overload Disorders**).

Gene/environment interactions: Certain dietary or environmental factors also may play a role in modifying disease expression, including the following:

1. **Amount of iron in the diet:** Dietary iron content may affect the amount of iron absorbed. This can be an important factor in certain populations, particularly in areas where meat intake is high.

2. **Medical iron compounds:** Occasional reports have described iron overload in persons who have ingested large amounts of medicinal iron over a long period.

3. **Alcohol:** Alcoholic beverages have been implicated as a source of dietary iron in some settings. Certain alcoholic beverages such as red wine may contain relatively large amounts of iron, as does the traditional beer consumed among sub-Saharan African populations (see section entitled **African Iron Overload**). In addition, it is thought that alcohol may enhance iron absorption, although the mechanism of this effect is unknown.

- **Minor degrees of iron overload in patients with alcoholic liver disease (ALD):** Hepatic siderosis sometimes is seen in patients with ALD, but the hepatic iron concentrations in such persons rarely approach the levels observed in hemochromatosis, and the total amount of excess storage iron does not exceed 2 g in most cases. The hepatic siderosis in patients with ALD is characterized by deposition of iron primarily in Kuppfer cells, however, in contrast to the predominantly parenchymal iron deposition seen in hereditary hemochromatosis. In addition, patients with ALD do not have an increased frequency of HLA A3, the antigen most commonly associated with the hereditary disease. These data suggest that in most cases the mild hepatic siderosis sometimes observed in ALD probably is not attributable to heterozygosity for hemochromatosis.

- **Major iron overload in patients with hereditary hemochromatosis who also have ALD:** The incidence of alcoholism among patients with clinically manifest hemochromatosis is higher than in the general population. As noted previously, alcohol may enhance iron absorption, thereby increasing the rate of iron accumulation in such patients. In addition, alcoholism lowers the threshold tissue iron concentration required for the development of fibrosis and cirrhosis, presumably through the additive effect of the combination of both alcohol and iron on the liver, thus leading to a more rapid development of cirrhosis in the combined presence of alcohol and excess iron.

Interactions between the Hemochromatosis Gene and Other Disorders that Affect Iron Metabolism

1. **Hereditary spherocytosis:** Most types of hemolytic anemia, including hereditary spherocytosis, characteristically do *not* cause iron overload; however, iron overload can occur in patients with hereditary spherocytosis who also are heterozygous carriers of the gene for hemochromatosis, suggesting that an interaction between the hemochromatosis carrier state and some other disorder that tends to promote iron absorption (in this case, increased erythropoiesis in response to hemolysis; see Chapters 2 and 4) may lead to a sufficiently high rate of absorption as to mimic the homozygous state.

2. **Sideroblastic anemia:** Sideroblastic anemia occurs in both inherited and acquired forms. Generally, the acquired form is a disease of older adults and is considered a myelodysplastic anemia (see Chapters 2 and 10). Heterozygous carriers of the hemochromatosis gene who suffer from hereditary or acquired sideroblastic anemia may develop severe iron overload, although it is not clear whether the hemochromatosis gene actually plays a role in this situation. Both the inherited and acquired forms are characterized by markedly increased ineffective erythropoiesis and increased intestinal iron absorption (see discussion of **iron overload associated with sideroblastic anemia** in the section entitled **Transfusional Iron Overload**). In addition, patients who are transfusion dependent accumulate excess iron from the transfused red blood cells.

3. **Thalassemia:** Nontransfusional iron overload of the same severity as in hereditary hemochromatosis has been observed in association with β-thalassemia minor, but this occurs only in patients who also are homozygous for hemochromatosis. The presence of the single β-thalassemia gene does not further potentiate the degree of iron overloading. In contrast, iron absorption may be increased in patients with β-thalassemia intermedia as a result of markedly increased ineffective erythropoiesis. This can lead to nontransfusional iron overload in the absence of a hemochromatosis gene (see discussion of the **thalassemia syndromes** in the section entitled **Transfusional Iron Overload**).

4. **Porphyria cutanea tarda (PCT):** Heterozygosity or homozygosity for C282Y has been implicated as a contributing factor in up to 40% of patients with the relatively mild hepatic iron overload seen in PCT. Patients with PCT have a deficiency of uroporphyrinogen decarboxylase (URO-D). Affected persons frequently suffer severe photosensitivity reactions, with bullous dermatitis involving sun-exposed areas of the skin, leading to scarring and hypertrichosis. The presence of an increased porphyrin level in the skin is responsible for the photosensitivity. The role of iron in the pathogenesis of PCT may be related, at least in part, to the ability of ferrous iron to inhibit URO-D. Removal of excess iron by phlebotomy leads to biochemical remission and relief of symptoms. The amount of excess storage iron in this condition usually is relatively modest (1.5–4.0 times normal in most cases); phlebotomy of as little as 1 to 3 U of blood over a period of a few weeks often is sufficient.

5. **Pyruvate kinase (PK) deficiency:** This autosomal recessive disorder is characterized by increased ineffective erythropoiesis and anemia, which may be severe and may require regular blood transfusion therapy. Increased iron absorption in PK deficiency may be attributable to the increased ineffective erythropoiesis (a mechanism that is discussed in greater detail in the section entitled **Transfusional Iron Overload**). One study suggested that patients who develop severe iron overload are also heterozygous carriers of the gene for hemochromatosis.

Etiology and Pathogenesis

The precise nature of the underlying metabolic defect in hereditary and hemochromatosis is still unknown. The recent discovery of the *HFE* gene has provided an opportunity to conduct functional studies of the normal and mutant HFE proteins. HFE is abundantly expressed in the crypt cells of the duodenal mucosa and may have a role in the regulation of iron absorption, although many unanswered questions remain about this process.

1. **Intestinal iron absorption:** Excessive intestinal iron absorption in hemochromatosis is fundamental to the pathogenesis of the disease. The normal mechanism for

regulation of iron absorption and the basis of the deranged control of this process in hemochromatosis remain poorly understood. Hemochromatosis patients absorb dietary iron at more than twice the normal rate from birth onwards, until body iron stores begin to approach toxic levels.

2. **Control of iron absorption by the intestinal mucosa:** No known active excretory pathway exists in humans to rid the body of unneeded iron. Thus, iron balance normally is maintained by regulation of intestinal iron absorption, and this control is mediated at the level of the duodenal mucosa:

- **Mucosal iron uptake:** Transport of nonheme iron across the brush border of the mucosal epithelium involves a different pathway from the transferrin-mediated uptake process for delivering iron to erythroid precursors (see Chapter 2). Recently, a transmembrane divalent metal transport (DMT1) localized to the brush border of absorptive enterocytes was identified as an essential component in uptake of dietary iron by mucosal epithelial cells.

- **Intracellular iron metabolism:** Some of the dietary iron taken up by the enterocyte is incorporated into the iron-storage molecule ferritin and is not transferred to the systemic circulation; instead, it is retained within the cytoplasm and subsequently removed from the body as the mucosal epithelial cells are sloughed into the gut lumen. Paradoxically, immunohistochemical studies of duodenal mucosal biopsies have shown only sparse ferritin deposits in the absorptive enterocytes of hemochromatosis patients, despite marked iron overload in other organs throughout the body. Indeed, there is even less ferritin in the duodenal enterocytes of patients with hemochromatosis than in patients with iron deficiency anemia. By contrast, patients with other (secondary) forms of iron overload (e.g., transfusional hemosiderosis) have markedly increased amounts of mucosal ferritin.

  Ferritin synthesis is controlled by iron regulatory proteins (IRPs) that bind to ferritin mRNA under conditions of decreased iron availability, thereby inhibiting translation. Recent studies showed that the IRP binding activity in mucosal biopsies of hemochromatosis patients is appropriate for the mucosal ferritin concentration. This finding suggests that the paucity of the ferritin deposits within the duodenal enterocytes of patients with hemochromatosis is a reflection of a paradoxically low intracellular iron concentration, which may offer a clue to the mechanism of the increased iron absorption in this disorder.

- **Transfer to the plasma:** Little is known about the mechanism of iron transport from the mucosal brush border through the cytoplasm and across the basolateral membrane. The latter process appears to be mediated at least in part by Ferroportin-1, (also called *Ireg1*), which is expressed on the basolateral surface. *In vivo* studies of iron absorption kinetics in patients with hemochromatosis indicated an increased rate of iron transfer from the mucosal epithelium to the plasma.

- **Relationship between intestinal iron absorption and systemic iron metabolism:** The rate of intestinal iron absorption normally is regulated to maintain body iron stores at a relatively constant level. It is not known how the body's iron status is communicated to the intestinal mucosa. One possibility is the supply of iron available to the mucosal epithelial cells in the crypts, transferrin receptors expressed in association with HFE on the basolateral membrane surface enable the crypt cells to acquire needed iron from plasma transferrin.

3. **Internal iron exchange and tissue iron distribution:** Storage iron distribution in hereditary hemochromatosis differs from that in other forms of iron overload. For example, patients with African iron overload have large amounts of iron in splenic macrophages, as well as the liver (see section entitled **African Iron Overload**), whereas patients with advanced hereditary hemochromatosis have relatively less iron in the spleen despite comparable hepatic iron levels.

4. **Comparative cellular iron distribution in hereditary hemochromatosis and other types of iron overload:**

- **Cellular iron distribution in hemochromatosis.** In addition to the aforementioned paucity of iron in splenic macrophages, patients with hemochromatosis also typically do not have conspicuous amounts of iron detectable elsewhere in the reticuloendothelial system (RES). For example, stainable iron in bone marrow macrophages usually is not markedly increased and may even be decreased or absent, despite the presence of heavy iron deposits in the parenchyma of many organs throughout the body. In the liver, iron is deposited initially in hepatocytes rather than Kupffer cells or sinusoidal lining cells. Generally speaking, significant amounts of iron can be detected in the RES only in advanced stages of the disease.

- **Cellular iron distribution in transfusional iron overload.** In contrast to the paucity of reticuloendothelial iron in hereditary hemochromatosis, transfusional iron overload is characterized by prominent reticuloendothelial iron deposition. Thus, bone marrow and splenic macrophages and hepatic Kupffer cells become iron-laden initially, and only later does a significant amount of iron begin to accumulate in hepatocytes and in parenchymal cells of other organs. In the end stages, the patterns of iron deposition in the liver in hereditary hemochromatosis and in transfusional iron overload may become morphologically indistinguishable, with heavy iron deposition in both parenchymal and RE cells.

5. **Reticuloendothelial iron metabolism:**

- **Iron content of macrophages.** The lack of heavy iron deposition in reticuloendothelial cells in hereditary hemochromatosis led some observers to suggest the existence of a defect in RES iron metabolism. Peripheral blood monocytes of iron-loaded patients with hemochromatosis also do not contain as much stainable iron as monocytes of comparably iron overloaded patients with transfusional iron overload or thalassemia, suggesting that monocytes may represent a useful model for the study of RES iron metabolism in this disease.

- **Macrophage iron traffic.** The normal pathway of iron transport within the RES begins with uptake of heme iron via phagocytosis of aged or damaged erythrocytes. The ingested erythrocytes are catabolized within the macrrophage, and iron is removed from the heme moiety in the presence of the enzyme heme oxygenase. Some of this iron may be incorporated into an intracellular storage pool within the macrophage in the form of ferritin or hemosiderin, but normally most of the iron is released to the plasma and bound by plasma transferrin. Transferrin-bound plasma iron is transported to cells throughout the body, with the largest proportion delivered to developing RBC precursors in the bone marrow to incorporate iron into hemoglobin.

Although the mechanism responsible for the enhanced release of iron by the RES in hemochromatosis is unknown, this phenomenon raises the possibility of a shared defect that promotes increased release (transfer) of iron from both the RES and the duodenal mucosal epithelium. Hence, it is plausible that, in hemochromatosis patients with a C282Y mutation, altered affinity of the transferrin receptor for transferrin may affect both duodenal enterocytes and macrophages in the same way.

Pathogenesis of Iron Toxicity and Organ Dysfunction

Organ damage in hemochromatosis is attributable to markedly increased tissue iron levels that exceed the capacity to store the iron safely in a nontoxic form.

1. **Iron storage in the RES:** The RES is involved not only in the breakdown of old RBCs but also in the storage of unneeded iron that is sequestered in ferritin and hemosiderin. Up to 4,000 to 5,000 iron atoms can be stored in each ferritin molecule, and very high concentrations seem to be relatively well tolerated in the RES. The ability of reticuloendothelial cells to store large amounts of iron in this relatively nontoxic form is consistent with the known importance of the RES in iron metabolism.

2. **Effects of iron accumulation in other tissues:** In contrast to the RES, other tissues, such as the heart and endocrine glands, normally contain relatively small amounts of storage iron. When the more limited capacity of these tissues to store iron in ferritin and hemosiderin becomes exhausted, tissue iron damage can occur. The threshold iron concentration for hepatocellular iron damage appears to be approximately six times higher than the upper limit of normal (see **Quantitavive determination of hepatitis iron concentration**).

3. **Mechanism of iron toxicity in chronic iron overload:** The toxic effect of excess iron storage is thought to be attributable to the generation of free radicals such as superoxide and hydroxyl iron. In chronic iron overload, increased amounts of these reactive oxygen species can damage cellular and subcellular membranes through lipid peroxidation.

4. **Manifestations of iron toxicity in hemochromatosis:** Screening for iron overload should be considered in patients who manifest any of the following disorders that may be associated with hemochromatosis:

- **Hepatotoxicity.** In hereditary hemochromatosis, iron is deposited in hepatocytes in a predominantly periportal distribution. When present, hepatic cirrhosis is of the micronodular type. Fibrosis and cirrhosis generally do not occur at iron concentrations less than about 250 µmol/g dry weight, whereas above a level of 350 µmol/g, such changes are common. The hepatic fibrosis and cirrhosis associated with advanced iron overload appear to represent a response to iron-induced cellular injury and cell death followed by liver regeneration.
- **Cardiac dysfunction.** In hemochromatosis, iron concentrations in the heart are considerably less than in the liver, and yet the heart is one of the major target organs for iron toxicity. This suggests that the threshold tissue iron concentration for cardiotoxicity is much lower than that for hepatotoxicity. Arrhythmias and congestive heart failure are common. Cardiac dysfunction may be the presenting manifestation in some patients. Patients initially respond to treatment with antiarrhythmic and inotropic agents but eventually become refractory unless iron-removal therapy is instituted. The frequency of cardiac symptoms reported in various studies ranges from 5% to 35% of symptomatic patients.
- **Endocrine system damage.** Iron also is deposited in glandular organs throughout the body, including sweat glands, pancreatic acinar cells and islets, and the anterior pituitary gland.
- **Endocrine pancreas.** Diabetes mellitus similar to type II diabetes may develop suddenly in up to 50% of symptomatic patients.
- **Anterior pituitary.** Manifestations of hypogonadism (impotence, amenorrhea) are found in 20% to 40% of symptomatic patients. Testosterone levels are low in men with impotence, as are estrogen levels in women with amenorrhea. Low levels of other pituitary hormones, including thyroid-stimulating hormone, have been reported, and hypothyroidism has been found in some patients.
- **Arthropathy.** Joint damage in hemochromatosis occurs in association with deposition of iron in the synovium. The arthritis may affect the hands, shoulders, knees, and hips. Arthropathy is present in about one half of symptomatic patients and is one of the most common presenting manifestations of hemochromatosis. Radiographic findings include bone cysts, condensation of the subchondral plate, irregular erosion of articular cartilage, and generalized chondrocalcinosis resembling pseudogout.
- **Increased susceptibility to infection.** An increased risk of infection has been observed in various types of iron overload, including hereditary hemochromatosis. Infecting microorganisms include *Yersinia enterocolitica, Listeria monocytogenes, Escherichia coli, Candida* species, and *Vibrio vulnificus,* a marine species found in some shellfish. This increased susceptibility to infection may be attributable to increased availability of iron for microbial growth in iron-overloaded patients who have increased transferrin saturation.
- **Central nervous system.** Neurologic symptoms have been described in patients with hemochromatosis, including weakness or fatigue, lethargy, somnolence, severe depression with psychomotor retardation, and, in some cases, frank disorientation or stupor. The pathogenesis of these nervous system manifestations is unknown.
- **Carcinogenesis.** As many as one-third of patients who have advanced hereditary hemochromatosis with hepatic cirrhosis eventually develop carcinoma of the liver (either hepatocellular carcinoma or cholangiocarcinoma). The frequent association of primary hepatic carcinoma with cirrhosis in patients with hemochromatosis has raised the question of whether iron in high concentrations has a direct carcinogenic effect. Hepatocellular carcinoma is rare in the precirrhotic stage of hemochromatosis, which emphasizes the importance of early diagnosis and treatment.

Non-HFE Hemochromatosis
A proportion of patients with clinical features of hemochromatosis have a wild-type *HFE* genotype (wt/wt; see discussion of **frequency of *HFE* mutations in patients with hemochromatosis and in the general population** in the section entitled **Disease Frequency and Origin**). This presentation is referred to as *non-HFE*

hemochromatosis. In most such cases, the genetic defect cannot be identified; however, a few patients have specific genetic defects involving other loci.

1. **Juvenile hemochromatosis** is a rare form of inherited iron overload associated with an accelerated rate of iron accumulation. Affected persons become symptomatic in the third decade of life or earlier. Presentation is characterized by a particularly high prevalence of cardiac manifestations and by hypogonadotropic hypogonadism. Both boys and girls are affected equally. The gene has been mapped to chromosome 1q but has not yet been identified. The rapid course of the disease suggests that the gene likely has major importance in the regulation of iron absorption. Early diagnosis and prompt treatment (see section entitled **Therapy and Prognosis**) are essential and potentially life-saving.

2. **Hemochromatosis associated with mutations of transferrin receptor 2 (TFR2):** The recent identification of TFR2, a transferrin receptor (TFRC) homolog, was followed by the discovery of mutations of TFR2 in several patients with non-*HFE* hemochromatosis. The normal role of TFR2 in iron metabolism is unknown, although it may function similarly to TFRC in mediating endocytosis of ferric transferrin. The gene has been mapped to chromosome 7q.

Diagnosis
No single laboratory test alone is pathognomonic of hemochromatosis. The diagnosis depends on a combination of tests of body iron stores. In addition, other possible causes of iron overload must be excluded. Genotyping to detect mutations associated with iron overload is also useful (see discussion of **genotyping for detection of *HFE* mutations**). The major tests and procedures used in the diagnostic evaluation of patients suspect of having hemochromatosis are summarized in Table 3.

Table 3. Screening for hemochromatosis and evaluation of iron overload

Test or procedure	Characteristic findings in hemochromatosis
Noninvasive screening tests[a]	
Transferrin saturation-calculated from serum iron (SI) and total iron binding capacity (TIBC)	Transferrin saturation >45%[b]
Serum ferritin (SF)	Generally >300 µg/dL (men) or 200 µg/dL (women); values from 1,000–5,000 µg/dL are typical (*Note:* SF may be in normal range in younger patients who have not yet accumulated a large amount of excess iron.)
Direct evaluation of tissue iron stores by liver biopsy[c]	Increased hepatocellular iron in a periportal distribution; usually 40% or more of hepatocytes involved in advanced cases. Quantitative measurement of tissue iron concentration is recommended (see text).

[a] For a discussion of the role of genetic testing, see **genotyping for detection of HFE mutations** in the section on **Diagnosis.**
[b] See discussion of **Interpretation** in the section on **Transferrin saturation**. Almost all (~98%) hemochromatosis patients have a transferrin saturation >45% on initial screening. Some experts recommend that, for confirmation, a slightly higher threshold (e.g., 50–55%) be used for the second determination (preferably with a fasting blood sample obtained in the morning).
[c] For a discussion of criteria for performing a liver biopsy, see section on **Liver biopsy for assessment of hepatic iron stores**. (The most definitive way to quantify total body iron stores is to remove all excess iron by serial phlebotomy therapy, as described in the discussion of **Quantitative phlebotomy** in the section on **Noninvasive approaches to evaluation of iron stores**.)

Screening tests include the following:

1. **Transferrin saturation.** Determination of transferrin saturation is the most sensitive single test for phenotypic detection of hereditary hemochromatosis. Transferrin saturation is calculated from the ratio of serum or plasma iron concentration to total iron-binding capacity (TIBC), as described later (see below). Often patients are identified by the incidental finding of high serum iron as part of automated serum chemistry panels, and many laboratories now routinely measure transferrin saturation in all samples.

The concentration of iron in the plasma is influenced by the state of body iron stores, recent dietary intake, and inflammatory disorders. Ideally, blood samples should be obtained in the fasting state to avoid any effect of recent dietary intake.

An alternative approach is to measure unbound iron binding capacity (UIBC), which can be determined by methods that are considerably less labor intensive than those required for TIBC. The methods for calculating transferrin saturation from both TIBC and UIBC are as follows:

Transferrin saturation is calculated by dividing serum iron (SI) by TIBC and multiplying by 100%. Thus,

$$\text{Transferrin saturation} = \text{SI/TIBC} \times 100\%$$

Typical units used in reporting results of SI and TIBC measurements are μg/dL or μmol/L. For example, assuming an atomic weight of 55.8 μg per μmol for iron (and rounding off to the nearest whole number), to calculate the transferrin saturation if SI = 201 μg/dL (36 μmol/L) and TIBC = 223 μg/dL (40 μmol/L), then

$$\text{Transferrin saturation} = \left(201\,\mu g/dL \div 223\,\mu g/dL\right) \times 100\% = 90\%$$

or

$$\text{Transferrin saturation} = \left(36\,\mu mol/L \div 40\,\mu mol/L\right) \times 100\% = 90\%$$

The upper limit of the reference range for transferrin saturation is about 50% in most laboratories. Thus, a saturation of 90% is clearly elevated and warrants further investigation. (The threshold value of transferrin saturation for identification of persons with possible iron overload is elaborated in the discussion of **interpretation** to follow).

Calculation of transferrin saturation using SI and UIBC is done by using the following formula:

$$\text{Transferrin saturation} = \text{SI} \div \left(\text{SI} + \text{UIBC}\right) \times 100\%$$

For example, if SI = 18 μmol/L and UIBC = 36 μmol/L, then

$$\text{Transferrin saturation} = 18\,\mu mol/L \div \left(18 + 36\right)\mu mol/L \times 100\% = 33\%$$

In this example, the transferrin saturation is normal.

Interpretation: Patients with hemochromatosis generally have transferrin saturations greater than 70% to 80%, and it is common to see values up to and even exceeding 100%. The average transferrin saturation among heterozygotes is slightly elevated compared with the average in the general population, but most have saturations within the normal range.

Some experts recommend using sex-specific thresholds for identification of possibly affected persons, such as 45% in women and 50% in men (or 50% and 55%, respectively). A value below the threshold level makes a diagnosis of hemochromatosis unlikely except in the presence of infection or other inflammatory disorder. Persons who have values above the threshold should have a second transferrin saturation measurement to confirm the initial elevated result.

Confirmation of an elevated transferrin saturation result: If the repeat test indicates a sustained elevation of transferrin saturation, the next step is to ascertain whether the patient has a history suggestive of other causes of iron overload or disorders known to give rise to an increased transferrin saturation (see section entitled **Other Iron-overload Disorders**). In the absence of any such condition, further investigation should be carried out to arrive at a diagnosis.

Effect of iron overload on TIBC: The TIBC usually is low when iron stores are significantly increased. This has the effect of magnifying the increase in transferrin saturation in iron overloaded hemochromatosis patients with increased SI. After excess body iron stores have been removed by phlebotomy (see section entitled **Therapy and Prognosis**), the serum iron and TIBC both return to normal.

2. **Serum ferritin:** If the patient has a sustained elevation of transferrin saturation, SF should be measured to assess iron stores. Unlike tissue ferritin, plasma ferritin contains little iron, and yet the plasma (or serum) ferritin concentration is proportional to total body iron stores (see Chapter 2, page 17) and serves as an index of *increased* iron stores in patients with iron-overload disorders, including hereditary hemochromatosis (Table 3). It is important to note that SF may be elevated in patients who have coexisting inflammatory conditions or liver disease, even when total body iron is normal. Therefore, it is advisable to determine the C-reactive protein level and evaluate liver function if the patient's SF is increased.

3. **Genotyping for detection of *HFE* mutations:** The identification of the gene for hemochromatosis has made it possible to test for *HFE* mutations in patients being screened for the disease. The advantages of *HFE* testing include early identification of individuals potentially at risk and possible avoidance of additional, more invasive, testing (i.e., liver biopsy; see subsequent section on **liver biopsy**).

Disadvantages include the facts that in the United States, 10% to 15% of patients with hemochromatosis have none of the common *HFE* mutations associated with iron overload, and yet they have clinical features indistinguishable from those who do have such mutations. Moreover, persons who are homozygous for the C282Y mutation may or may not have clinical expression of the disease. Thus, absence of the C282Y mutation does not rule out hemochromatosis, but homozygosity for C282Y does not necessarily mean that the patient is at risk for clinically relevant iron overload.

The place of genotyping in diagnosis and the optimal criteria for performing genetic testing have not been established. Ethical, legal, and social issues must be addressed; however, the potential diagnostic and prognostic benefits of genotyping outweigh such concerns, and the procedure is already commonly used by physicians involved in the care of patients with iron overload. Therefore, it is important to be able to interpret the results of *HFE* testing and to understand how to use such information in management.

Liver biopsy for assessment of hepatic iron stores: In the past, a liver biopsy generally was considered necessary to confirm the diagnosis of hemochromatosis. With the availability of *HFE* testing, a biopsy is no longer required in all cases. For C282Y homozygotes, the major indication for performing a liver biopsy is to detect the presence of fibrosis or cirrhosis, signs associated with a high risk for the eventual development of hepatocellular carcinoma. A biopsy is usually not necessary for homozygotes whose serum ferritin is below 1,000 µg per liter and who have no hepatomegaly or elevation of serum transaminases.

For patients who are not homozygous for C282Y despite strong evidence for iron overload, a liver biopsy is indicated for *diagnostic* purposes. The biopsy is informative concerning both the amount of storage iron and its distribution among different cell types within the liver. Such information about cellular iron distribution is particularly helpful in distinguishing different kinds of iron overload states. Increased hemosiderin deposits can be detected readily in hematoxylin and eosin (H & E) stains in patients with iron overload, but a specific stain for iron, such as Perl's Prussian blue, should be used to assess more accurately the degree of iron loading.

Hemosiderin deposits are identified by an intense blue staining, and this property aids in semiquantitative grading of hepatic iron stores (see the discussion on **estimation of iron stores by histologic grading**) that follows. A connective tissue stain also should be done to detect early fibrosis that may not be detectable by H & E stain.

Histologic assessment of hepatic iron stores:

- **Distribution of iron in the liver.** In hereditary hemochromatosis, iron is concentrated mainly in hepatocytes in a periportal distribution. In secondary iron overload (e.g., resulting from long-term transfusion therapy), the characteristic pattern is one of iron accumulation in a predominantly reticuloendothelial distribution involving Kupffer cells and sinusoidal lining cells. Patients with heavy iron deposits may have significant amounts of iron in parenchymal cells as well. Thus, in advanced stages, the pattern may be indistinguishable histologically from that seen in advanced hereditary hemochromatosis.

- **Estimation of iron stores by histologic grading.** Stainable iron should be graded on a semiquantitative scale according to the extent of hepatic parenchymal involvement (Table 4). Grades 0 to 1 are found in normal persons. Grade 2 can be seen in some homozygotes, particularly younger patients. Persons with grade 3 or 4 stainable iron must be considered to have hereditary hemochromatosis unless some other reason for iron overload is found.
- **Stainable iron index.** The hepatic iron level is age dependent in both normal subjects and in patients with hemochromatosis. To determine the stainable iron index, the stainable iron grade is divided by the patient's age in years. An index higher than 0.15 is considered to be consistent with hereditary hemochromatosis.

Quantitative determination of hepatic iron concentration. The hepatic iron concentration can be measured quantitatively after acid digestion followed by spectroscopic analysis. Normal persons have hepatic iron concentrations less than about 25 to 40 μmol of iron per gram of dry weight.

1. **Hepatic iron concentration in hemochromatosis.** Hepatic iron levels up to 900 μmol per gram and more have been reported. A liver iron concentration greater than 180 μmol per gram indicates iron overload consistent with hereditary hemochromatosis unless some other known reason for excess iron accumulation is evident. Younger, asymptomatic homozygotes may have concentrations below this level, however, and occasional heterozygotes may have concentrations as high as 200 μmol per gram.
2. **Hepatic iron index (HII).** Similar to the semiquantitative system for grading the amount of iron visualized by the Prussian blue reaction, the HII is calculated from the quantitative hepatic iron level by dividing the iron concentration in μmol per gram of dry weight by the age of the patient in years. An HII greater than 1.9 is consistent with the homozygous state and distinguishes homozygotes from either heterozygotes or patients with secondary iron overload.

Biopsy of other tissues: Although iron overload in hereditary hemochromatosis involves many other organs in addition to the liver, biopsy of other tissues is unnecessary. Little is gained from examination of the bone marrow because there is no significant increase in marrow iron stores in this disorder.

Table 4. Grading system for hepatic parenchymal stainable iron

Grade	Microscopic appearance[a]
0	No blue granules at high (400–450×) magnification
1	Blue granules in <5% of hepatocytes (or diffuse faint blue staining at high magnification)
2	Blue granules in 5% to 10% of hepatocytes in a periportal distribution
3	Abundant blue granules in up to 40% of hepatocytes (periportal with central sparing)
4	Abundant blue granules in >40% of hepatocytes, with relatively decreased load centrilobularly

[a] *Note:* The gross appearance of the iron-stained slide is purple to deep blue in grades 3 and 4, a phenomenon that can alert the examiner to the presence of iron overload; however, the actual grade assigned is based solely on the microscopic appearance.
Adapted from Witte DL, et al. *Practice parameters for hereditary hemochromatosis.* Northfield: College of American Pathologists, 1993.

Noninvasive approaches to evaluation of iron stores:

1. **Noninvasive estimation of hepatic iron concentration.** Approaches to non-invasive quantitation of hepatic iron stores currently under investigation include the following:

- **Magnetic susceptometry.** The paramagnetic property of nonheme iron, including tissue storage iron (ferritin and hemosiderin) has been exploited to measure hepatic iron concentration by magnetic susceptometry. Studies of patients having varying levels of storage iron have shown an excellent correlation between hepatic iron concentration measured by magnetic susceptibility and the chemically determined iron concentration in liver biopsy material. Unfortunately, such instruments are not widely available.

- **Computed tomography (CT).** Detection of increased hepatic iron stores with CT is possible by virtue of the relatively high electron density of iron compared with other body constituents. This technique is relatively insensitive and of value primarily only in patients with marked iron overload. Dual-energy CT (more sensitive) scanning is a better predictor of mild iron overload, but further development of this technique has been limited by the increasing availability of magnetic resonance imaging (MRI) which appears more promising.

- **MRI** is more sensitive than CT, although the threshold of iron detection is approximately twice the upper limit of normal. Widespread application of this method currently is limited by lack of standardization in reproducing results among different facilities.

2. **Quantitative phlebotomy:** The amount of iron removed with each phlebotomy can be estimated from the hematocrit and the volume of blood removed. A quick method for performing this calculation is based on the fact that 1 mL of packed red blood cells contains about 1 mg of iron. Serial phlebotomy to iron depletion is both therapeutic (see **Therapy and Prognosis**) and diagnostic.

Total body iron stores in hemochromatosis: Iron stores in patients with hereditary hemochromatosis typically amount to 10 to 12 g or more. The iron burden may be as high as 40 to 50 g in advanced cases. Removal of more than 4 g is considered consistent with the diagnosis of hemochromatosis, although it must be remembered that affected individuals identified at an early age may not have accumulated this much at the time of diagnosis (see **Therapy and Prognosis** on page 134).

Family studies: When a diagnosis of hereditary hemochromatosis has been established, the patient's family members should be screened to identify other affected persons. Siblings of the proband are at greatest risk because the disease is transmitted in an autosomal recessive manner. Children of affected persons also should be screened because the probability of homozygote–heterozygote matings is relatively high (see section entitled **Disease frequency and origin**).

1. **Initial screening tests for family members:** Siblings and children should be screened in the same way as other persons who are being evaluated for possible iron overload (see earlier discussion of **screening tests**). Those who show evidence of increased iron stores (increased transferrin saturation, increased SF) should be examined further. *HFE* genotyping is a valuable aid to diagnosis and should be done if the proband has *HFE* mutations (e.g., C282Y/C282Y). Relatives who are heterozygous (C282Y/wt) are not at risk for iron overload except in special circumstances (see section on **Interactions between the hemochromatosis gene and other disorders**). In families without *HFE* mutations, screening depends on the evaluation of iron status as in the past, before identification of the *HFE* gene.

2. **Management of relatives with equivocal initial screening results:** In relatives with marginal iron test results (e.g., increased transferrin saturation but normal SF), a repeat evaluation should be conducted in 3 to 5 years. Progressive iron overload evidenced by a continuous rise in SF indicates the need for treatment.

Population screening: It is now recommended that iron status be evaluated in patients having any of the manifestations of hemochromatosis, including liver disease, unexplained cardiac failure or arrhythmias, arthritis, type II diabetes, or gonadal dysfunction (e.g., impotence, amenorrhea). The feasibility of general population screening for hemochromatosis has yet to be determined, however, and the optimal approach to detection (i.e., testing for iron status vs. genetic testing or a combination of the two) is still under investigation.

Other Iron-overload Disorders

In hereditary hemochromatosis of Europeans, there is a primary defect of the regulation of iron absorption at the intestinal level. Some other forms of iron overload are associated with exposure to an exogenous source of excess iron or with disorders of iron metabolism that promote increased iron absorption as a secondary phenomenon. In addtion, recent evidence suggests that other iron-loading genes distinct from the gene for hereditary hemochromatosis may be present in some populations.

African Iron Overload

African iron overload is associated with consumption of a traditional beer brewed by natives of southern Africa using iron or steel containers. Iron overload in this setting has been attributed to the very high iron concentration in the beverage and the fact that most of the iron is in a readily absorbed state as divalent iron. Recent studies suggest that African iron overload may not be attributable entirely to dietary factors, however, but instead may represent an interaction between increased dietary iron availability and an iron-loading gene.

1. **Genetic studies:** The tendency to develop iron overload among drinkers of the traditional beer often runs in families, a manner consistent with an autosomal recessive inheritance pattern, suggesting the existence of an iron-loading gene in this population.

2. **Tissue iron distribution:** The distribution of iron among various organs in the body in African iron overload differs from that of hereditary hemochromatosis and is characterized by markedly increased iron deposition not only in the liver but also in the bone marrow and spleen. In hereditary hemochromatosis, iron in the bone marrow usually is not increased, and levels in the spleen are much lower than in the liver.

3. **Cellular iron distribution:** Iron is deposited both in the RES (including Kupffer cells in the liver and macrophages in the spleen and bone marrow) and in parenchymal cells (hepatocytes) in the liver.

4. **Clinical course:** Progressive iron accumulation eventually leads to a more marked degree of iron deposition in hepatocytes, approaching the amount seen in reticuloendothelial cells, with resultant liver damage and cirrhosis. Iron deposition in the pancreas and heart is less conspicuous than in hereditary hemochromatosis, however, and cirrhosis is the principal cause of morbidity and mortality in the African disease.

Autosomal Dominant Iron Overload

Observations suggest the existence of a distinct iron-loading gene in Melanesians, although the prevalence and precise etiology of the disorder have yet to be determined. The disease is not HLA-linked, although the pattern of iron deposition in affected persons is similar to that seen in hereditary hemochromatosis.

Medicinal Iron Overload

Iron overload caused by ingestion of medicinal iron compounds over a long period has been documented in a number of case reports. Persons who have taken medicinal iron for up to 10 years or more may develop severe hemosiderosis characterized by prominent reticuloendothelial iron deposition. In some cases, the extent of iron overload has resembled hemochromatosis; however, this form of iron overload appears to be relatively rare.

Transfusional Iron Overload

Transfusion of red blood cells in patients with bone marrow failure or chronic hemolytic conditions can lead to iron overload because, as the transfused red cells age and are removed from the circulation, iron accumulates in the RES. With continued iron accretion, parenchymal iron deposition develops as well, leading eventually to a condition resembling advanced hemochromatosis.

1. **Increased ineffective erythropoiesis:** In disorders associated with markedly increased *ineffective* erythropoiesis, the rate of erythropoiesis is so rapid that the demand may exceed the rate at which iron can be recycled via the RES, with the result that absorption of iron from the diet is accelerated. This increased iron absorption can add further to the iron burden in patients receiving frequent transfusions of RBCs.

- **The thalassemia syndromes.** Iron stores progressively accumulate as a result of the need for frequent transfusions and eventually reach toxic levels. Cardiac failure attributable to iron toxicity is the major cause of death for patients with thalassemia major treated in this way (see Chapter 6). Conspicuous iron deposits are also found in the pancreas and other endocrine glands, as well as in the spleen, liver, and bone marrow.
- Iron deposits can be detected in liver *parenchymal* cells in the earliest stages of iron accumulation and may be the result of increased iron absorption associated with the markedly increased ineffective erythropoiesis that characterizes this condition. Even patients with thalassemia intermedia who have not had transfusion often develop iron overload as a result of increased iron absorption alone.
- **Iron overload associated with sideroblastic anemia.** This group of disorders is characterized by the presence of ringed sideroblasts in the bone marrow and increased stainable iron in bone marrow macrophages. Iron overload in these conditions is a consequence, at least to some degree, of increased iron absorption, which in turn is probably attributable to markedly increased ineffective erythropoiesis. In addition, most patients require blood transfusions to maintain adequate hemoglobin levels, which also contribute to the development of iron overload.

2. **Other disorders often complicated by transfusional iron overload:**

- **Iron overload associated with hemoglobinopathies.** Patients with sickle cell anemia and related hemoglobinopathies characterized by sickling may develop iron overload as a result of repeated blood transfusions. Patients who have received in excess of 100 U of packed red blood cells are likely to have clinically relevant iron overload and may require iron-removal therapy as described in the section entitled **Therapy and Prognosis.**
- **Bone marrow failure.** Patients with aplastic anemia, pure red cell aplasia, or other bone marrow failure conditions may develop severe iron overload as a result of the frequent, long-term red blood cell transfusion support. As the number of units of red blood cells transfused approaches 100, reticuloendothelial iron stores begin to become saturated. Complications such as hepatic failure, diabetes, and cardiomyopathy may supervene and iron removal therapy should be considered for these patients before iron overload progresses to an abnormal advanced state.

Hereditary Atransferrinemia
This rare condition, thought to be transmitted in an autosomal recessive fashion, is characterized by a complete absence of plasma transferrin, hypochromic anemia, and severe iron overload involving the heart, pancreas, liver, and other organs. The bone marrow is devoid of iron.

Neonatal Iron Overload
A rare form of parenchymal iron overload affects some newborns who also suffer from severe, fatal liver disease. The condition tends to be familial, which suggests a possible genetic component. Unlike hereditary hemochromatosis, however, there is no linkage to the HLA locus.

Hereditary Hyperferritinemia Cataract Syndrome
This condition is the result of a mutation in the ferritin light-chain gene that causes an increased serum ferritin concentration despite the presence of normal body iron stores. The disorder is associated with premature cataract formation.

Therapy and Prognosis
The treatment for hereditary hemochromatosis consists of the removal of excess iron by serial phlebotomy. The loss of blood stimulates erythropoiesis, thereby promoting mobilization of iron from tissue stores. For patients with iron overload secondary to

Table 5. Iron removal therapy

Condition	Approach to therapy
Hereditary hemochromatosis	Removal of approximately 500 mL of blood by phlebotomy 1 to 2 times a week.[a] After iron stores have been depleted, maintenance phlebotomy (at less frequent intervals) must be continued for life.
Iron-loading anemias (e.g., thalassemia major, congenital sideroblastic anemia)	Continuous deferoxamine (DFO) infusion of 50 mg/kg/day, administered subcutaneously by portable pump over a 10- to 14-h period.[b]

[a] Before each phlebotomy, the hemoglobin (Hb) concentration or hematocrit (Hct) should be measured. Phlebotomy usually can be performed safely as long as the Hb concentration is ≥ 11 g/dL (Hct $\geq 33\%$), although generally, patients can maintain higher levels; see text.
[b] Ascorbic acid, 100 mg/day orally, may be given to increase the rate of iron metabolism after DFO therapy has been initiated.

blood transfusion therapy for anemia, however, this approach is not feasible. In such disorders, chelation therapy is necessary to promote iron excretion. The approaches to the treatment of iron removal are listed in Table 5.

Suggested Method for Phlebotomy to Iron Depletion
Although there is no universally agreed-on regimen for serial phlebotomy, the following approach is effective and is generally well tolerated.

Heavily iron-loaded patients with estimated iron stores of 10 g (SF approximately 800–1,000 µg/L) or more should be treated by phlebotomy of 450 to 500 mL at least once or twice a week until iron stores are depleted. For patients with lesser degrees of iron overload, phlebotomy needs to be performed no more than weekly. The hematocrit or hemoglobin concentration should be measured before each phlebotomy and generally should be above 40% (13 g hemoglobin/dL), as it is not necessary to render patients anemic during therapy. If the hematocrit is below this level, phlebotomy generally should be postponed unless the patient's usual baseline is lower to begin with (Table 5).

1. **Monitoring the course of phlebotomy therapy:** Serum ferritin decreases progressively during phlebotomy therapy but need not be monitored frequently. It is sufficient to monitor the hematocrit or hemoglobin concentration until the patient becomes anemic, although most physicians also measure SF periodically (e.g., once a month) during treatment. In most patients, depletion of iron stores is indicated by the observation that the hematocrit or hemoglobin remains below the usual level the patient has maintained during therapy, with failure to return to this baseline within 1 to 2 weeks. Iron depletion then can be verified by measuring SF, which should be in the iron-deficiency range (<20 µg/L). Patients with advanced disease may require removal of as many as 100 U (20–25 g of iron) or more over a period of up to 1 to 2 years. Most patients have lesser iron burdens (10–20 g), and the number of phlebotomies required is correspondingly fewer.

2. **Maintenance therapy:** Periodic phlebotomy must be continued for life; in most patients, a state of iron depletion can be maintained by phlebotomy three to five times per year. Measurement of SF periodically is helpful until a satisfactory phlebotomy schedule has been established, after which SF should be measured annually.

3. **Outcome of phlebotomy therapy and prognosis:** The response to phlebotomy therapy depends on the stage of the disease at the time treatment is initiated. Improvements in cardiac function are common, and reversal of fibrosis or partial reversal of hepatic cirrhosis have been reported. Progression of such disease manifestations may be prevented, and survival is prolonged. Removal of excess iron before development of organ damage competely prevents disease manifestations. Patients diagnosed and treated at this early stage have a normal life expectancy.

Chelation Therapy
Iron-removal therapy for patients suffering from transfusion-dependent conditions such as thalassemia major requires administration of the iron chelator deferoxamine (DFO) by continuous infusion, either intravenously or subcutaneously. The subcutaneous route is a more convenient approach and current standard of care.

The drug is infused using a portable ambulatory pump that is worn for 10 to 14 hours per day, 5 days a week (Table 5). Excess iron is mobilized from storage sites, presumably by chelation of iron in low-molecular-weight intracellular iron pools. This iron is excreted in the urine and via the biliary system through the gut.

The efficacy of chelation with DFO: DFO infusion therapy may prevent or retard the progression of cardiac damage in patients with thalassemia and can reduce hepatic iron levels. The therapy is cumbersome, expensive, and compliance often is not optimal. High doses of DFO can cause visual and auditory sensorineural toxicity.

Role of Ascorbic Acid (Vitamin C)
Concomitant administration of ascorbic acid enhances DFO-induced iron excretion and appears to act by expanding the body's chelatable iron pool; however, ascorbate in this setting may promote iron-induced lipid peroxidation, and in early studies the use of high doses was associated with increased cardiac dysfunction. More recently, however, it has been shown that lower, less toxic doses also are effective for augmenting iron excretion and can be administered safely once DFO therapy has been initiated (Table 5).

Splenectomy
The transfusion requirement in patients with thalassemia can be decreased by removing the spleen. The main factors responsible for anemia in thalassemic patients are increased ineffective erythropoiesis, which is discussed earlier (see section entitled **Transfusional Iron Overload**), and decreased red cell survival resulting from accelerated splenic destruction. Thus, by decreasing the rate of peripheral red cell destruction and thereby diminishing transfusion requirements, the rate of iron accumulation is decreased.

Suggested Readings

Barton JC, Edwards CQ, eds. *Hemochromatosis genetics, pathophysiology, diagnosis and treatment.* Cambridge: Cambridge University Press, 2000.

Brandhagen DJ, Fairbanks VF, Batts KP, et al. Update on hereditary hemochromatosis and the HFE gene. *Mayo Clin Proc* 1999;74:917–921.

Brittenham GM, Weiss G, Brissot P, et al. Clinical consequences of new insights in the pathophysiology of disorders of iron and heme metabolism. In: Hematology 2000. Washington, DC: American Society of Hematology, 2000:39–50 (available online, under "Educational Materials" at the American Society of Hematology website, www.hematology.org).

Britton RS, Tavill AS, Bacon BR. Mechanisms of iron toxicity. In: Brock JH, et al., eds. *Iron metabolism in health and disease.* Philadelphia: WB Saunders, 1994:311–351.

Brock JH. Iron in infection, immunity, inflammation and neoplasia. In: Brock JH, et al., eds. *Iron metabolism in health and disease.* Philadelphia: WB Saunders, 1994:353–389.

Burke W, Thomson E, Khoury MJ, et al. Hereditary hemochromatosis: gene discovery and its implications for population-based screening. *JAMA* 1998;280:172–178.

Cogswell ME, McDonnell SM, Khoury MJ, et al. Iron overload, public health, and genetics: evaluating the evidence for hemochromatosis screening. *Ann Intern Med* 1998;129:971–999.

Deugnier YM, Turlin B, Powell LW, et al. Differentiation between heterozygotes and homozygotes in genetic hemochromatosis by means of a histological hepatic iron index: a study of 192 cases. *Hepatology* 1993;17:30–34.

Edwards CQ, Griffen LM, Goldgar DE, et al. Prevalence of hemochromatosis among 11,065 presumably healthy blood donors. *N Engl J Med* 1988;318:1355–1362.

Felitti VJ, Beutler E. New developments in hereditary hemochromatosis. *Am J Med Sci* 1999;318:257–268.

Gordeuk VR, McLaren GD, Samowitz W. Etiologies, consequences and treatment of iron overload. *Crit Rev Clin Lab Sci* 1994;31:89–133.

Halliday JW, Ramm GA, Powell LW. Cellular iron processing and storage: the role of ferritin. In: Brock JH, Halliday JW, Pippard MH, et al., eds. *Iron metabolism in health and disease*. Philadelphia: WB Saunders, 1994:97–1212.

Hershko C. Iron chelators. In: Brock JH, Halliday JW, Pippard MH, et al., eds. *Iron metabolism in health and disease*. Philadelphia: WB Saunders, 1994:391–426.

Leggett BA, Halliday JW, Brown NN, et al. Prevalence of haemochromatosis amongst asymptomatic Australians. *Br J Haematol* 1990;74:525–530.

Lufkin EG, Baldus WP, Bergstralh EJ, et al. Influence of phlebotomy treatment on abnormal hypothalamic-pituitary function in genetic hemochromatosis. *Mayo Clin Proc* 1987;62:473–479.

Marciani MG, Cianciulli P, Stefani N, et al. Toxic effects of high-dose deferoxamine treatment in patients with iron overload: an electrophysiological study of cerebral and visual function. *Haematologica* 1991;76:131–134.

McDonnell SM, Witte DL, Cogswell ME, et al. Strategies to increase detection of hemochromatosis. *Ann Intern Med* 1998;129:987–992.

McDonnell SM, Phatak PD, Felitti V, et al. Screening for hemochromatosis in primary care settings. *Ann Intern Med* 1998;129:962–970.

McLaren CE, McLachlan GJ, Halliday JW, et al. Distribution of transferrin saturation in an Australian population: relevance to the early diagnosis of hemochromatosis. *Gastroenterology* 1998;114:543–549.

Phatak PD, Guzman G, Woll JE, et al. Cost-effectiveness of screening for hereditary hemochromatosis. *Arch Intern Med* 1994;154:769–776.

Pippard MJ. Secondary iron overload. In Brock JH, Halliday JW, Pippard MH, et al., eds. *Iron metabolism in health and disease*. Philadelphia: WB Saunders, 1994:271–309.

Press RD. Hereditary hemochromatosis: impact of molecular and iron-based testing on the diagnosis, treatment, and prevention of a common, chronic disease. *Arch Pathol Lab Med* 1999;123:1053–1059.

Wetterhall SF, Cogswell ME, Kowdley KV. Public health surveillance for hereditary hemochromatosis. *Ann Intern Med* 1998;129:980–986.

Witte DL, Crosby WH, Edwards CQ, et al. Practice guideline development task force of the College of American Pathologists: hereditary hemochromatosis. *Clin Chim Acta* 1996;245:139–200.

Worwood M. Laboratory determination of iron status. In: Brock JH, Halliday JW, Pippard MH, et al., eds. *Iron metabolism in health and disease*. Philadelphia: WB Saunders, 1994:449–476.

Zanella A., Berzuini A, Colombo MB, et al. Iron status in red cell pyruvate kinase deficiency: study of Italian cases. *Br J Haematol* 1993;83:485–490.

6. ABNORMALITIES OF HEMOGLOBIN

Sandra F. Schnall and Edward J. Benz, Jr.

Normal Hemoglobin Taxonomy
Hemoglobins
Hemoglobins are the oxygen-carrying elements in the body. They are heterogeneous proteins produced in developing erythroblasts. Each human hemoglobin (Hb) consists of a tetramer of 2α- and 2 "non"-α-globin chains bound to a single heme moiety. Heme contains one ferrous iron (Fe^{2+}) atom carried in a porphyrin ring.

Hemoglobins in Adult (Postneonatal) Red Blood Cells
1. The major adult hemoglobin is Hb A ($\alpha_2\beta_2$), constituting 96% to 98% of total hemoglobin content.
2. A minor hemoglobin Hb A_2 ($\alpha_2\delta_2$), constituting 1.5% to 3.0%.
3. Fetal hemoglobin, Hb F ($\alpha_2\gamma_2$) accounts for only 0.5% to 1.0% of hemoglobin in the adult.

Fetal Hemoglobin
The **major hemoglobin** produced *in utero,* Hb F, constitutes about 90% to 95% of total hemoglobin 8 to 35 weeks' gestation. Hb A then becomes the predominate hemoglobin due to the fetal to adult hemoglobin switch.

Embryonic Hemoglobins
1. Red cell production begins in the yolk sac of 19-day embryos.
2. By 6 weeks' gestation, the main site is the liver. Bone marrow production begins at 10 to 11 weeks' gestation.
3. The main embryonic globins are epsilon (ε, a non-α-chain) and zeta (α-like). These form the embryonic hemoglobins: Gower I ($\zeta_2\varepsilon_2$), Gower II ($\alpha_2\varepsilon_2$), and Portland ($\zeta_2\gamma_2$).
4. Embryonic hemoglobins are of no clinical importance after birth.

Normal Hemoglobin Genetics and Physiology
Alpha-like Globin Gene Cluster
Alpha gene loci are duplicated on chromosome 16, so diploid cells have four gene copies. Intergenic DNA and DNA sequences far upstream appear to be responsible for regulation (Fig. 1).

Non-α-like Globin Gene Cluster

1. Genes are clustered in a 60,000 base pair region on chromosome 11 in the following order: ε, $^G\gamma$, $^A\gamma$, δ, β; the order is the same as the order of developmental expression.
2. The genes are duplicated. $^A\gamma$ and $^G\gamma$ code for γ-globins, differing only at amino acid position 136 (alanine in $^A\gamma$glycerine in $^G\gamma$).
3. The β gene is present as a single copy. Patients thus inherit β-chain hemoglobinopathies in a simple mendelian fashion.
4. Positive and negative regulatory elements have been identified in the intergenic regions.

Regulation of Hemoglobin Synthesis
1. The synthesis of α- and non-α-globin chain production (i.e., equal amounts of each chain produced) is balanced in the normal human. The mechanism of regulation is unknown.
2. Hemoglobin tetramers are very soluble and can achieve their normal concentration in red blood cells (RBCs) without precipitating.

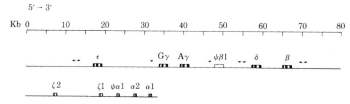

FIG. 1. The arrangements of the globin genes relative to one another on chromosomes 11 and 16. The upper bar shows the scale in kilobases (kb); 1 kb equals 1,000 base pairs. The genes are arranged in the direction of their transcription, that is, the direction in which they are copied into mRNA; the $5' \rightarrow 3'$ indicates the direction of transcription. The middle bar shows the rearrangements of the non-α-globin genes on chromosome 11, and the bottom bar, the α-like-globin genes on chromosome 16. The υα1 and υβ1 genes are pseudogenes, that is, remnants of genes that have been inactivated by mutations. The arrows scattered along the non-α-globin gene cluster indicate positions of much-repeated sequence elements and regions thought possibly to serve as enhancer elements that promote transcription. The dark portions of each gene indicate the portions that ultimately code for mRNA, whereas the lighter portions represent *introns,* which are portions of the gene transcribed into mRNA precursors but removed before the functional mRNA that codes for globin protein is transported to the cytoplasm for translation.

   3. Individual unpaired globin chains are highly insoluble. They precipitate, if allowed to accumulate, forming intracellular inclusion bodies leading to erythroblast death (ineffective erythropoiesis) and premature destruction of RBCs (hemolysis). α Chains are most insoluble; β chains are insoluble at high concentration.
   4. Posttranslation combination of globin chains with heme and with one another to form tetramers proceeds rapidly and spontaneously if globin chains are synthesized at normal rates and have normal structure.

Normal Hemoglobin Physiology
Hemoglobin is the major solute in RBCs. The properties of hemoglobin are adapted to the RBCs so that normal hemoglobin does not compromise size, shape, flexibility, or flow properties of the RBC. It is not surprising that mutations altering hemoglobin can have profound effects on RBC homeostasis. The critical elements of hemoglobin physiology from a clinical view are those altered by mutations causing disease:

   1. **Oxygen transport** (Fig. 2). Normal hemoglobins reversibly bind oxygen and release it so that adequate oxygen is delivered to the tissues at physiologically capillary-venous oxygen tension. The sigmoidal shape of the curve is critical to this function. Hemoglobin is also critical for pH and carbon dioxide regulation, but these aspects are not practically relevant to clinical features of hemoglobinopathies.
   2. **Solubility.** Precipitation of globin chains or hemoglobin tetramers causes ineffective erythropoiesis or hemolytic anemia by forming intracellular inclusion bodies (Heinz bodies), which disrupt cell metabolism.
   3. **Oxidation-reduction status.** The normal hemoglobin dissociation curve requires that the iron atoms be in the Fe^{2+} (ferrous or reduced) state. Methemoglobin is hemoglobin in which the iron is oxidized, or "ferric" (Fe^{3+}), it is brownish blue and binds oxygen too tightly to allow oxygen delivery to tissues at normal oxygen tensions.
   4. **Monomeric state.** Hemoglobin in RBCs is present at a very high concentration. Certain mutations, such as that causing sickle cell anemia, can cause hemoglobin to polymerize.

Hemoglobinopathies
Hemoglobinopathies are inherited disorders resulting from mutations in or near the globin genes that alter the structure (amino acid sequence) or the rate of synthesis of a particular globin chain. Hemoglobinopathies due to abnormal synthesis of globins are called

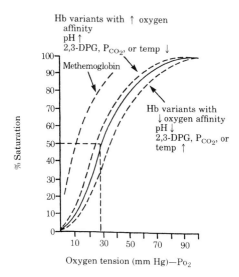

FIG. 2. Oxygen-binding properties of hemoglobin. The solid, sinusoidal, curved line indicates the normal oxygen-binding curve of hemoglobin. At increasing oxygen tensions, shown along the horizontal axis, hemoglobin binds progressively larger amounts of oxygen and thus becomes more fully saturated, as indicated by the saturation percentage value shown on the vertical axis. The curve is sigmoidal because the four subunits of hemoglobin operate in an autocatalytic, or cooperative, fashion, so that a small amount of oxygen binding begets more oxygen binding, thus increasing the affinity of hemoglobin for oxygen as the oxygen tension rises. The dashed rectangular lines that interact with the axes indicate the normal oxygen tension at which hemoglobin is 50% saturated with oxygen ($P_{50} = 28$ mm Hg). The dashed curved lines indicate the shifting of the position and shape of the oxygen-binding curve under various physiologic and pathologic conditions. Note the extraordinarily high oxygen affinity of methemoglobin. Hemoglobin Barts, seen in severe α-thalassemia *in utero,* has an oxygen affinity curve very similar to that of methemoglobin. Note that high levels of 2,3-diphospoglycerate (2,3-DPG), CO_2 or temperature reduce the affinity of hemoglobin for oxygen, as does acidemia. In contrast, alkalosis or reduced levels of 2,3-DPG, CO_2, or temperature increase the oxygen affinity curve.

thalassemias. Those due to abnormal globin structure are called *structural hemoglobinopathies.* The major clinically relevant hemoglobinopathies involve the α or β gene. Major dysfunctions of the ζ, ε, and γ chains are probably lethal in early gestation.

Major Mechanisms Producing Hemoglobinopathies

A change in the solubility or monomeric state of hemoglobin causes polymerization or precipitation of hemoglobin. For example, an amino acid substitution (β⁶ val glu)* results in sickle cell hemoglobin, which, in a deoxygenated state, polymerizes into fibrous polymers that alter the shape and stiffness of RBCs, producing the "sickle" cell and sickle cell anemia. Another substitution (β⁹⁸ val met) produces Hb Koln, a hemoglobin that is less soluble than normal. It precipitates in the circulating RBC, producing intraerythrocytic Heinz bodies that alter the RBC membrane and lead to phagocytosis of the RBC in the spleen (hemolytic anemia).

Alteration in oxygen affinity (Fig. 2) because of amino acid substitutions that alter the allosteric interaction of heme and globin chains necessary for normal oxygen affinity, are mutations that shift the oxygen dissociation curve. If the curve is shifted to the left (higher oxygen affinity) [e.g., Hb Zurich (β⁶³his arg)], tissue hypoxia results, and erythropoiesis is stimulated, producing erythrocytosis (polycythemia) (see Chapter 4). If the curve is shifted to the right (lower oxygen affinity) [e.g., Hb Kansas β^{102} asn thr)], the tissue requirement for oxygen can be satisfied at a lower hematocrit, producing a "pseudo" anemia. These low-affinity hemoglobins also can be desaturated at normal capillary oxygen, producing cyanosis.

   Methemoglobinemias are hemoglobins that contain their iron atoms in the Fe^{3+} (ferric) state. They can arise from mutations that impair the ability of the globin chain to maintain the iron atom in the reduced ferrous (Fe^{2+}) state [e.g., Hb MIwate [α^{87} his tyr)]. They also can arise from an inherited deficiency of enzyme called *methemoglobin reductase*. Acquired methemoglobin is the most common form. It arises from exposure to substances that oxidize the heme iron, notably nitrites and nitrates (Table 1). The color of methemoglobin causes the complexion of patients to resemble cyanosis, yet the arterial hemoglobin oxygen saturation percentage is usually normal, a key diagnostic indicator.

   An alteration in synthesis involves partial or complete deficiency in the synthesis of one of α- or β-globin chains; α-thalassemia results from deficient α-chain production; β-thalassemia results from reduced or absent β-chain production. These arise from mutations that impair production or translatability of globin messenger RNAs.

Structural Hemoglobinopathies
Sickle cell disorders are the most common hemoglobinopathies encountered in the United States (2).

Genetics and Pathophysiology
Sickle cell anemia results from a point mutation that changes the amino acid at position 6 on the β-globin chain from glutamic acid to valine. Hb S ($\alpha_2\beta_2{}^S$) behaves normally in the oxygenated state, but deoxy Hb S polymerizes. The homozygous state produces sickle cell amenia.

   Sickle trait (Hb AS) is the heterozygous state. Sickle cell trait occurs in 8% of African Americans in the United States. Its high frequency results from evolutionary selection. Hb S confers a protective advantage against falciparum malaria infection.

   Patients who inherit a β^S allele from one parent can inherit a different abnormal β allele [e.g., β-thalassemia or β^c (β^6 val leu)] from the other parent, producing a compound heterozygous state having unique features.

   The characteristic shapes of sickle cells arise from the deoxygenated Hb S polymers. These align in parallel, forming "tactoids" that distort the RBC into the classic sickle and oak leaf shapes. Sickle cells are also dehydrated, stiff, and viscous. They flow through capillaries poorly and have shortened life spans.

   Factors that promote increased sickling include low oxygen tension; low pH; increase in 2,3-diphosphoglycerate (2,3-DPG); reduction in RBC water content (i.e., increased serum osmolality); decreased nitrous oxide (NO); fever; and sluggish blood flow.

   Physiologic consequences are twofold:

1. Hemolysis of sickled cell due to membrane damage and fragility of deformed cell.
2. Hemolysis is usually brisk, but not life threatening.
3. Occlusion in microvascular circulation causing ischemia or infarction of tissues supplied by occluded vessels. This is the dominant cause of morbidity and mortality.

Table 1. Drugs that induce methemoglobinemia

Nitrites
Acetanilid
Phenacetin
Acetaminophen
Sulfonamides (see Table 2)
Nitroprusside
Local anesthetics (e.g., benzocaine, lidocaine)

Clinical Features

Vasoocclusive crisis, also called *painful* or *infarctive* crisis, is the most common form of morbidity; it results from periodic obstruction of small blood vessels by rigid, non-deformable sickled RBCs, leading to hypoxia and ultimately microinfarction (3). The chief clinical manifestation is pain, with or without fever, tachycardia, and leukocytosis. The most common precipitating factors include infection, fever, pregnancy, cold, dehydration, psychic stress, and surgery. The most common sites include bones, chest, abdomen, and spleen (see subsequent sections).

The **effects of sickling on the spleen** include the following:

1. Sequestration of sickled RBC occurs in all patients with Hb S; in early childhood, the spleen enlarges with entrapment of sickle cells. This can occur acutely in rare cases (splenic sequestration crisis) and can be a cause of death in infants less than 1 year of age.
2. In adults with Hb S, splenomegaly is rare because of repeated infarctions and fibrosis of the spleen leading to "autosplenectomy" and functional asplenia in early childhood.
3. Splenic function is usually lost at 1 to 2 years of age, before anatomic loss of the spleen is apparent. Patients are thus susceptible to infections and acute sepsis due to encapsulated organisms.

The **central nervous system** (CNS) and **retinal effects** (4) include the following:

1. Neurologic complications occur in up to 25% of patients with Hb S. Cerebrovascular accidents occur in up to 8% of patients with Hb S and 2% with Hb SC disease. Strokes are unusually common in children aged 5 to 12 years. Children at risk exhibit abnormal cerebral blood flow detectable by Doppler ultrasonography.
2. At least 65% of patients who suffer one stroke will suffer another. Those at more risk have more severe anemia, lower Hb F levels, higher white blood cell (WBC) counts, and higher homocysteine levels.
3. Proliferative retinopathy develops in an avascular site because of sickling in "watershed" areas, usually at the periphery of the retina; these vessels have an increased tendency to bleed after repeated occlusion and neovascularization, leading to retinal detachment and blindness.

Genitourinary effects (5) include the following:

1. *Priapism,* or painful engorgement of corpora cavernosa by sickle cells causing persistent erection of the penis, occurs in 7% to 40% of males with Hb S.
2. Proteinuria
3. Loss of ability to concentrate urine (hyposthenuria)
4. Painless hematuria, often spontaneous, especially in sickle cell trait
5. Distal renal tubular acidosis
6. Hypogonadism and underdeveloped genitalia (mechanism unclear)

Bone abnormalities include hand–foot syndrome (sickle dactylitis), a painful swelling of the hands and feet seen primarily in children. Aseptic necrosis of the femoral head occurs with infarction of the nutrient artery. Osteonecrosis also occurs in these patients.

Pulmonary effects (6,7) include acute chest syndrome (ACS) associated with fever, chest pain, pulmonary infiltrates, and rise in WBCs. It is a particularly severe complication, often requiring care in the intensive care unit; repeated ACS is associated with a worse prognosis. It is important to distinguish this event from infection. Reactive airway disease may be secondary to infection, bone infarction (ribs), or pulmonary embolus. Pulmonary hypertension is a late complication that can be fatal.

Leg and ankle ulcers are a common complication and may occur in up to 75% of patients, more commonly men. Stasis of blood flow plays a major role in their formation. Secondary infection contributes to their persistence. These ulcers also are seen in other chronic hemolytic states.

Hemolytic components include a shortened **RBC life span** in all varieties of sickle cell disorders (normal RBC, 120 days; Hb SS, 17 days; Hb SC, 28 days). There is, however, fluctuation in the amount of hemolysis seen in individual patients. Patients are rarely transfusion dependent, but they do exhibit other stigmata of hemolytic anemia (jaundice, hepatomegaly, increased cardiac output, bilirubin, gallstones, but no splenomegaly).

Aplastic crisis is an episode of acute and self-limited erythroid aplasia that lasts 5 to 10 days as a result of a common childhood pathogen, parvovirus B-19. Aplastic crisis occurs only once in most patients because immunity develops after the first infection. Thus, a true aplastic crisis is rare in adults. Because the RBC life span is so short in these patients, aplastic crisis can produce acute life-threatening anemia requiring immediate transfusion therapy. Key diagnostic findings in such patients are decreasing hematocrit and falling reticulocyte count. A rising reticulocyte count heralds recovery.

Hypoplastic "crisis" is not a true syndrome. Infection tends to suppress bone marrow activity in all individuals. Sickle cell patients with infection or inflammation who suffer some degree of bone marrow suppression experience an exaggerated transient decrease in hematocrit and reticulocyte count because of short RBC life span. The condition is rarely life threatening. Transfusions are indicated only on the basis of other symptoms.

Bilirubin stones, secondary to chronic hemolysis, may cause extrahepatic biliary obstruction and cholecystitis. Fifty percent of adult patients with Hb S have bilirubin gallstones. No completely reliable diagnostic criteria exist to distinguish among cholecystitis because of bilirubin gallstone, hepatic sickle cell crisis, or more rarely, early hepatitis. Indications for cholecystectomy remain a topic of extreme controversy.

Infections are among the most common causes of morbidity and mortality in this group. Sepsis, pneumonia, meningitis, and osteomyelitis are major sources of infection. It is best to regard patients with sickle cell syndromes as moderately immunocompromised and at great risk for infectious diseases.

Common bacterial organisms that cause infection in sickle cell patients include *Haemophilus influenzae, pneumococcus, Salmonella* (osteomyelitis), *Staphylococcus* (osteomyelitis), and *Mycoplasma pneumoniae.* Defenses against viruses and fungi are reasonably normal, but any infection can precipitate painful crisis.

Factors that contribute to the increased susceptibility to infections include functional asplenia, impaired antibody response, impaired complement activation, especially the alternate pathway, and abnormal chemotaxis and opsonization.

Patients with sickle cell syndromes are virtually the only group who get *Salmonella* osteomyelitis; however, *Salmonella* accounts for only a minority of the osteomyelitis seen in this group. *Staphylococcus* is the most common organism, as in the general population.

Diagnosis

In the homozygous state, diagnosis is usually apparent in a patient with repeated painful crises, infections, stigmata of hemolytic anemia, and abnormal red cell morphology characterized by the presence of sickle cells and oak leaf–shaped cells.

1. **Peripheral blood smear** is also notable for target cells (especially in Hb SC disease), Howell–Jolly bodies, nucleated RBC, RBC fragments, thrombocytosis, and frequent leukocytosis.

2. **Hemoglobin electrophoresis** is a routinely performed at alkaline pH; hemoglobin variants, including Hb S, can be detected by starch or agar gel electrophoresis.

3. **"Sickle prep"** test is performed by depriving RBCs of oxygen by using dithionite or metabisulfite compounds as reducing agents and placing a coverslip over a drop of blood on a glass slide. Cells sickle *in situ* and can be seen in the microscope as typical sickled cells. It is important to verify that a hemoglobin variant migrating in the position of Hb S by electrophoresis is really sickle hemoglobin by performing the sickle prep test. Some variants not associated with sickle cell anemia can comigrate with Hb S but are not associated with sickling of red cells.

4. Despite intensive efforts, there are no absolutely reliable tests to confirm or rule out the diagnosis of vasoocclusive crisis. Thus, this remains a diagnosis based largely on familiarity with the patient, clinical judgment, and intensive searches for other causes, such as infection.

Antenatal Diagnosis

The ability to detect sickle cell anemia in first- and second- trimester fetuses has been dramatically improved by the use of polymerase chain reaction (PCR) technology. DNA from amniotic fluid cells or chorionic villae allows a diagnosis to be made as early as 7 to 10 weeks' gestation. With PCR, a defined DNA sequence can be amplified *in vitro* many millions of times. This allows a rapid determination of normal and abnormal sequences at an earlier stage of pregnancy. Other methods include restriction analysis in allele specific hybridization and reverse dot blotting.

Treatment

Treatment of sickle cell syndromes is supportive, relying on hydration, oxygenation, and analgesia. Specific therapies to prevent sickling of red cells or to reduce the effects of sickled red cells on hemodynamics are being actively sought but, are not yet available for clinical use, except for the use of hydroxyurea.

When **vasoocclusive (infarctive) crises** occur, once a vessel is totally obstructed by sickle cells, infarction of downstream tissues is probably irreversible. Pain persists during healing, even after sickling has stopped. Fortunately, in most patients, these areas are small and scattered. Treatment is aimed toward relief of pain, prevention of further irreversible occlusions, and preservation of adjacent tissue:

1. **Adequate hydration,** including intravenous fluids at 100 to 200 mL per hour, especially if the patient is able to ingest several liters of oral fluids per day, is necessary. Daily fluid requirements must be individualized and adjusted for age and weight. Maintenance of a vigorous flow of urine should be a goal. Remember that sickle cell patients can neither concentrate nor dilute urine, so specific gravities do not provide a good guide of hydration status. Cardiovascular response to fluid must be monitored closely. Most young patients with sickle cell disease have reasonably vigorous cardiovascular systems, but overhydration must be avoided, especially in acute chest syndrome.

2. **Evaluate patient for infection.** Infections form the underlying basis of many crises; conversely, infections or inflammatory states such as arthritis must always be sought as the real cause of localized pain, fever, etc. Sickle cell crisis is a diagnosis of exclusion. Symptoms should be attributed solely to crisis only when the possibility of local or systemic infections has been thoroughly eliminated by the appropriate use of cultures and radiologic and scanning techniques. All infections should be treated vigorously in view of the immunocompromised status of sickle cell patients.

3. The efficacy of *oxygen therapy* remains poorly defined, but oxygen administration by nasal prongs is still used by many experts at a flow of 3 to 4 L per minute. A prior objection, namely that oxygen therapy suppresses erythropoiesis, is probably not germane in these patients. It is far more important to promote oxygenation at the pulmonary and arterial levels.

4. **Anticoagulation** does not play a role in most sickle cell crises.

5. **Analgesics (8,9).** Potent analgesia is frequently required to control the intense pain of sickle cell crisis. Analgesics should be prescribed on a regular basis during the early hours and days of the crisis, rather than as needed. Smaller doses at more frequent intervals are preferred to larger doses at long intervals. The latter provides intense swings between pain and the euphoric–analgesic effect of the drugs. Use of analgesics must be done judiciously because drug addiction is a significant problem among adult patients with sickle cell disease and histories of recurrent crises. Inadequate doses during peak periods of pain also can promote drug-seeking behavior, however. More recently, interest has been in using a "structured" analgesic regimen (i.e., a sustained-release morphine), such as that given to patients with malignancy, in patients with sickle cell pain. It is hoped that this will decrease admissions and length of hospital stays in these patients. Nonsteroidal, antiinflammatory agents (NSAIDs), surfactants that inhibit cell adherence, inhaled NO, and epidural anesthesia have been tried.

6. **Evaluate patient for other sources of pain.** This aspect of care is especially important in patients who repeatedly present with pain in the same tissue or area over a short period. For example, a repeatedly painful knee encountered over a period of a few

months may indicate the development of a sickle cell arthropathy rather than repeated crisis. It is important, again, to note that crisis is a diagnosis of exclusion.

7. **Exchange transfusion** is not recommended for typical crisis. Although it may offer an advantage over simple, chronic transfusions by decreasing the risk of alterations in viscosity and blood volume, the major role of exchange transfusion is in the management and prevention of life-threatening organ-related events, such as the acute chest syndrome, acute strokes, PaO_2 below 70 mm Hg, the need for blood volume (i.e., splenic sequestration), priapism, resistant leg ulcers, and retinal lesions.

Acute splenic sequestration requires exchange transfusion to maintain peripheral oxygen delivery. It may require splenectomy. It is usually seen in children 2 to 5 years of age. Most older patients have no anatomic or functional spleen.

CNS events are most effectively treated with exchange transfusion. Because of the high incidence of **recurrent** strokes, patients are placed on a chronic monthly exchange transfusion program to maintain a Hb S level of less than 30% to 40% for several years.

Retinal lesions are regarded as CNS lesions and treated with exchange transfusion. In addition, long-term management in conjunction with an ophthalmologist is required since these lesions do respond to laser photocoagulation or surgery.

Priapism is treated initially like sickle cell crisis; in addition, local therapy with ice packs is required to control pain and reduce further damage. Failure of the priapism to revolve in 24 hours may require exchange transfusions, using the criteria described in the description of CNS events in the section entitled **Structural Hemoglobinopathies.** Surgical intervention also be attempted, although this should be reserved for extreme cases because it can cause impotence. Recurrence may be decreased by administration of an α-adrenergic agent (oral or intravenous) (10).

Hematuria should be treated conservatively after investigation to rule out other causes. Coagulation-stimulating drugs, such as ε-aminocaproic acid, should be used with *extreme* caution due to the danger of stimulating massive thrombosis.

Pulmonary crises (11) require investigation to differentiate infection from infarction by using radiologic, microbiologic, and scanning technologies. Analgesics may be needed to prevent splinting and atelectasis. Empiric treatment for infections may be required while workup is in progress using antibiotics that cover the patient for common organisms, as described in **Structural Hemoglobinopathies.** It is extremely important to maintain proper pulmonary oxygenation because desaturation in the arterial circuit can be rapidly fatal as the result of massive total body sickling and bone marrow infarction with fat embolism. Intravenous hydration should not be excessive. Transfusion may be needed for worsening respiratory function and PaO_2 lower than 70 mg Hg.

Dactylitis and aseptic necrosis are treated like sickle cell crises once infection is ruled out. In extreme cases, exchange transfusion may be indicated.

Leg and ankle ulcers are best treated with conservative management, including rest, elevation of the limb, management of secondary infection, and zinc sulfate dressings or the equivalent. Exchange transfusion may be required in extreme cases (persistent ulcers). Hyperbaric oxygen, pentoxifylline, and erythropoietin are being evaluated.

Aplastic crisis is treated with red cell transfusions to maintain hematocrits in the range of 18% to 20%. These crises usually resolve in 7 to 10 days. There is no need to transfuse to a hematocrit higher than that present in the patient's chronic state.

Additional Measures and Prevention

1. **Folic acid** at a dose of 1 mg orally daily can be used as a supplement if nutrition is marginal.

2. **Vaccines** such as pneumovax and *Haemophilus influenzae* type B vaccines should be given to these functionally asplenic patients (12).

3. **Pregnancy.** In patients with sickle cell anemia, there is an increased rate of spontaneous abortion, intrauterine growth retardation (IUGR), stillbirth, toxemia/preeclampsia, and painful crisis in the mother. Patients with Hb SC disease or Hb S-β-thalassemia fare somewhat better during pregnancy. **Antenatal care** should

include folic acid and iron supplementation. The use of exchange transfusion is controversial. Exchange transfusion was once widely advocated, but no study has proved its usefulness. Results of the 1988 cooperative trial sponsored by the National Institutes of Health suggested that transfusion therapy is not routinely indicated except in high-risk situations (13). In terms of **contraception,** tubal ligation or use of mechanical barriers are probably safest; however, birth control pills can be used safely with low-dose estrogen agents (14).

Surgery and invasive diagnostic procedures: Before any invasive procedure (e.g., surgery, angiography), exchange transfusions to maintain Hb S at levels of 40% or less are advocated in many centers to prevent precipitation of an acute sickling event. In particular, contrast dyes tend to dehydrate RBCs and increase sickling. At the very least, great pains should be taken to make sure that sickle cell patients are fastidiously hydrated and oxygenated before and during use of any anesthesia or angiographic dyes.

Transfusion (15): Approximately 60% of patients with sickle cell disease have received blood products. Transfusions are used to prevent the effects of anemia, vasoocclusion, or both. Unfortunately, improvement in oxygen delivery may be counterbalanced by elevations in viscosity. An absolute indication for a blood transfusion is severe anemia associated with hypovolemia (e.g., splenic sequestration crisis, acute blood loss). Simple transfusion also should be considered in symptomatic anemias, severe aplastic crisis, and accelerated hemolysis. Chronic transfusions or exchange transfusions are used to suppress Hb S levels and maintain higher levels of Hgb A. A chronic transfusion program is absolutely indicated in patients who have had a cerebrovascular event. Other relative indications include severe debilitation, vasoocclusive symptoms, leg ulcers, and priapism (see preceding discussion).

Bone marrow transplantation (16): As yet, this is the only therapy that has been reported to "cure" sickle cell disease. Currently, the morbidity and mortality need to be further assessed before this can be considered to be a more standard approach, especially as patients live longer in the United States with conservative management.

Newer Therapeutic Modalities

1. **Antisickling agents:** Attempts have been made to treat sickle cell disease by modifying hemoglobin S, by modulating the response of red cells and red cell membrane to the sickling process, by elevating levels of fetal hemoglobin (Hb F), and by lowering the mean corpuscular hemoglobin concentration (MCHC) using techniques to swell red cells. None of these has achieved a clinical use.

2. **Induction of Hb F (17):** Hydroxyurea is a cell-cycle–specific agent that increases Hb F. Hydroxyurea is now regarded as a useful palliative agent. Sickle cell anemia is frequently milder in patients with high levels of Hb F. With the addition of hydroxyurea, Hb F levels may increase from 4% to 15%. This may decrease the frequency of pain, the severity of the anemia, and decrease the risk of acute chest syndrome. Short-term toxicity (cytopenias, mucositis) has been noted, but it is usually reversible. The concern for a leukemogenic effect is of special interest for children. Other ribonucleotide reductase inhibitors are in experimental trials. Hydroxyurea should be considered in patients with repeated severe crises (>3 per year) or ACS. It should be used in collaboration with a hematologist experienced with sickle cell anemia. The dose is usually titrated to maximize Hb F production while maintaining a polymorphonuclear (PMN) count above 2,000 to 2,500. Most patients experience a reduction in total white count, which can be beneficial.

3. **Butyrate compounds** appear to block the switch from fetal to adult hemoglobin. These compounds also may be able to increase the number of erythroblasts expressing γ-globin and possibly Hb F. The benefits are tempered by neurotoxicity, nausea, and vomiting. Regimens combining pulsed doses of butyrate and hydroxyurea have shown some promise.

4. **Vasoactive compounds** such as vasodilating agents have not proved effective. Nitrous oxide may increase O_2 affinity of sickle cells (18,19).

5. **Growth factors** such as erythropoietin have not been proven to have any major impact (20).

6. **Gene therapy** may provide promise in the future.

Other Sickle Cell Syndromes

Hemoglobin sickle cell disease: Hb C (β 6 glu lys) is found in 3% of African Americans. In Hb SC disease, patients have no normal β chains because they inherit a β S chain from one parent and the β C chain from the other.

Clinical features are similar to those in sickle cell anemia; however, these patients usually have higher hematocrits (less hemolysis), fewer painful crises and infections, and higher frequency of retinopathy and splenomegaly. Aseptic necrosis is no longer considered to be at higher frequency than in sickle cell anemia. The pathophysiology of the interaction between Hb S and C remains poorly understood. Hb C does tend to form crystals. The higher hematocrit increases blood viscosity and could promote sickling. Interestingly, Hb C homozygotes are clinically well.

Diagnosis is similar to that for Hb S. Hb C migrates in the position of Hb A_2 in routinely used gel electrophoretic systems, but clinical laboratories readily detect Hb SC disease by column and gel techniques.

A key diagnostic finding associated with Hb C is the presence of target cells on the peripheral smear with a normal mean corpuscular volume (MCV). Patients with Hb SC have many target cells as well as sickle forms.

Hemoglobin S-B thalassemia (S-thal disease) presents a very similar picture to sickle cell anemia. It results from inheritance of β^S allele from one parent and β-thalassemia from the other. Patients with β-globin thalassemia, who make no normal β0-globin, tend to be somewhat more severely affected (nearly identical to sickle cell anemia) than patients with Hb S-β+-thalassemia, who make 5% to 15% normal levels of β-globin. Hb S-thal patients may exhibit persistent splenomegaly, particularly Hb S-β+-thal. A key diagnostic feature is the presence of microcytosis or splenomegaly in patients with mild to moderately severe sickle cell syndrome, an elevated Hb A2, as well as microcytosis in one parent.

Hemoglobin SE, SD, S-α-thalassemia: Hb SD and Hb SE have generally clinically variable sickling because of coinheritance of Hb D or Hb E with Hb S, by analogy to Hb SC disease. α-Thalassemia is very common in African Americans (see the discussion of treatment in the section entitled **Methemoglobinemia**) and tends to reduce the severity of sickle cell anemia by reducing intracellular hemoglobin concentration. A key feature is microcytosis without elevated Hb A2. The effect on individual patients is unusually difficult to discern.

Unstable Hemoglobins (Hb Koln)

Unstable hemoglobins result from mutations that change the amino acid sequence of one of the globin chains in regions critical for solubility or binding of the heme moiety. More than a hundred mutations have been documented, most with mild instability.

Genetics and Pathophysiology

Inheritance is usually in an autosomal dominant fashion, although the rate of spontaneous mutations is high. Eighty percent affect the β chain. Fewer α-chain variants are detected because the genome contains four copies of the α gene. Inheritance of only one α allele for unstable hemoglobin may lead to a milder subclinical disorder, which is less readily detected. Abnormal hemoglobins tend to denature (precipitate) spontaneously in the RBC, forming aggregates called *Heinz bodies*.

Clinical Features (Highly Variable)

1. **Hemolytic anemia,** presenting often in childhood, associated with jaundice and splenomegaly. It is often episodic, precipitated by infection and oxidant drugs (Table 2).
2. Gallstones
3. Cyanosis, if mutation is also associated with methemoglobin, as a result of pleiotropic effect on solubility and heme–globin interaction

Diagnosis

Peripheral blood smear shows hypochromia, poikilocytosis, anisocytosis, and reticulocytosis. Usual stigmata of hemolytic anemia (i.e., lactic dehydrogenase, haptoglobin,

Table 2. Drugs that induce hemolysis in patients with unstable hemoglobins

Antimalarials	Sulfonamides	Others
Primaquine	Sulfacetamide	Acetanilid
Quinacrine	Sulfamethoxazole	Nalidixic acid
Pentaquine	Sulfanilamide	Nitrourantoin
Pamaquine	Sulfapyridine	Toluidine blue

indirect bilirubinemia, organomegaly). **Supravital stain** (1% methyl violet) demonstrates preexistent Heinz bodies but does not induce precipitation of unstable hemoglobins. Heinz bodies are often minimal or absent if the spleen is present. **Heat stability test** precipitates the unstable hemoglobin on exposure to 50°C in an appropriate buffer; it is detected as turbidity increases.

Hemoblobin electrophoresis is usually a poor "rule-out" test for unstable hemoglobins; the test is often normal due to an electrically neutral amino acid substitution, but it should be performed.

Treatment (Dependent on Severity)
1. **Folic acid,** 1 mg daily, administered orally.
2. **Oxidant drugs** (e.g., antimalarials) should be avoided (Table 2).
3. **Splenectomy** may be helpful in some patients to reduce symptoms.
4. **Transfusions** may be required, especially in infants, until splenectomy can be performed.

Hemoglobins with Altered Oxygen Affinity
Hemoglobins with altered oxygen affinity are due to amino acid substitutions that alter the α_2, β_2 interface with heme necessary for normal oxygen affinity. β-Chain variants are detected five times more often than are α-chain variants. There may also be mutations that alter 2,3-DPG binding.

High–Oxygen-Affinity Hemoglobins
These hemoglobins cause a left shift in the oxygen dissociation curve, resulting in less oxygen delivered to tissues at normal capillary PO_2 (Fig. 2).

1. Inheritance is autosomal dominant.
2. Patients are often asymptomatic.
3. Most have polycythemia with erythrocytosis.
4. Absence of splenomegaly is a key diagnostic finding (unless hemoglobin is also unstable, which is rare).
5. Diagnosis is made by the presence of *low* P_{50} and hemoglobin oxygen dissociation curve instead.
6. Treatment is rarely needed unless there is erythrocytosis (hematocrit >50–60) requiring phlebotomy.

Low-affinity Hemoglobins and Hb M
Low-affinity hemoglobins and Hb M have a shift to the right of the oxygen dissociation curve resulting in increased oxygen delivered, cyanosis, and pseudoanemia in some cases (Fig. 2).

1. Inheritance is autosomal dominant.
2. NADH diaphorase activity is normal (absent in methemoglobinemia).
3. Patients are often asymptomatic because tissue oxygen delivery is normal.
4. Some cases may be associated with a mild hemolytic anemia.
5. Diagnosis is made with an O_2 dissociation curve shifted to the right and a higher than normal P_{50}.
6. There is no effective therapy. Patients are not usually symptomatic.

Methemoglobinemia

Methemoglobinemia occurs when iron exits in the oxidized form (ferric) in greater than 1% of cells.

Genetics and Pathophysiology

Congenital types are inherited in autosomal dominant form (Hb M) because of an altered iron oxidation state resulting from mutation in globin chains. There is also an autosomal recessive form, quite rare, which is due to deficiency of methemoglobin reductase. Acquired methemoglobinemia states are most commonly encountered and are due to toxic exposures (Table 1). The **congenital disorder** occurs secondary to deficiency of NADH diaphorase, which is necessary for maintenance of hemoglobin in the ferrous state. **Acquired states** exist secondary to drugs or toxic substances that oxidize heme iron directly.

Clinical Features

Patients with congenital methemoglobinemia are cyanotic, which is primarily of cosmetic importance. It generally follows a benign course. In acquired states, cyanosis reflects acute alteration of tissue oxygen delivery. Methemoglobin has a very high affinity for oxygen and does not deliver oxygen well to tissues. Methemoglobin levels greater than 50% can be rapidly fatal. Patients present with hypoxia (i.e., cyanosis, headaches, dizziness, altered mental state) but *normal* arterial PO_2.

Laboratory Features

In the congenital disorder, the blood may appear chocolate brown. Laboratories can rapidly measure methemoglobin by optical absorption; a key finding is cyanosis with normal PO_2.

Treatment

For **congenital methemoglobinemia,** treatment is one of the following:

1. Ascorbic acid, 300 to 600 mg orally daily divided in three or four doses, or
2. Methylene blue, 60 mg orally three or four times daily, or
3. Riboflavin, 20 mg per day

Patients are usually not symptomatic.

For **toxic (acquired) methemoglobinemia,** promptly treat with methylene blue, 1 mg per kilogram of body weight, administered intravenously. Methylene blue must be used cautiously (only if methemoglobinemia is life threatening) in patients with G6PD deficiency in whom hemolysis can occur.

Thalassemia Syndromes

Definition (21,22)

The thalassemia syndromes are heterogeneous inherited disorders that arise from mutations in the globin genes that reduce or totally abolish synthesis of one or more of the globin chains. They result in hypochromia and microcytosis and, in the more severe forms, anemia. As a group, they compromise the most common single gene disorder known.

1. α-**Thalassemia:** Reduced (α^+-thalassemia) or absent (α^0-thalassemia) α-globin synthesis.
2. β-**Thalassemia:** Reduced (β^+-thalassemia) or absent (β^0-thalassemia) β-globin synthesis.
3. $\delta\beta$-**Thalassemia:** Both δ- and β-globin synthesis are reduced or absent.
4. **Hereditary persistence of fetal hemoglobin:** In these conditions, synthesis of elevated amounts of fetal hemoglobin persists in adult life. These conditions do not cause clinical disease but are important because they interact with thalassemias and sickle cell anemia to reduce severity.

Pathophysiology

Defective globin chain synthesis produces the following: First, inadequate hemoglobin tetramers are made, causing hypochromia and microcytosis. Second, synthesis of the unaffected globin chains continues at normal rates, resulting in accumulation of free (unpaired) globin chains. These either are insoluble, especially the α chains in β-thalassemia, or they form abnormal hemoglobins that have atypical properties, as occurs in α-thalassemia. The clinical syndromes are dominated by the adverse physiologic effects of the unpaired globin chains, even though the failure to synthesize hemoglobin produces the striking hypochromia and microcytosis that often provide the key diagnostic clues.

Clinical Importance

Severe forms of thalassemia are major health problems in many parts of the world but are seen rarely among the adult population in the United States. They are important disorders from a theoretic point of view because they are so well characterized at the molecular, genetic, and cellular levels. (The reader is referred to the References for this information, which does not yet impact directly on day-to-day diagnosis and treatment.) Severely affected thalassemic patients present complex management problems and should be referred to a specialist. For most general internists, the differential diagnosis of thalassemias and iron deficiency and recognition of severely affected thalassemic persons are the important considerations. Thalassemia is the most common genetic disorder in humans. Its high frequency is due to selective advantage of heterozygotes in areas where malaria is endemic.

α-Thalassemias

The most common forms of α-thalassemia result from deletion of one, two, three, or all four of the α-globin gene loci from the two copies of chromosome 16 present in normal humans. Analogous forms that do not involve gene deletion but arise instead from mutations that impair function of one or more copies of the gene, as well as mixed syndromes in which deletion and nondeletion forms are both present, also have been described. These are largely of research interest at the present time, however. α-Thalassemia is extremely common in Asia and the Mediterranean basin and in the indigenous African population.

Genetics and pathophysiology: The types of classic α-thalassemia are defined by the number of genes affected. **α-Thalassemia 2,** the "silent carrier" state, involves deletion of one of the four alleles. It is asymptomatic but transmissible as a trait that can add to the severity in offspring inheriting additional α-thalassemia alleles from the other parent.

A-Thalassemia 1 results from deletion of the two linked copies of the α-globin gene from the same chromosome (*in cis*). Mild hypochromic and microcytic changes are seen on smear with minimal anemia and can look like β-thalassemia trait but without elevation of Hb A_2 and usually with fewer dramatic changes.

Hemoglobin H disease involves inheritance of α-thalassemia 1(*cis*) from one parent and α-thalassemia 2 from the other, so that three out of the four α-globin alleles are missing. Only a small amount of Hb A is formed. Excess β chains accumulate in the adult, forming Hb H ($\beta4$), an abnormal hemoglobin that behaves like an unstable hemoglobin. These patients have moderate to moderately severe hemolytic anemia with usual stigmata, exacerbated by infections, drugs, and other oxidant stresses (much like patients with unstable hemoglobins and glucose-6-phosphate dehydrogenase [G6PD] deficiency). Free β-chains are more soluble than free α-chains, so that erythroblast precursors usually survive their development in the bone marrow, unlike in severe β-thalassemia. They can survive into adult life. It occurs most commonly in Asians, less so in Mediterranean people, and rarely in African Americans.

Hydrops fetalis with Hb Barts ($\gamma4$) involves inheritance of the α-thalassemia 2 chromosome from both parents, resulting in total absence of globin genes and therefore no fetal or adult hemoglobin synthesis. Only Hb Barts, consisting of γchains, accumulates. Hb Barts is moderately insoluble. More importantly, Hb Barts behaves like extremely high-affinity hemoglobin with a dramatically left-shifted oxygen dissociation curve, resembling that seen in carbon monoxide poisoning. There is no tissue oxygen delivery. Infants develop severe congestive heart failure (hydrops) and usually die *in utero*. There is an increased rate of polyhydramnios and maternal morbidity during early pregnancy.

α-Thalassemia in black populations: Deletion of one α-globin allele occurs in 10% to 30% of various African populations, so α-thalassemia 2 trait is extremely common. α-Thalassemia 2 tends to interact with sickle syndromes to reduce the severity slightly. Homozygous state for α-thalassemia 2 (i.e., one gene copy deleted from each chromosome "in trans") is also common, but α-thalassemia 1 chromosome is virtually nonexistent in these populations, so Hb H disease and hydrops are very rare.

α-Thalassemia with Hb Constant Spring arises from mutation in translation termination codon of α-globin gene; so ribosomes "read through" and incorporate an extra 31 amino acids onto the C-terminal end of the α-globin chain. In addition to this elongation of the α chain, production occurs at only 1% the normal rate; thus, the Constant Spring gene behaves like an α-thalassemia gene. Hb Constant Spring is very common in Asian populations, in whom α-thalassemia is common and interacts with α-thalassemia as though it were an α-thalassemia gene. Because Hb Constant Spring is always linked to a normal α allele on the same chromosome, hydrops fetalis does not occur.

Nondeletion α-thalassemia is more common in the Mediterranean than Asian populations, although both deletion and nondeletion forms are seen at high frequency in both populations (5%–15% gene frequency). For all practical purposes, it follows the same pathophysiologic scheme described in the discussion of classic types in the section on **α-Thalassemias (6).**

Diagnosis: α-Thalassemia trait is recognizable as microcytosis in patients with minimal or no anemia and a characteristic smear consisting of hypochromic microcytic populations with excessive numbers of target cells and anisocytosis. α-Thalassemia 2 trait may be completely silent with respect to laboratory findings and symptoms. Patients with Hb H disease present with evidence of hemolysis, sometimes with neonatal jaundice, because the α-globin gene defect is expressed *in utero.* Newborns have elevated levels of Hb Barts (absent from normal newborns) and, like their adult counterparts, have microcytic anemia with stigmata of hemolysis. Hb H is readily detectable by molecular hybridization technology. DNA studies or globin synthesis evaluation may confirm the diagnosis in utero. Hydrops fetalis is readily diagnosed by the presence of a hydropic infant in the absence of Rh or ABO immune incompatibility and predominance of Hb Barts by electrophoresis, as well as characteristic hypochromic microcytic smear findings.

Treatment and prevention: Hydrops fetalis, the only form of α-thalassemia for which prenatal intervention is currently recommended. It is readily detected as absence of a globin gene bands on Southern gene blot analysis of amniotic fluid DNA or chorionic villus sampling (CVS). It has become possible to carry out prenatal diagnosis with the PCR technique. The general approach is similar to that described for sickle cell anemia. α-Thalassemia trait requires no treatment other than genetic counseling of prospective parents. Hb H disease should be managed by principles similar to those for patients with unstable hemoglobins: avoidance of oxidant drugs, splenectomy for severe anemia, and judicious use of transfusion therapy. Hb H disease is usually compatible with survival into adult life.

β-Thalassemias: Nearly 50 forms of β-thalassemia have been described in various ethnic groups, each uniquely defined by the specific mutations identified using gene cloning methods. The condition is ubiquitous, but especially common in Mediterranean, Asian, and African populations. Malaria is thought to have some effect on gene frequency for various β-thalassemia syndromes, as in α-thalassemia, sickling syndromes, and other hemoglobinopathies. Clinical severity is very heterogeneous. A single β-globin gene means that β-chain abnormalities are inherited as simple mendelian traits: Patients are either heterozygous (β-thalassemia trait) or homozygous (β-thalassemia intermedia or β-thalassemia major). β-Thalassemia intermedia and β-thalassemia major differ from each other in that the patients with the latter syndrome require transfusions for survival, whereas β-thalassemia intermedia patients can survive without transfusion.

Pathophysiology: Forms of thalassemia arise in mutations that affect nearly every step in globin gene expression (i.e., transcription, translation, processing, and so on). Reduced or absent β-globin synthesis prevents adequate hemoglobin accumulation so that cells are hypochromic and microcytic. Free α-globin chains accumulate and precipitate during early erythroblast development because α-chains are so insoluble. α-Globin inclusions are highly toxic to erythroblasts, causing intramedullary destruction of erythroblasts (ineffective erythropoiesis). Few precursors survive to the reticulocyte erythrocyte stage, and those that do have shortened survival and circulation (hemolytic anemia). Anemia stimulates erythropoietin, which stimulates further ineffective bone marrow expansion, often to the point of invasion of bony cortex or, in some cases, formation of foci of extramedullary hematopoiesis, which presents clinically as space-filling masses resembling lymphomas.

Severely affected homozygous thalassemic patients exhibit a characteristic "mongoloid" facies because of marrow expansion into maxillary and skull spaces. They also exhibit profound anemia with congestive heart failure, stigmata of hemolysis, hepatomegaly, gallstones, excess iron absorption resulting from expanded erythron with subsequent iron overload, and a dramatic hypochromic and microcytic peripheral blood smear with many bizarre forms, nucleated RBCs, and massive erythroblastosis. Without transfusions, severely affected patients die in early childhood of congestive heart failure or infection.

The clinical severity is extremely heterogeneous. Coinheritance of α-thalassemia, common in the same populations, actually reduces the severity by reducing imbalance of α- and β-globin synthesis and, therefore, accumulation of free chains. Persistence of fetal hemoglobin into adult life at varying levels is also common in these populations. Hb F reduces severity by providing an alternative source of non-α-globin chains. In addition, the severity of β-globin synthetic lesion varies greatly according to the type of mutation inherited. Thus, some patients have relatively mild or moderate anemia that does not require transfusion or that requires transfusion only intermittently (β-thalassemia intermedia). Heterozygotes (β-thalassemia trait) are totally asymptomatic.

Diagnosis: β-Thalassemia trait is recognizable as significant hypochromia and microcytosis in a patient with mild or minimal anemia. The major differential diagnosis is iron deficiency. Iron, total iron-binding capacity (TIBC), and ferritin are normal in β-thalassemia trait. In general, patients with β-thalassemia trait have MCV less than 75 and hematocrit greater than 30. In contrast, iron-deficient patients rarely have MCV below 75 until the hematocrit has dropped below 30. A quantitative statement of this principle is the Mentzer index (MCV/RBC). If the MCV/RBC is greater than 13, it is compatible with iron deficiency; if less than 13, it is more compatible with β-thalassemia trait. Diagnosis is usually apparent from blood count and smear alone in about 70% to 80% of cases.

Hemoglobin electrophoresis reveals elevated Hb A_2 (usually >4%) in classic forms of β-thalassemia and provides a good confirmatory tool. The basis for an elevated Hb A_2 accumulation is unknown.

It is important to realize that a normal Hb A_2 does not rule out β-thalassemia trait. δβ-Thalassemia, a less common but not rare condition, is associated with elevated Hb F (usually in about 5%–10%) but normal or low Hb A_2. Other rare forms of thalassemia, such as Hb Lepore, have been described. These are readily recognized in most clinical laboratories. The reader is referred to the References for more extensive descriptions of these unusual hemoglobins.

In Southeast Asian populations, Hb E (β26 glu lys) is extremely common (10%–20% gene frequency). Hb E behaves normally in red cells but is synthesized in small amounts because the nucleotide substitution producing the structural change also affects metabolism of the mRNA precursor in the nucleus of developing erythroblasts. Hb E is thus a physiologically unusual but very common mild form of thalassemia in this population. Homozygous Hb E disease and Hb E trait are asymptomatic with microcytosis. Coinheritance of Hb E and β-thalassemia (Hb Eβ-thal) is also common because of the high frequency of β-thalassemia in these populations. This combination produces a thalassemia intermedia or thalassemia major phenotype. Hb E migrates like Hb A_2 on routine electrophoretic gels but is usually present at levels well above amounts seen for Hb A_2 (15%–30% for Hb E, 1%–7% for Hb A_2).

Diagnosis of thalassemia major is usually readily apparent in early childhood. Neonates are well at birth because production of fetal hemoglobin masks the phenotypic expression of mutation until well after birth.

Treatment and prevention: antenatal diagnosis of thalassemia using amniotic fluid or CVS is now more widely available by direct PCR-based DNA analysis. In

Europe and Asia, where only a few mutations predominate, prenatal diagnosis is routinely performed. In the United States, antenatal diagnosis is available through a number of reference laboratories. As a result, a diagnosis is often available in 3 to 7 days of fetal sampling. If parental samples are obtained, the mutation can be discovered in advance, and a fetal diagnosis sometimes can be obtained in 2 to 3 days.

β-Thalassemia trait requires no treatment except genetic counseling, avoidance of inappropriate iron therapy, and close monitoring during pregnancy for excessive drop in hematocrit. β-Thalassemia major requires treatment with regular transfusions or a protocol designed to maintain the hematocrit in the 30% to 35% range. Transfusion therapy usually relieves symptoms and allows more normal growth and development; however, iron overload and other complications from transfusions usually result in death in the second or third decade of life. Patients with β-thalassemia major should be managed at medical centers with capabilities for intensive iron chelation therapy and ready access to rapidly changing state-of-the-art approaches to this disease. Iron overload acts like other forms of hemochromatosis.

β-Thalassemia intermedia is the most difficult form of β-thalassemia to manage. It has variable presentations and severities. Decisions with respect to splenectomy, which can improve the anemia, institution of intermittent or permanent transfusion therapy, and use of iron chelators, are currently complex and controversial. Such patients should be managed only in close cooperation with a thalassemia expert.

Iron chelation therapy (23): Chelation therapy attempts to remove excess iron and prevent toxicity (cardiac, endocrine, etc.). Desferoxamine may be administered by a subcutaneous or intravenous infusion. Oral iron chelators are currently in trial use, and it is hoped that they will soon be widely available.

Bone marrow transplantation (24) may provide a hematologic cure for thalassemia. Allogeneic marrow transplantation may be a reasonable option for both children and adults who have a suitable donor.

Alternative forms of therapy (25), including manipulation of globin gene expression and gene therapy, are being actively pursued. Hydroxyrea and butyrate are also being evaluated in hopes of increasing Hb F production. As of this writing, Hb F manipulation has been much less successful in thalassemic than in sickle cell patients.

References

1. Bunn HF, Forget BG. *Hemoglobin: molecular genetic and clinical aspects.* Philadelphia: WB Saunders, 1986.
2. Embury SH, Vichinsky EP. Sickle cell disease. In: R. Hoffman et. al. (eds), *Hematology basic principles and practices.* New York: Churchill Livingstone, 2000: 510–553.
3. Hebbel RP, Yamada O, Moldow CF, et al. Abnormal adherence of sickle erythrocytes to cultured vascular endothelium: possible mechanism for microvascular occlusion in sickle cell disease. *J Clin Invest* 1980;65:154.
4. Balkaran B, Chan C, Morris JS, et al. Stroke in a cohort of patients with homozygous sickle cell disease. *J Pediatr* 1992;120:360.
5. Johnson C. Renal complications of sickle cell diseases. *American Society of Hematology education book,* 1999:44–50.
6. Castro O. Pulmonary complications of sickle cell disorders from an adult perspective. *American Society of Hematology education book* 1999:39–44.
7. Leong MA, Dampier C, Varlotta L, et al. Airway hyperactivity in children with sickle cell disease. *J Pediatr* 1997;131:278.
8. Eckman JR. Sickle cell anemia and the management of the adult patient with frequent pain. *American Society of Hematology education book* 1999:51–57.
9. Brookoff D, Polomano R. Treating sickle cell pain like cancer pain. *Ann Intern Med* 1992;116:364.
10. Virag R, Bachir D, Lee K, et al. Preventive treatment of priapism in sickle cell disease with oral and self-administered intracavernous injection of etileferie. *Urology* 1996;47:777.
11. Stuart MJ, Setty B. Sickle cell acute chest syndrome: pathogenesis and rationale for treatment. *Blood* 1999;94:1556.

12. Rao SP, RajKomar K, Schiffman G, et al. Antipneumococcal antibody levels three to seven years after first booster immunization in children with sickle cell disease, and after a second booster. *J Pediatr* 1995;127:590.
13. Koshy M, Burd L, Wallace D, et. al. Prophylactic red cell transfusion in pregnant patients with sickle cell disease: a randomized cooperative study. *N Engl J Med* 1998;319:1447.
14. Freie HMP. Sickle cell disease and hormonal contraception. *Acta Obstet Gynecol Scand* 1983;62:211.
15. Wayne AS, Kevy SV, Nathan BG. Transfusion management of sickle cell disease. *Blood* 1993;81:1109.
16. Kodish E, Lantos J, Stocking C, et al. Bone marrow transplantation for sickle cell disease. *N Engl J Med* 1991;325:1349.
17. Charache G, Dover GJ, Moore RD, et al. Hydroxyurea: effects of hemoglobin F production in patients with sickle cell anemia. *Blood* 1992;79:2555.
18. Rodgers GP, Roy MS, Noguchi CT, et al. Is there a role for selective vasodilation in the management of sickle cell disease? *Blood* 1998;71:597.
19. Atz AM, Wessel DL. Inhaled nitric oxide in sickle cell disease with acute chest syndrome. *Anesthesiology* 1997;87:988.
20. Goldberg MA, Brugnara C, Dover GJ, et al. Hydroxyurea and erythropoietin therapy in sickle cell anemia. *Semin Oncol* 1992;19:74.
21. Weatherall DJ. The thalassemias. In: Stamatoyannopoulos G, Nienhuis AW, Majerus PW, et al., eds. *Molecular basis of blood diseases,* 2nd ed. Phildelphia: WB Saunders, 1994:157.
22. Forget BG. Thalassemia syndromes. In: Hoffman R, et al., eds. *Hematology basic principles and practices.* New York: Churchill Livingstone, 2000:485–510.
23. Brittenham GN, Griffith PM, Nienhuis AW, et al. Efficacy of desferoxamine in preventing complications of iron overload in patients with thalassemia major. *N Engl J Med* 1994;331:567.
24. Lucarelli G, Giardini C, Baronciani D. Bone marrow transplantation in thalassemia. *Semin Hematol* 1995;32:294.
25. Beuzard Y. Towards gene therapy of hemoglobinopathies. *Semin Hematol* 1996; 33:43.

7. DISORDERS OF GRANULOCYTES: QUALITATIVE AND QUANTITATIVE

William R. Friedenberg

Granulocytes

Granulocytes consist of neutrophils, eosinophils, and basophils. These cells originate in the bone marrow and, under normal circumstances, participate in the host defense system and contribute to the inflammatory response.

Neutrophils

The most common abnormalities involve the neutrophils. The absolute number of neutrophils (ANC) is determined by multiplying the percentage of bands and segmented neutrophils (normal functioning cells) times the total leukocyte count (WBC). An ANC of less than 1,500 per milliliter (*neutropenia*) or greater than 8,000 per milliliter (*neutrophilia*) should be considered abnormal in white adults. Normal black patients may have ANCs as low as 1,000 per milliliter. Patients who develop an ANC of less than 1,000 per milliliter have an increased incidence of infection, and most patients with neutrophils less than 100 per milliliter are at high risk of developing an infection. The relative neutrophil count (percent of neutrophils in the WBC) is not as helpful as the ANC.

Normally, neutrophils are derived from pluripotent bone marrow stem cells, which mature through progenitor cells capable of producing colony-forming units (CFU-C). These progenitor cells then differentiate through the phases of myeloblast, promyelocyte, and myelocyte in a mitotic proliferating pool. They then go through a maturation and storage phase, during which they change from metamyelocytes into bands and polymorphonuclear neutrophils (PMNs), which are released into the circulation, where they have a half-life of approximately 6 hours (Fig. 1).

The storage pool consists of an emergency reserve that can release up to 10 times the number of normally circulating neutrophils given the appropriate stimulus. Granulocytopoiesis may be stimulated to generate new neutrophils within 48 hours. In the blood, neutrophils are equally distributed between a circulating and marginating pool. When neutrophils leave the circulation, they do not return to the blood but survive in body tissues for 4 to 5 days.

Cytoplasmic Granules

During the process of maturation, four types of cytoplasmic granules appear that remain present in PMNs. Azurophilic, or "primary" granules, are first seen in the promyelocyte. They are not formed after that stage, and so their number per cell diminishes. Myeloperoxidase, acid hydrolases, lysozyme, proteases, and bactericidal cationic proteins appear early in neutrophil development and are associated with azurophilic (primary) granules.

Beginning in the myelocyte stage, the specific or "secondary" granules are formed. Lysozyme, vitamin B_{12}–binding protein, and lactoferrin appear late in the granulocyte development and are associated with specific granules. Tertiary (gelatinase) granules and secretory vesicles also have been described. Alkaline phosphatase, as determined by a leukocyte alkaline phosphatase stain, is in secretory vesicles. The toxic granules seen on routine blood smears that appear in neutrophils during infection or inflammation are persistent primary granules.

The Pelger-Huët anomaly is the inheritance (dominant, non–sex-linked) of bilobed neutrophils, with no neutrophil dysfunction. The Alder–Reilly anomaly is a recessive disorder with granules that resemble toxic granules, whereas the May–Hegglin anomaly has neutrophil granules that resemble Döhle bodies, with mild thrombocytopenia. Neither of these disorders is associated with an increased incidence of infection.

Neutrophils frequently exhibit hypersegmentation in patients with uremia. Familial hypersegmentation of neutrophils occurs rarely and is not associated with an increased

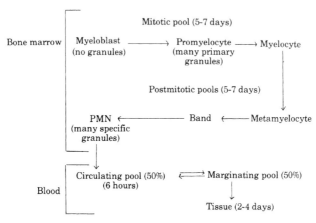

FIG. 1. Neutrophil kinetics.

risk of infection. Döhle bodies are sky-blue, discrete, round aggregates of rough endoplasmic reticulum and are seen with inflammation.

Defense against Infection
Neutrophils are critical in host defense against many microbial infections, including bacteria, fungi, and viruses (Fig. 2).

1. Neutrophils adhere to local blood vessel walls following damage to infected host cells.

2. Chemotactic factors may be released directly by the microorganism or by the damaged host cells, or they may be produced by antigen–antibody complexes or by enzymes that activate the complement system. Lymphocytes also respond to antigens by releasing chemotactic factors.

3. Neutrophils are deformable and can orient to the site of inflammation and move in the appropriate direction (chemotaxis) to arrive at the site of a foreign particle or microorganism.

4. To avoid killing normal host cells, the neutrophils must recognize the intruder. This recognition process is accomplished by opsonization, which is the coating of the microbe with complement C3b or immunoglobulin G (IgG) antibodies. The intruder attaches to neutrophils because of specific receptors for the opsonins on the neutrophil surface. When neutrophils encounter an opsonized foreign particle, they are capable of ingesting it by phagocytosis.

5. The neutrophil membrane encloses the particle within a piece of the plasma membrane, forming a phagosome, which then attaches to a lysosome, forming a phagolysosome.

6. Granules discharge their contents into the phagolysosome, destroying the microorganisms by enzymes in association with activation of the hexose monophosphate shunt, which provides reactive oxygen radicals for bactericidal activity.

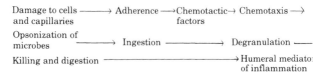

FIG. 2. Neutrophils in host defense.

7. Killing capacity is based on both oxidative and nonoxidative mechanisms. Enzymes and reactive oxygen radicals, along with myeloperoxidase and halide (chloride or iodide), form a powerful microbicidal system.

Neutropenia
Evaluation of the Patient with Neutropenia (Table 1)

A careful history and physical examination narrow the possible diagnoses considerably. A patient seen for a periodic examination who has mild (1,000–1,500/mL) absolute neutropenia may have an asymptomatic viral infection. All drugs should be stopped, if possible. In the absence of any etiologies on routine examination and laboratory testing, a repeat blood count should be done in 1 to 2 weeks, prior to an extensive evaluation, because some of these patients' counts will return to normal. A history of fatigue, mouth ulcers, malaise, and decreased appetite every 3 weeks is suggestive of cyclic neutropenia. The recent onset of symptoms such as fever, mouth sores, weight loss, and bone pain suggests acute leukemia and other bone marrow malignancies. Recent institution of a drug known to cause granulocytopenia, history of the patient's taking a drug for a long period, or recent exposure to a bone marrow toxin such as benzene is helpful in making a diagnosis. Prior illnesses such as rheumatoid arthritis may suggest Felty's syndrome or systemic lupus erythematosus as the cause of neutropenia. There may be a family history of other members having similar problems, or the patient may have had a history of neutropenia and recurrent infection since childhood, suggesting a congenital neutropenia.

During the physical examination, particular attention should be paid to any lymphadenopathy or hepatosplenomegaly as well as to signs of an underlying disease such as rheumatoid arthritis. Signs of superficial skin infections, particularly in the perineal and intertriginous areas, are helpful. Some patients have mouth ulcers or severe periodontal disease.

Patients with neutropenia may require extensive **laboratory testing** (Table 1). Patients who have severe neutropenia with no apparent reversible cause (e.g., drugs, viral illness) should have a bone marrow aspiration and biopsy. *In vitro* marrow culture may be of interest in some patients but is not necessary to determine the etiology of most neutropenias. Antinuclear antibody, rheumatoid factor, serum immunoelectrophoresis, serum folate and vitamin B_{12} levels, and antineutrophil antibodies may be helpful tests.

Table 1. Evaluation of neutropenia

History	Physical examination	Laboratory tests
Recent viral illness	Mouth ulcers	Examine peripheral smear for
Drugs	Lymphadenopathy	morphology and quantitate
Cyclical symptoms	Hepatomegaly	WBC count cell types
(10–35 days)	Splenomegaly	Bone marrow with biopsy
Recent versus	Skin abscesses	Antinuclear antibody, rheuma-
chronic symptoms	Deformed joints and	toid factor, direct Coombs' test
Constitutional	rheumatoid nodules	Serum immunoelectrophoresis
symptoms	Malar rash	Serum B_{12} and folate levels
Marrow toxins	Purpura	CSF assays
Prior illness	Periodontal disease	Epinephrine and prednisone
Family history		mobilization tests
History of infections		Neutrophil kinetics
		Antineutrophil antibodies
		Sequential ANC for cyclic
		neutropenia
		Evaluate splenic size—CT scan,
		ultrasound, liver–spleen scan

ANC, absolute neutrophil count; CSF, colony-stimulating factor; CT, computed tomography; WBC, white blood cell count.

Colony-stimulating factor (CSF) assays [granulocyte colony-stimulating factor (G-CSF), granulocyte-macrophage colony-stimulating factor (GM-CSF), interleukin-3 (IL-3)] in conjunction with *in vitro* bone marrow culture may be available in some centers. These tests are used to assess both intrinsically impaired myelopoiesis along with suppression of marrow by cytotoxic T cells or serum inhibitory factors.

Epinephrine and prednisone mobilization tests can provide a rough estimate of pool sizes and help determine the patient's risk of subsequent infection. These tests may be done in a single day by obtaining an ANC, injecting 0.3 mL of 1:1,000 epinephrine (adult dose) subcutaneously, and obtaining a second ANC 15 to 30 minutes later. Following this, 40 mg of prednisone is given orally, and another ANC is obtained 4 to 6 hours later.

Patients with pseudoneutropenia have an increase in their neutrophil count of more than 2,000 per milliliter with epinephrine but have less of a response to prednisone. Patients who have a good marrow reserve and an adequate storage pool increase their neutrophil count by more than 2,000 per milliliter with prednisone.

More extensive testing of mitotic pool size, postmitotic pool turnover, and blood turnover can only be done in selected patients at research centers with neutrophil labeling techniques. These techniques are cumbersome, expensive, and not necessary in most patients.

Diagnosis
Significant neutropenia (absolute neutrophil count < 1,500/mL) may be due to the several mechanisms (Table 2). The first of these are **disorders of decreased production of neutrophils,** including the following:

1. **Congenital defects.** Mutations of the gene encoding neutrophil elastase (ELA2) are a common cause of severe congenital neutropenia. **In reticular dysgenesis,** children may be born with severe granulocytopenia in addition to severe combined immunodeficiency (SCID) characterized by markedly reduced serum immunoglobulins, absent lymphoid and myeloid precursors in the bone marrow, lymphocytopenia, and thymic aplasia. These patients will die quickly without bone marrow transplantation. **Hereditary skin disorders (dyskeratosis)** may be associated with bone marrow hypoplasia. Some patients have anemia, neutropenia, thrombocytopenia, and other congenital defects suggesting **Fanconi anemia. Kostmann syndrome** is a moderate to severe congenital neutropenia sometimes associated with dysgammaglobulinemia, with normal granulocytic maturation up to the promyelocyte or myelocyte state and frequent chromosomal abnormalities. Marked bone marrow hypoplasia (**chronic hypoplastic neutropenia**) may be an isolated finding or may be associated with pancreatic insufficiency (**Schwachman–Diamond syndrome**). Initial symptoms may resemble fibrocystic disease, but the sweat test is negative. Children with this syndrome, as well as other congenital neutropenic states, may have short stature, skeletal abnormalities, mental retardation, and other congenital defects.

2. **Dysmyelopoiesis, aplastic anemia, and malignancies involving the bone marrow.** One of the most common causes of neutropenia is an acquired defect of all cell lines with anemia and thrombocytopenia in addition to neutropenia. A bone marrow examination is necessary to define these disorders, and treatment depends on the diagnosis.

3. **Drug-induced neutropenia.**
   - **Pathophysiology.** Bone marrow suppression and ineffective granulocytopoiesis are the most common mechanisms of neutropenia and often are induced by drugs. The chemotherapeutic agents used to treat malignancy are the most predictable, with the onset and severity of neutropenia depending on the dose and scheduling of the drugs. Other drugs may induce neutropenia by immunologic mechanisms, such as hypersensitivity reactions, antibodies, or hapten–antibody immune complexes.
   - **General concepts.** Patients with previous hypersensitivity reactions are more prone to drug-induced neutropenia, and idiosyncratic reactions seem to be more common in women and older patients. Neutropenia may occur with most classes of drugs. Even though a drug is not commonly associated with neutropenia and is not listed in either a standard textbook or in the *Physician's Desk Reference,* it should be suspected as the cause of the neutropenia and stopped unless it is critical to the

Table 2. Pathophysiologic diagnosis of neutropenia

Decreased production	Ineffective granulocytopenia	Abnormal distribution	Reduced survival	Combinations and miscellaneous causes
Congenital defects	Folic acid deficiency	Hypersplenism	Felty syndrome	Pseudoneutropenia
Reticular dysgenesis	B_{12} deficiency		Autoimmune neutropenia	Complement-activation neutropenia
Associated skin disorders	Drugs		Isoimmune neutropenia	Drugs
Kostman agranulocytosis	Bone marrow change		Systemic lupus erythematosus	Benign chronic neutropenia
Chronic hypoplastic neutropenia			Drugs	
Schwachman-Diamond Syndrome				
Acquired bone marrow damage (leukemia, myelodysplasia)				
Severe chronic neutropenia (idiopathic)				
Drug-induced				
Infections				
Cyclic neutropenia				
Suppressor T-cell induced				

patient's treatment. Drugs that have recently been instituted and associated with other side effects are more suspect than those that have been tolerated for a long time. There may be an increased incidence of adverse reactions in patients who have genetic variants of essential drug-detoxifying enzymes (slow acetylators).

- **Semisynthetic penicillins.** Although penicillin has been uncommonly implicated in causing agranulocytosis, the semisynthetic penicillins, when used at high doses for more than several weeks, have been associated with neutropenia.
- **Cephalosporins.** Although initially the cephalosporins were believed to be relatively safe, evidence suggests that neutropenia can occur with these agents (5%–15%).
- **Sulfonamides** may cause marrow suppression, but the combination of trimethoprim—sulfamethoxazole (Bactrim or Septra) is associated with the highest risk of neutropenia, especially in patients with sensitive bone marrows (e.g., following bone marrow transplant).
- **Phenothiazines** frequently cause neutropenia 2 to 8 weeks following initiation of treatment or after the dose of the phenothiazine has accumulated to more than 5 g; however, there is a significant amount of individual variation, depending on the patient's ability to compensate for phenothiazine-induced inhibition of DNA synthesis.
- **Phenylbutazone** and **oxyphenbutazone** are common causes of agranulocytosis, but other nonsteroidal antiinflammatory agents can also cause rapid granulocytopenia.
- **Gold.** In some patients, gold compounds seem to cause neutropenia by direct marrow suppression, whereas other patients may have an immune mechanism. Chelating agents to remove the gold may improve the neutropenia or thrombocytopenia.
- **Antithyroid drugs** may cause neutropenia in 10% to 15% of patients.
- **Cardiac antiarrhythmic drugs** such as quinidine and procainamide frequently cause neutropenia within the first 12 weeks of therapy unassociated with the development of the lupus syndrome.
- **Clozapine** is more effective than standard neuroleptic drugs in the treatment of severe schizophrenia but is associated with agranulocytosis in 0.80% of patients at 1 year and 0.91% at 1½ years. When clozapine was released in the United States in 1990, a special surveillance system monitoring weekly WBC counts was required. Agranulocytosis still occurs despite careful monitoring; the risk is increased in older patients, and the incidence decreases after 6 months of use. Patients who receive this drug require frequent monitoring and should discontinue the drug if the WBC count approaches or reaches 3,500 per milliliter.
- Patients who develop drug-induced agranulocytosis frequently have been taking the medication for a few days to a few weeks when they develop a sore throat, fever, and chills with or without other symptoms of infection. The ANC is usually less than 500 per milliliter, and the bone marrow is frequently hypocellular with a paucity of the late granulocytic forms and sometimes total absence of any myeloid elements. Bone marrow recovery may occur within a few days to several weeks following discontinuation of the medication. When the predominant mechanism of neutropenia is antibody induced, the bone marrow may be hypercellular with granulocytic hyperplasia, and the patient may recover within just a few days of discontinuing the offending medication. Occasionally, the count rises to quite high levels, and immature cells may be released, resembling acute leukemia; however, this should resolve quickly.

4. **Infections.** A protective role of neutrophils against bacterial infections is established, but it has also become apparent that they are important in protecting against viral and fungal infections as well. Infection is probably the most common cause of neutropenia, followed by drugs. Viral, fungal, and bacterial infections may cause marrow hypoplasia. Neutropenia also may be present secondary to immune complexes, antibodies, or hypersplenism. Endotoxin is known to cause peripheral margination of neutrophils, resulting in a decrease in the ANC. Patients may have a monocytosis with either normocellular or hypercellular bone marrows if sequestration of neutrophils is the dominant mechanism. Although the bone marrow frequently recovers rapidly, protracted neutropenia may occur on occasion.

5. **Cyclic neutropenia (CN)** is inherited as an autosomal dominant with variable expression and frequently presents in childhood but may not be diagnosed until late in adulthood. The genetic locus has been mapped to chromosome 19p13.3, which is the gene encoding neutrophil elastase (ELA2 gene). In about half the patients, a compensatory monocytosis occurs. There is usually a cyclic variation in monocytes, eosinophils, reticulocytes, and platelets. Bone marrow examinations during granulocytopenia usually show hypoplasia or an arrest in maturation at approximately the myelocyte stage. Patients who have symptoms suggestive of CN or who have variable neutropenia on several occasions should have ANCs done at least 3 times a week for 4 to 6 weeks to determine whether there is any periodic neutropenia. These patients typically develop symptoms (fatigue, malaise, mouth sores) every 21 days (10–35 days) and lasting 3 to 4 days. Patients may develop fever and infections during neutropenia, usually with pyogenic bacteria.

6. **Suppressor T-cell–induced neutropenia** is a syndrome of neutropenia and T-cell lymphocytosis this is sometimes associated with rheumatoid arthritis. Most of these patients have recurrent infections. Cyclic neutropenia, pure red cell aplasia, and thrombocytopenia also may occur. Monoclonal antibody studies have shown that these lymphocytes, which contain large granules, are phenotypically T-lymphocytes of the suppressor–cytotoxic type. Other studies have shown that some of these patients have a natural killer cell phenotype. Despite these various phenotypes, most patients have little cytotoxic or suppressor functional activity. Large granular lymphocyte proliferations may behave as a benign condition resembling Felty syndrome or a rapidly progressive, aggressive lymphoproliferative disease resembling a large cell lymphoma or an indolent disease acting like early chronic lymphocytic leukemia (CLL). The immunophenotype, cytogenetics, and T-cell receptor rearrangements may be useful in distinguishing these disorders.

Disorders of ineffective production of neutrophils include **megaloblastic anemia** secondary to either folic acid, or vitamin B_{12} deficiency which may cause ineffective myelopoiesis and neutropenia. In general, the neutropenia is not less than 1,000 per milliliter ANC, and associated macrocytosis of the red cells and thrombocytopenia are present. The absence of macrocytosis does not exclude B_{12} or folate deficiency because the patient may have concomitant iron deficiency normalizing the red cell indices. Vitamin B_{12} and folate levels should be checked in patients with unexplained mild neutropenia. **Drugs** can cause ineffective granulopoiesis and neutropenia without causing either anemia or thrombocytopenia. Some patients present with the appearance of ineffective granulocytopoiesis and eventually progress to severe bone marrow failure due to myelodysplasia, leukemia, or aplastic anemia.

Abnormal distribution of neutrophils: Hypersplenism is frequently associated with anemia or thrombocytopenia as well as neutropenia. Any combination is possible. An elevated reticulocyte count may suggest this diagnosis in the absence of palpable splenomegaly. Most patients have a palpable spleen, but on occasion, an enlarged spleen may require detection by other techniques (e.g., computed tomography, ultrasound). If the patient does not have liver disease or portal hypertension, a bone marrow examination should be done to exclude a disease that is causing infiltration of both the marrow and the spleen, such as a lymphoproliferative or myeloproliferative disorder. Depending on the results, further evaluation may be needed before considering splenectomy for diagnosis as well as treatment of the neutropenia (Tables 1 and 2).

Reduced survival: Felty's syndrome. Patients with rheumatoid arthritis, splenomegaly, and neutropenia have Felty's syndrome. This condition is an uncommon complication of advanced rheumatoid arthritis that has usually been present for many years. Splenomegaly is not always present but on occasion may be massive. Neither the degree of neutropenia nor the incidence of infection is directly related to splenic size. Neutrophil counts may be extremely low without associated symptoms. Rheumatoid nodules and high rheumatoid factors are invariably present. The exact pathophysiologic mechanism is controversial, but a shortened neutrophil survival with accelerated release of marrow neutrophils and an inadequate neutrophil response have been found. Serum inhibitory factors, increased suppressor T-cell activity, antineutrophil antibodies, and immune complexes all have been described.

Autoimmune and isoimmune neutropenia: Tests for neutrophil antibodies have improved. Some investigators appear to have reliable tests using various antibody assays to identify patients who have antibody-induced neutropenia analogous to immune hemolytic anemia and immune thrombocytopenia. In some cases where the bone marrow shows a deficiency of granulocyte precursors, it has been postulated that the antibody has affected neutrophil precursors similar to pure red cell aplasia. In most situations, the marrow is hyperplastic with adequate myeloid precursors except for mature neutrophils, with a marked neutropenia in the peripheral blood.

Isoimmune neutropenia: Infants may be born with severe neutropenia as a result of the transplacental passage of maternal IgG antineutrophil antibodies. This usually lasts for 6 to 12 weeks before the antibodies disappear. Neutrophil-specific antigens on fetal granulocytes move into the maternal circulation during pregnancy and stimulate the production of antibodies, which then cross into the fetal circulation. This resembles Rh-induced hemolytic anemia of the newborn. In one series, neutrophil antibodies were found in 119 of 121 patients, with 10% positive for the specific neutrophil antigens NA-1 and NA-2. This condition may be difficult to diagnose in the presence of sepsis because sepsis can induce severe neutropenia in infants. If antibiotics are ineffective, whole-blood exchange may be necessary.

Because multiparous women frequently have leukoagglutinins without causing neonatal neutropenia, it has been suggested that antineutrophil antibodies are not involved in the pathogenesis of neonatal neutropenia. These maternal leukoagglutinins are usually antibodies against antigens in the human leukocyte antigen (HLA) system rather than neutrophil-specific antigens and are absorbed by many tissues besides neutrophils. Therefore, they are probably insufficient in quantity to cause neonatal neutropenia.

Adults occasionally develop autoimmune neutropenia, and neutrophil-specific antibodies have been described. Some of these patients also have antibodies directed against red cells and platelets and respond to immunosuppression with steroids. In one study of 121 adult patients with chronic idiopathic neutropenia, 36% had antineutrophil antibodies.

Neutropenia occurs in about half the patients with systemic lupus erythematosus (SLE). Neutrophil-specific IgG antibodies have been demonstrated in the sera of some patients with SLE who have improved with glucocorticoids. A shortened granulocyte survival time has been demonstrated. Fewer than 5% of patients with SLE have severe neutropenia.

The **combination mechanisms and miscellaneous causes of neutropenia** includes **pseudoneutropenia.** Patients with significant neutropenia, no history of infections, and an underlying emotional disorder (e.g., chronic anxiety, anorexia nervosa) have been reported. These patients frequently have a dramatic response to epinephrine because they have a marked increase in their marginal pool and do not need further evaluation or treatment.

A transient spurious leukopenia may occur secondary to a cold agglutinin (IgM) directed against the WBC membrane, causing aggregation of leukocytes on blood smears. A diluted manual leukocyte count will correct the WBC count and avoids unnecessary evaluation.

Complement-activation neutropenia: Complement may be activated with sepsis, hemodialysis, and cardiopulmonary bypass. Activated complement (C5a) can cause granulocyte aggregation with neutropenia and pulmonary infiltration. This usually occurs within a few minutes of institution of dialysis or cardiopulmonary bypass and may be either ameliorated or prevented by the use of high-dose corticosteroids. Patients on hemodialysis who develop neutropenia may benefit from changing the dialysis membrane.

Benign chronic neutropenia (BCN) frequently begins within the first 2 years of life, and most children are asymptomatic. A variant of this disorder is ethnic neutropenia, in which African Americans and Yemenite Jews have mild to moderate neutropenia, with both total WBC count and ANC as low as 50% of normal. Patients with BCN have normal granulocyte reserve with stimulation tests and normal *in vitro* culture studies, suggesting that the neutropenia is related to the degree of marrow release. The bone marrow appears normal morphologically. Life expectancy is normal, and these patients do not have frequent infections.

Human immunodeficiency virus (HIV) infection is associated with both neutrophil dysfunction and neutropenia that is due to a variety of mechanisms, including G-CSF deficiency and the medications used to either treat acquired immunodeficiency syndrome (AIDS) or coexisting infections. Accelerated apoptosis of neutrophils occurs in patients with HIV infection.

Treatment of Neutropenia (Table 3)
General considerations include the following:

1. The likelihood of infection increases as neutropenia becomes more severe. Patients who have stable neutropenia and who have some ability to mobilize neutrophils from the bone marrow have a lower incidence of infection than patients with newly induced severe granulocytopenia (e.g., resulting from chemotherapy).

2. If at all possible, neutropenic patients should be managed at home because infections acquired in the hospital are often more difficult to eradicate. If additional immune defects are present, such as hypogammaglobulinemia or splenectomy, the risk of serious sepsis is even higher.

3. In addition to the severity of the neutropenia, the duration of the neutropenia is also a significant risk factor.

4. Most infections are caused by endogenous organisms, with a minority coming from external sources. Eating foods rich in gram-negative bacteria, such as fresh fruits, fresh vegetables, and black pepper, should be avoided.

5. Fresh flowers may contain fungi and should not be placed in the patient's room.

6. The water supply should be checked for growth of organisms such as *Legionella*.

7. Good handwashing should be practiced by all visitors before contact with the patient.

8. Patients are usually placed in private rooms to avoid contact with infected patients.

9. Invasive techniques may be necessary but should be limited to the extent possible.

10. Meticulous attention to sterile technique in handling long-term indwelling or central venous access catheters is important.

11. Laminar airflow rooms and other types of life islands have been designed to decrease environmental organisms by filtering air and removing particulate matter, including microbes. Such rooms may decrease the rate of infection, but they are expensive and difficult to maintain and have not proven to prolong survival in most studies. Other facilities use high-pressure rooms with some degree of air filtration [High-Efficiency Particulate Air (HEPA) filter] to try to decrease the burden of microorganisms while not removing them entirely.

12. Chemotherapy-induced neutropenia may be associated with significant stomatitis and intestinal ulceration. Techniques such as proctoscopy and endoscopy should be limited, and rectal temperatures and enemas should be avoided.

Table 3. Treatment of neutropenia: general measures

---

1. Manage at home if possible.
2. Avoid fresh fruits, fresh vegetables, and black pepper.
3. No fresh flowers in hospital room.
4. Check water supply *(Legionella),* and avoid humidifiers.
5. Good handwashing by hospital personnel and visitors.
6. Private hospital room.
7. Minimize invasive techniques.
8. Sterile technique with venous access devices.
9. Laminar airflow rooms, life islands, and high-pressure rooms with filtered air [High-Efficiency Particulate Air (HEPA) filter]
10. Selective microbial suppression—Bactrim-DS, fluconazole, nystatin, Mycelex-troche, quinolones.
11. Careful mouth and dental care.
12. Stool softeners and high-fiber diets.
13. Skin cleansing.
14. Venous access devices—Hickman, Quinton, etc.

---

13. Selective microbial suppression may be attempted with trimethoprim-sulfamethoxazole (Bactrim-DS), 1 tablet twice daily for adults, but this may prolong neutropenia and encourage the development of resistant organisms. Other problems associated with prophylactic antimicrobial regimens are increased cost and emergence of resistant bacteria. In some centers, quinolones (e.g., ciprofloxacin, norfloxacin) are being used.

14. Some centers use fluconazole, 400 mg daily, administered orally, to reduce fungal infection from *Candida*. Itraconazole is being evaluated for reduction of *Aspergillus* infections.

15. Systemic administration of antibiotics prophylactically, prophylactic granulocyte transfusions, and vaccines have not improved survival.

16. Patients should use a soft toothbrush and either mouthwashes or Water Piks to help clean their teeth.

17. Stool softeners and a high-fiber diet may decrease problems with hemorrhoids and perirectal abscesses.

18. Regular cleansing of the axillary and perineal areas with povidone–iodine and cleansing the skin with a germicidal soap may decrease the rate of infection.

19. For patients who are going to be neutropenic for considerable periods, multiple-lumen catheters may be useful but are frequently the source of serious infection and may require removal.

Treatment of infection: Despite all of the aforementioned maneuvers, fever frequently occurs. If it is a low-grade fever, that is, under 101°F (38°C), and possibly related to the recent administration of a blood product or associated with the underlying disease, a drug reaction, acute hemorrhage, or chemical-induced phlebitis, it is possible to obtain cultures and evaluate for possible infection without starting antibiotics. If the temperature is above 101°F (38°C) and is associated with shaking chills or other signs and symptoms of infection, cultures should be obtained and antibiotics instituted empirically. The severely neutropenic patient tends to tolerate infections poorly, and it is important to treat empirically and vigorously.

Because the patient does not have enough neutrophils to manifest a good inflammatory response, there is frequently a paucity of signs of inflammation in such sites as the skin, urinary tract, and lungs. Even with pulmonary infiltrates, neutrophils should not be expected in the sputum, and this should not be used as a guide to an adequate specimen. In addition, CSF and pleural fluid may be infected in the absence of neutrophils.

The general approach to fever in the neutropenic patient requires careful attention to the recent events and physical examination to determine any localized source of the fever (Table 4). Assuming no definite source is found, cultures should be obtained of the throat, blood, and urine. If any symptoms, signs, or chest radiographs suggest pneumonia, a sputum sample should be obtained. With abdominal pain or diarrhea, a stool should be obtained for enteric pathogens, ova, and parasites and *Clostridium difficile* toxin. Chest radiographs and sinus films should be performed routinely. If the fever persists, radiographs of the teeth (Panorex) may be necessary to uncover a periapical abscess. CSF should be examined if clinically indicated. Although bone marrow cultures occasionally reveal obligatory intracellular organisms such as fungi and mycobacteria, such tests are not recommended routinely. If the patient is febrile and no

Table 4. Considerations and guidelines in evaluating fever in the neutropenic patient

1. History of recent events and invasive procedures (e.g., peripheral or central venous catheter).
2. Physical examination.
3. Obtain cultures and radiographs from multiple sites and areas.
4. Serologies and cultures for viral diseases.
5. Initiate broad spectrum antibiotic therapy.
6. Initiate antifungal or antiviral therapy when appropriate.

source of the fever has been found, however, and a bone marrow aspirate or biopsy is performed to assess the status of disease, marrow cultures may be useful. Gallium scans and indium 111–labeled leukocytes occasionally can detect foci of infection but are not routinely efficacious and can be used when other studies and procedures have not proven fruitful. Other sources of infection such as viral diseases (cytomegalovirus and hepatitis), protozoan infections (toxoplasmosis), and fungal infections (candidiasis and aspergillosis) should be considered.

Most clinicians administer a combination of two antibiotics that are bactericidal for both gram-positive and gram-negative aerobic bacilli. A common regimen consists of an extended-spectrum penicillin plus an aminoglycoside. The empiric use of vancomycin to cover methicillin-resistant *Staphylococcus epidermis* is not recommended in the absence of a positive culture. Single-agent coverage with ceftazidime, cefepime, or imipenem is equally successful.

Patients are usually treated for several days after all signs of the infection have resolved and the neutrophil count rises to more than 500 per milliliter. If the patient remains febrile after 24 to 48 hours and no definite source of fever has been determined, amphotericin B should be added to the antimicrobial regimen. When a fungal infection has been documented, parenteral therapy with amphotericin B, 1.0 to 1.5 mg per kilogram, is given daily. Lipid formulations of amphotericin B have reduced toxicity with preserved efficacy. Infected neutropenic patients on multiple antibiotics need daily blood counts, chemistries, and careful attention to nutritional and metabolic needs.

The following are guidelines for the **treatment of specific diseases:**

Hypoplastic neutropenia. Patients with a possibly reversible cause of decreased neutrophil production such as acute leukemia or lymphoma should have treatment of the malignancy. **Growth factors**. G-CSF, and GM-CSF can be used to prevent or shorten the period of neutropenia expected after high-dose chemotherapy, with or without stem cell rescue. Growth factors can correct the neutropenia associated with AIDS, allowing tolerable doses of zidovudine, interferon, ganciclovir, and chemotherapy for malignancies. The function of neutrophils can be improved in patients with HIV infection treated with G-CSF along with increasing the neutrophil count.

Peripheral blood stem cells may be collected with growth factors and given following high-dose chemotherapy. **Stem cell rescue** should then be used, thus reducing neutropenic days, infectious complications, antibiotic use, and hospital days.

Severe chronic neutropenia (SCN), whether congenital, cyclic, or idiopathic, can be improved by G-CSF and other growth factors. In SCN, daily growth factors have been successful in resolving existing infections, decreasing the number of new infections, and decreasing oral ulcers or mucositis. The increased risk of myeloid leukemia or myelodysplasia is probably associated more with the underlying bone marrow disorder rather than with the use of growth factors.

Stem cell factor (SCF), also known as *c-kit-ligand, steel factor,* or *mast cell growth factor,* is the product of the steel locus (SL) in the mouse. SCF acts on primitive progenitors rather than the terminal differentiated cells stimulated by the currently available growth factors (G-CSF and GM-CSF), and it works synergistically with G-CSF and GM-CSF. Aplastic anemia, Fanconi anemia, and other pancytopenic conditions may be treated more effectively by the use of SCF along with other growth factors. SCF is currently undergoing clinical trials to assess its toxicity and efficacy.

Androgens. Patients with myelodysplasia or congenital hypoplastic neutropenia sometimes respond to androgens. Side effects include cholestatic jaundice, virilization, and salt and water retention.

Corticosteroids may be effective in increasing the neutrophil count. The neutrophil increase usually occurs within 4 to 6 hours and is caused by a release from the bone marrow storage pool and a decrease in granulocyte egress from the blood. The neutrophilia is not associated with a shift to the left in the peripheral white cells, and band forms remain in fewer than 6% of the total. This may be a helpful distinguishing feature in a patient on steroids who develops an infection. Glucocorticoids have profound immunologic and nonimmunologic side effects. Neutrophil function *in vivo* remains intact, but glucocorticoids cause a significant lymphocytopenia because of a redistribution of the circulating T-lymphocytes into lymphoid tissues. They also cause a depletion of monocytes and eosinophils and stimulate production of lipomodulin, which inhibits phospholipase-A, which blocks production of prostaglandin and leukotriene. Complement production and activity are unaffected. Large doses of glucocorticoids (30 mg/kg of methylprednisolone) prevent neutrophil aggregation. Glucocorticoids also have been implicated in accelerating osteoporosis, causing cataracts, exacerbating diabetes, contributing to hypertension, and increasing the risk of peptic ulceration. Because of the increased risk of infection and other side effects, glucocorticoids are not ideal drugs to stimulate neutrophils and prevent infection.

Although splenectomy has been tried in some patients with hypoplastic neutropenia, it has proven ineffective. If there is a component of hypersplenism (enlarged, palpable spleen), however, the neutrophil count may be improved.

Distribution disorders: hypersplenism. If hypersplenism is believed to be a component of the patient's illness, a splenectomy may improve the neutrophil count. Some patients may have bone marrow abnormalities in addition to hypersplenism, and it may be difficult to decide whether hypersplenism is playing a significant role in the patient's neutropenia. In this situation, the epinephrine and prednisone stimulation tests may be useful as well as more sophisticated neutrophil kinetics (if available).

Autoimmune neutropenia:

1. **Felty's syndrome.** Although 80% to 90% of patients respond to splenectomy, the response is frequently transient. At least 30% of patients relapse, and recurrent infections may persist in one third of cases despite normalization of the neutrophil count. Splenectomy should be performed only in patients with severe neutropenia who suffer recurrent infections. Corticosteroids and high-dose intravenous gamma globulin have not produced consistently good results. Growth factors have produced good results in isolated case reports. Gold therapy, cytotoxic agents, cyclosporin, D-penicillamine, and plasmapheresis have been used with some success. Lithium has not been sufficiently effective to outweigh potentially serious side effects associated with its use.

2. **Antibody-mediated** or **lymphocyte-induced neutropenia** may respond to glucocorticoids or other cytotoxic agents. Investigation of the value of specific cytotoxic agents is continuing.

3. Many patients with **autoimmune neutropenia** are relatively asymptomatic for long periods and should not be treated until they have significant symptoms or recurrent infections.

4. High-dose gamma globulin, danazol, vincristine, and plasmapheresis have been tried with occasional response.

5. Growth factors have been of benefit in a few case reports.

Complement-activation neutropenia: Patients with septic shock or who are undergoing hemodialysis or cardiopulmonary bypass have been shown to develop neutropenia because of activated complement (C5a), which causes granulocyte aggregation, neutropenia, and pulmonary infiltrates. When this occurs, large doses of glucocorticoids (methylprednisolone, 30 mg/kg, administered intravenously) may reduce granulocyte aggregation and improve pulmonary function. Patients on hemodialysis who regularly develop neutropenia may benefit from changing the dialysis membrane.

Neutrophilia
Mechanisms
Neutrophilia is commonly seen in clinical practice and may be due to several mechanisms. **Increased production by the bone marrow** may occur in infections or inflammatory conditions such as vasculitis, malignancies (especially with necrosis), myeloproliferative diseases, and in patients who take lithium. Chronic smokers frequently have a mild leukocytosis with neutrophilia.

Impaired egress of neutrophils from the peripheral blood into the tissues: Glucocorticoids increase ANC by impairing the egress of neutrophils into the tissue and by reducing margination as well as releasing neutrophils from the bone marrow storage pool.

Reduction in the percentage of neutrophils in the marginating pool with an increase in the circulating pool: Exercise induces neutrophilia just as exogenous epinephrine shifts cells from the marginating into the circulating pool.

"Leukemoid" Reactions

Very high white cell counts suggesting leukemia have been called *leukemoid* reactions (Table 5). Leukemoid reactions are associated with mature neutrophils consisting predominantly of PMN leukocytes with some bands, usually less than 10%. The neutrophil alkaline phosphatase levels are normal or increased but not decreased as in chronic granulocytic leukemia (CGL). Review of the peripheral smear fails to reveal any basophilia or eosinophilia suggestive of a myeloproliferative disorder. The platelets appear small, and they may be increased but are usually less than 600,000 per milliliter. Platelet aggregation tests do not show a dramatic abnormality unless the patient is taking antiplatelet agents. Bone marrow examination reveals myeloid hyperplasia with no other definitive abnormality. Patients with myeloproliferative disease may have myelofibrosis, confirming the process as a primary myeloproliferative disease and not a leukemoid reaction. Infections and underlying diseases such as vasculitis and cancer need to be excluded by a careful history and physical examination as well as the appropriate laboratory tests.

When a tumor invades the bone marrow, a typical "leukoerythroblastic picture" may be seen in the peripheral blood, consisting of a left shift in the myeloid series, with a total WBC that can be high, low, or normal, but without a predominance of blasts. Thrombocytopenia, nucleated red cells, schistocytes, and teardrop cells are common in the peripheral blood.

A chromosomal analysis of the bone marrow (karyotype) also may be useful to distinguish between a leukemoid reaction and a myeloproliferative disorder. The Philadelphia chromosome is present (90%) in CGL, and karyotypic abnormalities are sometimes evident in other myeloproliferative disorders.

In the absence of a cytogenetic abnormality, molecular probes for the *bcr-abl* rearrangement should be obtained. In some centers, X-linked inactivation techniques may be able to demonstrate clonality in the absence of other abnormalities.

Table 5. Differential diagnosis of severe neutrophilia

Leukemoid reaction	Myeloproliferative disease
Inflammatory disease recognized (pneumonia, necrotic tumor, vasculitis)	No other etiology identified including special examinations (CT scans)
Mature neutrophils: <10% bands; WBC usually <50,000/μL	Left shift with myeloid cells earlier than bands WBC count may be >100,000/μL
High LAP	LAP low in CGL; variable in other disorders
No basophilia, eosinphilia, or monocytosis	Frequently eosinphilia, basophilia, or monocytosis
Platelets are usually small and not >600,000–700,000/μL, with normal aggregation	Platelets frequently qualitatively abnormal, large, with abnormal aggregation and counts exceeding 1,000,000/μL
No thrombocytopenia	Thrombocytopenia may occur
Nucleated RBC not seen in peripheral blood; RBCs appear relatively normal	RBCs frequently nucleated on peripheral smear, with abnormal RBC morphology (teardrops, polychromatophilia)
No splenomegaly	Splenomegaly (25%–75%)
Bone marrow hyperplastic with normal karyotype; no clone demonstrated by X-linked inactivation techniques; no *bcr-abl* demonstrated by Southern blot or PCR	Bone marrow frequently abnormal with megakaryocytic and platelet clumping; possibly fibrosis Karyotype may be abnormal, especially in CGL with the Philadelphia chromosome; *bcr-abl* by Southern blot or PCR; clonality by X-linked inactivation techniques

CT, computed tomography; CGL, chronic granulocytic leukemia; LAP, leukocyte alkaline phosphatase; PCR, polymerase chain reaction; RBC, red blood cell count; WBC, white blood cell count.

Neutrophilia
Neutrophilia may be seen in a variety of other situations, including poisoning, bleeding, trauma (including surgery), seizures, and eclampsia or labor. Rarely, neutrophilia may be idiopathic or familial.

Qualitative Defects in Neutrophils
Just as adequate numbers of neutrophils are important in preventing infection, adequate function of neutrophils is also critical. Severe neutrophil dysfunction, although uncommon, may cause recurrent bacterial or fungal infection and should be suspected in patients who have adequate neutrophils numerically and normal immunoglobulins but develop unusual, persistent, or frequent bacterial or fungal infections. Typically, these patients have recurrent skin abscesses, sinopulmonary and ear infections, mucocutaneous candidiasis, and serious systemic or visceral infections.

Evaluation of Neutrophil Function
Screening tests are available in many clinical laboratories. If a defect is found or suspected, referral to a laboratory specializing in neutrophil function and dysfunction may be indicated. The ability of neutrophils to migrate into the tissues can be assessed by using skin windows or quantitative skin chambers (*in vivo* function) or by *in vitro* tests of neutrophil function (Table 6).

Diagnosis of Neutrophil Dysfunction
It is important to keep in mind that neutrophil dysfunction may be a **result** of a disease as well as the **cause** of an illness. Neutrophil dysfunction is common as a consequence of infections, drugs, burns, and transiently in the neonatal period. In addition, phagocytosis and bactericidal killing declines with advancing age. Because neutrophil function tests are biologic assays, they have a great degree of variability, based simply on the test itself, not even considering variation based on the status of the patient. The total absence of a specific neutrophil function, even in the face of an acute illness or in a patient receiving drugs, may be significant, but evidence of a partial deficiency requires improvement in the patient and repetitive assays to ensure that there is a consistent abnormality.

   Morphology: Cells more immature than bands and PMN leukocytes do not function normally and should not be included in the ANC. Neutrophils with toxic granules, Döhle bodies, hereditary diseases such as hypersegmentation of neutrophils, the Pelger-Huët anomaly, Alder–Reilly anomaly, and May–Hegglin anomaly have not been associated with recurrent infections. Patients with myeloproliferative or myelodysplastic disorders frequently have abnormal granulation or decreased segmentation of neutro-

Table 6. *In vitro* tests of neutrophil function

Function	Tests
Morphology	Phase microscopy, electron microscopy, shape changes
Adherence/aggregation	Adherence to glass or plastic with spreading; aggregation in an aggregometer; anti-CD18 and anti-sialyl-Lewis X positive neutrophils on flow cytometry
Locomotion	Random migration and chemotactic assays
Secretion	Lysosomal enzyme assays, lactoferrin, B_{12} binding protein
Bactericidal activity	Killing of *Staphylococcus aureus* or other microorganisms, chemiluminescence, nitroblue tetrazolium test, oxygen radical production
Phagocytosis	Uptake of microorganisms, latex beads, and assays of the hexose monophosphate shunt

phils (pseudo-Pelger-Huët anomaly) or hypersegmented polys, and these cells may function abnormally. Patients with the Cheéiak–Higashi anomaly have marked neutrophil dysfunction (see discussion of nondirected locomotion in this section).

Adherence and aggregation: Drugs such as corticosteroids, salicylates, ethanol, epinephrine, and colchicine affect the adherence of neutrophils *in vitro* and suppress inflammatory reactions *in vivo*. Some patients with frequent infections may have abnormal adherence to endothelial cells. A congenital defect in the integrin receptor molecules, leukocyte factor antigen-1 (LFA-1; common β subunit CD11/CD18), or the sialyl Lewis X ligand of E-selectin, have been reported as leukocyte adhesion deficiency types 1 and 2, respectively. Newborns may have decreased adherence as well as abnormal aggregation. Neonates and patients with diabetes mellitus may have difficulty with adequate deformability.

Nondirected locomotion (random migration): Neutrophils move without direction when they are not exposed to a chemotactic stimulus. This requires an intact actin–myosin system and intact structural elements (microtubules). These systems are localized at the leading edge of the cell and may be inhibited *in vitro* with cytochalasin B, which disrupts actin filaments. An infant has been described as having abnormal actin polymerization and impaired chemotaxis. Drugs such as colchicine and Taxol not only interfere with adherence but seem to inhibit microtubules, thereby inhibiting cell orientation, chemotaxis, and random locomotion. Functionally, patients with the Cheédiak–Higashi syndrome (recurrent pyogenic infections with abnormal giant lysosomal granules, abnormal chemotaxis, oculocutaneous albinism, nystagmus, and peripheral neuropathy) have leukocyte dysfunction similar to cells treated with colchicine. They have abnormal giant granules in monocytes and lymphocytes as well as neutrophils. **Kartagener syndrome** (chronic or recurrent upper respiratory infections in association with situs inversus) is an autosomal recessive disorder in which there is significant impairment of nondirected migration as well as chemotaxis.

Chemotaxis (directed migration): Patients may have either serum or cellular abnormalities causing abnormal chemotactic function:

1. **Serum abnormalities.** Complement deficiencies (C3 and C5 components), immunoglobulin deficiencies, and serum inhibitors of chemotactic factors or cellular chemotactic receptors may impair directed migration of neutrophils. Patients may acquire a C5a deficiency due to SLE, glomerulonephritis, or chronic dialysis. C5 may also be dysfunctional in Leiner disease (characterized by diarrhea, failure to thrive, recurrent gram-negative bacterial infections, and seborrheic dermatitis). Patients have been described as having an intrinsic cellular defect and appearing to have inhibitors of chemotaxis. This may be due to immune complexes, or the inhibitors may be derived from normal lymphocytes that inhibit either monocytes or neutrophils such as in the Wiskott–Aldrich syndrome. A naturally occurring inhibitor in human serum (carboxypeptidase) converts C5a into an inactive form that has no chemotactic activity. Chemotactic factor inhibitors (CFI) have been found in patients with sarcoidosis, Hodgkin disease, leprosy, SLE, and cirrhosis.

2. **Cellular defects:** (Table 7) Hyperimmunoglobulinemia E (hyper-IgE) syndrome (Job syndrome). Defective chemotaxis has been described in patients with severe eczema associated with hyperimmunoglobulinemia E and recurrent skin infections, frequently resulting from secondary *Staphylococcus aureus*. These patients have musculoskeletal abnormalities and associated mucocutaneous candidiasis. Recurrent pulmonary infections with lung abscesses and bronchiectasis are frequent. Incubation of normal leukocytes with serum from patients with the hyper-IgE syndrome does not impair their function. Many other diseases have been associated with impaired chemotaxis (Table 7). The impaired chemotaxis seen in patients with the Cheédiak-Higashi syndrome and Kartagener syndrome no doubt contributes significantly to their recurrent infections.

Abnormal degranulation: Several patients have been described who have neutrophil specific-granule deficiency. These patients have an autosomal recessive pattern of inheritance. Their neutrophils have abnormal nuclear morphology, frequently bilobed with nuclear blebs, clefts, and pockets. Specific granule-deficient neutrophils lack visual granules on Wright's stain, although myeloperoxidase stain reveals peroxidase-positive granules. Alkaline phosphatase may also be low, with specific-granule constituents

Table 7. Cellular defects of chemotaxis

Job syndrome (hyper-IgE syndrome)
Chédiak-Higashi syndrome
Kartagener syndrome
Severe malnutrition
Graft-versus-host disease
Dermatitis (atopic, ichthyosis, acrodermatitis, enteropathica)
Diabetes mellitus
Actin dysfunction
Hyperalimentation
Associated with neutropenia-Schwachman-Diamond syndrome, lazy leukocyte
    syndrome
Newborn infants
Drugs (colchicine, Taxol)
Bone marrow transplant
Down syndrome
Myotonic dystrophy
Infections (viral, bacterial, fungal)
Peridontal disease
Hypophosphatemia with decreased cellular adenosine triphosphatase
Zinc deficiency
Malignancies
Uremia

such as lactoferrin, vitamin B_{12}-binding proteins, and cytochrome B either absent or markedly reduced. The primary (azurophilic) granules may also be abnormal. Following burns and in neonates, specific or secondary granules have been shown to be deficient. In addition to absolute deficiency of these granules, there may be functional abnormalities of specific-granule release mechanisms. Bactericidal activity is usually deficient in neutrophils with specific-granule deficiency, whereas phagocytosis is normal.

Disorders of phagocytosis and killing include the following:

1. **Opsonization and phagocytosis** (Table 8). Deficiency in opsonic factors has been demonstrated in newborns who have low IgM antibody titers or reduced factor B with a decrease in generation of alternative complement components. Congenital disorders have been described, such as a deficiency in the third component of complement

Table 8. Disorders of opsonization and phagocytosis

Opsonization	Phagocytosis
Newborns-decreased IgM and factor B	Bone marrow damage-acute leukemia, myeloproliferative disorders, and myelodysplasia
Complement deficiencies (C3, C5, abnormal C5a)	Associated with neutropenia
Immunoglobulin (IgG) deficiencies, Bruton's agammaglobulinemia, common-variable immunodeficiency	Tuftskin deficiency Leukocyte adhesion deficiency (types 1 and 2)
Multiple myeloma, chronic lymphocytic leukemia (CLL), non-Hodgkin lymphoma	Actin dysfunction-impaired chemotaxis and ingestion secondary to inadequate polymerization of monomeric actin
Chronic liver disease—cirrhosis	
Sickle cell anemia	

(C3) and Bruton agammaglobulinemia. Acquired disorders such as multiple myeloma, CLL, and non-Hodgkin lymphoma have defective opsonization due to hypogamma-globulinemia. A decrease in opsonization has been found in chronic liver disease and sickle cell anemia. Acquired defects in phagocytosis may be seen in patients with damaged bone marrows such as in acute leukemia or aplastic anemia or associated with neutropenia. Tuftsin, a tetrapeptide derived from IgG, stimulates phagocytosis. In a few families and following splenectomy, tuftsin has been decreased, leading to defective phagocytosis. Primary defects in phagocytosis are rare; common secondary causes include infections, drugs, alcohol, and systemic illness. Patients with leukocyte adhesion deficiency and actin dysfunction may also have complement defects resulting in impaired antibody-induced phagocytosis.

2. **Defects in granule formation and degranulation.** The most common abnormality of neutrophil granules is myeloperoxidase deficiency. The congenital form is an autosomal recessive disorder associated with complete absence of myeloperoxidase from the primary granules. This disorder has an incidence of about 28 patients per 60,000 subjects but usually is not associated with severe clinical disease. Increased susceptibility to *Candida albicans,* usually associated with other diseases, has been reported. Defective granulation has been reported in patients with acute leukemia. Deficiency of secondary or specific granules is associated with abnormal chemotaxis and deficient bactericidal activity. Congenital defects of specific granules (lactoferrin) have been described as well as an acquired defect occurring approximately 2 weeks following thermal injury. The Chédiak–Higashi syndrome is a rare disorder associated with giant lysosomes in all cells that contain lysozymes. These represent fusion of the primary and secondary granules as well as microtubules. Neutrophils from these patients kill normal numbers of bacteria but at a decreased rate.

3. **Disorders of oxygen metabolism. Chronic granulomatous disease of childhood (CGD)** is a rare disorder characterized by defective oxidative metabolism with inability to generate hydrogen peroxide. Patients have an increased incidence of infections with catalase-positive microorganisms that destroy their own hydrogen peroxide. Infections are usually due to *Staphylococcus aureus, Escherichia coli, Serratia marcescens,* and certain fungi but not with catalase-negative bacteria, such as *Streptococcus pneumoniae.* Extensive inflammatory reactions with granuloma formation and draining lesions, particularly in the lymph nodes of the neck and axilla, are common. Surgery is frequently required for abscesses, even in the lung and liver, as well as drainage for osteomyelitis. Apparently, patients are unable to activate NADPH oxidase, leading to a deficiency in O_2^-.

There are four genetic forms of CGD. Almost two thirds of cases are caused by an X-linked recessive defect encoding the larger subunit (gp91[phax]) of flavocytochrome[b]558. The second most common mutation is an autosomal recessive abnormality encoding p22[phax], the smaller subunit of flavocytochrome[b]558. Rare autosomal recessive genetic defects exist in p47[phax] or p67[phax]. Gene therapy is under active investigation, but it has yet to be successfully applied. In addition to the many other defects in newborns, fetal neutrophils frequently have reduced oxygen metabolism, which can contribute to defective bactericidal activity. Glucose-6-phosphate dehydrogenase (G6PD) deficiency, glutathione reductase or synthetase deficiency, and vitamin E deficiency have been associated with impaired bactericidal activity and frequent pyogenic infections.

Treatment of Neutrophil Dysfunction
These patients have functional neutropenia even though they have normal or even increased numbers of neutrophils, and they should be treated as though they had significant neutropenia (see the discussion of **disorders of phagocytosis and killing** in this section), depending on the amount of neutrophil dysfunction.

Patients who develop clinical signs of infection should have early cultures obtained and aggressive antibiotic administration empirically before the specific organism is identified. Early surgical drainage of abscesses is indicated. Prophylactic antibiotics have been beneficial in some patients with neutrophil dysfunction. Trimethoprim–sulfamethoxazole has been beneficial in patients with CGD. A trial of this drug is indicated for all patients with CGD, but if infections continue, the drug should be discontinued. Patients with hyper-IgE syndrome can be treated with low doses of penicillinase-resistant antibiotics such as dicloxacillin with some benefit. Although pharmacologic manipulation of neutrophil function has been attempted by the use of ascorbic acid, levamisole, and with lithium only anecdotal benefit has been shown. *In vitro* chemotactic responsiveness has been improved by using levamisole in hyper-IgE patients, but patients given the drug tended to have more serious infectious complications than those given placebo in a double-blind clinical trial.

Correcting deficiencies such as a decreased serum zinc or phosphate level is indicated when possible. Bone marrow transplantation has been used in congenital defects and probably will be used more often as complications of graft-versus-host disease are ameliorated by improved techniques.

Granulocyte transfusions may be indicated in patients who do not have an adequate response to antibiotics, but prophylactic granulocyte transfusions are not indicated. Granulocyte transfusions may benefit newborn infants with sepsis because of their decreased marrow reserve.

The mainstay of treatments remains careful observation for infection and early and aggressive administration of appropriate antibiotics. Primary prevention may be possible if the carrier state can be detected, such as with CGD and leukocyte adhesion defects. If the pregnant woman is willing to consider abortion as an option, secondary prevention using various techniques prenatally are available for CGD, Chédiak-Higashi anomaly, and the leukocyte adhesion defects. It is hoped that gene therapy will be available in the future to ameliorate some of these disorders.

Eosinophils
Characteristics of Eosinophils
Eosinophils resemble neutrophils because they are nondividing granule-containing cells that arise in the bone marrow, have a limited life span in the circulation, and play an important role in host defense. The bone marrow maturation time is approximately 2 to 6 days, and the circulation half-life is between 6 and 12 hours. Eosinophils are end-stage cells containing large intracytoplasmic granules that stain orange or red with Wright's stain. Under an electron microscope, they have a characteristic crystalline core surrounded by an electron-dense matrix bound by a double-layered membrane.

The specific granules of eosinophils contain major basic protein (MBP), which makes up about 50% of the core, eosinophil cationic protein (ECP), peroxidase, and an eosinophil-derived neurotoxin (EDN). **MBP,** which has cytotoxic properties, may damage the endocardium and disrupt the integrity of the endothelial cells in patients with asthma. **ECP** can activate Hageman factor (factor XII) and plasminogen, contributing to the thromboembolic phenomenon seen in patients with the hypereosinophilic syndrome. **Eosinophilic peroxidase** is immunologically, structurally, and biochemically different from the myeloperoxidase of neutrophils and in the presence of iodide and hydrogen peroxide (H_2O_2) may contribute to the helminthotoxicity of eosinophils. **EDN,** similar to ECP, is a markedly cationic protein that has been implicated in mediating nervous system dysfunction in humans and in rabbits can cause cerebrocerebellar dysfunction (the *Gordon phenomenon*). Eosinophils have small granules that contain a variety of **lysosomal enzymes,** which may act as mediators of inflammation as well as having other functions. **Lysophospholipase** is an enzyme present in the eosinophil membrane that crystallizes to form the characteristic Charcot–Leyden crystals that closely parallel the number of eosinophils in the tissues. Eosinophils have the capacity to generate leukotriene via the lipooxygenase pathway and prostaglandins via the cyclooxygenase pathway.

Eosinophil Production and Function
The eosinophil concentration of blood is usually less than 450 per milliliter. A diurnal variation causes concentrations to vary approximately twofold, with a reciprocal relationship to plasma cortisol levels. Eosinophil counts peak in the evening. The proliferation, maturation, and release of eosinophils from the bone marrow are stimulated by GM-CSF, IL-3, and IL-5.

Helper T-lymphocytes (CD4) produce IL-5, but eosinophils produce GM-CSF, IL-3, and IL-5, suggesting an autocrine–paracrine mechanism in the pathogenesis of some hypereosinophilia syndromes. Glucocorticoids can inhibit this response.

Eosinophils adhere to endothelial cells and migrate through spaces into tissues via adhesion molecules (integrins and selectins) expressed on their surface [CD11a/CD18, CD11b/CD18, vanillacetic acid-4 (VLA-4), L-selectin], and endothelial cell [intercellular adhesion molecule-1 (ICAM-1), ICAM-2, vascular adhesion molecule-1 (VCAM-1), E-selectin, P-selectin]. Lymphocyte chemoattractant factor, IL-2, GM-CSF, IL-3, and IL-5 are powerful chemoattractants that promote migration of eosinophils into tissues.

If the parasite is too large for ingestion and phagocytic activity, a secretory response occurs, and granules are released and deposited in the extracellular space that contribute to digestion of the parasite.

Eosinophilia

An elevated eosinophil count (>450/mL) may be primary or secondary to a variety of etiologies (Table 9). The etiology of the eosinophilia can be apparent following a routine history and physical examination. In some patients, however, an extensive evaluation for parasites, vasculitis, lymphoma, or solid tumors may be necessary (Table 9). Eosinophilia may be prominent in certain subtypes of acute myeloid leukemia, that is, acute myelomonocytic leukemia (M4) characterized by a typical inversion of chromosome 16 and associated with a good prognosis.

Acute eosinophilic leukemia is a rare disease. It can be distinguished from hypereosinophilic syndrome (HES) by the increased number of immature eosinophils in the blood or bone marrow, increased myeloblasts in the bone marrow, infiltration of involved organs with immature cells, severe anemia and thrombocytopenia, poor response to prednisone, central nervous system infiltration with eosinophils, myeloblastomas, and malignant course. Patients with HES may be difficult to distinguish from those with chronic myeloproliferative disorders, including CGL. Basophilia, myelofibrosis, cytogenetic abnormalities (especially the Philadelphia chromosome), erythrocyte and platelet abnormalities, and poor response to prednisone support the diagnosis of a chronic myeloproliferative disorder.

Hypereosinophilia with limited organ involvement, such as eosinophilic pneumonia (PIE syndrome) or eosinophilic gastroenteritis, is not associated with cardiac, central nervous system, or other organ dysfunction.

The Churg–Strauss syndrome, a necrotizing vasculitis of small arteries and veins associated with extravascular granulomas, may be difficult to distinguish from HES in some patients because vasculitis may occur with HES. Bronchial asthma, migratory pulmonary infiltrates, paranasal sinus involvement, peripheral neuropathy, or mononeuritis multiplex necessitate muscle or sural nerve biopsy to evaluate for the characteristic vasculitis of Churg–Strauss syndrome.

Eosinophilic cellulitis, fasciitis, and other skin disorders can be separated from HES by the results of skin biopsy. Eczema, psoriasis, and T-cell lymphoproliferative disorders associated with erythroderma and increased IL-5 often are accompanied by eosinophilia.

The eosinophilic–myalgia syndrome caused by contaminated tryptophan can be excluded by the patient's history. This syndrome is similar to the toxic oil syndrome reported from Spain in 1981, in which dimeric L-tryptophan (peak E) contaminated a batch of L-tryptophan.

Before embarking on an extensive evaluation, any drug that may be implicated in causing the eosinophilia should be stopped. A follow-up blood count should be performed 1 to 2 weeks after discontinuation of the drug.

If all causes of secondary eosinophilia can be excluded, HES should be considered. The three criteria essential for the diagnosis are (a) sustained eosinophilia, (b) organ dysfunction, and (c) exclusion of other etiologies. In HES, eosinophilia is usually greater than 1,500 per milliliter, persists for at least 6 months, and eventually results in organ dysfunction. Usually, the total WBC is less than 25,000 per milliliter, with 30% to 70% eosinophils, although this count may exceed 90,000 per milliliter. The eosinophils may exhibit atypical morphology at the light microscopic or at the ultrastructural level. A mild degree of immaturity may be present, but the number of myeloblasts is not increased.

The syndrome is more common in men 20 to 50 years of age and has a 50% mortality rate within 1 year if left untreated. Patients with severe eosinophilia with no evidence of organ dysfunction may never become symptomatic and do not need treatment.

Table 9. Secondary eosinophilia

Allergic disorders
  Asthma
  Allergic rhinitis
  Hay fever
  Drug reactions

Infection
  Parasites—tissue invasive
  Bacteria—scarlet fever and tuberculosis
  Chlamydia
  Mycoses—coccidioidomycosis

Skin disorders
  Eczema
  Psoriasis
  Dermatitis herpetiformis
  Pemphigus vulgaris
  Pityriasis rubra
  Eosinophilic cellulitis (Well syndrome)
  Eosinophilic fascitis

Collagen-vascular disorder
  Vasculitis
  Rheumatoid arthritis
  Systemic lupus erythematosus
  Scleroderma
  Dermatomyositis

Hepatitis—cholestatic

Neoplasia
  Hodgkin disease
  Cutaneous T-cell lymphoma, T-cell lymphoblastic lymphoma and adult and T-cell
    luekemia/lymphoma (HTLV-I, II)
  Luekemia-acute myeloid
  Myeloproliferative syndromes, including chronic granulocytic leukemia
  Solid tumors

Immunodeficiencies
  Wiskott-Aldrich syndrome
  Job syndrome (hyper-IgE syndrome)
  Graft-versus-host disease
  IgA deficiency
  Cyclic neutropenia

Endocrine disease
  Addison disease
  Hypopituitarism

Renal disease—interstitial nephritis

Miscellaneous—postsplenectomy, following marrow suppression or viral illness

---

Hyper-IgE, hyperimmunoglobulinemia E; IgA, immunoglobulin A.

Symptomatic patients present with fatigue (26%), myalgias or angioedema (14%), cough (24%), dyspnea (16%), rash and low-grade fever (12%), and retinal lesions (10%). Sweating, pruritus, alcohol intolerance with abdominal pain, flushing, nausea, and diarrhea may occur.

A variety of tissues may be damaged in patients with HES, resulting in significant morbidity and mortality. Weight loss and anorexia are infrequent. HES may occur in patients with AIDS and may be secondary to human T-cell leukemia virus, type II (HTLV-II) infection.

Cardiovascular lesions with involvement of the heart are seen in 54% to 73% of patients with HES. Necrosis of the ventricular wall and intramural coronary endothelia occur early, resulting in thrombi, frequently followed by embolic sequelae. Later fibrosis of the posterior leaflets of the mitral and tricuspid valves may occur, resulting in mitral or tricuspid regurgitation and signs of left- or right-sided heart failure. Two-dimensional echocardiography may demonstrate endocardial fibrosis, myocardial damage, and intramural thrombi. The classic features of HES or echocardiography are mural thrombus, ventricular apical obliteration, and involvement of the posterior mitral leaflet. Angiography or endocardial biopsy may be necessary to confirm the diagnosis. Patients may benefit from standard therapy for congestive heart failure, arrhythmia, and valve replacement when indicated.

Mild anemia is associated with HES about 50% of the time. The bone marrow is usually hypercellular and contains 25% to 75% eosinophils. Myelofibrosis is uncommon. Thrombocytopenia occurs in 31% of patients, and hypersplenism may contribute to the anemia and thrombocytopenia.

Pulmonary complications are common in patients with HES, with pleural effusions resulting from either heart failure or thromboembolic disease secondary to cardiac involvement. Approximately one third of patients with HES have diffuse or focal pulmonary infiltrates without the peripheral predominance seen in chronic eosinophilic pneumonia.

Neurologic complications are seen in approximately 35% to 73% of patients with HES. Central nervous system symptoms include confusion, delusions, psychoses, ataxia, slurred speech, and coma. These symptoms may be secondary to thromboembolic disease or primary manifestations of HES. Peripheral neuropathy is evident in 50% of patients and may be either a pure sensory, motor, or mixed variety. Mononeuritis multiplex and radiculopathy may occur.

Cutaneous lesions are found in more than 50% of cases of HES. Patients with urticarial lesions or angioedema, and elevated IgE may be sensitive to corticosteroid therapy. Papulonodular lesions and blistering skin lesions may be associated with vasculitis and HES. Mucocutaneous lesions with severe mucosal ulcerations may be independent of other manifestations of HES.

Renal complications of HES are relatively uncommon, but an abnormal urine sediment may be seen in approximately 20% of patients. An occasional patient may develop azotemia in the absence of congestive heart failure.

Hepatomegaly is a common finding in HES (>80%) but usually is related to cardiac dysfunction or congestive heart failure. Only a small portion (15%) of these patients have significant elevation of liver function tests with eosinophilic liver infiltration.

Immunologic and rheumatologic manifestations of HES include arthralgias, large joint effusions, Raynaud phenomenon, digital necrosis, and rarely focal myositis or polymyositis. Patients with an increased IgE level (38%) respond to prednisone and have a good prognosis.

Gastrointestinal manifestations, including eosinophilic gastritis, enterocolitis, or colitis may occur. **Splenomegaly** is frequent (40%), and splenic infarcts are common.

Treatment of Eosinophilia

1. **Secondary eosinophilia:** Patients who have a known cause of their eosinophilia should have the underlying disease treated (Table 9).

2. **HES:** Patients with HES who have no organ dysfunction or symptoms should not be treated but should be followed at 3- to 6-month intervals. When patients become **symptomatic, oral corticosteroids** (prednisone, 1 mg/kg daily) should be administered until clinical improvement occurs, followed by alternate-day prednisone. If improvement continues, the dosage should be decreased gradually. If **organ dysfunction** increases with or without an increase in the eosinophil count, **chemotherapy** with hydroxyurea, cyclophosphamide, vincristine, 6-mercaptopurine, busulfan, chlorambucil, or etoposide (VP-16-213) is indicated. Hydroxyurea, because of its low incidence of leukemogenic effects and convenience of oral administration, is frequently begun at a dose of 1 to 2 g daily. Vincristine (1–2 mg administered intravenously) may reduce high eosinophil counts within a few days and improve thrombocytopenia worsened by hydroxyurea or alkylating agents. Interferon-α (IFN-α) and cyclosporin-A have been used successfully

in some patients. Although leukapheresis may provide a transient benefit, it is not useful for long-term control. Patients who develop **thromboembolic phenomenon** should be anticoagulated in conjunction with the treatment of the underlying disease. If the disease cannot be controlled, prevention of further thromboembolic complications may be difficult. Patients who appear to have their disease in good control but are symptomatic with congestive heart failure and valvular dysfunction may benefit from surgical correction of the lesion. Studies have shown that survival increased from 20% to 80% at 5 years with the use of aggressive medical and surgical treatment.

Basophilia

Basophils are rarely increased but are considered abnormal when greater than 50 cells per milliliter. To ensure accuracy, the absolute basophil count should be obtained by a direct basophil count. This is rarely necessary, however. Blood basophils can be mildly increased in certain allergic disorders, but the presence of basophilia is of practical value only in defining the myeloproliferative disorders and basophilic leukemia. Persistent basophilia may suggest the diagnosis of a myeloproliferative disease, and further evaluation is indicated. Symptoms of hyperhistaminemia indicate an increased turnover of basophils and may indicate a more accelerated phase of the myeloproliferative disease in the bone marrow before basophils increase in the peripheral blood. Some patients with CGL develop increasing numbers of basophils as the first manifestation of the accelerated phase or early blast crisis.

Mastocytosis

Mast cells and basophils are derived from CD34-positive hematopoietic stem cells, as are all the other hematopoietic cells. The most common form of mastocytosis is urticaria pigmentosa, characterized by patchy or widespread brownish, pigmented, flat or raised skin nodules densely infiltrated with mast cells. Trauma to the involved skin can produce urticaria or dermographism (Darier's sign) due to liberation of histamine from mast cells.

Frequently, a benign or transient disease of childhood, mastocytosis, can evolve into a systemic and progressive disease. When this occurs, mast cells may infiltrate multiple organs and tissues and produce locally destructive or fibrotic changes. Patients with an accelerated phase of the disease develop osteosclerotic changes and resemble patients with acute or subacute granulocytic leukemia.

Symptoms include episodes of erythematous flushing, urticaria, edema, pruritus, headache, hypotension, abdominal pain, and gastrointestinal symptoms, which may be precipitated by exposure to cold or use of alcohol or may occur secondary to fever. These vascular reactions appear to relate to the release of histamine from mast cells.

Treatment is as follows:

1. Patients who have symptoms related to excessive histamine release may benefit by agents that inhibit H_1 or H_2 receptors such as diphenhydramine, cimetidine, or others.
2. Cromolyn sodium, 200 mg four times a day by mouth or inhaled (Intal inhaler) may alleviate symptoms.
3. Low-dose prednisone may be helpful.
4. In acute and chronic myeloproliferative disorders, chemotherapy and radiation therapy may be effective in alleviating symptoms.
5. In systemic mastocytosis, IFN-α has been reported to be effective.

Suggested Readings

Adams DH, Shaw S. Leucocyte-endothelial interactions and regulation of leucocyte migration. *Lancet* 1994;343:831.

Altieri DC. Coagulation assembly on leukocytes in transmembrane signaling and cell adhesion. *Blood* 1993;81:569.

Alvir JMJ, Lieberman JA, Safferman AZ, et al. Clozapine-induced agranulocytosis. Incidence and risk factors in the United States. *N Engl J Med* 1993;329:162.

Anderson R. The immunostimulatory, anti-inflammatory and anti-allergic properties of ascorbate. *Adv Nutr Res* 1984;6:19.

Assa'ad AH, Spicer RL, Nelson DP, et al. Hypereosinophilic syndromes. *Chem Immunol* 2000;76:208.

Babior BM. Phagocytes and oxidative stress. *Am J Med* 2000;109:33.

Bain BJ. Eosinophilia—idiopathic or not? *N Engl J Med* 1999;341:1141.

Bain BJ. Hypereosinophilia. *Curr Opin Hematol* 2000;7:21.

Becker DJ, Lowe JB. Leukocyte adhesion deficiency type II. *Biochim Biophys Acta* 1999;1455:193.

Bonilla MA, Gillio AP, Ruggeiro M, et al. Effects of recombinant human granulocyte colony-stimulating factor on neutropenia in patients with congenital agranulocytosis. *N Engl J Med* 1989;320:1574.

Bowers TK, Eckert E. Leukopenia in anorexia nervosa: lack of increased risk of infection. *Arch Intern Med* 1978;138:1520.

Brown AE. Neutropenia, fever and infection. *Am J Med* 1984;76:421.

Butcher S, Chahel H, Lord JM. Ageing and the neutrophil: no appetite for killing? *Immunology* 2000;100:411.

Chan WC, Winton EF, Waldmann TA. Lymphocytosis of large granular lymphocytes. *Arch Intern Med* 1986;146:1201.

Chan WC, Gu LB, Masih A, et al. Large granular lymphocyte proliferation with the natural killer-cell phenotype. *Am J Clin Pathol* 1992;97:353.

Clark RA. The human neutrophil respiratory burst oxidase. *J Infect Dis* 1990;161:1140.

Corre F, Lellouch J, Schwartz D. Smoking and leucocyte counts. *Lancet* 1971;2:632.

Corssmit EPM, Trip MD, Durrer JD. Löffler's endomyocarditis in the idiopathic hypereosinophilic syndrome. *Cardiology* 1999;91:272.

Costa JJ, Weller PF, Galli SJ. The cells of allergic response: mast cells, basophils and eosinophils. *JAMA* 1997;278:1815.

Dale DC, et al. Comparison of agents producing a neutrophilic leukocytosis in man. *J Clin Invest* 1975;56:808.

Dale DC, et al. A randomized controlled phase III trial of recombinant human granulocyte colony-stimulating factor (Filgrastim) for treatment of severe chronic neutropenia. *Blood* 1993;81:2496.

Dale DC, Person RE, Bolyard AA, et al. Mutations in the gene encoding neutrophil elastase in congenital and cyclic neutropenia. *Blood* 2000;96:2317.

Denburg JA. Basophil and mast cell lineages *in vitro* and *in vivo*. *Blood* 1992;79:46.

Etzioni A, Frydman M, Pollack S, et al. Brief report: recurrent severe infections caused by a novel leukocyte adhesion deficiency. *N Engl J Med* 1992;327:1789.

Fauci AS, Harley JB, Roberts WC, et al. The idiopathic hypereosinophilic syndrome. *Ann Intern Med* 1982;97:78.

Friedenberg WR, Marx JJ, Hansen RL, et al. Hyperimmunoglobulin E syndrome: response to transfer factor and ascorbic acid therapy. *Clin Immunol Immunopathol* 1979;102:132.

Friedman GD, et al. Smoking habits and the leukocyte count. *Arch Environ Health* 21983;26:137.

Frigas E, Gleich GJ. The eosinophil and the pathophysiology of asthma. *J Allergy Clin Immunol* 1986;77:527.

Gallin JI. Leukocyte adherence-related glycoproteins LFA-1, Mol, and p150,95: a new group of monoclonal antibodies, a new disease and a possible opportunity to understand the molecular basis of leukocyte adherence. *J Infect Dis* 1985;152:661.

Gallin JI. Neutrophil specific granule deficiency. *Am Rev Med* 1985;36:263.

Gerson SL, Lieberman JA, Friedenberg WR, et al. Polypharmacy in fatal clozapine-associated agranulocytosis. *Lancet* 1991;2:262.

Gillio AP, Gabrilove JL. Cytokine treatment of inherited bone marrow failure syndromes. *Blood* 1993;81:1669.

Gleich GJ. Eosinophils, basophils, and mast cells. *J Allergy Clin Immunol* 1989;84:1024.

Gleich GJ, Leogering DA. Immunobiology of eosinophils. *Am Rev Immunol* 1984;2:429.

Haddy TB, Rana SR, Castro O. Benign ethnic neutropenia: what is a normal absolute neutrophil count? *J Lab Clin Med* 1999;133:15.

Hammond WP, Chatta WP, Chatta GS, et al. Abnormal responsiveness of granulocyte-committed progenitor cells in cyclic neutropenia. *Blood* 1992;79:2536.

Heinzelmann M, Mercer-Jones MA, Passmore JC. Neutrophils and renal failure. *Am J Kidney Dis* 1999;34:384.

Heit W, Heimpel H, Fischer A, et al. Drug-induced agranulocytosis: evidence for the commitment of bone marrow haematopoiesis. *Scand J Haematol* 1985;35:459.

Hetherington SV, Quie PG. Human polymorphonuclear leukocytes of the bone marrow, circulation and marginated pool: function and granule protein content. *Am J Hematol* 1985;20:235.

Iwakiri R, Inokuchi K, Dan K, et al. Marked basophilia in acute promyelocytic leukaemia treated with all-trans retinoic acid: molecular analysis of the cell origin of the basophils. *Br J Heamatol* 1994;86:870.

Kay AB. Biological properties of eosinophils. *Clin Exp Allergy* 1991;21:23.

Kay AB. Eosinophils as effector cells in immunity and hypersensitivity disorders. *Clin Exp Immunol* 1985;62:1.

Kluin-Nelemans HC, Jansen JH, Breukelman H, et al. Response to interferon a-2b in a patient with systemic mastocytosis. *N Engl J Med* 1992;326:619.

Kume A, Dinauer M. Gene therapy for chronic granulomatous disease. *J Lab Clin Med* 2000;135:122.

Kuritzkes DR. Neutropenia, neutrophil dysfunction, and bacterial infection in patients with human immunodeficiency virus disease: the role of granulocyte colony-stimulating factor. *Clin Infect Dis* 2000;30:256.

Kyle RA. Natural history of chronic idiopathic neutropenia. *N Engl J Med.* 1980;302:908.

Loughran TP Jr. Clonal diseases of large granular lymphocytes. *Blood* 1993;82:1.

Malech HL. Phagocyte oxidative mechanisms. *Curr Opin Hematol* 1994;19:123.

McEwen BJ. Eosinophils: a review. *Vet Res Commun* 1992;16:11.

Meuleman J, Katz P. The immunologic effects, kinetics and use of glucocorticosteroids. *Med Clin North Am* 1985;69:806.

Milbrandt EB, Byron W Jr, Davis B. Progressive infiltrates and eosinophilia with multiple possible causes. *Chest* 2000;118:230.

Ommen SR, Seward JB, Tajik AJ. Clinical and echocardiographic features of hypereosinophilic syndromes. *Am J Cardiol* 2000;86:110.

Pallister CJ, Lewis RJ. Effects of antimicrobial drugs on human neutrophil-microbe interactions. *Br J Biomed Sci* 2000;57:19.

Parulkar VG, Balsubramaniam P, Barua MJ, et al. Smoking and differential leucocyte (WBC) count. *J Postgrad Med* 1974;21:75.

Pisciotta AV, Konings SA, Ciesemier LL, et al. On the possible mechanisms and predictability of clozapine-induced agranulocytosis. *Drug Safety* 1992;7:33.

Pitrak DL. Neutrophil deficiency and dysfunction in HIV-infected patients. *Am J Health Syst Pharm* 1999;56:S9.

Pizzo PA, Hathorn JW, Hiemenz J. A randomized trial comparing ceftazidime alone with combination antibiotic therapy in cancer patients with fever and neutropenia. *N Engl J Med* 1986;315:552.

Potter MB, Fincher RK, Finger DR. Eosinophilia in Wegener's granulomatosis. *Chest* 1999;116:1480.

Quie PG. Phagocytic cell dysfunction. *J Allergy Clin Immunol* 1986;77:387.

Robbins SH, Conly MA, Oettinger J. Cold-induced granulocyte agglutination. *Arch Pathol Lab Med* 1991;15:155.

Roberts R, Gallin JI. The phagocytic cell and its disorders. *Ann Allergy* 1983;51:330.

Rohr LR, Rivers FM. Spurious automated leukopenia due to *in vitro* granulocyte aggregation. *Am J Clin Pathol* 1990;93:572.

Russof AH, Robinson WA, eds. Lithium effects on granulopoiesis and immune function. *Adv Exp Med Biol* 1980;27.

Sanderson CJ. Interleukin-5, eosinophils, and disease. *Blood* 1992;79:3101.

Schmidt K, Moser U. Vitamin C—a modulator of host defense mechanism, an overview. *Int J Vitam Nutr Res* 1985;27:363.

Schroeder JT, MacGlashan DW Jr. New concepts: the basophil. *J Allergy Clin Immunol* 1997;99:429.

Shastri KA, Logue GL. Autoimmune neutropenia. *Blood* 1993;81:1984.

Simon H, Plotz SG, Dummer R, et al. Abnormal clones of T cells producing interleukin 5 in idiopathic eosinophilia. *N Engl J Med* 1999;341:1112.

Snyderman R, Pike MC. Chemoattractant receptors on phagocytic cells. *Annu Rev Immunol* 1984;2:257.

Spry CJF. New properties and roles for eosinophils in disease: discussion paper. *J R Soc Med* 1985;78:844.

Strauss RG. Therapeutic granulocyte transfusions in 1993. *Blood* 1993;81:1675.

Thompson EI, Callihan TR, Mauer AM, et al. Prophylaxis in severe granulocytopenia. *Adv Intern Med* 1984;29:193.

Valent P, Bettelheim P. The human basophil. *Crit Rev Oncol Hematol* 1990;10:327.

Wallis WJ, Loughran TP, Jr., Kadin ME, et al. Polyarthritis and neutropenia associated with circulating large granular lymphocytes. *Ann Intern Med* 1985;103:357.

Walsh TJ, Finberg RW, Arndt C, et al. Liposomal amphotericin B for empirical therapy in patients with persistent fever and neutropenia. *N Engl J Med* 1999;340:764.

Weller PF. The immunobiology of eosinophils. *N Engl J Med* 324: 1110, 1991

Weller PF, Bubley GJ. The idiopathic hypereosinophilic syndrome. *Blood* 1994;83:2759.

Williams WJ, et al. *Hematology,* 3rd ed. New York: McGraw-Hill, 1983.

Wolach B, Baehner RL, Boxer LA. Review: clinical and laboratory approach to the management of neutrophil dysfunction. *Isr J Med Sci* 1982;18:897.

Yang KD, Hill HR. Neutrophil function disorders: pathophysiology, prevention, and therapy. *J Pediatr* 1991;119:343.

Yoon TY, Ahn GB, Chang SH. Complete remission of hypereosinophilic syndrome after interferon-α therapy: report of a case and literature review. *J Dermatol* 2000;7:110.

8. PLATELET DISORDERS: HEREDITARY AND ACQUIRED

Scott Murphy and A. Koneti Rao

Platelet Kinetics and Physiology

Platelets are produced as enucleate fragments of the cytoplasm of a giant cell in the bone marrow, the *megakaryocyte*. These cells are greatly outnumbered by myeloid and erythroid precursors, but their large size and characteristic morphology make them easy to identify. Once released, each platelet has the capacity to circulate for slightly more than 10 days, but because approximately 15% of the cells are used daily in ongoing hemostasis, actual mean platelet survival is 8 to 10 days. The normal platelet count, 150,000–400,000 per microliter, reflects a balance between production and destruction. In fact, it underestimates the total body platelet mass because one third of this mass is continuously sequestered in a pool of platelets in the spleen involved in free interchange with the circulation. This splenic pool provides a significant, although small, reserve at the time of massive hemorrhage.

Platelet Physiology
Following injury to the blood vessel, platelets adhere to exposed subendothelium by a process (*adhesion*) that involves the interaction of a plasma protein, von Willebrand factor (vWF), and a specific glycoprotein complex on the platelet surface, glycoproteins Ib-V-IX (GPIb-V-IX) (Fig. 1).

Adhesion is followed by recruitment of additional platelets, which form clumps, a process called *aggregation (cohesion)*. This process involves binding of fibrinogen to specific platelet surface receptors—a complex composed of glycoproteins IIb-IIIa (GPIIb-IIIa).

Activated platelets release the contents of their granules (secretion or release reaction), such as adenosine diphosphate (ADP) and serotonin from the dense granules, which cause recruitment of additional platelets. In addition, platelets play a major role in coagulation mechanisms; several key enzymatic reactions occur on the platelet membrane lipoprotein surface.

Numerous physiologic agonists interact with specific receptors on the platelet surface to induce responses, including a change in platelet shape from discoid to spherical (*shape change*), aggregation, secretion, and thromboxane A_2 (TxA_2) production. Other agonists, such as prostacyclin, inhibit these responses.

Ligation of the platelet receptors initiates the production or release of several intracellular messenger molecules, including Ca^{2+} ions, products of phosphoinositide (PI) hydrolysis by phospholipase C [diacylglycerol (DG), and inositol 1,4,5-triphosphate (InsP_3)], TxA_2, and cyclic nucleotides (cAMP)(Fig. 1). These induce or modulate the various platelet responses of Ca^{2+} mobilization, protein phosphorylation, aggregation, secretion, and liberation of arachidonic acid.

The interaction between the agonist receptors and the key intracellular effector enzymes (e.g., phospholipases A_2 and C, adenylyl cyclase) is mediated by a group of guanosine triphosphate (GTP)-binding proteins. As in most secretory cells, platelet activation results in a rise in cytoplasmic ionized calcium concentration; InsP_3 functions as a messenger to mobilize Ca^{2+} from intracellular stores. DG activates protein kinase C (PKC), and this results in the phosphorylation of a 47-kDa protein, pleckstrin. PKC activation is considered to play a major role in platelet secretion and in the activation of GPIIb-IIIa.

Another response to activation is the release from membrane phospholipids of free arachidonic acid, which is converted by cyclooxygenase to prostaglandins G_2 and H_2 and subsequently to TxA_2 by thromboxane synthetase. Numerous other mechanisms, such as activation of tyrosine kinases and phosphatases, also are triggered by platelet activation. Inherited or acquired defects in the above platelet mechanisms may lead to an impaired platelet role in hemostasis.

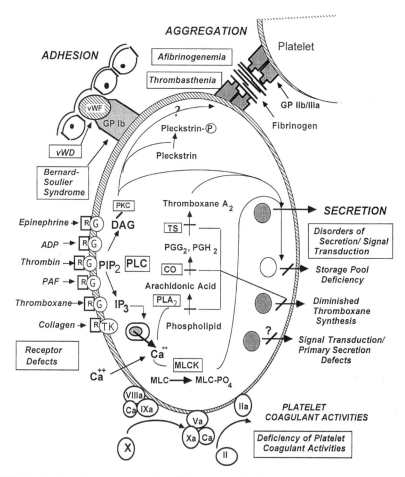

FIG. 1. A schematic representation of the normal platelet responses and the congenital disorders of platelet function. CO, cyclooxygenase; DAG, diacylglycerol; IP$_3$, inositoltrisphosphate; MLC, myosin light chain; MLCK, myosin light chain kinase; PIP$_2$, phosphatidylinositol bisphosphate; PKC, protein kinase C; PLC, phospholipase C; PLA$_2$, phospholipase A$_2$; TS, thromboxane syndrome; vWF, von Willebrand factor; vWD, von Willebrand disease.

Polymorphisms of platelet membrane glycoproteins are responsible for human platelet antigens (HPAs), which may result in alloantibody formation during pregnancy or after transfusion. The most important is HPA-1 (Pl^{A1}) due to a polymorphism on GPIIIa.

General Clinical Considerations

Platelets form aggregates at the site of blood vessel injury and are thus responsible for the primary arrest of bleeding. Abnormalities of their number (either too low or too high) or function may result in easy bruising, epistaxis, menorrhagia, bleeding from the gastrointestinal tract, and prolonged and excessive bleeding after surgery or dental work. With severe deficiencies, there may be spontaneous bleeding into the central nervous system and the urinary tract. All these manifestations may be produced by abnormalities of the plasma coagulation system as well, and these must be considered in the differential diagnosis. Patients with severe thrombocytopenia may develop the more specific manifestations of petechiae and coalescent petechiae referred to as purpura in the skin of dependent portions of the body. These are seen only rarely in patients with thrombocytosis, disorders of platelet function, or plasma coagulation; however, they may form in patients with small-vessel vasculitis and no platelet abnormality. Finally, some hemorrhagic manifestations, such as hemarthrosis, are seen only with coagulation factor disorders and not with platelet disorders. In this chapter, three major categories of disease are considered: thrombocytopenia, thrombocytosis, and disorders of platelet function.

Thrombocytopenia

The lower limit of the platelet count is generally considered to be 150,000 per microliter. Unless there is associated platelet dysfunction, few clinical manifestations occur in the range of 50,000 to 150,000 per microliter. Minor spontaneous bleeding and bleeding after surgery are seen in the range 20,000 to 50,000 per microliter, with more serious bleeding occurring as the platelet count falls below 20,000 per microliter. It should be remembered that cell counters report thrombocytopenia that is spurious in about 0.1% of patients. This is generally due to platelet clumping after drawing blood into the anticoagulant ethylenediaminetetraacetic acid. This can be confirmed by identifying platelet aggregates on blood smears and by testing the blood specimen immediately after phlebotomy. The classification of thrombocytopenic states is based on platelet kinetics: accelerated platelet destruction, impaired platelet production, and disorder of distribution (*hypersplenism*).

Accelerated Platelet Destruction

In contrast to patients who have the other two classes of thrombocytopenia, patients with accelerated platelet destruction generally have no abnormalities of leukocytes, erythrocytes, and bone marrow and have no splenomegaly. Accelerated platelet destruction as an isolated phenomenon is seen in idiopathic thrombocytopenic purpura (ITP). Other conditions mimic ITP, and it is useful to recognize and think in terms of the clinical picture of ITP. Once this is done, one must proceed with a clinical differential diagnosis as outlined in Table 1 because there are, with a few exceptions, no specific tests that separate these entities.

In **true ITP,** accelerated platelet destruction, predominantly in the spleen, is produced after sensitization of platelets by an autoantibody, which also may impair platelet production and function. In childhood, the disease usually presents acutely and runs a self-limited course in 3 to 6 months. This picture may be seen in adults, but a gradual onset is more common, and spontaneous remission occurs in only 10% to 15% of patients. In adults, it has long been thought that women in the childbearing years are most commonly affected, but the disease may occur in both sexes and all age groups. The patient has clinical manifestations of thrombocytopenia, no systemic toxicity, no enlargement of nodes or abdominal organs, normal blood count and smear except for thrombocytopenia, and normal bone marrow examination. Tests for antiplatelet antibody are of limited use.

Therapy for patients with platelet counts less than 30,000 per microliter traditionally has begun with corticosteroids, that is, prednisone at 1 mg per kilogram of body weight daily for platelet counts in the range of 10,000 to 30,000 per microliter without serious bleeding. For more severe thrombocytopenia and bleeding, 2 mg per kilogram of body weight can be used, along with gamma globulin administered intravenously, 1.0 g per kilogram of body weight is given each day for 2 days. In most treated patients, the platelet count rises in 2 to 7 days. Steroids then can be tapered to maintain the platelet count over 30,000 per microliter. If the dose of steroids is not excessive, they can be continued for 3 months to allow those patients who have spontaneous remission to do so. Splenectomy should be performed if steroids still are required after 3 months. If the patient does not respond to prednisone and gamma globulin within 2 weeks, splenectomy should be considered. Intravenous Rh(D) immune globulin (WinRho) is a new option for these patients if they are Rh(D) positive.

Table 1. Differential diagnosis of idiopathic thrombocytopenic purpura (ITP) and accelerated platelet destruction

Immunologic disorders	Nonimmunologic disorders	Useful studies
True ITP	Disseminated intra-	Blood studies
Drug-induced	vascular coagulation	Antinuclear antibody
Systemic lupus	Bacterial septicemia	HIV antibody
erythematosus	TTP-HUS	Fibrinogen
Lymphoproliferative	Ethanol-induced	Prothrombin time
disease	Massive blood loss	Partial thromboplastin time
HIV-1 associated	Hereditary conditions	Fibrinogen degradation
Posttransfusion		products
purpura		Blood culture
Sarcoidosis		Serum protein electrophoresis
Solid tumors		Other studies
Mononucleosis		Bone marrow aspiration and
Immunodeficiency		biopsy
Post marrow		Liver, spleen, and retroperito-
transplant		neal ultrasound or CT scan

CT, computed tomography; HIV-1, human immunodeficiency virus; TTP-HUS, thrombotic thrombocytopenic purpura and hemolytic uremic syndrome.

In some patients, 50 to 75 mg per kilogram of body weight given every few weeks, can raise the platelet count to safe levels, thus sparing the patient from the side effects of steroids and the need for splenectomy.

Therapy for patients with platelet counts greater than 30,000 per microliter: These patients generally have few symptoms, remain stable over many years, and do not require splenectomy or chronic therapy. Brief courses of prednisone may be used to raise the platelet count for dental work and surgery.

Splenectomy: If the patient responds to prednisone, a large enough dose should be given preoperatively to raise the platelet count to more than 50,000 per microliter. If the patient does not respond to steroids, gamma globulin or WinRho IV may be used. If the patient fails to respond to either of these measures, a platelet transfusion may be given at the time of intubation for anesthesia. These recommendations are perhaps overly conservative because an experienced surgeon often can perform extensive surgery, even in patients with severe thrombocytopenia, with only minor hemorrhage if the tissues are not inflamed or highly vascular. This is the situation in most splenectomies. Vaccination against encapsulated bacteria should be given prior to splenectomy. Splenic irradiation has produced remissions in patients with contraindications to surgery.

Splenectomy failures: After splenectomy, 50% of patients have a complete and permanent remission, whereas another 30% have an elevation of platelet count to the range of 30,000 to 150,000 per microliter, and the recommendations in the discussion of **therapy for true ITP** can be followed. Many of the remaining 20% of patients have platelet counts in the range of 10,000 to 30,000 per microliter. They may have few symptoms. These patients generally do not need chronic therapy, particularly considering the potential for long-term toxicity from therapies commonly used. Various therapies are available for the few patients who have severe thrombocytopenia and hemorrhage after splenectomy (Table 2).

The most reliable agents for obtaining an immediate, but generally transient, response are intravenous gamma globulin and vincristine. WinRho appears to be ineffective after splenectomy. Platelet transfusions may raise the platelet count immediately, but the count generally returns to baseline 24 hours later. Danazol azathioprine, cyclophosphamide, and a variety of other agents have been listed as effective in these cases. Combinations of parenteral chemotherapeutic agents have been recommended for severely affected patients.

Table 2. Therapy of ITP refractory to splenectomy and corticosteroids

Drug	Dosage
Intravenous gamma globulin	1.0 g/kg i.v. daily for 2 days
Vincristine	2 mg i.v. weekly for 3 doses
Danazol	200 mg p.o. q.i.d.
Azathioprine	2 mg/kg/day p.o.
Cyclophosphamide	2 mg/kg/day p.o. or 1.0–1.5 g i.v. every 3–4 wk
Combination chemotherapy	

ITP, idiopathic thrombocytopenic purpura; i.v., intravenous(ly); p.o., orally; q.i.d., four times daily.

Pregnancy: Circulating antiplatelet immunoglobulin G (IgG) is capable of crossing the placenta and producing neonatal thrombocytopenia. This is more common if the mother is thrombocytopenic at the time of delivery, but it may be seen after splenectomy or drug therapy has produced a remission in the mother. Some researchers believe the risk for serious bleeding in these newborns is very low, less than diagnostic or therapeutic interventions. Therefore, routine obstetric management should be used. Others are concerned that an occasional fetus will be severely thrombocytopenic and recommend percutaneous umbilical blood sampling to determine whether cesarean section is indicated to prevent fetal hemorrhage during vaginal delivery. It should be remembered that normal women may develop modest, apparently nonimmune thrombocytopenia (75,000/μL) as pregnancy progresses; the infants are not at risk for thrombocytopenia.

Immunologic disorders associated with the ITP clinical picture include the following:

When a patient presents with the clinical picture of ITP, any **drug** that the patient is using should be considered as a possible cause. If possible, such a drug should be stopped or replaced.

Quinidine and quinine, the sulfonamides, gold compounds, and heparin are the major offenders. For quinidine or quinine and sulfonamides, the diagnosis is generally confirmed by rapid improvement of the platelet count after drug withdrawal. In patients with gold-induced thrombocytopenia, gold and gold-related antibodies cannot be demonstrated in the plasma or associated with circulating platelets; apparently, however, gold induces an autoimmune state that responds to the measures used in treatment of true ITP. Steroids usually produce a prompt improvement that can be maintained until permanent remission occurs, generally in 6 to 12 months.

About 1% to 5% of patients who receive unfractionated heparin develop IgG antibodies against a complex of heparin and platelet factor 4. A subset of these patients will develop thrombocytopenia 5 to 14 days after the initiation of heparin therapy. A subset of the thrombocytopenic patients will develop life- and limb-threatening arterial and venous thrombosis. Sensitive assays are available to detect these antibodies, and heparin should be stopped in patients who develop thrombocytopenia. The risk for thrombosis remains high, however, and it is recommended that anticoagulation with recombinant hirudin (Lepirudin), argatroban, or Danaparoid, (but not warfarin or low-molecular-weight heparin) be administered.

Acute thrombocytopenia occurs in about 1% of patients treated with the humanized monoclonal antibody to GPIIb-IIIa, abciximab (ReoPro), and other GPIIb-IIIa inhibitors. The mechanism is believed to be immunological. Recovery occurs promptly when the drug is discontinued.

ITP picture associated with underlying illness: The clinical picture of ITP can occur in patients with systemic lupus erythematosus (SLE), Hodgkin disease, chronic lymphocytic leukemia, non-Hodgkin lymphoma, and a variety of infections. Because enlargement of the spleen or lymph nodes is not part of true ITP, such enlargement suggests occult SLE, or lymphoma in a patient who appears to have true ITP. The mechanism is believed to be immunologic, and the response to steroids and splenectomy is similar to the response in true ITP. Thus, one can use the same therapeutic approach to thrombocytopenia as in true ITP. The clinical picture of ITP, apparently on an immunologic basis, is also seen in sarcoidosis, solid tumors, mononucleosis, common variable immunodeficiency, and following allogeneic bone marrow transplantation.

Infection with human immunodeficiency virus (HIV): Patients with the acquired immunodeficiency syndrome (AIDS) and persons with HIV infection have an increased incidence of the clinical picture of ITP. Thus, the anti-HIV antibody test should be done in a patient with the clinical picture of ITP who is at risk for this infection. The initial treatment should be antiretroviral therapy for HIV, which is usually followed by an increase in platelet count. In addition, these patients respond to therapy with corticosteroids, intravenous gamma globulin, and splenectomy. These measures can be used in more severely affected patients who do not respond to antiretroviral therapy.

Posttransfusion purpura is a rare clinical syndrome in which marked thrombocytopenia occurs 5 to 10 days after a routine red cell transfusion. Most patients are women, and all have been previously pregnant or transfused. It is generally easy to demonstrate an antiplatelet antibody in their serum. In most patients, the antibody is specific for the platelet antigen HPA-1a (Pl^{A1}), and, on recovery (usually spontaneous in 10 days to 2 months), the patient's platelets lack HPA-1a (Pl^{A1}) antigen. Because 98% of the population are positive for HPA-1a (Pl^{A1}), demonstration of antibody with this specificity establishes the diagnosis. It is not known how the alloimmune reaction mediates destruction of the patient's antigen-negative platelets. Life-threatening bleeding occurs with some frequency. Therapy should be begun with intravenous gamma globulin as previously described. Plasmapheresis (exchange of 40 ml/kg of body weight daily) may be added in cases refractory to gamma globulin.

Nonimmunologic disorders that mimic true ITP include the following:

1. **Disseminated intravascular coagulation (DIC) and sepsis.** DIC results from activation of coagulation in the vascular tree. Accelerated platelet consumption is almost always seen. DIC can be distinguished from immune thrombocytopenia by finding prolongation of the prothrombin and partial thromboplastin times, decreased plasma fibrinogen, and elevated plasma fibrin–fibrinogen split products. DIC can be seen with infections (e.g., viral, Rickettsial, bacterial, malarial infections); obstetric catastrophes (abruptio placentae and the retained dead fetus syndrome); malignancies; trauma; and vascular abnormalities such as giant hemangiomas and aortic aneurysms. Generally, the cause is obvious, and treatment should be directed toward correcting the underlying cause. Support with plasma and platelet transfusions may be required for bleeding complications until the cause has been corrected. In some bacterial infections, there may be accelerated platelet destruction and lowering of the platelet count, even to the range of 20,000 to 30,0000 per microliter, without major abnormalities of plasma coagulation factors. The thrombocytopenia gradually resolves as the infection is controlled.

2. **Thrombotic thrombocytopenic purpura (TTP)** and **hemolytic uremic syndrome (HUS):** TTP is a clinical syndrome that probably is caused in most patients by endothelial damage in microscopic blood vessels, resulting in microscopic thrombi. These thrombi are composed primarily of platelets that are rapidly consumed by the process. It has been proposed that antibody-mediated deficiency of a vWF-cleaving protease may allow the accumulation of large vWF multimers, which facilitate platelet agglutination. The disease usually has a fulminant or subacute onset. The following findings are seen in various combinations: thrombocytopenia with normal or increased megakaryocytes in the marrow; microangiopathic hemolytic anemia characterized by marked red cell poikilocytosis on the peripheral blood smear (e.g., fragments, helmet cells, burr cells) and elevated serum lactate dehydrogenase (LDH); fluctuating central nervous system deficits consistent with intermittent ischemia; renal failure; and fever. In adults, it is likely that HUS and TTP are similar, if not identical, illnesses with prominent renal failure in the former. The TTP–HUS syndrome may be idiopathic or associated with (a) drugs such as quinidine, ticlopidine, clopidogrel, mitomycin C, and cyclosporine; (b) allogeneic bone marrow transplantation; (c) HIV infection; and (d) pregnancy and the postpartum period. A related illness, seen at the end of a pregnancy

complicated by preeclampsia or eclampsia, is the HELLP syndrome, characterized by hemolysis with poikilocytosis, elevated liver enzymes (including LDH), and low platelet count. Most of these patients recover spontaneously after delivery, but some with persistent disease are treated in the same way as the TTP–HUS syndrome is treated. Initial therapy is plasma exchange (removal of 40 mL/kg of body weight and replacement with an equal volume of fresh frozen plasma). This treatment should be performed daily until the platelet count has risen to more than 100,000 per microliter, and there is clear evidence for a fall in LDH, reflecting improvement in hemolysis. Once improvement has occurred, the frequency of plasma exchange should be gradually reduced over 1 to 2 weeks. The course of the disease is variable, but the most patients obtain and maintain a remission with treatment. Plasmapheresis should be reinstituted promptly if any of the features of the disease recur. Splenectomy is effective for the minority of patients who respond suboptimally to plasma exchange or who continue to require it after 4 to 6 weeks.

3. **Ethanol-induced thrombocytopenia:** "Binge" drinkers may develop severe thrombocytopenia with platelet counts in the range of 10,000 to 20,000 per microliter because of direct suppression of platelet production and shortening of platelet life span by ethanol. Megakaryocytes are present in the marrow. Usually, the platelet count begins to rise as soon as alcohol is withdrawn and becomes normal within 5 to 10 days.

4. **Thrombocytopenia due to massive blood loss and replacement with banked blood:** Red cell transfusions contain few viable platelets. Therefore, if massive, acute blood loss is replaced with only red cells, thrombocytopenia develops because platelet reserves are too small to keep up with the external losses. Typically, the platelet count is in the range of 50,000 to 100,000 per microliter after 10 to 20 U of red cells have been infused. Platelet transfusion is not routinely indicated in these patients, but it can be used if the thrombocytopenia appears to be contributing to continued bleeding (see Chapter 17).

5. **Hereditary thrombocytopenia:** A few patients who appear to have ITP have thrombocytopenia on a hereditary basis. The index of suspicion should be raised by thrombocytopenia in a family member, a history in the patient of thrombocytopenia dating back to childhood without the spontaneous remission that is typical of childhood ITP, failure to respond to steroid therapy and splenectomy, and marked decrease or increase in platelet size on peripheral smear or by electronic counter. Platelet counts should be obtained for all family members. Most of these patients have an autosomal dominant mode of transmission, moderate thrombocytopenia (platelet counts in the range of 30,000–100,000/μL), normal platelet size, and no associated defect in platelet function and rarely have severe bleeding problems. They do not improve with steroid therapy or splenectomy and need no therapy other than an occasional platelet transfusion for bleeding associated with surgery or trauma.

Exceptions include the following:

- **The Wiskott–Aldrich syndrome.** More severe thrombocytopenia and hemorrhagic symptoms are associated with an X-linked, recessive mode of transmission, small platelets on peripheral blood smear, eczema, and an increased susceptibility to infection. The thrombocytopenia generally improves after splenectomy, but there is a high rate of life-threatening bacterial sepsis after surgery, and lifelong penicillin prophylaxis is mandatory.

- **The Bernard–Soulier syndrome.** Thrombocytopenia is associated with giant platelets and a defect in platelet function (see section entitled **Congenital Disorders of Platelet Function**).

- **May–Hegglin anomaly.** Moderate thrombocytopenia inherited as an autosomal dominant trait is associated with huge platelets and the presence of pale-blue inclusions known as Döhle bodies in the cytoplasm of granulocytes. Circulating platelet mass is commonly normal, and there is no defect in platelet function. These patients rarely have difficulty with severe hemorrhage, and therapy is generally not required.

- **Autosomal recessive thrombocytopenia with normal platelet function.** These patients have giant platelets, but platelet function is normal. Therefore, hemorrhagic symptoms are mild compared to the Bernard–Soulier syndrome.

Impaired Platelet Production
By definition, there is a bone marrow abnormality that is almost always reflected by a morphologic abnormality when bone marrow smears and biopsies are examined. In general, megakaryocytes are decreased in number. Furthermore, a deficit in platelet production is rarely seen without abnormalities in the production of white cells and red cells.

Classification (see Chapters 2, 10, 11, and 15 for an extensive discussion of these entities):

   1. **Marrow panhypoplasia** is most commonly seen as an expected pharmacologic response after marrow suppressive chemotherapy or radiotherapy for malignancy but may be seen as an idiosyncratic reaction to hepatitis or to drugs such as chloramphenicol, phenylbutazone, gold compounds, phenytoin, and sulfonamides or as idiopathic aplastic anemia. In approximately 2% to 5% of patients with acquired aplastic anemia, there may be severe thrombocytopenia with decreased megakaryocytes in the marrow and only minor abnormalities of the white cell and red cell series. In addition, there is an autosomal recessive hereditary disorder in which a marked depletion of megakaryocytes occurs with no associated abnormality of the red or white cell series. Because the radii are commonly absent in these patients, the syndrome has been called thrombocytopenia with absent radius (TAR) syndrome. If the patient survives the first year, the prognosis is good; platelet transfusions are only rarely needed for surgery.
   2. **Malignant invasion.** Leukemias, lymphomas, and carcinomas (particularly breast, lung, stomach, renal, and prostate) can produce thrombocytopenia by this mechanism.
   3. **Dysmyelopoietic syndromes.** Megaloblastic anemia secondary to deficiency of folic acid or vitamin B_{12} may produce severe thrombocytopenia as part of a general pancytopenia, and so may the idiopathic dysmyelopoietic syndromes (see Chapter 10). Normal or increased numbers of megakaryocytes may be present in these marrows, indicating ineffective thrombopoiesis as the cause for the thrombocytopenia.

   Nonspecific therapy for thrombocytopenia (see Chapters 2, 10, 11, and 15 for specific therapy for these marrow diseases) includes platelet transfusions and epsilon-aminocaproic acid (Amicar).

   Platelet transfusions are administered as pooled random-donor platelet concentrates (PC) or as single-donor platelets. A random-donor PC is obtained by differential centrifugation of a routine blood donation and contains, on average, 0.7 to 0.9 × 10^{11} platelets and approximately 10^9 contaminating leukocytes in 50 mL of plasma. Under optimal circumstances, 1 PC should raise the platelet count of an average 70-kg adult by 15,000 per microliter. Thus, pools of 4 to 6 PC are administered. Single-donor platelets are obtained by plateletpheresis of an individual donor to obtain approximately 4 × 10^{11} platelets in 300 to 500 mL of plasma. Thus, on average, a single-donor product is equivalent to five random donor PCs.

   Indications for platelet transfusion in patients with bone marrow failure: Patients with platelet counts above 20,000 per microliter rarely have significant spontaneous bleeding and do not need to be transfused unless they have an anatomic bleeding lesion (e.g., an ulcer) or unless surgery is planned. In such patients, enough platelets should be administered to raise the platelet count to the range of 60,000 to 80,000 per microliter, at which point the prolonged bleeding time secondary to thrombocytopenia is substantially corrected. Patients with platelet counts consistently below 10,000 per microliter frequently have episodes of serious bleeding and prophylactic platelet transfusion is indicated. If a patient whose platelet count is in the range of 10,000 to 20,000 per microliter and this patient is not bleeding, platelet transfusion is optional. In this range, one leans toward prophylactic transfusion if there is fever, active infection, an anatomic lesion that has the potential for bleeding, a high leukemic blast cell count, or an associated plasma clotting factor abnormality or if drugs that inhibit platelet function are being administered. Prophylactic platelet transfusions under these circumstances generally need to be repeated every 2 to 3 days.

Leukoreduction of platelet preparations: After support for 2 to 8 weeks with pooled random donor platelets, some patients develop alloantibodies to contaminating leukocytes, resulting in febrile reactions. Alloantibodies to human leukocyte antigens (HLAs) also can prevent the rise in platelet count expected after a platelet transfusion. Primary HLA alloimmunization requires exposure to both class I and class II antigens, which are present only on monocytes and B lymphocytes. It is less likely to occur if the patient is exposed only to the class I antigens on platelets. Furthermore, when cytomegalovirus (CMV) is transmitted by transfusion, it is carried by leukocytes contaminating the transfusions. For all these reasons, platelet transfusions should be leukoreduced either prior to storage or by filtration during bedside infusion.

Evaluation of patients who are having poor platelet count increments to transfusion: Coexistent conditions such as infection, fever, bleeding, DIC, and splenomegaly often shorten platelet survival time, so that no increment is observed 18 to 24 hours after transfusion. In these patients, platelet counts should be obtained 10 to 60 minutes after transfusion. If there is no increase in the count at that time, the patient probably is alloimmunized and will likely benefit from a switch to single-donor platelets obtained from donors who are HLA compatible or who are losely matched. If there is an acceptable increment at 10 to 60 minutes, the patient may not be alloimmunized. Evaluation of these patients should include a lymphocytotoxic antibody screen for HLA antibodies. Patients who lack such antibodies generally do no better with matched platelets than with randomly selected platelets.

Epsilon-aminocaproic acid (Amicar): The extent of bleeding at an anatomic site reflects a balance between hemostatic factors (platelets and plasma clotting factors) and fibrinolysis induced by plasmin. Amicar inhibits plasmin and often slows thrombocytopenic bleeding at mucosal surfaces where fibrinolytic activity is high, such as in the nose, mouth, and gastrointestinal and urinary tracts. Therefore, for thrombocytopenic patients who fail to respond to platelet transfusions, therapy with Amicar may be begun with 5 g intravenous push followed by 1 g per hour administered intravenously as a continuous infusion. Hemostasis can be maintained with oral therapy at a dosage of 3 g every 6 hours.

Disorders of Distribution (Hypersplenism)
As discussed in the section entitled **Platelet Kinetics and Physiology,** the total body platelet mass is divided between the circulating pool and a pool sequestered in the spleen in excess of what would be predicted based on splenic blood volume. Both pools are freely exchangeable with one platelet in the spleen for every two in the circulation. In patients with marked splenomegaly, the splenic pool is increased, with a decrease in the circulating pool, resulting in platelet counts in the range of 30,000 to 100,000 per microliter. Often there is an associated leukopenia with a normal white cell differential and a nearly normal hemoglobin. In nontropical areas, the most common causes of hypersplenism are portal hypertension secondary to liver disease and lymphoproliferative involvement of the spleen.

Splenectomy corrects the thrombocytopenia but is rarely necessary because hypersplenism alone causes only a moderate thrombocytopenia; however, splenectomy may be helpful if there are additional thrombocytopenic mechanisms such as marrow involvement with lymphoma, with the combination leading to severe thrombocytopenia. In some patients in whom the etiology of the splenomegaly is not known, splenectomy can be both diagnostic and therapeutic.

Thrombocytosis

An elevated platelet count is commonly seen as a response to acute or chronic illness (*reactive thrombocytosis*). Common causes are malignancies and chronic inflammatory conditions such as rheumatoid arthritis. Generally, the elevation is in the range of 500,000 to 1,000,000 per microliter, but it may be higher. Other causes are iron deficiency, anemia, and splenectomy. In addition, the platelet count may be elevated because of a primary increase in production in the myeloproliferative diseases (MPD): polycythemia vera, chronic myelocytic leukemia, essential thrombocythemia (ET), and agnogenic myeloid metaplasia (see Chapter 9). There may be associated platelet dysfunction, as discussed in the section to follow entitled **Acquired Disorders of**

Platelet Function. Finally, thrombocytosis may be seen in myelodysplastic syndromes, particularly acquired sideroblastic anemia and the 5q-syndrome.

Differential Diagnosis
Generally, the distinction between reactive thrombocytosis and thrombocytosis in MPD is not difficult. In reactive thrombocytosis, manifestations of the responsible illness are obvious. If MPD is responsible for the thrombocytosis, there are generally other findings such as polycythemia, leukocytosis, a leukoerythroblastic reaction with poikilocytosis in the peripheral blood, or splenomegaly on physical examination. No laboratory tests make a definitive distinction, however. When the distinction is not clear, the physician can look for other nonspecific manifestations of chronic inflammatory disease and malignancy, such as an increase in the sedimentation rate and fibrinogen and lowering of the serum iron and iron-binding capacity. The bone marrow biopsy shows increased megakaryocytes in both disorders, but in MPD, megakaryoctyes are greatly increased and dysplastic. Increased reticulin or even fibrosis may be apparent.

Prognosis and Treatment
Reactive thrombocytosis is generally harmless and needs no therapy, with one exception. When a splenectomy is done for anemia secondary to hemolysis or ineffective erythropoiesis and the anemia is not completely corrected, the postsplenectomy thrombocytosis generally persists indefinitely. This contrasts with splenectomy done under other circumstances, in which postoperative thrombocytosis generally resolves in 6 to 18 months. These chronically anemic patients with thrombocytosis have an increased incidence of venous thromboembolism and may be candidates for indefinite oral anticoagulation.

    Essential thrombocythemia frequently is complicated by thrombotic or hemorrhagic events, which improve when the platelet count is lowered with myelosuppressive therapy (see Chapter 9). Thrombotic complications often reflect intermittent or permanent occlusion of arterial vessels and consist of transient cerebral and ocular ischemic episodes that may progress to infarction and peripheral arterial occlusive disease associated with "erythromelalgia." The latter condition manifests by intermittent, painful erythema and cyanosis of the fingers and toes. Patients with these thrombotic manifestations should be treated with low-dose aspirin, 80 ("baby" aspirin) to 300 mg daily, with a future consideration of myelosuppressive therapy. Aspirin usually produces dramatic improvement in many patients.

    Hemorrhagic complications of essential thrombocytosis include bleeding after surgery and spontaneous upper gastrointestinal bleeding. Aspirin and nonsteroidal antiinflammatory agents (NSAIDs) contribute to these hemorrhagic events.

    Some would disagree, but many hematologists believe that asymptomatic patients should not be treated with myelosuppressive therapy unless they are elderly or have underlying occlusive vascular disease. There is concern in young patients for long-term complications of myelosuppressive therapy, such as induction of malignancy. Selected young patients with only thrombotic complications can be managed chronically with aspirin alone. The choice among myelosuppressive therapies is discussed further in Chapter 9.

Disorders of Platelet Function
Disorders of platelet function are characterized by highly variable mucocutaneous bleeding and excessive hemorrhage following surgery or trauma. Most patients, but not all, have a prolonged bleeding time. *In vitro* platelet aggregation and secretion studies provide evidence for the defect but are not always predictive of the severity of clinical manifestations. Defects in platelet function may be inherited or acquired; the latter are far more common. The platelet dysfunction in these patients arises by diverse mechanisms.

Congenital Disorders of Platelet Function
Table 3 provides a **classification** based on the platelet functions or responses that are abnormal (Fig. 1).

Table 3. Classification of congenital disorders of platelet function

1. Defects in platelet-vessel wall interaction (disorders of adhesion)
   a. von Willebrand disease (deficiency or defect in plasma vWF)
   b. Bernard–Soulier syndrome (deficiency or defect in GPIIb-IIIa)
2. Defects in platelet–platelet interaction (disorders of aggregation)
   a. Congenital afibrinogenemia (deficiency of plasma fibrinogen)
   b. Glanzmann thrombasthenia (deficiency or defect in GPIIb-IIIa)
3. Disorders of platelet secretion and signal transduction
   a. Abnormalities of granules
      i. Storage pool deficiency
      ii. Quebec platelet disorder
   b. Signal transduction defects (primary secretion defects)
      i. Defects in platelet-agonist interaction (receptor defects); receptor defects: thromboxane A_2, collagen, ADP, epinephrine
      ii. Defects in G-protein activation: Gαq deficiency
      iii. Defects in phosphatidylinositol metabolism: phospholipase C-β_2 deficiency
      iv. Defects in calcium mobilization
      v. Defects in protein phosphorylation (pleckstrin)
   c. Abnormalities in arachidonic acid pathways and thromboxane A_2 synthesis
      i. Impaired liberation of arachidonic acid
      ii. Cyclooxygenase deficiency
      iii. Thromboxane synthase deficiency
   d. Defects in cytoskeletal regulation
      Wiskott-Aldrich syndrome
4. Disorders of platelet coagulant–protein interaction
   Defect in factor Va-Xa interaction on platelets (Scott syndrome)

GP, glycoprotein; vWF, von Willebrand factor.

In patients with **defects in platelet-vessel wall interactions,** adhesion of platelets to subendothelium is abnormal. The two disorders in this group are vWD, due to a deficiency or abnormality in plasma vWF, and the Bernard–Soulier syndrome, where platelets are deficient in GPIb membrane complex (and GPV and IX) and the binding of vWF to platelets is abnormal. In the latter, the bleeding time is markedly prolonged; the platelet count is decreased; and on the peripheral smear, the platelets are increased in size. In platelet aggregation studies, the responses to ADP, epinephrine, thrombin, and collagen are normal, but the response to ristocetin is decreased, a feature shared with vWD.

Abnormalities of platelet-platelet interaction (aggregation) arise because of a severe deficiency of plasma fibrinogen (congenital afibrinogenemia) or because of a quantitative or qualitative abnormality of the platelet membrane GPIIb–IIIa complex (Glanzmann thrombasthenia). Thrombasthenia is a rare autosomal, recessive disorder characterized by markedly impaired platelet aggregation to most agents tested, a prolonged bleeding time, and relatively more severe mucocutaneous bleeding manifestations than some of the other platelet function disorders. The primary abnormality may be a defect in GPIIb or GPIIIa genes, resulting in decreased expression of the complex on the platelet membrane surface. Because of this, fibrinogen binding to platelets on activation and aggregation are impaired. Congenital afibrinogenemia also is characterized by an absence of platelet aggregation. In this disorder, however, both prothrombin time (PT) and activated partial thromboplastin time (APTT) are markedly prolonged, whereas they are normal in thrombasthenia.

Defects in platelet secretion and signal transduction are a heterogeneous group of defects "lumped together" for convenience of classification rather than on the basis of an understanding of the specific underlying abnormality. The major common characteristic is an inability to release intracellular dense granule contents on activation of platelet-rich plasma with agonists such as ADP, epinephrine, and collagen.

In aggregation studies, the second wave of aggregation is blunted or absent. Patients with these characteristics constitute the majority of patients encountered with mucocutaneous bleeding manifestations and defective platelets. A small portion of these patients have a deficiency of dense granule stores (**storage pool deficiency**). The term *storage pool deficiency* (SPD) refers to patients with deficiencies in platelet content of dense granules (δ-SPD), α-granules (α-SPD), or both types of granules (αδ-SPD). The **Quebec platelet disorder** is an autosomal dominant disorder associated with abnormal proteolysis of α-granule proteins, deficiency of platelet α-granule multimerin (a factor V binding protein), and markedly impaired aggregation with epinephrine. In other patients, the impaired secretion results from aberrations in signal transduction events such as interaction of agonists with specific platelet receptors, G-protein activation, and activation of effector enzymes such as phospholipase C and phospholipase A$_2$ (Fig. 1).

Lastly, there are patients who have an abnormality of the interactions of platelets with proteins of the coagulation system related to a decreased surface expression of phosphatidylserine following platelet activation. The best described is the **Scott syndrome,** in which the bleeding time, platelet aggregation responses, PT, and partial thromboplastin time (PTT) are normal; however, the serum PT has been abnormally short.

The **approach to diagnosis of congenital platelet function defects** is as follows: In patients suspected to have a platelet function defect, laboratory studies should include a platelet count, the bleeding time, and studies to assess platelet aggregation and secretion responses *in vitro*. The platelet studies usually are performed using a platelet-rich plasma harvested from anticoagulated blood, and responses are monitored to various agonists including ADP, epinephrine, collagen, a TxA$_2$ analog U46619, thrombin receptor peptides, and ristocetin. The patterns of responses provide clues to the nature of the underlying platelet defect, although specific techniques, largely available in research laboratories, are required to delineate the precise platelet mechanisms that are altered (Fig. 1). Patients with classic thrombasthenia have absent primary and the secondary waves of aggregation in response to all the commonly used agonists, except ristocetin. Impaired response to ristocetin but normal response to other agonists suggests von Willebrand disease or the Bernard–Soulier syndrome. In the latter, the platelet count is decreased, platelet size is increased, and plasma levels of vWF and factor VIII are normal. Patients with impaired granule secretion or diminished dense granule contents (SPD) generally show a diminished or absent second wave of aggregation in response to ADP and epinephrine, blunted responses to other agonists (collagen, TxA$_2$ analog), and decreased release of granule contents.

Therapy for congenital platelet function defects: Patients with vWD and afibrinogenemia are managed by methods aimed at elevating the deficient factor levels in plasma and are discussed elsewhere. Platelet transfusions and 1-desamino-8D-arginine vasopressin (DDAVP) are the mainstays of therapy of patients with inherited platelet defects. Because of the wide disparity in bleeding manifestations, therapeutic approaches need to be individualized. Platelet transfusions are effective in controlling bleeding manifestations but come with potential risks associated with blood products, including alloimmunization. Patients with thrombasthenia may develop antibodies against GPIIb–IIIa that compromise the efficacy of subsequent platelet transfusions. In preparation for surgery or invasive procedures, platelet transfusions should be administered only if severe bleeding has occurred in the past, if the procedure is "blind" (i.e., the surgeon cannot achieve hemostasis mechanically), or if the surgery is at a site where a sudden bleed could produce irreversible damage before a transfusion could be administered, such as in the eye or central nervous system. In other scenarios, surgery may be performed with platelets readily available to transfuse if bleeding should occur. A viable alternative to platelet transfusions is intravenous DDAVP, which shortens the bleeding time in a substantial number of patients, particularly those with disorders of platelet secretion and relatively mild bleeding symptoms. The mechanisms by which DDAVP enhances hemostasis in patients with platelet defects are unclear, but its administration induces a rise in plasma vWF, factor VIII, and tissue plasminogen activator. The abnormal *in vitro* platelet aggregation or secretion responses in patients with platelet defects are not corrected by DDAVP. The beneficial effect on the bleeding time lasts about 4 to 5 hours; depending on the nature of surgery and the initial response, a second dose of DDAVP can be administered 12 hours after the first one. The response to DDAVP appears to be dependent on the abnormalities leading to the platelet dysfunction. Most patients with thromboasthenia have not responded to DDAVP with a shortening of the bleeding time. Responses in patients with storage pool deficiency have been variable, with shortening of the bleeding time in some patients but not others. It is feasible to manage selected patients undergoing surgical procedures with intravenously administered DDAVP alone, but this approach needs to be individualized and platelet transfusions need to be ready available. However, it is unknown whether DDAVP improves hemostasis in these patients despite a lack of shortening of the bleeding time.

Acquired Disorders of Platelet Function

Alterations in platelet function occur in many acquired disorders (Table 4). In most cases, the specific biochemical and pathophysiologic aberrations leading to platelet dysfunction are poorly understood. In several disorders, abnormalities have been described in multiple aspects of platelet function, including adhesion, aggregation, secretion, and the platelet coagulant activities. In MPDs, there is production of intrinsically abnormal platelets by the bone marrow. In others, the dysfunction results from interaction of platelets with exogenous factors, such as pharmacologic agents, artificial surfaces (cardiopulmonary bypass), compounds that accumulate in plasma because of impaired renal function, and antibodies.

Myeloproliferative diseases: Bleeding tendency, thromboembolic complications, and qualitative platelet defects are recognized in all MPDs, which include ET, polycythemia vera (PV), agnogenic myeloid metaplasia (AMM), and chronic myelogenous leukemia (CML). The platelet abnormalities most likely result from their development from an abnormal clone of stem cells, but some may be secondary to enhanced platelet activation *in vivo.* Platelet aggregation is diminished in response to several agonists, particularly epinephrine. Platelet defects are demonstrable even in asymptomatic patients, and bleeding and thrombotic events may occur in the same patient. Bleeding appears more prevalent in AMM, whereas patients with other MPD are more prone to thrombosis. The risk of spontaneous hemorrhage may be increased with platelet counts in excess of 1,000,000 per microliter. The management of these disorders is discussed in Chapter 9.

Uremia: Although the incidence of major bleeding in uremia has clearly declined with adequate dialysis, it is a serious concern in patients undergoing surgery or invasive procedures. Usually, it is mucocutaneous and believed to be due to platelet dysfunction and impaired platelet–vessel wall interaction. These problems can be attributed to accumulation in the plasma of inhibitory and dialyzable molecules. A consistent laboratory abnormality is prolongation of the bleeding time. Intensive dialysis

Table 4. Disorders in which acquired defects in platelet function are recognized

Myeloproliferative disorders
  Essential thrombocythemia
  Polycythemia vera
  Chronic myelogenous leukemia
  Agnogenic myeloid metaplasia
Uremia
Acute leukemias and myelodysplastic syndromes
Dysproteinemias
Cardiopulmonary bypass
Acquired von Willebrand disease
Acquired storage-pool deficiency
Antiplatelet antibodies
Liver disease
Drugs and other agents

(either hemodialysis or peritoneal) corrects the bleeding diathesis in some patients but is only partially effective in others. Elevation of the hematocrit with packed red cells or recombinant erythropoietin can shorten the bleeding time, improve platelet adhesion, and correct mild bleeding in uremic patients. Other treatments for uremic patients with significant bleeding include DDAVP, cryoprecipitate, and conjugated estrogens. The role of platelet transfusions in uremia is limited because of the availability of other modalities and the possibility that the transfused platelets acquire the uremic defects *in vivo*.

Acute leukemias, myelodysplastic syndromes, and dysproteinemias: The most common cause of bleeding in these conditions is thrombocytopenia. In patients with normal or elevated platelet counts, however, it may be the result of platelet dysfunction. In patients with dysproteinemias, excessive bleeding appears to be related to multiple mechanisms including platelet dysfunction, specific coagulation abnormalities (e.g., factor X deficiency), hyperviscosity, the acquired form of vWD, and alterations in blood vessels resulting from amyloid deposition. Acute bleeding episodes can be managed by lowering the paraprotein levels by plasmapheresis, and chronic bleeding may be controlled by chemotherapy aimed at reducing the concentration of the abnormal protein in patients with dysproteinemias.

Acquired storage pool disease: In general, this defect reflects *in vivo* release of platelet dense-granule contents resulting from activation or a hematopoietic abnormality with abnormal platelets produced by the marrow. Acquired SPD may therefore, occur in diverse clinical states including in patients with antiplatelet antibodies, collagen vascular disease, disseminated intravascular coagulation, idiopathic thrombocytopenic purpura, multiple congenital cavernous hemangioma, MPDs, or cardiopulmonary bypass.

Drugs that inhibit platelet function: Many drugs affect platelet function. For several drugs, the effects have been established largely *in vitro,* and the relevance of such findings to the drug levels achieved in clinical practice is not well established.

Aspirin irreversibly acetylates and inactivates the platelet cyclooxygenase, leading to the inhibition of endoperoxide (prostaglandins G_2 and H_2) and TxA_2 synthesis. Aspirin prolongs the bleeding time in many normal persons. Its antithrombotic effect is not dose related in the range of 30 mg to 1,300 mg daily; however, the gastrointestinal toxicity is dose-related. In otherwise normal subjects taking aspirin who need to undergo elective surgery, aspirin should be discontinued 7 to 10 days prior to the procedure; however, this is often not feasible in many patients. If excessive perioperative hemorrhage is encountered, it is usually responsive to platelet transfusions. Moreover, DDAVP infusion shortens the prolongation in bleeding time with aspirin.

Like aspirin, most NSAIDS inhibit both forms of cyclooxygenase (cyclooxygenase-1 and-2). The two selective cyclooxygenase-2 inhibitors, celexocib (Celebrex) and rofecoxib (Vioxx), have no antiplatelet activity.

Several newer classes of antiplatelet agents, including the thienopyridine drugs (ticlopidine and clopidogrel) and the GPIIb–IIb antagonists (abciximab, tirofiban, eptifibatide) prolong the bleeding time and may induce clinically significant hemorrhage.

β-Lactam antibiotics, including penicillins and cephalosporins, inhibit platelet aggregation responses, and some induce a bleeding diathesis at high doses. These include carbenicillin, penicillin G, ticarcillin, ampicillin, nafcillin, cloxacillin, mezlocillin, oxacillin, and piperacillin. The patients at particular risk of bleeding appear to be those with concurrent illnesses, including sepsis, malnourishment, thrombocytopenia, and malignancy. The typical setting is the intensive care unit. A host of other agents, including β-blockers, heparin, thrombolytic agents, dextrans, and ethanol, may affect platelet responses. Their role in causing a clinically significant platelet defect remains to be clarified.

Suggested Readings

Aster RH. Drug-induced immune thrombocytopenia: an overview of pathogenesis. *Semin Hematol* 1999;36:2–6.

Bishop JF, McGrath K, Wolf MM, et al. Clinical factors influencing the efficacy of pooled platelet transfusions. *Blood* 1988;71:383–387.

Bussel JB, Pham LC, Aledort L. Maintenance treatment of adults with chronic refractory immune thrombocytopenic purpura using repeated intravenous infusions of gamma globulin. *Blood* 1988;72:121.

Figueroa M, Gehlsen J, Hammond D, et al. Combination chemotherapy in refractory immune thrombocytopenic purpura. *N Engl J Med* 1993;328:1226.

Frederiksen H, Schmidt K. The incidence of idiopathic thrombocytopenic purpura in adults increases with age. *Blood* 1999;94:909.

George JN, Raskob GE, Shah SR, et al. Drug-induced thrombocytopenia: a systemic review of published case reports. *Ann Intern Med* 1998;129:886–890.

George JN, Woolf SH, Raskob GE, et al. Idiopathic thrombocytopenic purpura: a practice guideline developed by explicit methods for the American Society of Hematology. *Blood* 1996;88:3.

Bierling P, Bettareb A, Oksenhendler E. Human immunodeficiency virus-related immune thrombocytopenia. *Semin Thromb Hemost* 1995;21:68–75.

Mannucci PM. Hemostatic drugs. *N Engl J Med* 1998;339:245–253.

McMillan R. Therapy for adults with refractory chronic immune thrombocytopenic purpura. *Ann Intern Med* 1997;126:307.

Mueller-Eckhardt C. Annotation: post-transfusion purpura. *Br J Haematol* 1986;64:419.

Murphy S. Hereditary thrombocytopenia. *Clin Haematol* 1972;1:359.

Preiksaitis JK. The cytomegalovirus-"safe" blood product: is leukoreduction equivalent to antibody screening? *Transfus Med Rev* 2000;14:112.

Rao AK. Congenital disorders of platelet secretion and signal transduction. In: Colman RW, Hirsh J, Marder VJ, et al., eds. *Hemostasis and thrombosis: basic principles and clinical practice*. Philadelphia: JB Lippincott, 2001:893–904.

Rao AK. Acquired qualitative platelet defects. In: Colman RW, Hirsh J, Marder VJ, et al., eds. *Hemostasis and thrombosis: basic principles and clinical practice*. Philadelphia: JB Lippincott, 2001:905–920.

Rao AK, Ghosh S, Sun L, et al. Effect of mechanism of platelet dysfunction on response to DDAVP in patients with congenital platelet function defects: a double-blind placebo-controlled trial. *Thromb Haemost* 1995;74:1071–1078.

Rebulla P, Finanzi G, Marangoni A, et al. The threshold for prophylactic platelet transfusions in adults with acute myeloid leukemia. *N Engl J Med* 1997;337:1870.

Roberts, I. Review: management of thrombocytopenia in neonates. *Br J Haematol* 1999;105:864.

Scaradavou A, Woo B, Woloski BMR, et al. Intravenous anti-D treatment of immune thrombocytopenic purpura: experience in 272 patients. *Blood* 1997;89:2689.

TRAP Study Group. Leukocyte reduction and ultraviolet B irradiation of platelets to prevent alloimmunization and refractoriness to platelet transfusions. *N Engl J Med* 1997;337:1861.

Warkentin TE, Chong BH, Greinacher A. Heparin-induced thrombocytopenia: towards consensus. *Thromb Haemost* 1998;79:1.

9. MYELOPROLIFERATIVE DISEASES

Ayalew Tefferi

The current classification of the chronic myeloproliferative disorders (CMPD) includes the following:

- Polycythemia vera (PV)
- Agnogenic myeloid metaplasia (AMM)
- Essential thrombocythemia (ET)

These three disorders are considered separate from chronic myeloid leukemia and the myelodysplastic syndrome. The diagnosis of chronic myeloid leukemia requires the demonstration, in the bone marrow or peripheral blood, of the Philadelphia (Ph[1]) chromosome or its molecular equivalent (*bcr/abl* fusion gene). Trilineage myeloid dysplasia and peripheral monocytopenia, bicytopenia, or pancytopenia characterize the myelodysplastic syndrome, whereas the CMPD usually are associated with erythrocytosis, thrombocytosis, or granulocytosis. The CMPD, for the most part, are clonal stem cell processes with variable propensity to evolve into acute leukemia; in addition, PV and ET are characteristically associated with an increased risk of thrombosis. The respective incidences of PV, AMM, and ET are approximately 2.3, 1.3, and 2.5 per 100,000 population. Median age at diagnosis is similar among the CMPDs, about 60 years. There is a slight preponderance of males in PV and AMM and of females in ET.

Polycythemia Vera
Pathogenesis
Both early and recent studies in PV, based on X chromosome-associated enzyme and DNA analysis, have shown clonal myeloproliferation that involves multiple lineages. Erythrocytosis in PV is independent of the erythroid growth factor, erythropoietin (EPO). Furthermore, the EPO receptor and certain components of the EPO-receptor–associated downstream signal transduction pathway are structurally and functionally intact. Alternatively, EPO-independent erythroid viability in PV may be facilitated by an abnormal expression of apoptosis-inhibiting oncoproteins or augmented stimulatory signal transduction. The latter possibility is consistent with the observation that erythroid progenitors in PV are hypersensitive to a variety of cytokines, including insulin-like and myeloid growth factors (stem cell factor, granulocyte-monocyte colony stimulating factor, interleukin-3).

Diagnosis
Most physicians use the PV study group (PVSG) criteria to diagnose PV (Table 1); however, these criteria are not based on biologic characteristics of the disease and lack diagnostic sensitivity and specificity. The current availability of disease-specific biologic tests may obviate measurement of red cell mass and allow identification of early or atypical cases. In general, an increased hemoglobin concentration (or hematocrit) may represent (a) the upper tail end distribution among normal persons, (b) a relative polycythemia (normal red cell mass with decreased plasma volume), or (c) absolute erythrocytosis. Absolute erythrocytosis may result from autonomous proliferation of red cells (PV), EPO-mediated proliferation (secondary erythrocytosis), or an EPO receptor mutation, which is extremely rare. We currently pursue further evaluation of "erythrocytosis" in the presence of the following:

1. A hemoglobin level greater than 18 g per deciliter in a white male or the corresponding sex- and race-adjusted value
2. A documented and persistent increase in hemoglobin concentration of greater than 2 g per deciliter, regardless of the absolute value
3. A high-normal hemoglobin value (16–18 g/dL) along with a PV-associated feature (Table 2)

Table 1. The Polycythemia Vera Study Group (PVSG)
diagnostic criteria for polycythemia vera[a]

Major criteria	Minor criteria
Increased red cell mass Males ≥36 mL/kg Females ≥32 mL/kg	Platelets >400,000/μL Leukocytes >12,000/μL
Normal arterial oxygen saturation, ≥92% Splenomegaly	Leukocyte alkaline phosphatase >100 or vitamin B_{12} >900 pg/mL or unbound B_{12} binding capacity >2,200 pg/mL

[a]Diagnosis of polycythemia vera requires the presence of all three major criteria or the presence of the first two major criteria and any two minor criteria.
From Tefferi A, Silverstein MN. Myeloproliferative diseases. In: Goldman L, Bennett JC, eds. Cecil textbook of medicine, 21st ed. Philadelphia: WB Saunders, 2000:935–941, with permission.

Our diagnostic evaluation starts with a serum EPO (sEPO) determination. A diagnosis of PV is considered only if the sEPO value is low or normal. If a repeated value confirms low sEPO, a bone marrow biopsy is performed to evaluate for morphologic evidence of PV, including bone marrow hypercellularity, atypical megakaryocytic hyperplasia and clustering, and decreased bone marrow iron stores. If the findings are not confirmatory, immunohistochemical studies with the thrombopoietin receptor (cMpl) are done to determine whether there is decreased megakaryocyte expression of cMpl as is characteristic of PV. Endogenous erythroid colony formation may be used to evaluate difficult cases.

Clinical Features
Approximately 20% of patients present with thrombotic events, including stroke, transient ischemic attack, retinal artery or venous occlusion, coronary artery ischemia, pulmonary embolism, hepatic or portal vein thrombosis, deep vein thrombosis, and digital ischemia. Bleeding complications are both less frequent and less serious compared with thrombosis and have been significantly associated with the use of aspirin. Leukemic conversion occurs in fewer than 5% of patients with PV who are treated with phlebotomy alone. Treatment with certain agents increases the risk of acute leukemia. In contrast, specific therapy may or may not modify the risk of fibrotic transformation of the bone marrow, which occurs in 10% to 30% of patients with PV who have been followed for 10 to 25 years. Aquagenic pruritus is a characteristic manifestation of PV that is difficult to treat.

Prognosis
Age and a history of previous thrombosis are the most powerful predictors of recurrent thrombosis. In addition to advanced age and a positive history of thrombosis, treatment with phlebotomy alone has been associated with an increased risk of thrombosis. In contrast, neither the degree of thrombocytosis nor the presence of platelet function abnormalities has been correlated with thrombotic risk. Patients with PV,

Table 2. Polycythemia vera–related clinical and laboratory features

Persistent leukocytosis
Persistent thrombocytosis
Microcytosis secondary to iron deficiency
Splenomegaly
Generalized pruritus (post bath)
Unusual thrombosis (portal or hepatic vein, etc.)
Erythromelalgia (acral dysesthesia and erythema)

similar to those with ET, may be stratified into defined risk groups that are managed differently (Table 3).

Treatment
Fatal thrombotic complications limit survival to less than 2 years in patients with untreated PV. With phlebotomy alone, survival is improved to a median of more than 12 years. To date, no other or additional therapy has been shown to offer a survival advantage over treatment with phlebotomy alone. Treatment of PV with phlebotomy alone, however, is associated with an increased rate of early thrombosis. When either chlorambucil or ^{32}P was added to phlebotomy, survival was significantly compromised because of an increased incidence of acute leukemia. In a nonrandomized study by the PVSG, treatment with hydroxyurea in addition to phlebotomy was associated with a lower incidence of both early thrombosis and acute leukemia. Therefore, we currently add hydroxyurea treatment (starting dose, 500 mg orally twice a day) in the presence of increased thrombosis risk (Table 3). The use of high doses of aspirin may not improve thrombosis risk but instead may increase the risk of gastrointestinal bleeding. More recent studies have suggested that lower doses of aspirin (40–100 mg/day) may be safe in both PV and ET. Their benefit is not known, however. Current evidence is not conclusive in implicating hydroxyurea as being leukemogenic in the treatment of PV when it is used alone. If this becomes a concern, however, interferon-α has been effective in PV and may be considered an alternative.

Therapeutic agents reportedly successful for PV-associated pruritus have included interferon-α, histamine H_2-receptor antagonists, and photochemotherapy. Tables 4 and 5 show a treatment algorithm for PV and information on the treatment agents used, respectively.

Agnogenic Myeloid Metaplasia (AMM)
Pathogenesis
Trilineage myeloproliferation in AMM has been shown to be monoclonal by analysis of X chromosome inactivation patterns at both the enzyme and the DNA levels. In addition to this clonal myeloproliferation, the bone marrow in AMM is characterized by an increased stromal reaction that includes collagen fibrosis, neoangiogenesis, and osteosclerosis. This stromal reaction is currently considered a reactive process mediated by fibrogenic and angiogenic cytokines that may be abnormally secreted by clonal megakaryocytes or monocytes.

Diagnosis
The diagnosis of AMM is usually suspected when the peripheral blood smear shows teardrop-shaped red blood cells, nucleated erythrocytes, and granulocyte precursors (myelocytes, metamyelocytes, and blasts). This is generally referred to as a *myelophthisic* or *leukoerythroblastic* blood picture. A similar blood picture also may result from bone marrow infiltration by metastatic cancer or infectious granulomas.

Table 3. Risk stratification in essential thrombocythemia and polycythemia vera

Low risk
  Age <60 yr,
  No history of thrombosis,
  Platelet count <1.5 million/µL, and
  No cardiovascular risk factors (smoking, obesity)
High risk
  Age ≥60 yr or
  A previous history of thrombosis
Intermediate risk
  Neither high risk nor low risk

From Tefferi A. Chemotherapy of chronic myeloproliferative disorders. In: Perry MC, ed. *The chemotherapy source book*, 3rd edition. Philadelphia: Lippincott Williams & Wilkins, 2001: 857–863, with permission.

Table 4. Treatment algorithm in polycythemia vera

Risk category	Age <60 yr	Age ≥60 yr	Women of childbearing age
Low risk	Phlebotomy alone[a] or with low-dose aspirin[b]	Not applicable	Phlebotomy alone[c] or with low-dose aspirin[b]
Intermediate risk (platelet count <1.5 million/µL)	Phlebotomy alone[a] or with interferon-α[b] and/or low-dose aspirin[b]	Not applicable	Phlebotomy alone[c] or with low-dose aspirin[b]
Intermediate risk (platelet count >1.5 million/µL)	Phlebotomy alone[a] or with interferon-α[d]	Not applicable	Phlebotomy alone[c]
High risk	Phlebotomy + Hydroxyurea[d] or interferon-α[d] + Low-dose aspirin[b]	Phlebotomy + Hydroxyurea[d] + Low-dose aspirin[b]	Phlebotomy + Interferon-α[c,d] + Low-dose aspirin[b]

[a] Recommendation supported by a randomized study.
[b] Recommendation not supported by good evidence.
[c] Recommendation supported by anecdotal reports of safety during pregnancy.
[d] Recommendation supported by a nonrandomized prospective study.
From Tefferi A, Solberg LA Jr, Silverstein MN. A clinical update in polycythemia vera and essential thrombocythemia. *Am J Med* 2000;109:141–149, with permission.

Therefore, a bone marrow biopsy is required both to show the presence of collagen fibrosis and to rule out other causes of bone marrow fibrosis (Table 6). In AMM, the bone marrow fibrosis is associated with atypical megakaryocytic hyperplasia and thickening and with distortion of the bony trabeculae (osteosclerosis). In some patients, the bone marrow is markedly hypercellular, with scant fibrosis (cellular phase of AMM).

Clinical Features
In 20% of patients, the disorder may be discovered incidentally in an asymptomatic phase. Most patients with AMM have anemia and marked splenomegaly. The marked splenomegaly in AMM usually is associated with early satiety and hypercatabolic symptoms, including severe fatigue, low-grade fever, night sweats, and weight loss. Occasionally, severe left upper quadrant pain may result from splenic infarction. The major cause of hepatosplenomegaly is extramedullary hematopoiesis. Hepatomegaly often is associated with markedly elevated levels of alkaline phosphatase, a fraction of which comes from the bone as a result of associated osteosclerosis. Many other organs also may be involved with extramedullary hematopoiesis, including lymph nodes, the peritoneum (ascites), pleura (pleural effusion), and paraspinal and epidural spaces (cord compression). Portal hypertension in AMM may develop as a result of either massive splenomegaly (increased splanchnic blood flow) or intrahepatic obstruction (presinusoidal extramedullary hematopoiesis, portal fibrosis, thrombotic obliteration of small portal veins). Osteosclerosis that accompanies the bone marrow fibrosis in AMM may cause severe bone and joint pain that is difficult to treat.

Prognosis
The median survival in AMM is between 3 and 5 years. Risk factors for decreased survival include advanced age (> 60 years), hepatomegaly, weight loss, anemia (hemo-

Table 5. Clinical properties of platelet-lowering agents

	Hydroxyurea	Anagrelide	Interferon-α
Drug class	Antimetabolite	Imidazoquinazolin	Biologic response modifier
Mechanism of action	Not genotoxic, impairs DNA repair by inhibiting ribonucleotide reductase	Interferes with terminal differentiation of megakaryocytes	Myelosuppressive
Specificity	Affects all cell lines	Affects platelet production only	Affects all cell lines
Pharmacology	Half-life ≅4 h; renal excretion	Half-life ≅1.5 h; renal excretion	Kidney is main site of metabolism
Starting dose	500 mg p.o. b.i.d. or t.i.d.	0.5 mg p.o. t.i.d or q.i.d.	3–5 million units s.c. 3–5 days/wk
Onset of action	≅3.5 days	≅6–10 days	3–26 wk to achieve remission
Side effects observed in >10% of patients	Neutropenia, anemia, oral ulcers, hyperpigmentation, rash, nail changes	Headache, forceful heart beat, palpitations, diarrhea, fluid retention	Flulike syndrome, fatigue, anorexia, weight loss, lack of ambition, alopecia
Side effects observed in <10% of patients	Leg ulcers, lichen planus-like lesions of the mouth and skin, nausea, diarrhea	Congestive heart failure, arrhythmias, anemia, light-headedness, nausea	Confusion, depression, autoimmune thyroiditis or arthritis, pruritus, myalgia

b.i.d., twice a day; q.i.d., four times a day; s.c., subcutaneously; t.i.d., three times a day; p.o., by mouth, orally.

From Tefferi A. Chemotherapy of chronic myeloproliferative disorders. In: Perry MC, ed. The chemotherapy source book, 3rd edition. Philadelphia: Lippincott Williams & Wilkins, 2001:857–863, with permission.

Table 6. Causes of bone marrow fibrosis

Myeloid disorders
Chronic myeloproliferative diseases
Myelodysplastic syndrome
Acute myelofibrosis
Acute myeloid leukemia
Mast cell disease
Malignant histiocytosis

Lymphoid disorders
Lymphoma
Hairy cell leukemia
Multiple myeloma

Nonhematologic disorders
Metastatic cancer
Connective tissue disease
Infections
Vitamin D deficiency rickets
Renal osteodystrophy
Gray platelet syndrome

From Tefferi A, Silverstein MN. Chronic myeloproliferative disorders. In: Wachter RM, Goldman L, Hollander H, eds. *Hospital medicine*. Philadelphia: Lippincott Williams & Wilkins, 2000, with permission.

globin <10 gm/dL), leukocytosis (white count >30,000/μL), leukopenia (white count <4,000/μL), circulating blasts 2% or more, male sex, thrombocytopenia (platelet count <150,000/μL), and abnormal karyotype. Low-risk patients (hemoglobin ≥10 g/dL), a white count between 4,000 and 30,000 per microliter, and no hypercatabolic symptoms) may expect a median survival of 8 to 10 years. The presence of any two of the aforementioned risk factors may compromise survival to less than 3 years.

Treatment
    1. **Allogeneic hematopoietic stem cell transplantation (allo-HSCT):** Allo-HSCT has a "curative" potential in AMM. A recent collaborative study of 55 patients with AMM who received allo-HSCT reported an engraftment rate of 91% and a 5-year survival rate of 47%. The substantial risk of mortality and morbidity associated with the procedure, however, limits its use to young patients with poor risk factors.
    2. **Androgen therapy:** The combination of an androgen preparation, fluoxymesterone (Halotestin), 10 mg administered orally twice daily, and a corticosteroid (prednisone), 30 mg orally per day, improves anemia in approximately 25% of the patients. After 1 month of therapy, treatment with fluoxymesterone is continued in responding patients and the corticosteroid is tapered. All patients treated with androgens should have periodic monitoring of liver function tests, and male patients should be screened for prostate cancer (digital rectal examination and measurement of prostate-specific antigen) before therapy is initiated. In our experience, treatment with EPO has not been successful.
    3. **Cytoreductive therapy:** Hydroxyurea (starting dose 500 mg administered orally twice a day) may result in reduction of spleen size and control of thrombocytosis and leukocytosis in some patients. Unfortunately, anemia may worsen with hydroxyurea therapy, and thrombocytopenia may develop.
    4. **Splenectomy:** When hydroxyurea fails to control splenomegaly-associated complications (mechanical discomfort, refractory anemia, hypercatabolic symptoms, portal hypertension), surgical removal of the spleen is considered. At experienced centers, the mortality rate with the procedure should be less than 10%. Postsurgical complications include intraabdominal bleeding, subphrenic abscess, sepsis, large-vessel thrombosis, extreme thrombocytosis, and accelerated hepatomegaly. Laboratory evidence of dis-

seminated intravascular coagulation before splenectomy may increase the risk of perioperative bleeding, and it is recommended that the operation be postponed until the abnormalities abate. After splenectomy, almost all patients experience improvement in hypercatabolic symptoms and portal hypertension. In addition, approximately half of patients with refractory anemia may benefit from splenectomy.

5. **Splenic irradiation:** In poor surgical candidates, the alternative to splenectomy is splenic irradiation (200–300 cGy delivered in 10–15 daily fractions), which usually provides a transient (3–6 months) benefit. Radiation therapy is most useful in the management of extramedullary hematopoiesis.

Essential Thrombocythemia
Pathogenesis
Recent studies suggested pathogenetic heterogeneity in ET by demonstrating a clonal stem cell process in some patients and polyclonal hematopoiesis in others. On the other hand, neither thrombopoietin (TPO) nor its receptor (c-Mpl) has been implicated in the pathogenesis of ET. Similarly, serum TPO levels in ET are either normal or mildly elevated and do not differ significantly from serum TPO levels in the control population or in those with reactive thrombocytosis.

Diagnosis
At present, ET is not a cytogenetically or morphologically defined disease entity, and the diagnosis refers to a chronic nonreactive thrombocythemic state that is not accounted for by another chronic myeloid disorder.

Other subsets of chronic myeloid disorder that may mimic ET in their clinical presentation include chronic myeloid leukemia, the "cellular phase" of AMM, and myelodysplastic syndrome. Therefore, a clinical diagnosis of ET requires the exclusion, first of conditions associated with reactive thrombocytosis (Table 7) and, second, of other chronic myeloid disorders. When a cause for reactive thrombocytosis is not readily apparent, demonstration of increased acute-phase reactants (C-reactive protein), fibrinogen, and erythrocyte sedimentation rate may be used as evidence for the presence of an occult inflammatory process. Once reactive thrombocytosis is considered to be an unlikely cause, a bone marrow examination with cytogenetic studies is required to exclude the presence of AMM, myelodysplastic syndrome, or chronic myeloid leukemia.

Clinical Features
Thirty to 50% of patients are asymptomatic. Vasomotor symptoms occur in a third of patients and include headache, lightheadedness, syncope, atypical chest pain,

Table 7. Causes of reactive thrombocytosis

Acute
  Immediate postsurgical period
  Bleeding
  Hemolysis
  Infections
  Tissue damage (acute pancreatitis, myocardial infarction, trauma, burns)
  Coronary artery bypass grafting
  Rebound effect from chemotherapy or immune thrombocytopenia
Chronic
  Iron deficiency anemia
  Surgical or functional asplenia
  Metastatic cancer, lymphoma
  Inflammations (rheumatoid arthritis, vasculitis, allergies)
  Renal failure, nephrotic syndrome

From Tefferi A. The Philadelphia chromosome negative chronic myeloproliferative disorders: a practical overview. *Mayo Clin Proc* 1998; 73:1177–1184, with permission.

acral paresthesia, visual disturbances, livedo reticularis, and erythromelalgia, the last-named referring to burning pain of the hands or feet associated with erythema and warmth. Thrombosis occurs in 9% to 22% of patients and includes cerebrovascular accident, myocardial infarction, portal or hepatic vein thrombosis, deep vein thrombosis, pulmonary embolism, peripheral artery occlusion, transient ischemic attack, and angina. Hemorrhage (3%–37% of patients) includes gastrointestinal bleeding, epistaxis, and retinal hemorrhage. Splenomegaly occurs in about 25% of patients.

Prognosis
In a study of 74 young women with follow-up of up to 26 years, we observed disease transformation into PV, myelofibrosis with myeloid metaplasia, and acute myeloid leukemia in 2.7%, 4%, and 1.4%, respectively. Others have reported leukemic conversion in 0.6% to 5% of cases. Leukemic conversion in ET has also occurred in the absence of previous therapy, suggesting that the event may be a natural sequela of the disease, that is, depending more on disease biology and duration than on specific therapy. Currently accepted risk factors for thrombosis in ET include (a) a history of thrombosis and (b) age over 60 years.

The role of cardiovascular risk factors or extreme thrombocytosis (platelet count >1–2 million/μL) in the overall risk of thrombosis in ET is debated. Nonetheless, on the basis of aforementioned variables, patients with ET may be stratified into clinically practical risk categories (Table 3). Although the risk of bleeding may be high in the presence of extreme thrombocytosis, supporting evidence for this is not strong.

Treatment
Table 8 is a treatment algorithm in patients with ET. Information on treatment agents is detailed in Table 5. In general, life expectancy in ET may not differ significantly from that of the age- and sex-matched control population. Furthermore, in a nonrandomized but prospective study, low-risk patients with ET (Table 3) were shown to have a thrombotic risk similar to that of the control population. Therefore, such patients may not require any specific therapy. In contrast, a randomized study demonstrated a reduced risk of thrombosis in high-risk patients with ET who were treated with hydroxyurea. Consequently, we recommend the use of a platelet-lowering agent in high-risk patients.

Table 8. Treatment algorithm in essential thrombocythemia

Risk category	Age <60 yr	Age ≥60 yr	Women of childbearing age
Low risk	No treatment[a] or low-dose aspirin[b]	Not applicable	No treatment[c] or low-dose aspirin[b]
Intermediate risk (platelet count <1.5 million/μL)	No treatment[a] or anagrelide[b] or low-dose aspirin[b]	Not applicable	No treatment[c] or low-dose aspirin[b]
Intermediate risk (platelet count >1.5 million/μL)	No treatment[c] or anagrelide[b]	Not applicable	No treatment[c]
High risk	Hydroxyurea[d] or anagrelide[a] + low-dose aspirin[c]	Hydroxyurea[d] + low-dose aspirin[c]	Interferon α[e] + low-dose aspirin[c]

[a] Recommendation supported by a nonrandomized prospective study.
[b] Recommendation not supported by good evidence.
[c] Recommendation supported by a retrospective cohort study.
[d] Recommendation supported by a randomized study.
[e] Recommendation supported by the anecdotal reports of safety during pregnancy.
From Tefferi A, Solberg LA Jr, Silverstein MN. A clinical update in polycythemia vera and essential thrombocythemia. *Am J. Med* 2000;109:141–149, with permission.

There is growing concern regarding potential leukemogenicity associated with the long-term use of hydroxyurea. The reported incidence rates of acute leukemia in ET when this drug was used alone is 0%–5%, however, have not differed significantly from the previously cited general incidence figures. In any case, anagrelide is a reasonable alternative in young patients with ET who require therapy.

In patients who fail to respond to both hydroxyurea and anagrelide, interferon-α and ^{32}P provide additional treatment choices. Because ^{32}P has shown delayed leukemogenicity in PV, it is usually not used in ET unless the anticipated life expectancy is less than 10 years. In women of childbearing age, interferon-α is considered the safest of the available agents.

Suggested Readings

Asimakopoulos FA, Hinshelwood S, Gilbert JG, et al. The gene encoding hematopoietic cell phosphatase (SHP-1) is structurally and transcriptionally intact in polycythemia vera. *Oncogene* 1997;14:1215.

Barosi G, Berzuini C, Liberato LN, et al. A prognostic classification of myelofibrosis with myeloid metaplasia. *Br J Haematol* 1988;70:397.

Berk PD, et al. Treatment of polycythemia vera: a summary of clinical trials conducted by the Polycythemia Vera Study Group. In: Wasserman LR, Beck PD, Berlin NI, eds. *Polycythemia vera and the myeloproliferative disorders*. Philadelphia: WB Saunders, 1995:166–194.

Berlin NI. Diagnosis and classification of the polycythemias. *Semin Hematol* 1975;12:339.

Birgegard G, Wide L. Serum erythropoietin in the diagnosis of polycythaemia and after phlebotomy treatment. *Br J Haematol* 1992;81:603.

Cerutti A, Custodi P, Duranti M, et al. Thrombopoietin levels in patients with primary and reactive thrombocytosis. *Br J Haematol* 1997;99:281.

Cervantes F, Pereira A, Estevev J, et al. Identification of 'short-lived' and 'long-lived' patients at presentation of idiopathic myelofibrosis. *Br J Haematol* 1997;97:635.

Cervantes F, Tassies D, Salgado C, et al. Acute transformation in nonleukemic chronic myeloproliferative disorders: actuarial probability and main characteristics in a series of 218 patients. *Acta Haematol* 1991;85:124.

Cortelazzo S, Finazzi G, Ruggeri M, et al. Hydroxyurea for patients with essential thrombocythemia and a high risk of thrombosis. *N Engl J Med* 1995;332:1132.

Cortelazzo S, Viero P, Finazzi G, et al. Incidence and risk factors for thrombotic complications in a historical cohort of 100 patients with essential thrombocythemia. *J Clin Oncol* 1990;8:556.

Cotes PM, Dore CJ, Yin JA, et al. Determination of serum immunoreactive erythropoietin in the investigation of erythrocytosis. *N Engl J Med* 1986;315:283.

Dupriez B, Morel P, Demory JL, et al. Prognostic factors in agnogenic myeloid metaplasia: a report on 195 cases with a new scoring system. *Blood* 1996;88:1013.

Elliott MA, Chen MG, Silverstein MN, et al. Splenic irradiation for symptomatic splenomegaly associated with myelofibrosis with myeloid metaplasia. *Br J Haematol* 1998;103:505.

Fairbanks VF, Klee GG, Wiseman GA, et al. Measurement of blood volume and red cell mass: re-examination of ^{51}Cr and ^{125}I methods. *Blood Cells Mol Dis* 1996;22:169.

Fruchtman SM, Mack K, Kaplan ME, et al. From efficacy to safety: a Polycythemia Vera Study Group report on hydroxyurea in patients with polycythemia vera. *Semin Hematol* 1997;34:17.

Guardiola P, Esperou H, Cazals-Hatem D, et al. Allogeneic bone marrow transplantation for agnogenic myeloid metaplasia: French Society of Bone Marrow Transplantation. *Br J Haematol* 1997;98:1004.

Harrison CN, Gale RE, Machin SJ, et al. A large proportion of patients with a diagnosis of essential thrombocythemia do not have a clonal disorder and may be at lower risk of thrombotic complications. *Blood* 1999;93:417.

Michiels JJ, Abels J, Stekatee J, et al. Erythromelalgia caused by platelet-mediated arteriolar inflammation and thrombosis in thrombocythemia. *Ann Intern Med* 1985; 102:466.

Najean Y, Rain JD. Treatment of polycythemia vera: the use of hydroxyurea and pipobroman in 292 patients under the age of 65 years. *Blood* 1997;90:3370.

Najean Y, Rain JD. Treatment of polycythemia vera: use of ^{32}P alone or in combination with maintenance therapy using hydroxyurea in 461 patients greater than 65 years of age: the French Polycythemia Study Group. *Blood* 1997;89:2319.

Nand S, Stock W, Godwin J, et al. Leukemogenic risk of hydroxyurea therapy in polycythemia vera, essential thrombocythemia, and myeloid metaplasia with myelofibrosis. *Am J Hematol* 1996;52:42.

Quesada JR, Talpaz M, Rios A, et al. Clinical toxicity of interferons in cancer patients: a review. *J Clin Oncol* 1986;4:234.

Raskind WH, Fialkow PJ. The use of cell markers in the study of human hematopoietic neoplasia. *Adv Cancer Res* 1987;49:127.

Regev A, Stark P, Blickstein D, et al. Thrombotic complications in essential thrombocythemia with relatively low platelet counts. *Am J Hematol* 1997;56:168.

Reilly JT. Pathogenesis of idiopathic myelofibrosis: present status and future directions. *Br J Haematol* 1994;88:1.

Rozman C, Giralt M, Feliu E, et al. Life expectancy of patients with chronic non-leukemic myeloproliferative disorders. *Cancer* 1991;67:2658.

Ruggeri M, Finazzi G, Tosetto A, et al. No treatment for low-risk thrombocythaemia: results from a prospective study. *Br J Haematol* 1998;3:772.

Shibata K, Shimamoto Y, Suga K, et al. Essential thrombocythemia terminating in acute leukemia with minimal myeloid differentiation—a brief review of recent literature. *Acta Haematol* 1994;91:84.

Silva M, Richard C, Benito A, et al. Expression of Bcl-x in erythroid precursors from patients with polycythemia vera. *N Engl J Med* 1998;338:564.

Silver RT. Interferon alfa: effects of long-term treatment for polycythemia vera. *Semin Hematol* 1997;34:40.

Sterkers Y, Preudhomme C, Lai JL, et al. Acute myeloid leukemia and myelodysplastic syndromes following essential thrombocythemia treated with hydroxyurea: high proportion of cases with 17p deletion. *Blood* 1998;91:616.

Tefferi A. Myelofibrosis with myeloid metaplasia. *N Engl J Med* 2000;342:1255.

Tefferi A. The Philadelphia chromosome negative chronic myeloproliferative disorders: a practical overview. *Mayo Clin Proc* 1998;73:1177.

Tefferi A, Elliot MA, Solberg LA Jr., et al. New drugs in essential thrombocythemia and polycythemia vera. *Blood Rev* 1997;11:1.

Tefferi A, Ho TC, Ahmann GJ, et al. Plasma interleukin-6 and C-reactive protein levels in reactive versus clonal thrombocytosis. *Am J Med* 1994;97:374.

Tefferi A, Mesa RA, Nagorney DM, et al. Splenectomy in myelofibrosis with myeloid metaplasia: a single-institution experience with 223 patients. *Blood* 2000;95:2226.

Tefferi A, Silverstein MN, Petitt RM, et al. Anagrelide as a new platelet-lowering agent in essential thrombocythemia: mechanism of action, efficacy, toxicity, current indications. *Semin Thromb Hemost* 1997;23:379.

Tefferi A, Solberg LA Jr, Silverstein MN. A clinical update in polycythemia vera and essential thrombocythemia. *Am J Med* 2000;109:141.

Tefferi A, Yoon S-Y, Li CY. Immunohistochemical staining for megakaryocyte *c-mpl* may complement morphologic distinction between polycythemia vera and secondary erythrocytosis. *Blood* 2000;96:771–772.

Zanjani ED, Lutton JD, Hoffman R, et al. Erythroid colony formation by polycythemia vera bone marrow *in vitro:* dependence on erythropoietin. *J Clin Invest* 1977;59:841.

10. MYELODYSPLASTIC SYNDROMES

Kenneth B. Miller

The myelodysplastic syndromes (MDS) are a heterogenous group of clonal stem cell disorders characterized by impaired proliferation and maturation of hematopoietic progenitor cells resulting in symptomatic anemia, leukopenia, or thrombocytopenia. Morphologic and functional abnormalities involving one or more cell lines are common. The clinical course is very variable, ranging from a chronic, stable, mildly symptomatic disorder, to one that progresses rapidly to acute leukemia. Infections and bleeding are most frequent causes of morbidity and mortality. Whereas the evaluation of patients with MDS and the acute leukemias is similar, their clinical course, prognosis, and treatment approaches are very different. The treatment of patients with MDS is controversial and should be individualized based on the patient's MDS subtype, age, and prognostic variables.

Incidence and Epidemiology

Most commonly, MDS affects elderly patients and is unusual in persons younger than 50 years of age. The overall incidence is 3.5 to 12.6 per 100,000 per year. In people over the age of 70 years, the incidence is between 15 and 50 per 100,000 per year, an incidence similar to that of other common hematologic malignancies in this population. The overall incidence of MDS may be much higher, however, as the result of difficulties in diagnosis, classification, and recording.

Approximately 25% to 30% of patients with MDS will transform to acute myelogenous leukemia (AML). The transformation to AML varies by subtype from 10% to 60% for the low-risk and high-risk groups, respectively. Most patients with MDS die as a result of the disease without progressing to AML. The major causes of mortality in MDS are the effects of the impaired maturation and function of platelets, red cells, and neutrophils, resulting in infections and bleeding.

Etiology

The etiology of the MDS in most patients is unknown; however, several factors are associated with an increased risk for the development of MDS.

Cytotoxic Chemotherapy

A prior exposure to alkylating agents (cyclophosphamide, chlorambucil, and melphalan) is associated with increased risk of MDS. The risk is related in part to the dose and duration of treatment and generally occurs 3 to 7 years after exposure. MDS occurring after chemotherapy exposure is called *secondary* or *therapy-related MDS* and has a poor prognosis.

Patients who received the **combination** of radiation therapy plus chemotherapy have an increased risk of MDS. Patients who have received total body irradiation administered as part of the preparation regimen for an autologous stem cell transplantation are at higher risk for MDS. The incidence of MDS is increased in patients who have been exposed to benzene and related compounds.

Pathogenesis

Myelodysplastic syndrome is an acquired clonal stem cell disorder characterized by ineffective and dysplastic hematopoiesis. The dysplasia usually involves more than a single cell line and is the result of impaired maturation and proliferation of an abnormal clone of stem cells that replaces normal hematopoietic progenitors.

The cellular and molecular events in the pathogenesis MDS are poorly understood. The clinical manifestations of MDS are due to impaired and abnormal cellular maturation. An alteration of progenitor cell survival may be one of the underlying mechanisms to explain the ineffective hematopoiesis and cytopenias that are characteristic of MDS.

Apoptosis, an active process that controls programmed cell death, is increased in MDS progenitor cells. The increased levels of apoptosis could explain the ineffective hematopoiesis in the bone marrow of MDS patients. The bone marrow is typically hypercellular with increased hematopoietic activity but with peripheral cytopenias because of the impaired and abnormal maturation within the bone marrow.

Abnormal oncogene expression in progenitor cells and deregulation of cell cycle kinetics has been implicated in MDS. Alterations in N-*ras* oncogenes, *p53* expression, tumor suppressor genes, and transcription factors have been described in MDS progenitors cells.

Immunoregulatory abnormalities manifest as impaired T-cell, natural killer (NK) cell, and B-cell function occur in patients with MDS. MDS is associated with a number of autoimmune disorders, including immune hemolytic anemia and immune thrombocytopenia.

Classification
FAB Classification
The FAB (French–American–British) group defined five subtypes of MDS (Table 1). These subtypes are based on the morphology and the percent of myeloblasts in the bone marrow and peripheral blood. This morphologic classification is useful in categorizing patients and broadly assessing prognosis.

1. **Refractory anemia** constitutes 30% to 40% of all cases of MDS. Patients usually present with a macrocytic anemia and a low reticulocyte count. Usually, one or more cell lines will be abnormal. Red cell abnormalities include *anisocytosis* (abnormalities in size), *poikilocytosis* (abnormalities in the shape), and basophilic stippling. The bone marrow aspirate and biopsy are typically hypercellular for the patient's age with dysplastic erythropoiesis. Bone marrow blasts are fewer than 5%, and there are fewer than 1% blast forms in the blood.

2. **Refractory anemia with ringed sideroblasts (RARS):** RARS constitutes 15% to 25% of all MDS cases. Patients usually present with signs and symptoms of anemia. The red cells are usually macrocytic, but they can be normocytic, with dysplastic changes in the bone marrow and blood. Ringed sideroblasts (erythroid precursors with iron staining in the mitochondria forming a necklace around the nucleus) account for more than 15% of all nucleated cells in the bone marrow of patients with RARS.

3. **Refractory anemia with excess blasts (RAEB):** RAEB constitutes 15% to 25% of MDS cases. Patients usually present with signs and symptoms of anemia or bruising. Cytopenias usually involve two or more lineages and dysplastic changes in all three lineages with fewer than 5% circulating blast forms. The bone marrow is hypercellular with increased blast forms: more than 5% but fewer than 20% blasts in the bone marrow.

4. **Refractory anemia with excess blasts in transformation (RAEB-T):** RAEB-T constitutes 5% to 10% of MDS cases. This category includes patients with 5% blasts in the blood and between 21% to 30% blasts in the bone marrow. Auer rods may be present (aggregates or lysozymes appearing as thin rods in the cytoplasm of immature myeloid cells). More than 50% of patients will transform to AML. The World Health Organization (WHO) proposed that 20% blasts should be the dividing line between MDS and AML. The RAEB-T MDS subtype would be classified as AML with multilineage dysplasia in the WHO classification.

5. **Chronic myelomonocytic leukemia (CMML)** constitutes 15% of MDS cases. CMML has features of both a myeloproliferative disorder and MDS. The peripheral blood demonstrates a monocytosis ($>1 \times 10^9$/L). Many patients will present with prominent splenomegaly and an elevated total white blood cell count. Immunologic abnormalities are most common in this subtype. About half the patients demonstrate autoantibodies and 5% to 10% will have a monoclonal antibody.

Special Subtypes Not Defined by the FAB Group
The **5q-syndrome** is a favorable prognostic subtype of MDS defined by specific cytogenetic abnormalities: the loss of all or part of the long arm of chromosome 5. The q, or long arm, of chromosome 5 contains the genes that encode for a number of growth

Table 1. The myelodysplastic syndromes French–American–British (FAB) classification and survival

FAB subtype	Bone marrow blasts	Blood blasts	Auer rods	Monocyte $>1 \times 10^9$L	Ring sideroblast	Survival (median mo)	AML
RA	<5%	<1%	Absent	No	None	48	10–15%
RARS	<5%	<1%	Absent	No	>15%	72	5–10%
RAEB	5–20%	<5%	Absent	No	Rare <15%	12	30–45%
RAEB-T	21–30%	>5%	Present	No	Rare <15%	6	50–60%
CMML	<20%	<5%	Absent	Yes	Rare	30	25–35%

CML, chronic myelomonocytic leukemia; RA, refactory anemia; RAEB, refactory anemia with excess blasts; RAEB-T, refactory anemia with excess blasts in transformation; RARS, refactory anemia with ringed sideroblasts.

factors, including interleukin 3 (IL-3), IL-5, IL-9, and granulocyte macrophage–colony-stimulating factor (GM-CSF). How the loss of these factors contributes to the development of this syndrome is unclear. The 5q-syndrome is frequently associated with morphologic features of refractory anemia. Most patients present with a refractory macrocytic anemia, mild neutropenia, and thrombocytosis (a platelet count >400,000 m³). The megakaryocytes are of normal size but are nonlobulated. The 5q-syndrome is more common in elderly women (70%) and rarely transforms to AML. Most patients are red cell transfusion dependent; therefore, particular attention should be paid to managing and preventing iron overload.

Pediatric MDS is uncommon in children. MDS is much higher in Down syndrome. Abnormalities of chromosome 7, monosomy 7, and 7q-are more frequent in pediatric MDS. Unlike in adult patients, however, this cytogenetic abnormality is not associated with an adverse prognosis. The rate of AML progression is higher in the pediatric population. Juvenile chronic myelomonocytic leukemia, one of the most common pediatric MDSs, has features of both MDS and a myeloproliferative disorders.

Hypoplastic MDS: Most patients with MDS present with a hypercellular or normal cellular bone marrow with ineffective hematopoiesis. A subset of patients will present with hypocellular bone marrow (<15% cellularity on bone marrow biopsy) and minimal dysplasia. Hypocellular MDS must be differentiated from aplastic anemia and hypocellular AML. A characteristic MDS cytogenetic abnormality helps to define this disorder (i.e., −5, −7, +8, 20q-). The course and treatment of these patients are similar to those for patients with aplastic anemia.

Myelodysplasia with bone marrow fibrosis: MDS with bone marrow reticulin deposition generally is associated with a poor prognosis. MDS with myelofibrosis must be differentiated from the M7 subtype of AML and myelofibrosis with myeloid metaplasia. In this MDS subtype, patients present with trilineage dysplasia, <30% blast forms in the bone marrow, and an absence of hepatomegaly or prominent splenomegaly.

Therapy-related MDS: MDS that occurs following exposure to certain cytotoxic chemotherapy or ionizing radiation is referred to as *secondary* or *therapy-related* MDS. Trilineage dysplasia is common, and the prognosis of therapy related MDS is generally worse than *de novo* MDS.

1. For **alkylating agent related** MDS, the prognosis is generally poor. The latency period is 3 to 7 years. This condition is associated with abnormal cytogenetics involving loss or deletions of chromosome 7 or 5.

2. **Topoisomerase II inhibitors,** including epipodophyllotoxins and anthracyclines, has a latency period of 18 months to 3 years after exposure. This condition is associated with a balanced translocation involving chromosome bands 11q23 and 21q22.

Myelodysplastic syndromes and myeloproliferative disorders (MDS/MPD): The MPDs are clonal stem cell disorders characterized by increased but effective hematopoiesis resulting in the increase peripheral blood levels of one or more cell lines. The bone marrow is typically hypercellular without dysplasia. Patients typically present with hepatosplenomegaly. The MDS/MPD subtype is an overlap disorder characterized by features of both MDS and MPD. Patients present with a clinical picture that demonstrates both increased proliferation and maturation but ineffective maturation. The MDS/MPD category includes patients with juvenile myelomonocytic leukemia, subtypes of chronic myelomonocytic leukemia, and atypical chronic myelogenous leukemia (Philadelphia chromosome negative). The bone marrow and the blood show evidence of both effective, increased hematopoiesis with maturation and dysplasia or ineffective hematopoiesis. MDS/MPS disorders resembles both a chronic MPD and a syndrome of ineffective and impaired maturation and function. The MDS/MPD disorders have a variable course but a generally poor prognosis and an increased incidence of leukemic transformation.

Prognostic Features
The International Prognostic Scoring System (IPSS)
The International Prognostic Scoring System (IPSS) is a risk-based scoring system that was developed by the International MDS Risk Analysis Workshop (Table 2). The scor-

Table 2. International prognostic scoring system (IPPS)
for myelodysplastic syndromes

	IPPS score value				
Variable	0	0.5	1	1.5	2
Marrow blasts (%)	<5	5–10		11–20	21–30
Karyotype[a]	Good	Intermediate	Poor		
Cell lines[b]	0–1	23			

[a] Good, normal, 5q-, 20q-; Poor, >3 Abnormalities, -7, multiple; intermediate, all others.
[b] Neutrophils <1,800 cmm; platelets <100,000 cmm; hemoglobin <10 g/dL.

ing system assigns a point score for the number of bone marrow blast forms, karyotypic abnormalities, and number of cell lines affected (cytopenias). The combined score determines the risk category: low (score 0), intermediate 1 (score 0.5–1.0), intermediate 2 (1.5–2.0), and high (score >2.5). The risk score reflects the overall survival and frequency of transformation to AML.

The prognostic scoring system is helpful in planning treatment. For instance, patients with fewer than 5% blasts in the bone marrow and favorable cytogenetics have a median survival of greater than 5 years and infrequently evolve to AML. In contrast, patients with a marrow blast count greater than 11% and unfavorable cytogenetics have a median survival of less than 2 years and frequently progress to AML.

1. **Cytogenetics:** Favorable cytogenetics include normal cytogenetics, deletion of the Y chromosome, deletion of 5q or 20 q. Poor prognostic cytogenetics include complex karyotypic changes (i.e., three or more defects) and abnormalities of chromosome 7; the intermediate prognostic group included all other karyotypic changes, including abnormalities of chromosome 8.

2. **Cytopenias:** Defined as hemoglobin of less than 10 g per deciliter, absolute neutrophil count below 1,800/mm^3. The percentage of marrow blasts is divided into four prognositc groups: <5%, 5% to 10%, 11% to 20%, and 20%.

Age: Age is an important prognostic indicator. Patients younger than 60 years of age have a better survival for all risk categories (Table 3).

Clinical and Laboratory Findings
General
1. Most patients present with a macrocytic anemia [mean corpuscular volume (MCV) >102] and a low reticulocyte count.
2. Pancytopenia is present in about 50%.
3. Prominent splenomegaly and leukocytosis are uncommon except in CMML.
4. Risk of infection and bleeding risk is increased because of neutrophil and platelet dysfunction.

Table 3. International prognostic scoring system

	Median survival	
Score	Age <60 yr	Age >60 yr
Low (0)	11.8	4.8
Intermediate 1 (0.5–1.0)	5.2	2.7
Intermediate 2 (1.5–2.0)	1.8	1.1
High (>2.5)	0.4	0.5

5. Serum B$_{12}$ and folic acid levels are normal.
6. White blood count is usually low or normal.
7. The platelet count is normal or low, but patients may give a history of excessive bleeding after minor trauma or procedures, even with a normal platelet count reflecting the platelet dysfunction in MDS.
8. Dysplastic changes in one or more cell lines in the peripheral blood.

Specific Cell Line Abnormalities on Peripheral Smear
In **red cells,** these abnormalities include oval macrocytosis, basophilic stippling (red cell inclusions composed of ribonucleoprotein and mitochondrial remnants), nuclear binding, poikilocytosis (abnormal shape), anisocytosis (abnormal size), and teardrop-shaped red blood cells.
  In **white cells,** abnormalities include the following:

1. Neutrophils are hypogranulated and hyposegmented.
2. Pseudo Pelger–Huet abnormality (an acquired defect in the shape of neutrophils). The neutrophils are hyposegmented with one or two lobes instead of the usual three to five. Hyposegmented neutrophils may be confused with band forms on peripheral smear.
3. Nuclear fragmentation.
4. Impaired function–decreased myeloperoxidase activity.

  In **platelets,** thrombocytopenia, giant platelets, megakaryocytic fragments may be seen in peripheral blood smear and impaired function occur.

Cytogenetic Abnormalities
  1. Abnormal cytogenetics in 60% to 80% of patients.
  2. Most common cytogenetic abnormalities include monosomy 5, 5q-, monosomy 7, trisomy 8, deletion 20q, loss of X or Y chromosomes.
  3. Fluorescence *in situ* hybridization (FISH) uses specific DNA probes to identify individual chromosomal abnormalities. FISH can be performed on interphase and metaphase cells, and FISH analysis can be performed on either bone marrow or peripheral blood smears. FISH analysis does not depend on dividing cells and is a rapid technique to identify marker chromosomal abnormalities in MDS patients; however, FISH is restricted to established cytogenetic abnormalities.

Bone Marrow Findings
A bone marrow aspirate and biopsy are essential to diagnosis and define the MDS subtype. Bone marrow cytogenetics should be performed to assign prognosis and differentiate MDS from other disorders:

1. Bone marrow is usually hypercellular for age.
2. Micromegakaryocytes–mononuclear megakaryocytes are reliable markers of dysplasia.
3. Megaloblastic changes (nuclear:cytoplasm asynchrony).
4. Increased blast forms (>5%).
5. Increased ringed sideroblasts (>15%).

Differential Diagnosis
Patients with MDS usually present with impaired production of one or more cell lines. The finding on peripheral smear may be nonspecific and similar to other disorders that impair bone marrow function:

1. Aplastic anemia
2. Early AML-hypoplastic AML
3. Congenital dyserythropoietic syndromes
4. Anemia of chronic disease
5. Effects of chemotherapy are transient, reversible
6. Megaloblastic anemia (B$_{12}$, folic acid deficiency).

Treatment

Myelodysplastic syndromes are a heterogeneous group of disorders with a variable clinical course and prognosis. Treatment should be individualized based on the patient's age, subtype, percent blasts in the marrow, and cytogenetics. Most MDS patients are elderly and tolerate intensive chemotherapy poorly. Moreover, standard therapies did not result in a cure, and their impact on survival is unclear. Therefore, any potential benefits of treatment must be weighed against the side effects and the patient's overall prognosis. The standard of care for most patients with MDS remains supportive care. Whereas several therapeutic options are available for MDS patients, none, other than an allogeneic stem cell transplantation, has been shown to be better than supportive therapy with regard to both overall survival or leukemic transformation.

The therapeutic options for patients with MDS include the use of hematopoietic growth and trophic factors, immunosuppressive agents, low-intensity cytoreductive chemotherapy, intensive chemotherapy, and allogeneic stem cell transplantation.

Supportive Therapy

Supportive therapy represents the standard of care for most patients. Red cell and platelet transfusions are administered symptomatic treatment of the anemia and thrombocytopenia.

1. **Red cell transfusions:** Patient may require multiple transfusion over many years. The potential for iron overload secondary to transfusions should be addressed early in the patient's course. Chelation therapy with desferrioxamine to prevent progressive iron overload should be considered for stable patients who will receive greater than 20 U of packed red cells.

2. **Platelet transfusions for symptomatic bleeding:** Platelet dysfunction is common, and patients may bleed even with an adequate platelet count. Patients who have a normal platelet count may require platelet transfusions before surgery and other procedures.

Trophic Agents

1. **Recombinant growth factors:** Recombinant human erythropoietin (rHuEPO), granulocyte-colony stimulating factor (G-CSF) and granulocyte-macrophage colony stimulating factor (GM-CSF) have a role in managing the anemia and neutropenia in selected patients with MDS. Symptomatic anemia is observed in the majority of individuals with MDS. Recent studies suggest a role for r-HuEPO in increasing red cell production and reducing transfusion requirements in patients with MDS. Approximately 30% of patients will respond to treatment with rHuEPO. G-CSF and GM-CSF may be synergistic with EPO and increase the response rate in selected anemic patients. Patients should have adequate iron stores prior to starting rHuEPO (transferrin saturation at least 20% and serum ferritin > 100ng/ml).

Best responses to r-HuEPO are observed in patients with endogenous EPO level < 200 U, and transfusion requirement less than 2 units/month. The response rate is 30–50%: refractory anemia, RA, and RAEB (but with <10% blasts) subtypes respond best to treatment. The starting dose of rHuEPO is 150–300 U/Kg three times weekly. The median duration of response is 11–26 plus months. Low doses of G-CSF (1mcg/kg) or GM-CSF (adjusted to maintain a WBC of 2000–5000 cmm) may be synergistic with EPO.

2. **Danazol** is an attenuated, synthetic, androgen that has been used in the treatment of immune-mediated thrombocytopenia (ITP). Danazol may increase the platelet count in low-risk MDS patients who are thrombocytopenic. The mechanism of action is unclear, but some patients with MDS have immune-mediated thromocytopenia, which may respond to danazol. Danazol, 200 mg administered orally three times weekly, is generally well tolerated and associated with an increase in platelets in 10% to 46% of treated patients. The duration of response to danazol is variable, 2 to 26-plus months, and is maintained only while the drug is administered.

Low-dose Chemotherapy

1. **Low-dose cytarabine (Ara-C)** has been frequently used for the treatment of elderly patients with high-risk, symptomatic MDS. Cytarabine is administered daily by

either continuous infusion or bolus subcutaneous injections at doses of 10 to 20 mg/m^2 for 14 to 21 days. Patients with RAEB and RAEB-T have the highest response rates: 20% to 35% complete remission plus partial remission. The median duration of response is 8 to 15 months. The effect of treatment with low-dose cytarabine on overall survival, compared with supportive therapy alone is unclear.

2. **5-Azacytidine (5-Aza)** is a pyrimidine analog that inhibits DNA methyltransferase activity, which leads to hypomethylation of cytosine residues. The response to low-dose 5-azacytidine is 20% to 66%. The duration of response is short. The effect on survival is unclear.

Immunosuppressive Therapy
Immunosuppressive therapy is effective in a subgroup of MDS patients who present with a hypocellular marrow (<15% cellularity) and minimal dysplasia. Selected patients who received immunosuppressive regimens similar to those used in aplastic anemia have had durable responses. The use of antithymocyte globulin (ATG) resulted in some complete remissions. Cyclosporine alone or in combination with ATG also resulted in durable clinical responses in selected patients.

Intensive Chemotherapy
Combination antileukemic type induction chemotherapy should be considered for younger patients who present with poor-prognosis MDS. Selected patients with high-risk features who are younger than 60 years of age are candidates for intensive combination chemotherapy. Newly diagnosed patients with RAEB-T without a prior history of MDS appear to respond in a similar fashion as *de novo* AML to standard induction chemotherapy. Patients with an antecedent or evolving MDS generally respond poorly to intensive AML induction chemotherapy. Few patients attain a complete remission, and the responses of those who do are of short duration. Intensive chemotherapy should be reserved for selected younger patients who are progressing to acute leukemia.

Allogenic Transplantation
Allogenic stem cell transplantation should be considered for young patients who have a human leukocyte antigen (HLA)-compatible donor. Allogeneic transplantation is the only potentially curative therapy for patients with MDS; however, patients with MDS appear to have an increased incidence of transplant-related complications, peritransplant mortality, and relapse rate compared with AML. Timing of the transplant remains controversial for good-risk patients. For the younger patient with a good performance status and a suitable HLA-matched donor, an allogeneic stem cell transplant should be considered.

Suggested Readings

Bennett JM, Catovsky D, Daniel MT, et al. Proposals for the classification of the myelodysplastic syndromes. *Br J Hematol* 1982;51:189–199.

Bernstein SH, Brunetto VL, Davey FR, et al. Acute myeloid leukemia-type chemotherapy for newly diagnosed patients without antecedent cytopenias having myelodysplastic syndrome as defined by French-American-British criteria: a Cancer and Leukemia Group B Study. *J Clin Oncol* 1996;14:2486–2494.

Greenberg P, Cox C, LeBeau MM, et al. International scoring system for evaluating prognosis in myelodysplastic syndromes. *Blood* 1998;91:1100–1110.

Harris NL, Jaffe ES, Diebold J, et al. The World Health Organization classification of hematological malignancies report of the Clinical Advisory Committee Meeting, Airlie House, Virginia, November 1997. *Mod Pathol* 2000;13:193–207.

Heaney ML, Golde DW. Myelodysplasia. *New Engl J Med* 1999;340:1649–1660.

Hellstrom-Lindbeg E, Negrin R, Stein R, et al. Erythroid response to treatment with G-CSF plus erythropoietin for the anemia of patients with myelodysplastic syndrome: proposal for a predictive model. *Br J Haematol* 1997;99:344–351.

Italian Cooperative Study Group for rHuEPO in Myelodysplastic Syndromes. A randomized double-blind placebo-controlled study with subcutaneous recombinant human erythropoietin in patients with low-risk myelodysplastic syndromes. *Br J Haematol* 1998;103:1070–1074.

Miller K. Erythropoietin, with and without granulocyte-colony stimulating factor (G-CSF), in the treatment of myelodysplastic syndrome (MDS) patients. *Leuk Res* 1998;22:13–16.

Miller K, Kyungmann K, Morrison FS, et al. The evaluation of low dose cytarabine in the treatment of myelodysplastic syndromes: a phase III intergroup study. *Ann Hematol* 1980:65;162–168.

Molldrem JJ, Caples M, Mavroudis D, et al. Antithymocyte globulin for patients with myelodysplastic syndrome. *Br J Haematol* 1997:99;699–705.

Thompson JA, Gilliland DG, Prchal JT, et al. Effect of recombinant human erythropoietin combined with granulocyte/macrophage colony-stimulating factor in the treatment of patients with myelodysplastic syndrome. *Blood* 2000;95:1175–1179.

Wattel E, Cambier N, Caulier MT, et al. Androgen therapy in myelodysplastic syndromes with thrombocytopenia: a report on 20 case. *Br J Haematol* 1994; 87:205–208.

Wattel. E, De Botton S, Luc Jai J, et al. Long-term follow-up of de novo myelodysplastic syndromes treated with intensive chemotherapy: incidence of long-term survivors and outcome of partial responders. *Br J Haematol* 1997:98;983–991.

Wihermans PW, Krulder JWM, Hujgens PC, et al. Continuous infusion of low dose 5-aza-2-deoxycytidine in elderly patients with high risk myelodysplastic syndrome. *Leukemia* 1997;11:19–23.

11. ACUTE LEUKEMIAS IN ADULTS

Jacob M. Rowe and Irit Avivi

The acute leukemias are a heterogeneous group of disorders of the pluripotent stem cell that express themselves either as disorders of the hematopoietic system [acute myelogenous leukemia (AML)] or as the lymphoid system [acute lymphoblastic leukemia (ALL)].

Incidence and Epidemiology
The incidence of acute leukemia in adults is approximately 2.4 cases per 100,000 population per year, and it increases progressively with age, to a peak of 12.6 per 100,000 adults aged 65 years or older. Acute leukemia accounts for approximately 10% of all human cancers and is the leading cause of cancer deaths in adults younger than 35 years of age. In adults, the incidence of AML is much higher than that of ALL, which is the reverse of the incidence pattern in childhood (Fig. 1).

Etiology
Although the cause of acute leukemia remains unknown in the majority of patients, several risk factors related to an increased incidence have been identified: Leukemia following radiation exposure has been documented by the Atomic Bomb Casualty Commission in Hiroshima and Nagasaki. Leukemogenesis has also been observed after therapeutic irradiation for such diseases as ankylosing spondylitis and Hodgkin disease. Benzene exposure has been closely associated with the subsequent development of leukemia, and chemical leukemogens have been identified in animal models. Exposure to phenylbutazone, arsenic, thorotrast, and chloramphenicaol may be related to the future development of leukemia. In most cases, bone marrow aplasia caused by drug exposure is the initial event, and acute leukemia evolves later.

Cytotoxic therapy, especially with alkylating agents such as melphalan, chlorambucil, and cyclophosphamide, increases the risk for leukemia 4 to 7 years later. The risk seems to be related to the total dose of the alkylator agents that are received. Furthermore, there is a causal relationship between treatment with topoisomerase II inhibitors and the development of secondary leukemia (6–24 months later).

The combination of alkylating therapy and radiation therapy, which was frequently administered in the past to patients with Hodgkin disease, confers the highest risk for subsequent development of acute leukemia, almost invariably AML. Therapy-related leukemias, or secondary leukemias, have a poorer prognosis than de novo leukemias not associated with prior cytotoxic therapy.

There is evidence implicating RNA viruses in the etiology of animal leukemia. A similar etiologic agent has not yet been defined in the pathogenesis of human leukemia, except in the case of adult T-cell leukemia, which is endemic in the Caribbean area and associated with human T-cell leukemia virus type I (HTLV-I). Congenital factors and immunologic deficiencies may also be important in the pathogenesis of leukemia, but these are usually more important in the acute leukemias of childhood.

Pathogenesis and Molecular Genetics in Acute Myelogenous Leukemia
Acute leukemia is a clonal disorder that is a consequence of acquired somatic mutation in the hematopoietic progenitor cells that confers a proliferative growth advantage. In many leukemias, the mutation involves a balanced reciprocal chromosomal translocation, resulting in the creation of a new fusion gene. These translocations involve genes that normally have a major role in the maturation and differentiation of hematopoietic progenitor cells. By transferring these genes and fusing them with other genes, their function is distorted, and a block in maturation and differentiation can occur. It is worth noting that progression to acute leukemia may require multiple genetic events until the transformed phenotype is able to be expressed.

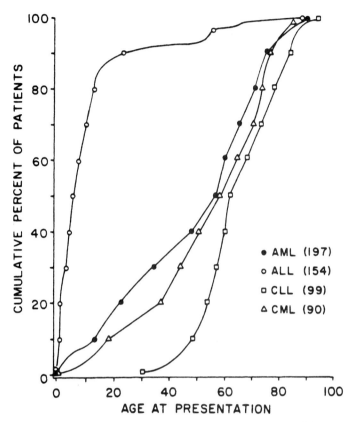

FIG. 1. Cumulative percentage of subjects of a given age at the time of diagnosis with acute myeloid (AML), acute lymphocytic (ALL), chronic lymphocytic (CLL), and chronic myeloid (CML) leukemias. Number of patients with each type of leukemia shown in parentheses. (From Rowe JM. Clinical and laboratory features of the myeloid and lymphocytic leukemias. *Am J Med Technol* 1983;49:103, with permission.)

Acute Myelogenous Leukemia

Acute myelogenous leukemia is a disease of the myeloid or hematopoietic stem cell (Fig. 2). As a result, all cell lines are likely to be qualitatively defective irrespective of the actual cell count. In reality, the origin of the leukemia often goes back to the pluripotent stem cell with a clinical expression that may predominate in the myeloid or hematopoietic stem cell line. It is not surprising, however, that many patients with so-called AML present with subtle features traditionally associated with ALL, especially when analyzed for leukemia-specific immunophenotype. In the past, these leukemias often were termed *biphenotypic* leukemias. It is now recognized that these are AML with lymphoid markers and should be treated as typical AML. True biphenotypic leukemia is rare.

Clinical and Laboratory Features

Most patients with AML present with progressive fatigue and commonly have evidence for infection or bleeding diathesis. The white blood cell (WBC) count is usually elevated but many be normal or low. It is not necessary for leukemic blasts to be present in the

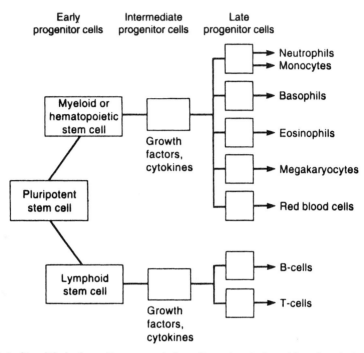

FIG. 2. Simplified schematic representation of hematopoiesis and lymphopoiesis. The pluripotent stem cell differentiates into hematopoietic and lymphoid stem cells, and intermediate and late progenitors develop under the influence of growth factors and cytokines. Acute leukemias usually originate from clonal abnormalities at the stem cell level, which explains the various clinical expressions of these malignancies.

peripheral blood for the diagnosis of AML to be made. In fact, the term *leukemia* is a misnomer in this instance because the diagnosis can be made on the presence of leukemic cells in the bone marrow. Anemia is present and is often profound. Thrombocytopenia is also common, and patients may present with petechiae, ecchymoses, hematuria, or gastrointestinal bleeding.

Hemorrhage in the central nervous system (CNS) is a rare but often a fatal complication of acute leukemia. It occurs most commonly in patients who present with very high WBC counts. Disseminated intravascular coagulation presents with petechiae, gingival bleeding, or even life-threatening bleeding. It is seen most often in patients with promyelocytic leukemia, but it also can occur in myelomonocytic and in monocytic leukemia. In the monocytic and myelomonocytic variants, signs of extramedullary involvement, including gingival hypertrophy, skin infiltration (leukemia cutis), or meningeal leukemia, may be seen.

Rarely, a solid tumor mass, known as a *chloroma* or *granulocytic sarcoma,* may be the only presenting sign of AML. Examination of the peripheral blood smear may reveal dysplastic changes in the red cells, granulocytes, and platelets. Myeloid immaturity is usually present, and the diagnosis may be based on the presence of typical blast cells in the peripheral blood. Blast cytoplasm frequently contains Auer rods (azurophilic granules within lysosomes). The rapid turnover of leukemic blasts produces a hypermetabolic state with increased levels of lactate dehydrogenase (LDH) and uric acid. The bone marrow is usually hypercellular and often is replaced by leukemic blast cells.

Uncommonly, the bone marrow may be hypocellular. In this case, the diagnosis may be somewhat more difficult to establish and depends on very precise morphologic delineation of the cells that are present. Ideally, immunophenotypic and cytogenetic analysis is used for confirmation.

Electrolyte imbalances, such as hypokalemia and hypophosphatemia, are common features at presentation. Care must be taken to distinguish several laboratory abnormalities because of the ongoing metabolism or lysis of blast cells in the collected specimen before laboratory processing.

Pseudohyperkalemia may be present, usually in patients with very high WBC, and may be confirmed by checking an anticoagulated plasma specimen. Pseudohypoglycemia occurs as a result of glucose utilization by blast cells. The rapid oxygen consumption by large numbers of leukocytes, also known as *leukocyte larceny,* leads to pseudohypoxemia, which may make it impossible to determine the arterial blood oxygen accurately.

Classification
The traditional classification of AML is based on morphologic and histochemical characterization of the peripheral blood and bone marrow cells. This is the most rapid way of making the diagnosis of AML and historically has been the most consistent. New technologies, including flow cytometric studies with immunophenotypic analysis, cytogenetic testing, and analysis at the molecular level, in many instances surpassed the value of morphologic classification in terms of prognosis and the specific use of therapy-directed modalities for subtypes of AML. Although certain cell types may predict particular clinical features, such as the increased incidence of disseminated intravascular coagulation (DIC) with the promyelocytic variant or the increased incidence of extramedullary leukemia in the monocytic leukemias, it must be pointed out that all subtypes of AML have overlapping clinical syndromes. They fundamentally represent the same disease and respond to identical therapy. Based on the fact that the traditional morphologic classification correlates rarely with treatment outcome and cytogenetic markers, the World Health Organization (WHO) proposed a new classification.

Morphologic Classification
One of the most widely used morphologic classifications [described by the French–American–British (FAB) Group] relates the morphology of leukemia cells to their presumed hematopoietic counterparts. Several types of AML (M0–M7) (see Appendix H) have been described: Patients with M0 have no visible myeloid features; M1 is undifferentiated myeloblastic leukemia; the M2 variant is undifferentiated myeloblastic leukemia with classic myeloblasts and Auer rods; M3 is the promyelocytic leukemia; M4 is myelomonocytic leukemia; M5 is the classic monocytic (or Schilling) leukemia; and M6 describes erythroleukemia or DiGuglielmo syndrome. M7 refers to megakaryoblastic leukemia or what was formerly often termed *acute myelofibrosis.*

Two types of cytochemical stains are used to characterize leukemic cells and aid in the morphologic diagnosis: enzymatic (e.g., peroxidase and the esterases: chloroacetate esterase and nonspecific esterases) and nonenzymatic [e.g., Sudan black, and periodic acid Schiff (PAS)]. The peroxidase and esterase stains are particularly useful for the diagnosis and accurate morphologic classification of AML. Unequivocal peroxidase positivity is generally diagnostic of AML. The esterases are often helpful in cases in which the peroxidase staining is negative (see Appendixes J and K). It must be emphasized that a negative peroxidase or esterase stain may still be consistent with AML.

New WHO Classification
According to this classification, AML patients can be categorized into four groups (see Appendix H):

1. AMLs with recurrent cytogenetic balanced translocations including t (8;21), t (15;17), inv 16 and AML with 11q23 abnormalities
2. AML with multilineage dysplasia
3. AML and myelodysplastic syndrome, therapy related
4. AML not categorized by 1 or 3, classified by immunologic and morphologic classifications according to the FAB subtypes

Cytogenetics
Clonal cytogenetic abnormalities, defined using sensitive banding techniques, are present in the most patients with newly diagnosed AML. Certain cytogenetic abnormalities may be found in both AML and ALL, but some are found exclusively in AML. These include t (8;21), (q22;q22), and 16q22. Although the application of such information to the management of individual patients may be difficult, these defects have been associated with better overall prognosis. Other cytogenetic abnormalities often seen in AML are t(15;17), classically associated with promyelocytic leukemias; trisomy 8; and 11q23, which is often associated with monoblastic morphology.

Abnormalities of chromosomes 5 and 7 (del 5q, del 7q) are commonly seen in alkylating agent–related AML or in elderly patients with *de novo* AML. These variants often are associated with a more resistant form of the disease, with a somewhat lesser likelihood of attaining a complete remission with therapy.

Many of these alkylating agent-related AMLs are preceded by a more indolent form of leukemia that often is referred to as *myelodysplasia* or *oligoblastic* leukemia. Topoisomerase II inhibitor–related AML tends to develop without a preleukemic phase and involve mainly the 11q23 chromosome.

In general, patients with a normal karyotype have a better prognosis than patients with a single karyotypic abnormalities, who, in turn, have a better prognosis than patients with multiple or complex cytogenetic abnormalities. Exceptions are those with inversion 16, t (8;21), t (15;17); these patients will have a better prognosis than patients with a normal karyotype.

Immunophenotypic Analysis
Immunophenotypic analysis often provides a valuable tool for the detection of acute leukemia and may be especially useful for detection of minimal residual disease. It may be especially useful in patients with a normal karyotype. Myeloid blasts are characterized by the presence of CD13 and CD33 on 20% or more blasts. It is very useful to recognize typical myeloid antigens, which often are identified with leukemic blast expression such as CD9, CD11b, CD13, CD14, CD15, CD33, CD34, or CD117 (which can be found in lymphoid progenitors, too). The immunophenotype is especially useful in cases where the morphology and cytochemical staining are not diagnostic. AML, M_0, M_5 may present with undifferentiated peroxidase-negative cells, and immunophenotyping may help determine the diagnosis. AML blasts may simultaneously express both myeloid and lymphoid associated antigens, which may include CD2, CD5, CD7, CD10, and CD19. Terminal deoxynucleotidyl transferase (TdT), typically a marker commonly associated with lymphoblasts, has been reported in an increasing number of patients with AML. Its prognostic significance is still being debated.

Prognostic Factors
Adverse prognostic factors include the following:

1. Unfavorable karyotype
2. Age greater than 60 years
3. Poor performance status
4. Secondary AML
5. Multidrug resistance (MDR)
6. High WBC at diagnosis

Although all these are important prognostic factors in univariate analysis, in multivariate analysis, only the karyotype is truly predictive of outcome.

Treatment
Induction therapy most commonly consists of an anthracycline, such as daunorubicin, idarubicin, or mitoxantrone, together with cytosine arabinoside. A typical proven induction regimen for AML consists of daunorubicin, 45 to 60 mg/m² for 3 days, together with cytosine arabinoside, 100 to 200 mg/m² continuous infusion for 5 to 7 days. Results from cooperative group trials revealed an overall remission rate using such a regimen to be approximately 65% with more patients under the age of 40 years obtaining complete remission.

Typically, a bone marrow sample is obtained on day 10 to day 14 and examined. If the marrow is not hypocellular and there is unequivocal residual leukemia, a second course of therapy with similar doses is administered. As many as 25% to 40% of patients require two courses of induction chemotherapy to attain a complete remission, and this may be an adverse prognostic factor for such patients. The length of hospitalization for induction chemotherapy is 4 to 6 weeks, during which time the patient has a 2- to 4-week period of absolute pancytopenia. During this period, the patient requires multiple transfusions with red cells and platelets and multiple antibiotics and is placed in isolation for life-threatening neutropenia. The induction therapy for acute promyelocytic leukemia is different and is based on the combination of anthracylines and all trans retinoic acid (ATRA) (discussed separately).

Postremission therapy: Clinical trials indicate that the results of induction chemotherapy for adult AML have not changed dramatically over the past 15 years. It has now been established that once a patient has entered a complete remission, the only hope of long-term survival rests with some form of postremission therapy. Clinical trials also confirmed an almost 100% rate of relapse in patients subjected to observation-only postinduction. Therefore, efforts have been directed at improving postremission therapy on the assumption that more intensive postremission therapy may lead to more prolonged remissions and perhaps a higher rate of cure. The best mode of postremission chemotherapy has yet to be determined, but several treatment modalities are now being used.

Conventional consolidation or postremission chemotherapy typically consists of high doses of cytosine arabinoside with or without an anthracycline or other antileukemic agents. Regimens may involve 106 complete cycles of high-dose chemotherapy. At present, there is no clear evidence that one form of consolidation therapy is better than any other treatment. Another commonly used alternative consolidation regimen includes mitoxantrone and etoposide, and other intensive consolidation regimens appear to be as effective as high doses of cytosine arabinoside.

Allogeneic bone marrow transplantation (BMT) is a form of therapy that is most effective in the first complete remission for younger patients who have a histocompatible sibling. Allogeneic BMT offers patients younger than 50 to 55 years of age a 50% chance of long-term, disease-free survival. Relapse rate following transplantation is low, in the order of 15% to 20%, but the peritransplant mortality, primarily from graft-versus-host disease (GVHD) and interstitial pneumonitis, may be as high as 25% to 30% (see Chapter 19).

Autologous BMT is a procedure that offers an alternative avenue for postremission therapy. The advantage of such a procedure is that it uses the patient's own marrow for reinfusion. Clinical trials simply demonstrate that such therapy has added curative potential. Autologous BMT can be offered to patients up to age 65 to 70 years, and the procedural mortality is considerably lower than with allogeneic transplant. The overall mortality for AML patients who undergo transplantation in first remission is now less than 5% (see Chapter 19).

The disadvantage of this procedure compared with allogeneic transplantation is the absence of the immunologic effects of graft-versus-leukemia, which is now recognized to have major antileukemic properties. Another disadvantage is the potential for reinfusion of leukemic cells, although most evidence suggests that most patients have a relapse after autotransplantation because of residual leukemia as a result of failure to eradicate the disease rather than reinfusion of contaminated bone marrow.

Many methods of cleansing or "purging" of bone marrow with monoclonal antibodies or cytotoxic agents such as 4-hydroperoxycyclophosphamide (4-HC) can be used, and mafosfamide is more commonly used in Europe. At present, data that demonstrate unequivocally that bone marrow purging is of value in the therapy of AML are not available.

Because of the absence of the major complications typically associated with allogeneic BMT, such as GVHD or interstitial pneumonitis, it may be better to think of autologous BMT as the most intensive form of consolidation therapy. At present, the best form of postremission therapy has not been determined. Major clinical trials over the past decade prospectively evaluated the role of autologous BMT by comparing it to a more conventional established consolidation regimens using chemotherapy alone.

The results from these trials are confusing and have not helped to define clearly the best postremission therapy. It seems, however, that autologous BMT is associated with the best antileukemic effect and a prolonged disease-free survival compared with conventional consolidation therapy.

With the use of peripheral blood as the source of the autologous stem cell, the morbidity and mortality rates have been further lowered, and this form of therapy is gaining widespread acceptance, although there have been no prospective clinical trials to date that have unequivocally demonstrated a prolonged overall survival.

Relapsed and refractory AML: Unfortunately, most patients with AML have a relapse. Once relapse has occurred, the only therapy with curative potential is allogeneic BMT. Usually, the first step is reinduction into a second complete remission. No evidence at this time shows that maintenance chemotherapy increases the likelihood of cure in these patients.

If the first remission lasts for more than 6 to 12 months, there is a 50% to 65% chance of obtaining a second complete remission by using a standard regimen for relapse such as mitoxantrone, 12 mg/m^2, together with VP-16, 100 to 150 mg/m^2 for 5 days, or high doses of cytosine arabinoside, 2–3 mg/m^2 given in 8 to 12 doses.

Allogeneic BMT probably will cure 30% to 40% of patients who undergo transplantation during a second complete remission. Evidence indicates that autologous BMT is also beneficial; a significant number of cures, in the order of 10% to 25% of patients, may be effected for patients who undergo autotransplantation during a second complete remission. These data have been reported irrespective of whether the patient's bone marrow has been purged with pharmacologic or immunologic agents.

Patients who have a relapse after a short first remission or refractory AML patients who never attained a complete remission following standard therapy, known as *primary treatment failures,* are best entered into experimental clinical trials. These trials may be able to determine the efficacy of newer agents as well as combination of established agents to evaluate the best regimen for these patients. Agents being studied include intensive combinations of cytosine arabinoside, etoposide and mitoxantrone, and carboplatin (used singly or in combination) as well as the addition of high-dose cyclophosphamide to standard induction regimens. Currently, it is possible to reinduce into complete remission only 20% to 30% of such refractory patients. Another optional treatment regimen for refractory patients is allogeneic BMT if a compatible sibling donor is available.

Interesting experimental studies are being performed to determine whether agents that modulate the multidrug resistance gene. For example, high doses of cyclosporin A or PSC-833 may overcome an inherent or acquired drug resistance and help induce patients with such resistance into complete remission by using conventional doses of anthracyclines and often etoposide. The results to date have been disappointing, but new agents and studies are ongoing.

Treatment of AML in older patients is important because more than 50% of patients with AML are older than 65 years. Unfortunately, in this age group, cytogenetic factors, drug resistance, and antecedent myelodysplasia—all known to be adverse prognostic factors—are very frequent.

Older patients tolerate chemotherapy surprisingly well, assuming they do not have major organ dysfunction when starting therapy. They do not tolerate prolonged aplasia, however. Previously, lower doses of therapy with palliative intent only or attenuated attempts at induction therapy were offered to many patients over the age of 60. Improved supportive care led to the administration of intensive induction chemotherapy to patients in older age groups, and routine treatment of older adults with low doses of cytosine arabinoside is no longer recommended.

Many centers are now using fairly intensive induction regimens for older patients, including those over the age of 70 years, knowing that the best opportunity of getting such patients into remission is with the first induction chemotherapy course. Patients with a poor performance status or multiple adverse prognostic factors may be treated with investigational protocols studying new agents or modalities. There may be some evidence that low-dose maintenance chemotherapy, after the induction of remission, can delay the onset of relapse.

Acute promyelocytic leukemia (APL): All trans-retinoic acid therapy (ATRA). Over the past few years, major advances have been reported in the treatment of APL. It has been observed that these leukemias are strikingly sensitive to trans-retinoic acid (ATRA, tretinoin). This observation was followed closely by the discovery of a specific molecular genetic abnormality in the retinoic acid receptor. These observations provided major scientific insight about leukemogenesis and resulted in alterations of the treatment management in patients with this disease. Patients with acute promyelocytic leukemia respond to ATRA at a dose of approximately 45 mg/m^2 given in divided doses over a period of 30 to 60 days. ATRA has been extremely useful in ameliorating some of the major hemorrhagic complications associated with this disorder. It is clear now that treatment with ATRA and chemotherapy concurrently improves outcome compared with chemotherapy alone and enables the achievement of molecular or cytogenetic remission. Maintenance ATRA, with or without chemotherapy, appears to reduce the relapse rate in APL. The response to ATRA in APL only occurs if the cytogenetic t (15;17) or molecular PML-RARα defect has been unequivocally demonstrated.

Immunotherapy: Evidence for a significant role of immunologic mechanisms in the therapy of AML is increasing. The most important data are derived from results of allogeneic BMT, which indicate and increased risk of relapse for patients transplanted from identical twins (syngeneic transplants) compared with histocompatible allogeneic donors. Furthermore, patients in whom donor cells are depleted of T cells in an attempt to ameliorate the graft-versus-host reaction also have been reported in most studies to have an increased rate of leukemia relapse. Similarly, patients who have survived allogeneic transplant and have had acute and GVHD have a better likelihood of long-term survival than patients who have similarly survived BMT but have not had GVHD. Taken together, these immunologic mechanisms are thought to be responsible for the graft-versus-leukemia effect seen in allogeneic BMT. Attempts are being made to induce or stimulate such immunologic responses, either following autologous BMT or chemotherapy. At present, clinical trials are under way to evaluate agents such as the interleukins, primarily interleukin-2 (IL-2), cyclosporin A, and roquinimex, all of which are thought to be responsible for significant immunomodulation in patients with leukemia. These clinical trials added an exciting dimension to the therapy of AML, although preliminary data from these trials have not been overly promising.

The use of monoclonal antibodies to deliver chemotherapeutic agents to myeloid leukemia has received increasing attention. Leukemia blast cells express the CD33 antigen in most patients with AML, and clinical trials have shown that unmodified anti-CD33 monoclonal antibodies can produce molecular response in occasional patients. By combining the anti-CD33 monoclonal antibody with the chemotherapeutic agents, with calicheamicin (CMA-676), or with radioisotopes, a much higher response rate can be achieved. Promising results already have been reported with gemtuzumab ozogamicin CMA-676, and more data are expected over the next few years. It does not appear, however, to be very useful in refractory patients.

Supportive Care

Major improvements have occurred over the last two decades in the supportive care of patients with acute leukemia. These developments are responsible, in part, for the improved results in the therapy of AML. Infections remain the main threat to absolutely neutropenic patients. The management of febrile neutropenic patients must be empiric because infections in such patients are life threatening, and delaying therapy until results of cultures are available is not possible in most cases. When absolutely neutropenic patients become febrile, even without an obvious source, they must be placed on broad-spectrum antibiotics that provide effective coverage against gram-negative organisms. Traditionally, two antibiotics are used, usually a semisynthetic penicillin with an aminoglycoside. Alternative regimens are based on a single broad-spectrum antibiotic, such as imipenem, ceftazidime, or ciprofloxacin. The empiric addition of specific antistaphylococcal antibiotics is recommended by some authorities because nearly all leukemic patients now have central venous access catheters, and more than 50% of initial fevers are the result of gram-positive infections. Treatment delay while awaiting positive blood cultures is much more likely to be fatal in the case of gram-negative infections than in gram-positive infections, however. For this reason, many catheters do not treat empirically with the optimal antibiotics for gram-positive coverage before the results from cultures are available. These are considered "opportunistic infections" and occur primarily in immunosuppressed patients.

Antimicrobial therapy: With the advent of superior broad-spectrum antibiotics, fewer patients are dying of bacterial sepsis. A major cause of death, especially in young adults with acute leukemia, is fungal infection with either *Candida* or *Aspergillus mucor,* although a less common fungal pathogen is especially important in diabetic patients.

Therapy of fungal infections represents a unique challenge. If treatment is deferred until cultures demonstrate systemic fungal infection, the outcome is likely to be fatal. Therefore, if the patient remains febrile 24 to 72 hours after institution of broad-spectrum antibiotics, coverage with amphotericin B, an antifungal agent, should be initiated. Certain circumstances increase the likelihood of invasive fungal infections, and, in these instances, *prophylactic* amphotericin B should also be considered. At present, there is no equivocal evidence that antifungal prophylaxis delays the onset or prevents the occurrence of invasive fungal infection. Patients who have had prior therapy with high-dose corticosteroids, protracted granulocytopenia prior to admission to the hospital, and previous fungal sepsis during the preceding few months are in definite high-risk groups.

Clinical trials are under way to evaluate the role of prophylactic amphotericin B or other agents such as liposomal amphotericin B, fluconazole, or itraconazole in the management of patients with AML. No equivocal evidence supports the use of either prophylactic antimicrobial therapy before the patient becomes febrile. Similarly, gut-sterilizing antibiotics or sterilized food products have not been beneficial. The mainstay of prophylaxis rests with placing patients in reverse isolation with meticulous handwashing by all health care personnel involved with the patient's care.

Transfusion therapy: Management of profoundly pancytopenic patients requires repeated red cell and platelet transfusion. With multiple platelet transfusions, patients develop alloimmunization and become progressively more refractory to subsequent platelet transfusion. Alloimmunization may be reduced by using special leukocyte filters for both red cells and platelets, special washing of platelets, or, if necessary, using platelets from ABO-compatible donors or leukocyte antigen (HLA)-matched donors.

The use of white cell transfusions remains controversial. Variations in the white cell product itself are marked, and administration is usually fraught with adverse reactions. The ability of blood banks to deliver the product to the patient within a few hours of collection from the donor varies as well. White cell transfusions should be considered only in life-threatening conditions such as documented gram-negative infections with hemodynamic compromise, resistance to standard antimicrobial therapy, or invasive candidiasis or aspergillosis.

Because many patients subsequently undergo BMT, it is critically important to administer blood products that are negative for cytomegalovirus (CMV) to those patients who are CMV negative at presentation. All blood products (except fresh frozen plasma and cryoprecipitable) should be irradiated to avoid GVHD.

Hematopoietic growth factors: The use of hematopoietic growth factors, such as granulocyte-macrophage colony-stimulating factor (GM-CSF) or granulocyte colony-stimulating factor (G-CSF), has been evaluated in several progressive clinical trials to determine whether these recombinant cytokines can reduce the period of neutropenia and the mortality and morbidity related to infections. Multiple trials have demonstrated that CSFs given at the nadir following induction chemotherapy are safe and do not stimulate leukemic clone proliferation significantly. Results from several prospective clinical trials also demonstrate that growth factors shorten the period of neutropenia. In most of these studies, there was no reduction in the number of documented infections, although in some the duration of fevers and infection was shortened. Growth factors therefore have a significant role in the supportive care of patients with AML and should be administered to all patients with a high risk of therapy-related morbidity and mortality. Data also indicate that cytokines given following BMT are safe and can shorten the period of neutropenia. Another role of growth factors is mobilizing stem cells from the bone marrow or peripheral blood. Stem cells collected from the peripheral blood after mobilization with cytokines have accelerated the rate of hematopoietic engraftment.

Miscellaneous support therapy: Cell lysis from cytotoxic therapy produces a large amount of uric acid that must be excreted by the kidneys and may cause acute renal failure. To prevent this complication, all patients with a high leukemic burden should be started on allopurinol and receive vigorous intravenous hydration before the initiation of and during cytotoxic therapy.

The following are unusual complications that can occur:

1. **DIC** may develop in patients with any acute leukemia, but it is more likely with promyelocytic leukemia. If not present initially, DIC may develop during therapy, when cells are lysed, and release thrombogenic material. Optimal management of DIC in promyelocytic leukemia remains controversial, but a useful guideline follows:

- ATRA treatment reduces DIC dramatically. It is recommended that ATRA be given before or concurrent with chemotherapy.
- Frequent monitoring of coagulation parameters is necessary.
- If there is no evidence of clinical bleeding and only mild coagulation abnormality is present, close observation without the addition of prophylactic heparin is appropriate.
- If evidence of clinical bleeding or severe DIC is apparent, platelet cryoprecipitate and fresh frozen plasma should be instituted according to the laboratory coagulation results.
- Only in life-threatening bleeding, unresponsive to treatment as mentioned already, should low doses of heparin, 300 to 500 U per hour by continuous infusion, be considered.

2. **Hyperleukocytic leukemias.** These leukemias often require emergent therapy, especially if signs of leukostasis are present. Clinical features include dyspnea and CNS signs and symptoms as well as funduscopic findings of distended vessels, blurred disk margins, and hemorrhagic infiltrates. Leukapheresis should be used to relieve signs of leukostasis and to avoid complications related to massive tumor lysis. Patients are offered leukapheresis until the blast count is less than 50,000 per microliter, at which point standard antileukemic therapy is given. It is worth noting that with the hyperleukocytic leukemias, several spurious laboratory observations may be noted, and clinicians need to be aware of these. Pseudohyperkalemia, pseudohypoglycemia, and pseudohypoxemia are common. In fact, with the normal systems available for measuring arterial oxygenation, it may be impossible to obtain a true reading in these patients. Unless the clinician is aware of possible laboratory aberrations, inappropriate therapeutic intervention can ensue, causing additional problems and complications. True potassium levels are measured simply by obtaining plasma levels.

3. **Meningeal leukemia:** This type of leukemia most commonly occurs in the lymphoblastic leukemias and the monocytic variants of AML (m-5). Unless patients have CNS signs or symptoms, cerebrospinal fluid should not be examined until the blasts have cleared from the peripheral blood. This fluid may become contaminated with leukemic blasts from the peripheral blood, especially during a traumatic spinal tap. If meningeal leukemia is present, therapy consists of methotrexate, 12 to 15 mg, or cytosine arabinoside, 30 to 50 mg, given by lumbar puncture or via an Omaya reservoir. Intrathecal therapy is given every 3 to 4 days until the cerebrospinal fluid is clear on at least two or three occasions. Although the cerebrospinal fluid can be successfully cleared and patients may attain a complete peripheral remission, the CNS remains a site of potential relapse. The use of cranial irradiation in uncomplicated meningeal leukemia is not considered standard therapy in AML.

Acute Lymphoblastic Leukemia

Unlike ALL of childhood, of which most children can be cured, long-term survival for adult patients with ALL remains dismal. Established poor diagnostic factors include a high white count at presentation (>25,000–30,000/μL), the presence of the Philadelphia (Ph) chromosome with the 9;22 translocation, pure B-cell ALL, long duration to attain initial complete remission (> 4 weeks), and adult age. Clinical and laboratory features are similar to the presenting characteristics for AML.

Classification
The morphologic classification for ALL is less useful than it is for AML. For practical purposes, it is far better to base therapeutic decisions on the immunophenotypic and cytogenetic analysis. The lymphoblasts of ALL are negative for commonly used histochemical stains, including myeloperoxidase, naphthol choloroacetate, and Sudan black. Lymphoblasts often contain large blocks of periodic acid Schiff–staining material.

Cytogenetics
Technically, cytogenetic analysis in ALL is more difficult than in the other leukemias, primarily as a result of the morphology of leukemic metaphases, which consist of poorly spread chromosomes that often fail to produce a clearly defined banding system. Nevertheless, because of the major importance of chromosome studies in ALL, an increased effort by cytogeneticists to detect clonal changes has resulted in the ability to detect cytogenetic abnormalities in approximately 80% of patients tested.

The most common cytogenetic abnormality in adult ALL, the presence of the Ph chromosome, is also the one that confers the poorest prognosis. The percentage of patients who are positive for this abnormality may be increased by about 5% to 10% when very sophisticated techniques that use the polymerase chain reaction are included in the molecular analysis.

The Ph chromosome, t(9;22)(q34;q11), can be found in approximately 25% to 30% of newly diagnosed patients with ALL. The Ph chromosome is found most commonly in the early B-lineage ALL, and it is rarely found in T-cell ALL. It tends to occur in older adults and always expresses early B-lineage–associated antigens in the immunophenotypic analysis. This may be one of the reasons why T-cell ALL in adults does not appear to be an adverse prognostic factor as it is in childhood ALL. A very small fraction of patients may present in a lymphoid blast crisis of chronic myelogenous leukemia (CML) without known antecedent abnormalities in the blood counts.

The molecular analysis may be particularly useful in distinguishing between Ph chromosome–positive ALL and the lymphoid blast crisis of CML because the typical molecular gene rearrangement is usually in different positions in the two disorders and different protein products result.

Other common cytogenetic abnormalities in ALL are t(4;11) q(21;q23), t(1;19) (q23;p13), and t(8;14) (q24;q32). The t(1;19) (q23;p13) is associated with a pre-B phenotype, whereas the t(8;14) (q24;q32) abnormalities appear to be most specific for the rare B-cell ALL. The T-cell ALL often exhibits the t(11;14) (p13;q11) abnormality. Other, more frequent chromosomal findings in ALL have no known significant prognostic significance in ALL in adults, although they are commonly observed. Many of these changes can occur singly or in conjunction with other abnormalities and include rearrangement of the short arm of chromosome 9 and 12 and deletions of the long arm of chromosome 6.

Immunophenotypic Analysis
Eighty percent of adult ALL patients express early B lineage in their phenotype as indicated by positivity for CD19 and CD22. Most of these ALL patients with B lineage express CD10 ("common ALL antigens," or CALLA) and are named pre-B ALL. Cases of B-lineage ALL that lack CD10 and cytoplasmic immunoglobulin heavy-chain expression are called pre-pre-B or pro-B ALL. About 50% to 60% of patients with ALL synthesize cytoplasmic heavy chains, and these leukemias are termed pre-B ALL.

Uncommonly, a few patients with B-lineage ALLs express mature surface immunoglobulin (usually IgM), and these leukemias are called pure B-cell ALL. Unlike most other patients with B-lineage ALLs, these patients show immunophenotypic features typical of mature B cells, such as strong CD20 and CD37 expression.

In contrast with most other B-lineage ALL, these with mature B cell ALL patients do not usually demonstrate the presence of the intracellular enzyme TdT. The morphology of most of these patients resembles that of a typical Burkitt lymphoma or the L3 by the FAB classification (see Appendix K). These patients also possess a typical chromosomal translocation of the t(8;14), t(8;22) t(8;2).

T-cell ALL cases make up approximately 20% of adult ALLs and usually express positivity for CD7 and CD3. Confirmation of the T-cell immunotype can be elegantly performed by T-cell receptor gene receptor rearrangements or deletions. Most of these patients present with typical mediastinal mass.

Induction Therapy

Irrespective of the phenotype or cytogenetic abnormality, all patients with ALL receive identical induction regimens that usually contain prednisone, vincristine, an anthracycline, and L-asparaginase. A significant number of patients may go into remission using prednisone and vincristine alone, but other drugs are added to increase the proportion of complete remitters.

A typical regimen for induction of ALL involves two phases: Phase I consists of daunorubicin, 45 to 60 $\mu g/m^2$ given on days 1, 8, 15, and 22; vincristine, 1.4 mg/m given days 1, 8, 15 to 22; and prednisone given twice daily at a dose of approximately 60 mg/m^2 for a total of 28 days. L-asparaginase, 5,000 to 10,000/m^2 units is usually added for 7 to 12 days beginning on day 15 to 17 of phase I. Phase II, which is administered very soon after completion of phase I, usually includes cyclophosphamide, cytarabine, and 6-mercaptopurine as well as prophylaxis with intrathecal methotrexate or cytosine arabinoside.

Induction therapy in ALL yields an 80% to 85% complete remission rate and must be followed by additional therapy. If CNS leukemia is present, methotrexate usually is given intrathecally or by Omaya reservoir weekly at a dose of 12 to 15 mg until blasts have cleared in the cerebrospinal fluid. Craniospinal irradiation is usually administered concurrently with phase II of the induction therapy.

Postremission Therapy

Following induction therapy, patients require prolonged maintenance therapy for 9 to 24 months. This therapy utilizes alternating regimens of several effective drugs, including anthracyclines, cytosine arabinoside, cyclophosphamide, methotrexate, L-asparaginase, vincristine, and prednisone. Most such maintenance programs can be administered on an outpatient basis.

Central Nervous System (CNS) Prophylaxis

Even if no meningeal involvement was documented at presentation, CNS treatment is mandated. Although administration of CNS prophylaxis may not be critical at induction, it is used throughout most intensification and maintenance regimens. Cranial irradiation, intrathecal prophylaxis, or systemic therapy appears to provide satisfactory CNS prophylaxis, thus preventing late CNS relapses, when used with high-dose cytosine arabinoside or high-dose methotrexate.

Bone Marrow Transplantation (BMT) (see Chapter 19)

Experience with BMT—both allogeneic and autologous—for ALL is much more limited than it is for AML. Results of allogeneic transplants in adults for ALL in first remission have shown long-term, disease-free survival rates in the order of 50% to 60%, much like those in AML.

The data for autologous transplantation as postremission therapy for adults with ALL, which are far more limited than in AML, are the subject of an ongoing international clinical trial. This international trial recognizes the value of allogeneic transplants in ALL. For this reason, all patients under the age of 50 years who have a histocompatible sibling are assigned to allogeneic transplantation following initial induction and intensification therapy. Opinions differ on allogeneic transplants. Some investigators maintain that certain groups of adult patients, especially those between the ages of 15 and 20 years who lack any of the adverse prognostic features, may be treated with standard therapy alone and allogeneic transplantation should be reserved for relapse. Information on the precise role of BMT in ALL should become clearer over the next decade as the results of clinical trials become known. As in AML, there is no evidence that purging is superior to autotransplants performed without purging.

The one group of patients about whom there is a consensus that they should be referred for allogeneic transplantation are those who present with the Ph-1 chromosome. This group of patients has a uniformly poor prognosis, and multiple clinical trials have demonstrated that the long-term outcome is dismal using current therapy.

Early trials with BMT have shown that approximately one third of these patients may have durable long-term survival with this modality of therapy.

Relapse

Most patients with ALL have a relapse, and the success of reinduction therapy depends on the duration of the first remission. Patients who have a first remission of 18 months or longer have an almost equal likelihood of achieving a second remission as they did at presentation. In such patients, it is not necessary to use a new cross-resistant regimen for reinduction; however, patients who have a relapse after a brief first remission or while receiving maintenance chemotherapy are likely to require the use of non–cross-resistant-agents; achieving a second remission is often difficult.

Once patients have had a relapse, irrespective of the duration of the first remission, the outcome is always fatal without BMT. Patients who have suffered relapses should be referred for allogeneic transplantation after a second subsequent remission has been attained. If no donors are available, they probably should be referred to centers that have trials using autologous BMT or transplant centers offering experimental treatment with matched unrelated or mismatched related donors.

Supportive Care

Supportive care for patients with ALL is similar to that used in AML and will not be repeated here. Additional risks for ALL patients include steroid exposure and the tumor lysis syndrome.

Induction therapy includes high doses of corticosteroids, which increase the incidence for opportunistic infections such as *Pneumocystis carinii* and may delay diagnosis and treatment of infection by masking fever and other such symptoms. Fungal infections also are probably more common in ALL patients receiving high doses of corticosteroids.

Tumor lysis syndrome may occur in ALL patients with high cell counts when treatment with corticosteroids is instituted. Thus, it is important to begin hydration and to administer allopurinol and bicarbonate before initiating the therapy.

The most common laboratory abnormalities are hypocalcemia, hyperkalemia, hyperphosphatemia, hyperuricemia, elevated creatinine, blood urea nitrogen, and LDH. Leukapheresis is often used to reduce high cell counts before beginning chemotherapy.

Patients should be started on allopurinol, 300 to 600 mg daily, administered orally. For those at significant risk for development of tumor lysis syndrome, vigorous hydration with urinary alkalinization is used.

Summary

Acute leukemias have been and remain among the most aggressive and lethal malignancies in adults. Despite the high initial response rate following optimal therapy, most adults with acute leukemia die from the disease. Improvements in therapy and long-term outcome have been based on using better agents to achieve and prolong remission, improving supportive care measures, and using both allogeneic and autologous BMT. New therapies, including immunologic therapies and biologic modifiers, should be more precisely defined in the coming decade.

Suggested Readings

Bloomfield CD, ed. *Chronic and acute leukemias in adults.* Boston: Martinez Nijhoff, 1985.

Burnett AK, Goldstone AH, Stevens RM, et al. Randomized comparison of addition of autologous bone-marrow transplantation to intensive chemotherapy for acute myeloid leukemia in first remission: results of MRC AML 10 trial. *Lancet* 1998;351:700.

Cassileth PA, Begg CB, Silber R, et al. Prolonged unmaintained remission after intensive consolidation therapy in adult acute non-lymphocytic leukemia. *Cancer Treat Rep* 1987;71:137.

Cassileth PA, Harrington DP, Appelbaum FR, et al. Chemotherapy compared with autologous or allogeneic bone marrow transplantation in the management of acute myeloid leukemia in first remission. *N Engl J Med* 1998;339:1649.

Champlin R, Gale RP. Acute myelogenous leukemia: recent advances in therapy. *Blood* 1987;69:1551.

Estey EH. How to treat older patients with AML. *Blood* 2000;96:1670.

Feld R. Vancomycin as a part of initial empirical antibiotic therapy for febrile neutropenia in patients with cancer: pros and cons. *Clin Infect Dis* 1999;29:503–507.

Foon KA, Todd RF. Immunologic classification of leukemia and lymphoma. *Blood* 1986;68:1.

Forman SJ, Blume KG. Allogeneic bone marrow transplantation for acute leukemia. *Hematol Oncol Clin North Am* 1990;4:515.

Gassmann W, Loffler H, Thiel E, et al. Morphological and cytochemical findings in 150 cases of T-lineage acute lymphoblastic leukemia in adults. *Br J Haematol* 1997;97:372.

Harris NL, Jaffe ES, Diebold J, et al. World Health Organization classification of neoplastic diseases of the hematopoietic and lymphoid tissues. *J Clin Oncol* 1999;17:3835.

Hiddemann W, Kern W, Schoch C, et al. Management of acute myeloid leukemia in elderly patients. *J Clin Oncol* 1999;17:3569.

Hoelzer D, Thiel D, Loffler H, et al. Prognostic factors in a multi-center study for treatment of acute lymphoblastic leukemia. *Blood* 1988;71:123.

Hussein KK, Dahlberg S, Head D, et al. Treatment of acute lymphoblastic leukemia in adults with intensive induction, consolidation and maintenance chemotherapy. *Blood* 1989;73:57.

Mayer RJ. Allogeneic transplantation versus intensive chemotherapy in first remission acute leukemia: is there a "best" choice? *J Clin Oncol* 1988;6:1532.

Scheper RJ, Broxterman HJ, Scheffer GL, et al. Overexpression of a M(r) 110,000 vascular protein in non-P-glycoprotein-mediated multidrug resistance. *Cancer Res* 1993;53:1475.

Sievers EL, Appelbaum FR, Spielberger RT, et al. Selective ablation of acute myeloid leukemia using antibody targeted: a phase I study of an anti-CD33 calicheamicin immunoconjugate. *Blood* 1999;93:3678.

Rowe JM. Treatment of acute myelogenous leukemia in older adults. *Leukemia* 2000; 14:480.

Tallman MS. Therapy of acute promyelocytic leukemia: ALL trans retinoic acid and beyond. *Leukemia* 1998;12:S37–S40.

Thomas ED, Buckner CD, Banaji M, et al. One hundred patients with acute leukemia treated by chemotherapy, total body irradiation, allogeneic bone marrow transplantation. *Blood* 1977;49:511.

Westbrook CA, Hooberman AL, Spino C, et al. Clinical significance of the BCR-ABL fusion gene in adult acute lymphoblastic leukemia: a cancer and leukemia group B study (8762). *Blood* 1992;80:2983.

Yeager AM, Kaizer H, Santos GW, et al. Autologous bone marrow transplantation in patients with acute non-lymphocytic leukemia using [ex vivo] marrow treatment with 4-hydroxyperoxycyclophosphamide. *N Engl J Med* 1986;315:141.

12. CHRONIC LEUKEMIA

Chronic Lymphoid Leukemias

Kenneth A. Foon

Epidemiology and Etiology
Incidence
Chronic lymphocytic leukemia (CLL) is the most common type of leukemia in Western countries, accounting for 0.8% of all cancers and 30% of leukemias. The disease is rare in Asians; 90% of patients are older than 50 years of age. Men are affected more often than women are by a ratio of 2:1.

Etiology
1. **Genetic factors:** Familial clusters of CLL have been described. The incidence in relatives of patients with leukemia is twofold to threefold greater than that of the general population. The great majority of cases are sporadic.
2. **Immunologic factors:** Inherited and acquired immunodeficiency syndromes are often associated with CLL and other lymphoproliferative neoplasms. These observations suggest that defective immunosurveillance may result in proliferation of malignant cell clones and increased susceptibility to potential leukemogens, such as viruses.
3. **Chromosomes, oncogenes, and viruses:** Viruses have not been demonstrated to play a direct role in CLL leukemogenesis. A variety of chromosome abnormalities have been described in patients with CLL. Using *in situ* hybridization, interphase cytogenetic techniques, and improved methods to induce metaphases in CLL cells, abnormalities of 13q14-23.1 are the most common. This is followed in order by trisomy 12, then deletion of 11q22.3-23.1 deletion of 6q21-23, and deletions or mutations of 17q13 involving the *p53* tumor suppressor gene.
4. **Radiation:** Populations exposed to radiation do not have an increased incidence of CLL.
5. **Environmental factors:** Currently, there is no association known between CLL and exposure to solvents, pesticides or sunlight.

Pathology and Natural History
Pathology
Chronic lymphocytic leukemia is a clonal disease of immunologically incompetent long-lived lymphocytes that express high levels of antiapoptotic proteins, including BCL-2 and bcl-x_L and lower levels of the proapoptotic protein bax or bcl-xs. All cases involve CD5-B lymphocytes, which represent about 10% of normal B-lymphocytes and appear to play a major role in autoimmunity.

Natural History
Immunologic abnormalities: CLL is associated with hypogammaglobulinemia, low complement levels, altered expression of major histocompatibility complex class II antigens on the CLL cells, impaired granulocyte function, defects in T cells with likely impaired T helper cell type 1 immunity. CLL cells downmodulate expression of the CD-40 ligand (CD154) on activated T cells, inhibiting their ability to interact with antigen presenting cells, and may account for the inability of B-cell clone to produce immunoglobulin G (IgG). CLL cells generate immune suppressive factors. The leukemia cells have low levels of surface immunoglobulin and display a single heavy-chain class, typically μ; some cells display both μ and δ. Less commonly, α, σ, or no heavy-chain determinant is found. The leukemia cells display either κ or λ light chains, but never both.
Surface membrane antigens include the B-cell antigens CD19 and CD23 and low levels of CD20. The CD11c and CD25 antigens are found on cells in half of cases. CD5 is always present on CLL cells.

Monoclonal paraproteins are not routinely identified; however, when one uses more sensitive techniques, it appears that most patients with CLL secrete small amounts of paraproteins (usually IgM). These paraproteins rarely produce symptoms of hyperviscosity.

Coombs'-positive warm antibody hemolytic anemia occurs in about 10% of patients and immune thrombocytopenia in about 5%. Immune neutropenia and pure red blood cell aplasia are rare. Compared with the general population, the incidence of skin carcinoma is increased eightfold and visceral cancers twofold in patients with CLL.

Clinical course: The natural history of CLL is highly variable. Survival is closely correlated with the stage of disease at diagnosis. Because most patients are elderly, more than 30% die of diseases unrelated to their leukemia.

Manifestations: In 25% of patients, CLL is first recognized at routine physical examination or by a routine complete blood count (CBC). Clinical manifestations develop as the leukemia cells accumulate in the lymph nodes, spleen, liver, and bone marrow or reticuloendothelial system:

1. Osteolytic lesions and isolated mediastinal involvement are unusual and suggest a diagnosis other than CLL.
2. Pulmonary leukemic infiltrates and pleural effusions are common late in the course of disease.
3. Renal involvement is common in CLL, but functional impairment is unusual in the absence of obstructive uropathy, pyelonephritis, or hyperuricemia secondary to tumor lysis from therapy.
4. Skin involvement is rare.
5. Transformation into a diffuse large cell lymphoma (Richter syndrome) or "prolymphocytoid" leukemia occurs in fewer than 5% of patients.

Progressive disease is accompanied by deterioration of both humoral and cell-mediated immunity:

1. Herpes zoster is the cause of 10% of infections in CLL patients.

2. Bacterial pathogens associated with hypogammaglobulinemia include *Streptococcus pneumoniae, Staphylococcus aureus,* and *Haemophilus influenzae.*

3. *Pneumocystis carinii* may be the causative infectious agent in patients with pulmonary infiltrates.

4. As the disease progresses, patients develop progressive pancytopenia, persistent fever, and inanition. During the latter stages of disease, cytotoxic chemotherapy is generally ineffective, and dosages are restricted because of pancytopenia. Death usually is caused by infection, bleeding, or other complications of the disease.

Diagnosis

Symptoms and Signs
Patients with CLL that was discovered by chance are usually asymptomatic. Chronic fatigue and reduced exercise tolerance are the first symptoms to develop. Advanced, progressive disease is manifested by severe fatigue out of proportion to the degree of the patient's anemia, fever, bruising, and weight loss. Lymphadenopathy, splenomegaly, and hepatomegaly should be assessed carefully. Edema or thrombophlebitis may result from obstruction of lymphatic or venous channels by enlarged lymph nodes.

Laboratory Studies
A hemogram measures the following:

1. **Erythrocytes.** Anemia may be caused by lymphocyte infiltration of the bone marrow, hypersplenism, autoimmune hemolysis, and other factors. Red blood cells are usually normocytic and normochromic in the absence of prominent hemolysis.

2. **Lymphocytes.** The absolute lymphocyte count typically ranges from 10,000 to 200,000 per microliter but may exceed 500,000 per microliter. Morphologically, lymphocytes are usually mature appearing and have scanty cytoplasm and clumped nuclear chromatin. When blood smears are made, the cells are easily ruptured, producing typical "basket" or "smudge" cells.

3. **Granulocytes.** Absolute granulocyte counts are normal or increased until late in the disease.

4. **Platelets.** Thrombocytopenia may be produced by bone marrow infiltration, hypersplenism, or immune thrombocytopenia.

Other useful studies that should be obtained in patients with CLL include the following: (a) renal and liver function tests; (b) Coombs' (antiglobulin) tests; (c) serum protein electrophoresis; (d) chest radiographs; and (e) computed tomography (CT) scans, which can be used to evaluate retroperitoneal, abdominal, and pelvic lymph nodes.

Bone marrow examination is usually not necessary to establish the diagnosis in patients with persistent lymphocytosis. The bone marrow of all patients with CLL contains at least 30% lymphocytes. The pattern of bone marrow infiltration is an important prognostic factor (see the discussion of **prognostic factors** in the section entitled **Staging and Prognostic Factors**). The indications for bone marrow aspiration and biopsy include the following: (a) borderline cases of lymphocytosis when the diagnosis is in doubt; (b) thrombocytopenia, to distinguish immune thrombocytopenia from severe bone marrow infiltration; and (c) Coombs' negative, unexplained anemia.

Establishing the diagnosis of CLL: The National Cancer Institute (NCI) Working Group on CLL has established useful guidelines for the minimum diagnostic requirements for this disease, which are as follows: (a) absolute lymphocytosis (5,000/μ or more) with mature-appearing lymphocytes that is sustained; (b) characteristic immunophenotype of monoclonal B cells, including the expression of pan-B cell antigens (CD19, CD20, and CD23), the coexpression of CD5 on the leukemic B cells, and surface immunoglobulin of low-intensity (most often IgM).

Differential Diagnosis

Benign causes of lymphocytosis in adults include viral infections, especially hepatitis, cytomegalovirus, and Epstein-Barr virus (EBV). Lymphadenopathy and hepatosplenomegaly are absent or mild in elderly patients who have infectious mononucleosis. The presence of fever, liver function tests compatible with hepatitis, and positive EBV serologies should distinguish mononucleosis from CLL. Other causes are brucellosis, typhoid fever, paratyphoid, and chronic infections; autoimmune diseases; drug and allergic reactions; thyrotoxicosis and adrenal insufficiency; and postsplenectomy.

Hairy cell leukemia (HCL) must be differentiated from CLL because management of the two disorders is different. Diagnosis depends on recognizing the pathognomonic hairy cells.

Cutaneous T-cell lymphomas are suspected if skin involvement is extensive. Differentiation from CLL is made by identifying the convoluted nuclei and helper T cells (with immunohistochemistry and flow cytometry) that are characteristic of this disease.

The leukemic phase of non-Hodgkin lymphoma (NHL) usually is distinguished from CLL morphologically and immunologically. Follicular center cell NHL (FCC) cells are often cleaved, whereas CLL cells are never cleaved. In addition, FCC NHL cells demonstrate intense surface immunoglobulin without the CD5 antigen, and the opposite is generally true for CLL cells. Mantle cell NHL cells express CD5, but they do not express CD23 and typically have higher intensity surface immunoglobulin and CD79a than CLL cells.

Prolymphocytic leukemia is characterized by large lymphocytes with prominent nucleoli. Lymphadenopathy is minimal; splenomegaly is massive.

Large granular lymphocyte leukemia (LGLL) has a characteristic morphology with abundant pale to clear, sharply defined cytoplasm and multiple distinct azurophilic granules of varying size. The cells are true T cells, and most correspond to natural killer cells. The immunophenotype is positive for CD3, CD8, CD16, and CD57. LGLL is indolent and almost uniformly associated with neutropenia. Rheumatoid arthritis is peculiarly present in about one third of patients.

Staging System and Prognostic Factors
Prognostic Factors

Routine CBCs may detect asymptomatic cases of CLL, but this has no bearing on the overall survival of these patients. If survival has been improved (and it is not clear that it has), effective treatment of complicating infections in CLL probably has been more responsible for the improvement than cytotoxic agents.

Clinical staging is helpful for determining prognosis and deciding when to initiate treatment. Anemia and thrombocytopenia adversely affect prognosis when they are due to leukemic infiltration ("packing") of the bone marrow but not when due to autoimmune destruction of red blood cells or platelets. The pattern of bone marrow infiltration also appears to affect prognosis. Patients with nodular or interstitial patterns of bone marrow involvement have longer survival times than patients with diffuse ("packed") involvement.

Other adverse prognostic factors appear to be a lymphocyte doubling time of less than 12 months, elevated serum β_2 microglobulin level, high serum levels of soluble CD23, blood leukocytic count greater than 30,000 per microliter, which is atypical morphology, complex karyotypes including trisomy 12, and expression of CD38 and nonmutated IgV genes.

Staging System
The *modified Rai classification* of CLL (see section III.C for differences with the NCI Working Group criteria) is shown in Table 1.

Management
Indication for Treatment
Chronic lymphocytic leukemia is usually indolent. Treatment of asymptomatic stable disease is not warranted. The blood lymphocyte count does not indicate the need to start therapy and generally is not useful to monitor therapy. The indications for instituting therapy in CLL areas follow:

1. Persistent or progressive systemic symptoms (fever, sweats, weight loss)
2. Lymphadenopathy that causes mechanical obstruction or bothersome cosmetic deformities
3. Progressive enlargement of the lymph nodes, liver or spleen
4. Stage III or IV (high-risk) disease that results from the replacement of bone marrow with lymphocytes
5. Immune hemolysis or immune thrombocytopenia
6. Rapid lymphocyte doubling time

Chemotherapy
Fludarabine is superior to alkylating agents in its associated complete response rate and duration of response but not overall survival. Fludarabine may be the initial treatment

Table 1. The modified Rai classification of chronic lymphocytic leukemia

Stage	Extent of disease	Risk	Median survival (yr)
0 1	Lymphocytosis of bone marrow (≥40% lymphocytes) and blood (>5,000/μL)	Low	0
I	Stage 0 plus lymphadenopathy	Intermediate	7
II	Stage 0 or I plus splenomegaly and/or hepatomegaly	Intermediate	7
III	Stage 0, I, or II plus anemia (hemoglobin <11.0 g/dL)[a]	High	2
IV	Stage 0, I, or II plus thrombocytopenia (platelets <100,000/μL)[a]	High	2

[a] Excluding anemia or thrombocytopenia caused by immunologic destruction of cells.

of choice for patients who would benefit from a rapid and sustained remission, such as cases designated for further aggressive therapy. Prolonged treatment with fludarabine and other nucleoside analogs (such as cladribine), however, is also associated with marked immunosuppression and an increased risk for opportunistic infections and autoimmune hemolysis.

Guidelines for chemotherapy are the following:

1. The initiation of therapy should be timed according to the clinically assessed pace of disease. Complete remission is not a necessary goal. Treatment is discontinued when the inciting problem has been controlled (after a few weeks to several months).

2. Immune hemolysis or thrombocytopenia should be treated with prednisone alone, 60 mg orally daily, which is then tapered after achievement of control of blood cell counts.

3. Resistant disease should be treated with alkylating agents if a nucleoside was first-line therapy. Third-line therapy includes combination chemotherapy regimens, such as CVP (cyclophosphamide, vincristine, and prednisone) or CHOP (cyclophosphamide, hydroxydaunomycin, Oncovin, and prednisone) (see Chapter 21).

4. Differential staining cytotoxicity (DiSC) to assess the sensitivity of CLL cells to fludarabine and other drugs *in vitro* may predict *in vivo* response but is not standardly used.

Drugs include the following:

1. Alkylating agents. Chlorambucil, 0.1 to 0.2 mg per kilogram of body weight administered orally daily for 3 to 6 weeks as tolerated; the dose is usually tapered to 2 mg daily until the desired effect is achieved. Alternatively, 15 to 30 mg/m^2 may be given orally for 1 day (or divided over 4 days) every 14 to 21 days; the dose is adjusted to tolerance. Cyclophosphamide, 2 to 4 mg per kilogram of body weight administered orally PO daily for 10 days; the dose is then adjusted downward for continued therapy until the desired effect is achieved.

2. Nucleosides. Fludarabine, 25 to 30 mg/m^2 administered intravenously daily for 5 consecutive days every 4 weeks. Cladribine (2-chlorodeoxyadenosine, 2-CdA), either 0.10 mg per kilogram of body weight daily administered by continuous intravenous infusion for 7 days or 0.12 mg per kilogram of body weight daily administered intravenously over 2 hours for 5 consecutive days every 4 weeks. Pentostatin, 4 mg/m^2 administered intravenously every other week.

3. Combination chemotherapy. Combinations of cyclophosphamide, mitoxantrone, cytarabine, and cisplatin with any of the nucleoside agents are under investigation.

4. Rituximab is a humanized monoclonal antibody that binds to the human CD20 and generates responses in 50% of FCC NHL patients but in considerably fewer CLL patients, possibly related to the low density of CD20 on CLL cells. Patients with CLL are being studied at higher than the standard rituximab dose of 375 mg/m^2 weekly for 4 consecutive weeks. Patients with greater than 50,000 per microliter circulating CLL cells are at risk for a cytokine-release syndrome secondary to the release of tumor necrosis factor-α and interleukin-6 (IL-6) with fever, chills, nausea, vomiting, hypotension, and dyspnea.

5. CAMPATH-1H is a humanized monoclonal antibody that binds to CD52. Patients treated with 30 mg intravenously three times weekly for 12 weeks experienced a 42% response rate, primarily in the blood and bone marrow, with minimal effect on enlarged nodes and spleen.

6. Lym-1 is a murine monoclonal antibody that binds to a major histocompatability class II antigen. Clinical responses were reported in 50% of NHL patients treated with iodine-131 (^{131}I)-labeled Lym-1. Considerably fewer responses were reported in CLL patients.

7. Stem cell transplantation using either autologous or allogeneic stem cells led to responses in most cases. Autologous transplant responses are relatively short, but the procedure has a significantly lower mortality rate. Nonmyeloblative regimens to harness the graft-versus-leukemia effect of allogeneic transplant are currently being explored.

Radiation Therapy
Local irradiation is recommended only for reduction of lymph node masses that threaten vital organ function and that have responded poorly to chemotherapy. Splenic irradiation may result in improvement of disease elsewhere and may improve temporarily the signs of hypersplenism; however, the clinical usefulness of splenic irradiation has not been established. Total-body irradiation remains investigational and potentially dangerous.

Surgery
Splenectomy is indicated in CLL patients who have immune hemolytic anemia or thrombocytopenia that either fails to respond to corticosteroid therapy or must be treated with corticosteroids chronically. Splenectomy also may be helpful in patients with problematic hypersplenism.

Special Clinical Problems
Richter Syndrome
About 5% of patients with CLL develop a diffuse large cell lymphoma with rapid clinical deterioration and death occurring within 1 to 6 months. The clinical features include fever, weight loss, increasing localized or generalized lymphadenopathy, lymphocytopenia (as well as other cytopenia), and dysglobulinemia. Combination chemotherapy with CHOP (see Appendix A2) is usually tried but is rarely effective.

Prolymphocytic Leukemia
Prolymphocytic leukemia is a rare variant of CLL. The main clinical features are massive splenomegaly without substantial lymph node enlargement. Leukocytosis usually exceeds 100,000 per microliter and is characterized by large lymphoid cells with single prominent nucleoli. Tissue sections show almost no mitotic figures despite the immature appearance of the leukemic cells. Fludarabine or cladribine used as single agents or combination therapy with CHOP may be useful.

Eighty percent of cases involve B cells that have different surface markers than typical CLL (the B cells of prolymphocytic leukemia show intense surface immunoglobulin, the CD19 and CD20 B-cell antigens, but typically not the CD5 antigen). Twenty percent of cases are T cell, usually with the helper phenotype (CD3 and CD4 positive). A small percentage of CLL patients develop a "prolymphocytoid" transformation, whereby more than 30% of the peripheral blood cells are prolymphocytic. This differs from *de novo* prolymphocytic leukemia in that the cells maintain the immune features of CLL and the clinical course resembles typical CLL, albeit in a late stage of the disease.

Other Chronic Lymphoid Leukemias
A variety of lymphoproliferative disorders distinct from CLL that are distinguished by unique clinical features and cellular morphology and phenotype have been described. Derived from both the B- and T-lymphocyte at various stages of maturation, they each present a unique array of characteristics (Table 2).

Hairy Cell Leukemia
Epidemiology and Etiology
Hairy cell leukemia (HCL; leukemic reticuloendotheliosis, lymphoid myelofibrosis) accounts for about 2% of all leukemias. The incidence in men outnumbers women 5:1. The median age of patients is 55 years; patients younger than 30 years of age are unusual. The etiology is unknown.

Pathology and Natural History
   1. Pathology: The pathognomonic hairy cell can be identified in the peripheral blood, bone marrow, liver, and spleen of affected patients. The hairy cells are B-lymphocytes in virtually every case.
   2. Natural history: The natural history is extremely variable, ranging from a relatively fulminant course to a waxing and waning course of exacerbations and spontaneous improvements, and to prolonged survival measured in decades. Most patients

Table 2. Lymphoid malignancies

	Median age at diagnosis (yr)	Male; female ratio	Leukocyte count ($\times 10^9$L)	Lymph nodes	Spleen	Skin	Other
B-lymphocytes							
Chronic lymphocytic leukemia	60	2:1	10 to >200	50	50	<5	Autoimmune hemolytic anemia thrombocytopenia, and neutropenia, hypogamma-globulinemia
Prolymphocytic leukemia	65	4:1	100 to >500	<25	>90	<5	
Waldenström's macroglobulinemia	50	1:1	Normal to 50	30	30	<5	Elevated IgM
Leukemic phase of lymphoma	50	2:1	Normal to >100	90	75	5	
Hairy cell leukemia	50	5:1	<1–100	30	>75	<5	Pancytopenia, splenomegaly
T-lymphocytes							
Adult T-cell leukemia/ leukemia/lymphoma	40	M > F	Normal to >150	90	>50	>50	HTLV-1, hypercalcemia, lytic bone lesions
Prolymphocytic leukemia	60	M > F	100 to >500	25	>90	10	
Large granular lymphocytic leukemia	50	2:1	Normal to >100	10	30		
Cutaneous T-cell lymphoma (Sézary cell leukemia)	50	M > F	Normal to >150	50	10	100	

HTLV-1, human T-cell leukemia virus type 1; IgM, immunoglobulin M.

are able to function normally throughout most of their illness. Patients with HCL usually present with an insidious development of nonspecific symptoms, splenomegaly, and pancytopenia. Progression of disease is manifested by bleeding because of thrombocytopenia, anemia requiring transfusions, and recurrent infections. Death is caused by severe infection in more than half the cases and (uncommonly) by hemorrhage.

Diagnosis

Symptoms and signs: Weakness and fatigue are the presenting complaints in about 40% of cases. A bleeding diathesis, recent infection, or abdominal discomfort is present in about 20% of patients. Splenomegaly occurs in 95% of patients and is severe in most. Hepatomegaly is seen in about 50% of patients and is usually mild. Peripheral lymphadenopathy is rarely present; however, CT scans of the abdomen may reveal retroperitoneal lymphadenopathy.

Preliminary laboratory studies include the following:

1. CBC. Anemia and thrombocytopenia occur in 85% of patients. About 60% of patients have leukopenia with granulocytopenia; 20% have increased hairy cells with a leukocytosis in the peripheral blood, usually associated with an absolute granulocytopenia.

2. Blood chemistries. Only 10% to 20% of patients have abnormal liver or renal function tests. Polyclonal hyperglobulinemia or decreased normal immunoglobulin concentrations occurs in 20% of patients.

Special diagnostic studies: The diagnosis of HCL is made by identifying the pathognomonic mononuclear cells in the peripheral blood or bone marrow. The cells have irregular and serrated borders with characteristic slender, hairlike cytoplasmic projections and round, eccentric nuclei with spongy chromatin. The cytoplasm is sky blue without granules.

1. Immune flow cytometry demonstrates a characteristic pattern of CD19, CD20, CD22, CD11c, CD25, and CD103 positivity. Hairy cell variants may be CD25 or CD103 negative and typically do not have as good a prognosis as classic HCL.

2. Phase-contrast microscopy with supravital staining of fresh preparations is extremely valuable for demonstrating the cellular characteristics because the cytoplasm of hairy cells is often poorly preserved in films mixed with Wright's stain.

3. Tartrate-resistant acid phosphatase (TRAP): HCL cells have a strong acid phosphatase activity, which is resistant to inhibition by 0.05 molar tartaric acid (because of the presence of isoenzyme 5 of acid phosphatase); the acid phosphatase in leukocytes from most patients with lymphomas and CLL is sensitive to tartrate. A strongly positive TRAP study is present in most patients with HCL but is not required for the diagnosis and can be detected in patients with other lymphoid malignancies.

4. Bone marrow aspiration frequently is unsuccessful ("dry tap"): Marrow biopsy shows a characteristic loose and spongy arrangement of cells, even with extensive infiltration with hairy cells. Fibrosis of the marrow with reticulin fibers is also characteristic in areas of HCL infiltration and accounts for the high frequency of dry taps.

5. Splenic morphology. The spleen is the most densely infiltrated organ in HCL. The red pulp of the spleen may contain a unique vascular lesion: pseudosinuses lined by hairy cells.

Differential Diagnosis

It is important to distinguish HCL from other diseases because management is substantially different. HCL is most often confused with CLL, malignant lymphoma, histiocytic medullary reticulosis, myelofibrosis, or monocytic leukemia. Differentiation is made by identifying the pathognomonic cell, the characteristic immune profile, TRAP test, and pathologic findings of the bone marrow biopsy.

Staging System and Prognostic Factors

The natural median survival time for HCL appears to be 5 to 10 years, but this has been dramatically altered by current therapies.

Management
The decision to treat: Many cases tend to have an indolent course, and these patients have excellent survival times without therapy. Therapy may be deferred for asymptomatic patients until at least one of the following problems develops:

1. Anemia (hemoglobin <10g/dL)
2. Granulocytopenia (< 1,000/µL)
3. Severe thrombocytopenia (< 100,000/L)

Splenectomy has achieved at least a partial response in 75% of patients and historically had been the standard therapy for HCL.

Cladribine is now the treatment of choice for HCL. The drug is given by continuous intravenous infusion *once only* at a dose of 0.09 mg per kilogram per day for 7 consecutive days. More than 95% of patients respond to treatment, and 80% are complete responders. If the patient does not respond to the initial course of cladribine, it is unlikely they will benefit from additional courses. Twenty percent of patients may relapse, and most respond to an additional course of cladribine. Toxicity has been limited to transient fevers that are usually associated with neutropenia.

Interferon-α (IFN-α) is a highly effective agent in reversing the pancytopenia and splenomegaly in HCL. Dosages of IFN ranging from 2 to 4 million U daily or three times weekly for 1 year achieve responses in 90% of patients with HCL. Complete responses with disappearance of hairy cells from the bone marrow, however, are unusual. Immune parameters, such as natural killer cells and cell-surface markers, normalize in association with the reversal in the hematologic parameters.

Pentostatin (2'-deoxycoformicin) is also highly effective therapy for HCL. Most patients not only have normalization of their CBC but also have a complete response with disappearance of hairy cells from their bone marrow (rarely seen with IFN-α). Complications include skin rash and neurotoxicity. The dosage is 4 mg/m^2 IV every 2 weeks for 3 to 6 months.

Prolymphocytic Leukemia
Morphology
These large cells have abundant cytoplasm and a prominent nucleolus. They likely represent activated cells.

Immunophenotype
The cells typically have high-density immunoglobulin (higher than CLL) with the B-cell antigens CD19, CD20, and CD22 (typically absent or reduced in CLL), and no CD5. Rearrangement of heavy- and light-chain genes are routinely seen.

Cytogenetics
There is no classic cr consistent chromosomal abnormality.

Clinical Features
Patients with prolymphocytic leukemia usually have extremely high blast counts and splenomegaly but often lack significant lymphadenopathy.

Treatment
There exists no standard therapy. Treatment is with single-agent nucleosides such as fludarabine and cladribine or with combination chemotherapy: CHOP, which includes cyclophosphamide (750 mg/m administered intravenously on day 1), doxorubicin (50 mg/m^2 given intravenously on day 1), vincristine (2 mg intravenously on day 1), and prednisone (100 mg given orally on days 1–5) at 3-week intervals.

T-cell prolymphocytic leukemia represents 20% of total cases and tends to be more aggressive than the B-cell variety. The cells express the CD3 and CD4 antigens (sometimes CD8) with rearrangement of the β-T-cell receptor gene. Inversion of chromosome 14 is commonly seen. Treatment with pentostatin may be effective.

Waldenström Macroglobulinemia (See Chapter 13)
Morphology
The B-lymphocytes of Waldenström macroglobulinemia are larger and more plasmacytoid morphologically than are the cells of CLL. An eccentrically placed nucleus with

abundant periodic acid Schiff (PAS)-positive cytoplasm and a well-developed endoplasmic reticulum characterize these cells. Both cytoplasmic and surface IgM are easily detectable; increased amounts of IgM paraprotein are typically found in the plasma, appearing as a monoclonal spike on the serum protein electrophoresis pattern. Not infrequently, this increase in IgM paraprotein can cause a "hyperviscosity syndrome" that is characterized by signs and symptoms of decreased central nervous system perfusion (CNS). The bone marrow in Waldenström macroglobulinemia is usually hypercellular and contains increased numbers of large plasmacytoid lymphocytes and plasma cells.

Clinical Features
The peak incidence of this disorder occurs during the sixth and seventh decades, and the disease typically progresses slowly and resembles malignant lymphoma in some aspects because of the prominent lymphadenopathy and hepatosplenomegaly that can be present. In contradistinction to multiple myeloma, lytic bone lesions and renal failure are infrequent. Lightheadedness, fullness in the head, decreased visual acuity with engorgement of the retinal veins, and decreased hearing acuity are sometimes experienced by patients and are part of the hyperviscosity syndrome. Bleeding manifestations due to abnormalities of the clotting factors, caused by the high plasma levels of IgM, are occasionally seen.

Treatment
Treatment with chlorambucil or other alkylating agents may be effective. Fludarabine and cladribine are also effective.

Adult T-cell Leukemia
Morphology
The cells are typically large and have a distinct cloverleaf nucleus.

Immunophenotype
The cells have the CD3 and CD4 antigens typical of helper T-cell lymphocytes but function as inducers of suppressor T cells. They always express CD25 and display rearrangement of the T-cell receptor β.

Clinical Features
A range of disease, from a smoldering, low-grade leukemia or lymphoma to a very aggressive disease with high white blood cell counts, skin infiltration, hypercalcemia, and lytic bone lesions may be seen. This disease is commonly found in southern Japan and the Caribbean, but it may occur in the southeastern United States and Europe.

Etiology
The human T-cell leukemia virus-1 (HTLV-1), an RNA retrovirus, is the cause of this disease.

Treatment
Typically, CHOP will lead to a rapid response, but unfortunately, relapse is inevitable. Studies using fludarabine, cladribine, and other agents are under way.

Large Granular Lymphocytic Leukemia
Morphology
The characteristic cell is a large granular lymphocyte.

Immunophenotype
The most common immunophenotype is CD3, CD8, CD16, CD56, and CD57. Approximately 20% of patients do not express the CD3 (T-cell receptor) and have the classic immunophenotype of a natural killer cell CD16, CD56, and CD57.

Clinical Features
The classic presentation is that of an indolent lymphoma with severe neutropenia. The neutropenia is thought to be secondary to antigranulocyte antibodies or direct cellular cytotoxicity of myeloid precursors. Patients typically have a moderately elevated white

blood cell count, tumor infiltration (but not replacement) of the bone marrow, and modest splenomegaly without lymphadenopathy or cutaneous lesions.

Treatment
Therapy with chemotherapy has been largely ineffective, although some patients have responded to methotrexate and others to prednisone. Increased neutrophils are reported following treatment with cyclosporin or granulocyte–colony-stimulating factor.

Suggested Readings
Chronic Lymphocytic Leukemia
Delannoy A, Martiat P, Gala JL, et al. 2-chlorodeoxyadenosine (CdA) for patients with previously untreated chronic lymphocytic leukemia (CLL). *Leukemia* 1995;9:1130–1135.

Dighiero G, Maloum K, Desablens B, et al. Chlorambucil in indolent chronic lymphocytic leukemia. *N Engl J Med* 1998;338:1506.

Dohner H, Stilgenbauer S, Benner A, et al. Genomic aberrations and survival in chronic lymphocytic leukemia. *N Engl J Med* 2000;343:1910–1916.

Foon KA, Thiruvengadam R, Saven A, et al. Genetic relatedness of lymphoid malignancies. *Ann Intern Med* 1993;119:63.

Johnson S, Smith AG, Loffler H, et al. Multicentre prospective randomized trial of fludarabine versus cyclophosphamide, doxorubicin and prednisone (CAP) for the treatment of advanced-stage chronic lymphocytic leukemia. *Lancet* 1996;347:1432.

Keating MJ, O'Brien S, Lerner S, et al. Long-term follow-up of patients with chronic lymphocytic leukemia (CLL) receiving fludarabine regimens as initial therapy. *Blood* 1998;92:1165.

Robak T, Blasinska-Morawiec M, Krykowski E, et al. Intermittent 2-hour intravenous infusions of 2-chlorodeoxyadenosine in the treatment of 110 patients with refractory or previously untreated B-cell chronic lymphocytic leukemia. *Leuk Lymphoma* 1996;22:509–514.

Saven A, Lemon RH, Kosty M, et al. 2-Chlorodeoxyadenosine activity in patients with previously untreated chronic lymphocytic leukemia. *Journal of Clinical Oncology* 1995;13(3):570–574.

Seymour JF, Cusack JD, Lerner SA, et al. Case control study of the role of splenectomy in chronic lymphocytic leukemia. *J Clin Oncol* 1997;15:52.

Sorensen JM, Vena DA, Fallavollita A, et al. Treatment of refractory chronic lymphocytic leukemia with fludarabine phosphage via the group C protocol mechanism of the National cancer Institute: five-year follow-up report. *J Clin Oncol* 1997;15:458.

Hairy Cell Leukemia
Cheson BD, Sorensen JM, Vena DA, et al. Treatment of hairy cell leukemia with 2-chlorodeoxyadenosine via the group C protocol mechanism of the National Cancer Institute: a report of 979 patients. *Clin Oncol* 1998;16:3007.

Hoffman MA, Janson D, Rose E, et al. Treatment of hairy-cell leukemia with cladribine: response, toxicity, and long-term follow-up. *J Clin Oncol* 1997;15:1138.

Johnston JB, Eisenhauer E, Wainman N, et al. Long-term outcome following treatment of hairy cell leukemia with Pentostatin (Nipent): a National Cancer Institute of Canada study. *Semin Oncol* 2000;27(Suppl 5):32–36.

Saven A, Burian C, Koziol JA, et al. Long-term follow-up of patients with hairy cell leukemia after cladribine treatment. *Blood* 1998;92:1918.

Tallman MS, Hakimiar D, Rademaker AW, et al. Relapse of hairy cell leukemia after 2-chlorodeoxyadenosine: long-term follow-up of the Northwestern University experience. *Blood* 1996;88:1954.

Large Granular Lymphocytic Leukemia
Lamy T, Loughran TP Jr. Current concepts: large granular lymphocyte leukemia. *Blood Rev* 1999;13:230–240.

Loughran TP Jr. Large granular lymphocytic leukemia: an overview. *Hosp Pract* 1998;133.

Prolymphocytic Leukemia
Shvidel L, Shtalrid M, Bassous L, et al. B-cell prolymphocytic leukemia: a survey of 35 patients emphasizing heterogeneity, prognostic factors and evidence for a group with an indolent course. *Leuk Lymphoma* 1999;33:169–179.

Chronic Myelogenous Leukemia

Joseph J. Mazza

Chronic myelogenous leukemia (CML) is a myeloproliferative disease characterized by a proliferation of myeloid cells without loss of their capacity to differentiate. Cytogenetic and isoenzyme studies have provided evidence that this is a clonal hematopoietic stem cell disorder arising from a single cell. Clinically, there is a chronic stable phase of the disease during which patients are asymptomatic and show no evidence of an evolving leukemic process. After a variable period in the chronic stable phase, virtually all patients evolve into an acute or blast phase that is usually refractory to standard chemotherapy and die as a direct result of their leukemia. Recently, because of the unique cytogenetic abnormalities associated with CML, attempts to induce complete durable remissions by ablating the leukemic clone have led to better understanding of the clonal proliferative nature of this disease and have provided ways of monitoring the effects of therapy.

Etiology
Radiation
Factors that may have direct etiologic implications are not apparent in most patients with CML; however, the increased incidence of this disorder in certain groups of persons who have been exposed to excessive amounts of ionizing radiation seems to be a factor of major importance. People exposed to high levels of radiation in Hiroshima and Nagasaki at the time of and subsequent to the atomic bomb explosions in 1945 have shown an increased incidence of CML and other hematologic disorders.

Chemicals and Drugs
Exposure to certain organic solvents, such as benzene, has been associated with CML and other hematologic malignancies. Evidence associating CML with other factors, such as drugs and organic chemicals, seems to be mounting, but most studies indicate that the development of leukemia on exposure to such agents results in acute leukemia rather than CML.

Heritability
There is no convincing evidence that CML is an inherited disease, and children born to affected mothers are not affected.

Epidemiology
Chronic myelogenous leukemia accounts for approximately 20% of all cases of leukemia in the Western countries, and its incidence in the United States is approximately 1.4 per 100,000. The death rate per year is approximately 1 per 100,000 population. The peak incidence occurs during the fourth and fifth decades of life, with a slightly higher incidence in men. The clinical features and course of CML appear to be identical in both sexes, but there is some evidence that would indicate better survival in women than in men.

Clinical Features
Usually, the signs and symptoms of CML develop insidiously and frequently are vague and nonspecific. In contrast to chronic lymphocytic leukemia, it is unusual to make the diagnosis of CML in an asymptomatic patient. When such situations occur, it is usually only a matter of weeks or months before overt manifestations of the disease are detectable. Generalized weakness, malaise, weight loss, and decreased exercise tolerance are common early symptoms of the disease process. Left upper-quadrant fullness and discomfort with early satiety are common symptoms associated with an enlarged spleen and become more symptomatic as the disease progresses. Bleeding manifestations caused by quantitative and qualitative abnormalities of platelets are seen occasionally (i.e., petechiae, purpura, and mucous membrane bleeding). Features of hypermetabolism, such as warm, moist skin and fever, are not uncommon early symptoms

of CML and usually parallel the severity of the disease as measured by the degree of the anemia, leukocytosis, and splenomegaly.

Clinical Course

Chronic myelogenous leukemia is characterized clinically by a prolonged, chronic stable phase that eventually proceeds to an accelerated phase and finally a blastic transformation (*blast crisis*). The timing of the blast transformation is not predictable in an individual patient and may occur 1 to 5 years subsequent to the initial diagnosis. Usually, however, the chronic stable phase lasts 3 to 5 years. Factors that have been associated with a shorter chronic stable phase or a more accelerated course are as follows:

1. Older patients (>60 years of age)
2. Male sex
3. Persistent anemia
4. Thrombocytopenia or thrombocytosis
5. Increased number of basophils and circulating blasts or excessive immature cells in the peripheral blood

At initial presentation, the manifestations of CML usually respond promptly to therapy and are easily controlled by appropriate adjustments in the dosage of myelosuppressive therapy. **The progression to accelerated phase** may occur gradually or abruptly and usually is accompanied by a constellation of clinical and hematologic changes; however, accelerated phase without blast transformation may occur.

1. Anemia usually ensues.
2. Thrombocytopenia or in some instances thrombocytosis is present.
3. Leukocytosis is accompanied by an increase in the degree of immaturity on the differential count. Basophilia may also be present. The hematologic picture may become more characteristic of a "subacute" leukemia.
4. Duration of the accelerated phase may be quite variable.
5. Refractoriness to therapy usually accompanies progression to accelerated phase.

Blast crisis occurs when there is a transformation to an acute leukemia. The blast phase may occur in a matter of weeks and may be myeloid or lymphoid. Once this phase of CML occurs, numerous complications commonly seen in other acute leukemias ensue, but certain features unique to blast phase CML deserve emphasis:

1. The complete remission rate in patients with acute-phase CML or blast crisis is significantly lower than in other acute nonlymphocytic leukemias (<10%), and the duration of the complete remission is considerably shorter (< 3 months).
2. Approximately 20% to 30% of patients who develop the acute blast phase of their disease have a lymphoid transformation, which can be confirmed by using special histochemical stains and immunologic marker (immunophenotyping) studies. Usually, the lymphocytes are pre-B cells and are terminal deoxynucleotidyl trasnsferase (TdT) and common acute lymphocytic leukemia antigen (CALLA) positive (CD10⁺).
3. Most patients who transform from the accelerated phase of their disease to the blast phase become increasingly refractory to therapy and die as a result of the acute leukemia; however, a significant number of patients die as a direct result of the complications (i.e., infection and hemorrhage) associated with intensive multidrug chemotherapy.

Cytogenetics

Philadelphia Chromosome

A wide spectrum of chromosomal abnormalities have been shown to exist in myeloproliferative diseases, and with the advent of a new banding technique, complex chromosomal rearrangements, breaks, and deletions have been more easily demonstrable. The most consistent abnormality that has become the hallmark of CML is the Philadelphia (Ph) chromosome, which is detectable in more than 90% of patients with CML. The Ph chromosome is present during the blast phase of the disease and throughout the entire course of CML.

The Ph chromosome consists of a reciprocal translocation of chromosomal material between chromosomes 9 and 22 [t (9; 22)]. This chromosomal abnormality appears to be unique for CML but has been found in some cases of acute lymphocytic leukemia (ALL) and rarely in other myeloproliferative diseases [e.g., polycythemia rubra vera (PRV)]. Other complex translocations may occur in approximately 5% of cases of CML. The Ph chromosome can be detected at any stage of the disease and persists throughout the chronic stable phase, when the patient is asymptomatic and the bone marrow and peripheral blood appear normal. As the patient enters the accelerated or blast phase of the disease, the Ph chromosome persists, but additional chromosomal abnormalities are frequently seen and include trisomy 9, 19, or 21, isochromosome 17, double Ph, or the deletion of the Y chromosome.

Philadelphia Chromosome Negative

A small percentage of patients with CML are Ph-negative and run a clinical course that differs significantly from their Ph-positive counterparts. Ph-negative patients respond less favorably to therapy, and evolution into an accelerated-phase or blast-phase CML occurs more rapidly, resulting in shorter survival.

Cytotoxic Findings

Cytotoxic findings in CML would suggest that this is a clonal disease, that is, arising from a single cell with an acquired chromosomal abnormality. Findings of lymphocyte phenotype markers and positive Ph chromosomes in lymphoid cells in CML suggest that the pluripotential stem cell has sustained the malignant transformation.

The c-abl Protooncogene

This protooncogene is situated at a specific breakpoint on chromosome 9 (C9), called the *breakpoint cluster region* (BCR); it is translocated to the long arm (q) of chromosome 22 (C22) to form the Ph chromosome. This translocation of genetic material results in an abnormal fusion gene (BCR/abl) that encodes for an abnormal gene product, the BCR/abl oncoprotein (210 kDa) that has tyrosine specific protein activity. This product may play a major role in the expansion of the altered stem cell clone and the pathogenesis of CML. It is not yet known, however, what role this abnormal fusion gene may play in the initiating events of the myeloproliferative process characteristic of the early stages of CML and the frequent progression of stable phase CML to an acute leukemia.

Laboratory Studies

Peripheral Blood

A moderate to marked increase in the white blood cell (WBC) count is the hallmark of CML. The leukocytosis may vary from 50 to 300×10^3 per microliter. An occasional blast cell may be present on the peripheral smear, but significant numbers are not found at the time of diagnosis. Early granulocytic cells are present with polys and band forms predominating the differential count. There is no leukemic hiatus.

The platelet count may be decreased in the early stage of CML, but more often it is normal to slightly increased, and in some cases may be significantly increased (>500,000/m^3). Mild to moderate anemia is almost always present at diagnosis and is usually normochromic normocytic. Evidence of hemolysis is usually not apparent, and the reticulocyte count is usually normal. A mild increase in the percentage of basophils and eosinophils on a differential count at diagnosis is frequently evident; this often increases as the disease progresses.

Bone Marrow

The bone marrow is characteristically hypercellular with marked proliferation of all granulocytic elements. Megakaryocytes are frequently prominent and increased on the marrow aspirate smears, and increased numbers of eosinophils and basophils are also characteristic features of CML. Mild fibrosis of the marrow, best appreciated on the bone marrow biopsy sections, is not uncommon and present in approximately 10% to 15% of patients at diagnosis.

Other Laboratory Abnormalities

A low leukocyte alkaline phosphatase (LAP) is a unique laboratory finding in CML and helps in the differential diagnosis of the leukocytosis from other myeloproliferative diseases. Although LAP levels rise once patients enter the chronic stable phase of the disease with therapy, they are a consistently reliable finding at the time of the initial diagnosis and workup. Hyperuricemia is commonly found at diagnosis and reflects increased cell turnover.

An elevated serum B_{12}-binding protein (predominantly TC-I), which is synthesized by the granulocytes, is invariably present at the time of the initial workup. The level seems to correlate well with the degree of leukocytosis.

Treatment

The treatment of CML has become more controversial in the recent past with the onslaught of biotherapy. Currently, three agents are capable of inducing and maintaining a chronic stable phase of the disease: busulfan, hydroxyurea, and α-interferon (IFN-α).

Once the diagnosis is established and myelosuppressive therapy is instituted, patients should be followed closely with frequent blood counts and examinations to monitor the efficacy of therapy. The two most commonly used myelosuppressive agents in the treatment of CML are busulfan (Myleran) and hydroxyurea (Hydrea). Only recently has IFN-α come into vogue and has been shown to be an effective treatment agent for CML.

Busulfan, an alkylating agent, at a dosage of 6 to 8 mg per day orally, usually lowers the WBC count and decreases the size of the spleen in 4 to 6 weeks. This drug is usually well tolerated by patients and is not associated with any side effects at the time of its ingestion. The dosage of busulfan should be decreased by 50% when the WBC count is decreased by 50% from its pretreatment level. Busulfan should be temporarily discontinued when the WBC approximates the upper limit of normal range or is less than 15,000 per microliter. It is important to adjust and titrate maintenance therapy for each patient. Frequently, intermittent busulfan may be all that is necessary for maintaining patients in the chronic stable phase of the disease. Low-dose busulfan also can be used as maintenance therapy; frequently as little as 2 to 4 mg weekly maintains a normal WBC. Because of the potent myelosuppressive properties of busulfan, pancytopenia and marrow hypoplasia are the most common adverse effects associated with its use. Like all other alkylating agents, busulfan has been associated with inducing myelodysplasia and acute myeloid leukemia when given over an extended period. Therefore, frequent blood counts while patients are being treated are imperative and cannot be overemphasized. Other adverse effects associated with long-term busulfan therapy include hyperpigmentation and pulmonary fibrosis.

Hydroxyurea, an inhibitor of deoxynucleotide synthesis, used in a similar manner as busulfan, is equally effective in lowering the WBC and platelet counts and improving the hemoglobin in CML. Several studies have shown a survival advantage for patients treated with hydroxyurea rather than busulfan. An initial dosage of hydroxyurea of 1,000 to 1,500 mg daily or 30 mg per kilogram of body weight daily administered orally is usually sufficient to improve the hematologic parameters within 2 to 6 weeks. As with busulfan, careful frequent monitoring of blood counts is advocated (every 2 weeks) until there is a significant fall in the WBC count, at which time the dosage can be decreased or discontinued. Appropriate timely adjustments in the dosage of hydroxyurea can be made as the disease comes under control and when the WBC count approximates normal. Bone marrow hypoplasia and the adverse effects seen with long-term busulfan therapy are not usually seen with hydroxyurea.

Although there is some evidence in the literature to suggest that the length of the chronic stable phase of CML is longer when patients are treated with hydroxyurea than with busulfan, there is no large randomized series currently available in the literature comparing these two agents. Hydroxyurea is considered the more desirable of the two drugs because of the possible induction of second malignancies with long-term use of alkylating agents. This complication, however, is of little clinical significance in CML because of the relatively short life expectancy of patients with this disease.

IFN-α, a naturally occurring cytokine with antiviral and antiproliferative properties, has been introduced as a new and promising alternative to chemotherapy for conservative management of CML. Numerous recent studies have demonstrated the potential of IFN-α to induce hematologic and cytogenetic remissions.

Evidence has been accumulated through clinical trials that suggests that, compared with hydroxyurea or busulfan, IFN-α can increase life expectancy, with a 5-year survival rate of 50% to 59%, compared with 29% to 44% in those treated with hydroxyurea or busulfan.

Because of an associated chronic flu-like syndrome and high cost, some clinicians are reluctant to use IFN-α to treat CML. Frequently, treatment must be discontinued because of these problems.

IFN-α must be given parenterally (subcutaneously) on a regular basis, but dose and frequency of administration range from 3 to 15 mU per day, depending on the tolerance or adverse effects elicited. Although IFN-α has been demonstrated to have potent antiproliferative properties, its mode of action in CML has not been clearly elucidated. IFN-α is not an effective therapy for patients in accelerated stage and blast phase of CML.

Responses to IFN-α in patients with CML appear to be longer than with conventional chemotherapy. Patients with a significant cytogenetic response (decrease of the Ph-positive cell clone) appear to have a longer duration of response and survival. Recent studies suggested that IFN-α used in combination with other chemotherapeutic agents, such as cytarabine or hydroxyurea, may further add to the survival benefit in patients with CML but with increased toxicity.

Intensive Chemotherapy

In stable-phase CML, intensive chemotherapy has been shown to be effective in reducing significantly the percentage of Ph chromosome–positive metaphases in the bone marrow. In a few studies, these patients have shown improved survival compared with patients who have not shown similar cytogenetic response to chemotherapy. It is difficult to say whether these intensive therapy regimens alter the course of the disease or merely select high- and low-risk patients according to their cytogenetic response. Despite these encouraging results from a few institutions using intensive chemotherapy programs, none has been curative, nor has any substantially improved overall survival. With increased toxicity and greater expense plus longer hospitalization time, there seems to be little justification for intensive chemotherapy for patients with CML in the chronic phase.

Gene Therapy

In recent years, attempts have been made to use uniquely designed nucleotide sequences, antisense molecules, against the BCR/abl and MYB genes to interfere with the important genes responsible for the synthesis of the gene products necessary for CML. This has met with limited success thus far and work continues in this area.

Signal Transduction Inhibitors

Signal transduction inhibitor STI-571 has emerged as an effective representative of a new class of drugs used in the treatment of CML. This compound has proven capable of inducing both hematologic as well as cytogenetic remissions in CML patients. These agents act selectively on the BCR/abl fusion gene product, an intracellular protein with elevated tyrosine kinase activity necessary for the transforming ability of the BCR/abl gene and the proliferation of the leukemic clone.

In a recently published clinical trial using STI-571, complete hematologic responses were achieved in more than 90% of patients treated within the first 3 weeks of therapy. Cytogenetic responses have been achieved in 45% of patients, with a complete cytogenetic response in 10% of patients and confirmed by molecular analysis.

Radiation Therapy

Radiation therapy to the spleen has a limited role in the treatment of CML. It has been used as an effective means of achieving rapid regression of an enlarged symptomatic spleen and to control the progression of the disease from the stable chronic phase. Radiation therapy, however, is no more efficacious than busulfan or hydroxyurea in causing regression of the splenomegaly in CML.

Splenectomy

In chronic-phase CML, a splenectomy may improve tolerance for chemotherapy during the later stages of the disease, but it is clear that splenectomy does not change the incidence of blast transformation or the overall survival of patients with CML. Splenectomy may be useful in the patient with refractory hypersplenism.

Leukophoresis
When leukocytosis is extreme (>300 × 10³ μL) is an effective means of lowering the WBC count and improving blood flow. Central nervous system (CNS) symptoms as a result of leukostasis usually improve promptly after the first apheresis. Twice weekly apheresis is recommended to decrease the WBC count while myelosuppressive therapy is being administered. This mode of therapy is expensive and temporary in its efficacy, and it should not be used as a long-term means of therapy.

Bone Marrow Transplantation (BMT) (See Chapter 19)
The only curative treatment of CML thus far demonstrated is high-dose chemotherapy plus total body irradiation, followed by allogeneic bone marrow transplantation (BMT) rescue with marrow from a human leukocyte antigen (HLA)-identical sibling. Allogeneic BMT has been used mainly for patients in the chronic stable phase. Its use in accelerated and blast-phase disease has met with much less success.

Conditioning regimens used for BMT have been able to ablate the malignant cell clone completely, as is evident by the absence of the Ph chromosome following marrow engraftment, an achievement that has not been consistently accomplished with standard myelosuppressive chemotherapy.

At present, allogeneic BMT must be considered the treatment of choice for young patients (<45 years of age) with chronic-phase CML who have an HLA-identical sibling donor. Recent follow-up studies of this group of patients showed more than 60% disease-free survival at 3 years.

Mortality and morbidity rates in BMT patients remain high, and the main causes of death are attributable to interstitial pneumonia, infection, recurrent leukemia, and graft-versus-host disease. Because of the long, indolent, symptom-free clinical course that many patients are able to achieve with simple outpatient oral chemotherapy, it is difficult to determine which patients should receive transplantation and when the procedure should be done.

Autologous Bone Marrow Transplantation
This procedure has become increasingly more popular in its use for treating a variety of hematologic malignancies, including CML. Autologous BMT has obvious and distinct advantages over allogeneic BMT (see Chapter 19): It applies to a larger number of patients for two reasons: It does not require an HLA-matched donor, and it is better tolerated by older patients who would otherwise be excluded from consideration of receiving an allogeneic BMT. The overall toxicity and cost of the procedure are considerably less than with allogeneic BMT. Autologous BMT is not associated with graft-versus-host disease toxicity, a common major complication of allogeneic BMT.

The efficacy of autologous BMT in CML has been addressed in a recent analysis of more than 200 ABMTs performed at eight centers throughout the world. The results showed that ABMT could provide prolonged survival in chronic or accelerated phase patients compared with conventional therapy. In a multicenter analysis of 200 patients, survival probability of chronic phase patients at 6 years is greater than 50%. These data suggest that autologous BMT therapy for CML can provide prolonged survival exceeding that associated with conventional therapy.

Further studies are needed to determine the optimal time to perform transplantation in patients who are in a stable chronic phase, whether peripheral stem cell harvesting has advantages over bone marrow, and whether *ex vivo* purging or treatment of stem cells before reinfusion is beneficial or improves the results of this procedure.

Matched Unrelated Donor Marrow
For patients who are considered good candidates for an allogeneic BMT but who do not have an HLA-matched sibling donor, an unrelated HLA-matched donor may be identified through the National Marrow Donor Registry (NMDR) Program. Other registries in other countries have led to a worldwide network, allowing for a greater possibility of a patient–donor match. This procedure shows similar survival as a matched sibling

donor group in children and young adults, but experience is limited and toxicity associated with this program has been a major impediment to this option.

Recent analysis of a large group of patients who received an unrelated donor marrow transplant through the NMDR Program showed that the combined beneficial effects of critical, favorable, prognostic variables (age < 35 years, transplantation within the first year of chronic stable phase of disease) yielded a 5-year disease-free survival rate of 64%.

Blast Phase

The treatment of the blast phase of CML leaves much to be desired, and thus far there have been no effective agents or combination of agents capable of improving the dismal complete remission rate and short duration of survival. The subgroup of patients who develop the lymphoid blast crisis, however, has shown much better response rates (>50%) and improved survival with standard ALL induction treatment programs using vincristine, prednisone, and doxorubicin. Thus, it is important to identify this subgroup of patients in blast crisis who have a lymphoid transformation by histochemical and immunologic marker studies.

Suggested Readings

Allan NC, Richards SM, Shepherd PC. UK Medical Research Council randomised, multicentre trial of interferon-alpha n1 for chronic myeloid leukaemia: improved survival irrespective of cytogenetic response. The UK Medical Research Council's Working Parties for Therapeutic Trials in Adult Leukaemia. *Lancet* 1995;345: 1392.

Armitage JO, et al. Marrow transplantation for stable-phase chronic granulocytic leukemia. *Exp Hematol* 1984;12:717.

Auclerc G, et al. Post-therapeutic acute leukemia. *Cancer* 1979;44:2017.

Bhatia R, et al. Autologous transplantation therapy for chronic myelogenous leukemia. *Blood* 1997;89:2623.

Bolin RW, et al. Busulfan versus hydroxyurea in long-term therapy of chronic myelogenous leukemia. *Cancer* 1982;50:1683.

Buckner CD, Stewart P, Clift RA. Treatment of blastic transformation of chronic granulocytic leukemia by chemotherapy, total body irradiation and infusion of cryopreserved autologous marrow. *Exp Hematol* 1978;6:96.

Champlin R. Allogeneic, syngeneic, and autologous bone marrow transplantation for chronic myelogenous leukemia. *Leukemia* 1993;7:1084.

Champlin R, et al. Allogeneic bone marrow transplantation in chronic myelogenous leukemia in chronic or accelerated phase. *Blood* 1982;138.

Coulombel L, et al. Long-term marrow culture reveals chromosomally normal hematopoietic progenitor cells in patients with Philadelphia chromosome–positive chronic myelogenous leukemia. *N Engl J Med* 1983;308:1493.

Cunningham I, et al. Results of treatment of Ph[1] chronic myelogenous leukemia with an intensive treatment regimen (L-5 protocol). *Blood* 1979;53:375.

Druker BJ, et al. Clinical efficacy and safety of an ABL specific tyrosine kinase inhibitor as targeted therapy for CML. *Blood* 1999;94:368a.

Druker BJ, Lydon NB. Lessons learned from the development of an abl tyrosine kinase inhibitor for chronic myelogenous leukemia. *J Clin Invest* 2000;105:3.

Fialkow PG, et al. Evidence for a multistep pathogenesis of chronic myelogenous leukemia. *Blood* 1981;58:158.

Freund M, et al. Combination of chemotherapy and interferon alfa-2b in the treatment of chronic myelogenous leukemia. *Semin Hematol* 1993;30(Suppl 3):11.

Gamis AS, et al. Unrelated-donor bone marrow transplantation for Philadelphia chromosome-positive chronic myelogenous leukemia in children. *J Clin Oncol* 1993;11:834.

Gewirtz AM, et al. Oligodeoxynucleotide therapeutics for human myelogenous leukemia: interim results. *Blood* 1996;88:270a.

Goldman JM, Lu DP. New approaches in chronic granulocytic leukemia—origin, prognosis, treatment. *Semin Hematol* 1982;19:241.

Goldman JM, et al. Marrow transplantation for patients in the chronic phase of chronic granulocytic leukaemia. *Lancet* 1982;2:623.

Goto T, Nishikori M, Arlin Z. Growth characteristics of leukemia and normal hematopoietic cells in Ph[1] positive chronic myelogenous leukemia and effects of intensive treatment. *Blood* 1982;59:793.

Guilhot F, et al. Interferon alfa-2b combined with cytarabine versus interferon alone in chronic myelogenous leukemia: French Chronic Myeloid Leukemia Study Group. *N Engl J Med* 1997;337:223.

Hehlmann R, Hockhaus A. The changing nature of conventional therapy in CML. In: Talpaz M, Kantarjian H, eds. *Medical management of CML*. New York: Marcel Dekker (*in press*).

Hehlmann R, et al. Randomized comparison of busulfan and hydroxyurea in chronic myelogenous leukemia: prolongation of survival by hydroxyurea: the German CML Study Group. *Blood* 1993;82:398.

Hehlmann R, et al. Randomized comparison of interferon-alpha with busulfan and hydroxyurea in chronic myelogenous leukemia: the German CML Study Group. *Blood* 1994;84:4064.

Hester JP, et al. Response of chronic myelogenous leukemia patients to COAP-splenectomy: a Southwest Oncology Group study. *Cancer* 1984;54:1977.

The Italian Cooperative Study Group on Chronic Myeloid Leukemia. Results of a prospective randomized trial of early splenectomy in chronic myeloid leukemia. *Cancer* 1984;54:333.

The Italian Cooperative Study Group on Myeloid Leukemia. Interferon alfa-2a as compared with conventional chemotherapy for the treatment of chronic myeloid leukemia. *N Engl J Med* 1994;330:820.

Kantarjian HM, et al. Intensive combination chemotherapy (ROAP 10) and splenectomy in the management of chronic myelogenous leukemia. *J Clin Oncol* 1985;3:85.

Koeffler HP, Golde DW. Chronic myelogenous leukemia—new concepts. *N Engl J Med* 1981;201.

Marks SM, Baltimore D, McCaffrey R. Terminal transferase as a predictor of initial responsiveness to vincristine and prednisone in blastic chronic myelogenous leukemia. *N Engl J Med* 1978;298:812.

McGlave PB. Unrelated donor and autologous marrow transplant therapy of CML. *Leukemia* 1993;7:1082.

McGlave PB, et al. Successful allogeneic bone-marrow transplantation for patients in the accelerated phase of chronic granulocytic leukemia. *Lancet* 1982;2:625.

McGlave PB, et al. Therapy for chronic myelogenous leukemia with unrelated donor bone marrow transplantation: results in 102 cases. *Blood* 1990;75:1728.

McGlave PB, et al. Unrelated donor marrow transplantation for chronic myelogenous leukemia: 9 years' experience of the National Marrow Donor Program. *Blood* 2000;95:2219.

Medical Research Council's Working Party of Therapeutic Trials in Leukemia. Randomized trial of splenectomy in Ph[1] positive chronic granulocytic leukemia, including an analysis of prognostic factors. *Br J Haematol* 1983;54:415.

Miescher PA, Jaffé ER, eds. Interferon in the treatment of chronic myeloid leukemia. *Semin Hematol* 1993;3:1.

Rowley JD. Ph[1] positive leukemia including chronic myelogenous leukemia. *Clin Haematol* 1980;9:55.

Sokal JE. Evaluation of survival data from chronic myelocytic leukemia. *Am J Hematol* 1979;1:493.

Speck B, et al. Occasional survey: allogeneic bone marrow transplantation for chronic myelogenous leukemia. *Lancet* 1984;11:665.

13. MULTIPLE MYELOMA AND RELATED MONOCLONAL GAMMOPATHIES

Robert A. Kyle

Each monoclonal protein (M protein, paraprotein) consists of two heavy-chain polypeptides of the same class and subclass and two light-chain polypeptides of the same type. The different monoclonal proteins are designated by capital letters that correspond to the class of their heavy chains, which are designated by Greek letters: γ in immunoglobulin G (IgG), α in IgA, μ in IgM, δ in IgD, and ε in IgE. Their subclasses are IgG1, IgG2, IgG3, and IgG4, or IgA1 and IgA2, and their light-chain types are kappa (κ) and lambda (λ). A monoclonal protein is characterized by a narrow peak (like a church spire) (Fig. 1) or a localized band on electrophoresis and by a localized band on immunofixation. The differential diagnosis of monoclonal gammopathies is shown in Table 1. The distribution of patients with monoclonal gammopathies seen at the Mayo Clinic in 1999 is shown in Fig. 2.

In contrast to a monoclonal protein, a polyclonal protein consists of one or more heavy-chain classes and *both* light-chain types. A polyclonal protein is characterized by a broad peak or band, usually of γ mobility on electrophoresis (Fig. 3) and by the absence of a localized band with appropriate antisera on immunofixation. The differential diagnosis of polyclonal gammopathies is shown in Table 2. It is important to differentiate monoclonal from polyclonal increases in immunoglobulins because the former are associated with a neoplastic or potentially neoplastic process, whereas the latter are associated with an inflammatory or reactive process.

Monoclonal proteins have long been considered abnormal proteins, but studies during the past several years indicate that they are only excessive quantities of normal immunoglobulins. Monoclonal proteins are individual antibodies and are products of a single clone of plasma cells. Although some monoclonal proteins represent known antibodies, most do not. The one-cell, one-immunoglobulin concept is supported by the fact that nearly all individual plasma cells contain either κ or λ light chains but not both.

Recognition of Monoclonal Proteins

Analysis of the serum or urine for monoclonal proteins requires a rapid, dependable screening method and a specific assay to identify the heavy-chain class and light-chain type of the protein. Electrophoresis on agarose gel is advised for screening. After screening with agarose gel, immunofixation should be used to confirm the presence of a monoclonal protein and determine its heavy-chain class and light-chain type.

Electrophoresis

Serum protein electrophoresis should be done in all patients in whom multiple myeloma, macroglobulinemia, or amyloidosis is known or suspected. Electrophoresis also is indicated in any patient with unexplained weakness or fatigue, anemia, elevation of the erythrocyte sedimentation rate, back pain, osteoporosis, osteolytic lesions or fractures, immunoglobulin deficiency, hypercalcemia, Bence Jones proteinuria, renal insufficiency, or recurrent infections. Because the presence of a localized band or spike is strongly suggestive of primary amyloidosis, serum protein electrophoresis also should be performed in adults with unexplained peripheral neuropathy, carpal tunnel syndrome, refractory congestive heart failure, nephrotic syndrome, orthostatic hypotension, or malabsorption.

Constituents of the major components of the serum electrophoretic pattern are listed in Table 3. A large peak in the α_2-globulin area may represent free hemoglobin–haptoglobin complexes resulting from hemolysis. Large amounts of transferrin in patients with iron-deficiency anemia may produce a peak in the β region. Fibrinogen is seen as a discrete band between β and γ peaks. The specimen should be examined for a clot, and if there is none, thrombin should be added to the sample. If evidence of fibrinogen is not found, immunofixation is indicated because the β–γ band may repre-

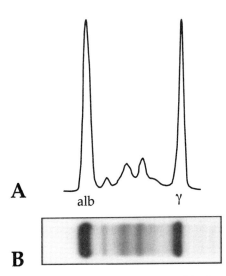

FIG. 1. A: Monoclonal pattern of serum protein as traced by densitometer after electrophoresis on agarose gel: tall, narrow-based peak of γ mobility. **B:** Monoclonal pattern from electrophoresis of serum on agarose gel (anode on left): dense, localized band representing monoclonal protein of γ-mobility. (From Kyle RA, Katzmann JA. Immunochemical characterization of immunoglobulins. In: Rose NR, Conway de Macario E, Folds JD, et al., eds. *Manual of clinical laboratory immunology,* 5th ed. Washington, DC: American Society for Microbiology, 1997:156–176, with permission.)

sent a small monoclonal protein. Hypogammaglobulinemia (<0.7 g/dL) is seen in nearly 10% of patients with multiple myeloma and in approximately one fourth of patients with primary systemic amyloidosis. It also may be congenital; associated with nephrotic syndrome, chronic lymphocytic leukemia, lymphoma, protein-losing enteropathy, or malnutrition; or caused by corticosteroid therapy.

A monoclonal protein may be present even when the total serum protein concentration, β- and γ-globulin peaks, and quantitative immunoglobulins are all normal. The agarose gel must be examined visually because the densitometer tracing may not detect a small monoclonal protein. A small monoclonal protein also may be concealed among the β or γ components. A monoclonal light chain (Bence Jones proteinemia) is rarely seen on the agarose gel. A localized band occasionally is seen in μ heavy-chain disease, but it is never seen in α heavy-chain disease. In γ heavy-chain disease, a broad band rather than a sharp, localized band often is seen on electrophoresis. A monoclonal protein may appear as a rather broad band and may be mistaken for a polyclonal increase in immunoglobulins. Hence, immunofixation is necessary to identify a monoclonal protein.

A densitometer tracing of the serum protein electrophoretic pattern is preferred for following the size of a monoclonal protein. Quantitation of immunoglobulins by rate nephelometry is also satisfactory, but the nephelometry value for IgM and occasionally IgG or IgA is much higher than the value obtained with a densitometer tracing of serum protein electrophoresis. Consequently, either electrophoresis or nephelometry must be used throughout the course of the patient's illness rather than alternating the techniques.

Immunofixation
Immunofixation should be performed in all cases in which a sharp peak or localized band is found on electrophoresis or in which myeloma, macroglobulinemia, amyloidosis, or a related disorder is suspected. An immunofixation pattern of a monoclonal protein is

Table 1. Differential diagnosis of monoclonal gammopathies

I. Malignant monoclonal gammopathies
  A. Multiple myeloma (IgG, IgA, IgD, IgE, and free light chains)
    1. Overt multiple myeloma
    2. Smoldering multiple myeloma
    3. Plasma cell leukemia
    4. Nonsecretory myeloma
    5. Osteosclerotic myeloma (POEMS syndrome)
  B. Plasmacytoma
    1. Solitary plasmacytoma of bone
    2. Extramedullary plasmacytoma
  C. Malignant lymphoproliferative diseases
    1. Waldenström (primary) macroglobulinemia
    2. Malignant lymphoma
  D. Heavy-chain diseases (HCDs)
    1. γ-HCD
    2. α-HCD
    3. μ-HCD
  E. Amyloidosis
    1. Primary
    2. With myeloma (secondary, localized, and familial amyloidosis have no monoclonal protein)
II. Monoclonal gammopathies of undetermined significance
  A. Benign (IgG, IgA, IgD, IgM, and, rarely, free light chains)
  B. Biclonal gammopathies
  C. Idiopathic Bence Jones proteinuria

Ig, immunoglobulin; POEMS, polyneuropathy, organomegaly, endocrinopathy, M protein, skin changes.
From Kyle RA. Classification and diagnosis of monoclonal gammopathies. In: Rose NR, Friedman H, Fahey JL, eds. *Manual of clinical laboratory immunology,* 3rd ed. Washington, DC: American Society for Microbiology, 1986: 152–167, with permission.

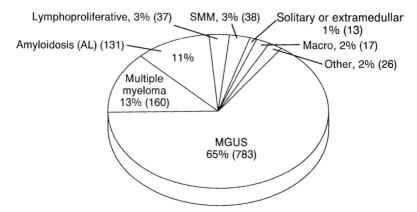

FIG. 2. Diagnosis of monoclonal gammopathies at Mayo Clinic, 1999. MGUS, monoclonal gammopathy of undetermined significance; SMM, smoldering multiple myeloma.

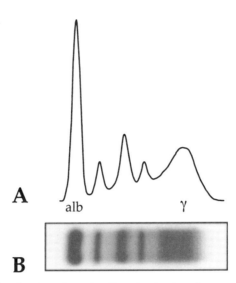

FIG. 3. A: Polyclonal pattern from densitometer tracing of agarose gel: broad-based peak of γ mobility. **B:** Polyclonal pattern from electrophoresis of agarose gel (anode on gel). Band at right is broad and extends throughout the γ area. (From Kyle RA, Katzmann JA. Immunochemical characterization of immunoglobulins. In: Rose NR, Conway de Macario E, Folds JD, et al., eds. *Manual of clinical laboratory immunology,* 5th ed. Washington, DC: American Society for Microbiology, 1997:156–176, with permission.)

shown in Figure 4. All sera with a monoclonal free light chain should be screened with Ouchterlony immunodiffusion for IgD or IgE monoclonal proteins.

Immunofixation may detect a small monoclonal protein in (a) suspected primary amyloidosis, (b) apparently solitary plasmacytoma or extramedullary plasmacytoma, (c) treated myeloma or macroglobulinemia when the localized band has disappeared on electrophoresis, or (d) the presence of a polyclonal increase in immunoglobulins.

Immunofixation is also helpful in recognition of a **biclonal gammopathy** (Fig. 5). The κ:λ ratio obtained from nephelometry has been used in the detection of the light-chain type of large monoclonal gammopathies, but small monoclonal proteins have a normal ratio and are not recognized. This approach is not recommended; immuno-fixation is necessary.

Quantitation of Immunoglobulins
Rate nephelometry is the preferred method for quantitation of immunoglobulins because it is not affected by the molecular size of the antigen. The degree of turbidity produced by antigen–antibody interaction is measured in the near ultraviolet region by nephelometry. Nephelometry measures 7S IgM, polymers of IgA, or aggregates of IgG accurately, unlike radial immunodiffusion, which is not recommended. Quantitation of

Table 2. Differential diagnosis of polyclonal gammopathies

Chronic liver disease, especially chronic active hepatitis
Connective tissue (autoimmune) diseases
Chronic infections
Lymphoproliferative diseases
Normal persons

Table 3. Constituents of the major components of the serum electrophoretic pattern[a]

| + (Anode) ◄─────────────────────────────────────► – (Cathode) | | | | |
Albumin	α_1-Globulin	α_2-Globulin	β-Globulin	γ-Globulin
Albumin	α_1-Antitrypsin	α_2-Macroglobulin	β_1-Lipoprotein	IgG
	α_1-Lipoprotein	α_2-Lipoprotein	Transferrin	IgA
	α_1-Acid	Haptoglobin	Plasminogen	IgM
	glycoprotein	Ceruloplasmin	Complement	IgD
	(orosomucoid)	Erythropoietin	Hemopexin	IgE

[a]Immunoglobulins may migrate from the slow gamma to the α_2-globulin area.
From Kyle RA, Greipp PR. Immunoglobulins and laboratory recognition of monoclonal proteins. In: Wiernik PH, Canellos GP, Kyle RA, et al., eds., *Neoplastic diseases of the blood.* New York: Churchill Livingstone, 1985:431–459, with permission.

immunoglobulins is more useful than immunofixation for the demonstration of hypogammaglobulinemia.

Analysis of Urine for Monoclonal Proteins

When patients with gammopathies are studied, analysis of urine is essential. Sulfosalicylic acid is superior to dipsticks for detection of monoclonal proteins because dipsticks often do not recognize Bence Jones protein. The heat test is not worthwhile for the detection of Bence Jones protein. The recognition of Bence Jones proteinuria depends on the demonstration of a monoclonal light chain by immunofixation of an adequately concentrated urine specimen.

Electrophoresis
Electrophoresis should be performed in all cases with a monoclonal serum protein or with the diagnosis or suspicion of multiple myeloma, macroglobulinemia, amyloidosis,

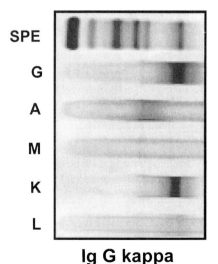

Ig G kappa

FIG. 4. Immunofixation of serum with antisera to immunoglobulin G (IgG), IgA, IgM, κ and λ shows a localized band of IgG and κ antisera, indicating an IgG κ monoclonal protein (Sebia 4 IF). Serum protein electrophoresis (SPE) is on top.

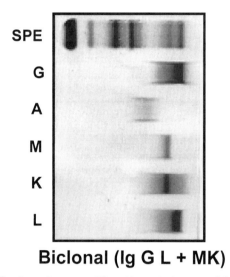

Biclonal (Ig G L + MK)

FIG. 5. Immunofixation of serum with antisera to immunoglobulin G (IgG), IgA, IgM,κ, and λ shows a discrete IgG band with a similar λ band and a discrete IgM band with a similar κ band, indicating a biclonal gammopathy consisting of IgG λ (IgGL) and IgM κ (MK) monoclonal proteins. (Sebia 4 IF). SPE, serum protein electrophoresis (SPE) is on top.

or related diseases. First, a 24-hour collection of urine must be made for determination of the total amount of protein excreted each day. This is important when following the course of a patient who has a monoclonal light chain in the urine because the amount of protein correlates directly with the size of the plasma cell burden. A urinary monoclonal protein is seen as a dense, localized band on agarose gel or as a tall, narrow, homogeneous peak on the densitometer tracing. The amount of monoclonal protein (Bence Jones protein) is calculated from the size of the spike on the densitometer tracing and the total 24-hour urine protein content.

Immunofixation
Immunofixation should be performed on the urine of patients with monoclonal gammopathy of undetermined significance (MGUS) who have a serum monoclonal protein greater than 1.5 g per deciliter. It also should be done for patients who have a known or suspected myeloma, amyloidosis, or plasmacytoma, even if the result of the sulfosalicylic acid test is normal, and who have no globulin spike demonstrated on electrophoresis of urine. The test also should be performed on the urine of every adult older than 40 years in whom a nephrotic syndrome of unknown cause develops. Most patients with a nephrotic syndrome and monoclonal light chain in the urine have primary systemic amyloidosis (usually λ) or light-chain deposition disease (usually κ) (Fig. 6).

Multiple Myeloma
Multiple myeloma (plasma cell myeloma, myelomatosis, or Kahler disease) is characterized by a neoplastic proliferation of a single clone of plasma cells engaged in the production of a monoclonal protein (IgGκ, IgGλ, IgAκ, IgAλ, IgDκ, IgDλ, IgEκ, IgEλ, free κ, and free λ). Multiple myeloma accounts for about 1% of all types of malignant diseases and slightly more than 10% of hematologic malignancies. The incidence is approximately 4 per 100,000 persons per year. The cause of multiple myeloma is unknown. Radiation, exposure to industrial or agricultural toxins, or a genetic element may have a role in some cases.

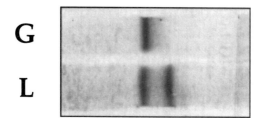

FIG. 6. Immunofixation of urine with antisera to IgG and λ. There are two λ bands. A discrete IgG band corresponds to one of the λ bands. The findings indicate a λ monoclonal protein plus an IgG λ fragment. (From Kyle RA, Katzmann JA. Immunochemical characterization of immunoglobulins. In: Rose NR, Conway de Macario E, Folds JD, et al., eds. *Manual of clinical laboratory immunology,* 5th ed. Washington, DC: American Society for Microbiology, 1997:156–176, with permission.)

Clinical Features

Multiple myeloma has a peak incidence in the seventh decade of life. Only 2% of patients are younger than 40 years. Bone pain, particularly in the back or chest, is present in more than two thirds of patients at diagnosis. The pain is usually aggravated by movement. Weakness and fatigue are common and often are associated with anemia.

Renal insufficiency occurs in about half the patients. This is often due to "myeloma kidney," in which the distal and collecting tubules become obstructed by large laminated casts consisting mainly of Bence Jones protein. Hypercalcemia is also a common, preventable cause of renal insufficiency.

Neurologic involvement is most often manifested by root pain from compression of the nerve. Compression of the spinal cord or cauda equina occurs in about 5% of patients. Leptomeningeal infiltration by myeloma cells occurs infrequently.

Patients with multiple myeloma often have increased susceptibility to bacterial infections, particularly pneumococcal pneumonia. The incidence of gram-negative infections and herpes zoster is increased in myeloma. Bleeding may occur from thrombocytopenia, qualitative platelet abnormalities, or inhibition of coagulation factors from the monoclonal protein. Pallor is the most frequent physical finding. The liver is palpable in about 20% of patients and the spleen in 5%. Extramedullary plasmacytomas are more common in the late stages of the disease.

Laboratory Features

A normocytic, normochromic anemia is present in two thirds of patients at diagnosis but eventually occurs in nearly all patients with multiple myeloma. Increased plasma volume from the osmotic effect of large amounts of monoclonal protein may produce a spurious decrease of hemoglobin and hematocrit values.

Serum protein electrophoresis reveals a tall, sharp peak or localized band in 80% of patients, hypogammaglobulinemia in 10%, and no apparent abnormality in the remainder. A monoclonal protein is detected in the serum in about 90% of patients. Approximately 60% are IgG, 20% IgA, 10% light chain only (Bence Jones proteinemia), and 1% IgD.

Immunofixation of the urine reveals a monoclonal protein in 75% of patients (Fig. 6). Almost all (98%) patients with multiple myeloma have a monoclonal protein in the serum or urine at diagnosis. The serum creatinine level is increased in about half of the patients, and hypercalcemia is present in 20% at diagnosis.

Conventional radiographs reveal abnormalities consisting of punched-out lytic lesions, osteoporosis, or fractures in about 75% of patients. The vertebrae, skull, thoracic cage, pelvis, and proximal humeri and femurs are the most frequent sites of involvement. Technetium-99m bone scans are inferior to conventional radiographs for detecting lesions in myeloma. Magnetic resonance imaging or computed tomography is helpful in patients with myeloma who have skeletal pain but who have no abnormality on radiographs. Magnetic resonance imaging is too expensive for routine use.

The peripheral blood of patients with myeloma shows a reduction in CD4+ (helper T-lymphocytes) cells and an increase in CD8+ (suppressor T lymphocytes) cells. The demonstration of the monoclonal-protein idiotype and the production of the patient's monoclonal protein by peripheral blood lymphocytes indicate that these cells are part of the malignant clone.

Differential Diagnosis
Bone pain, anemia, and renal insufficiency constitute a triad that is strongly suggestive of multiple myeloma. The diagnosis depends on the demonstration of increased numbers of plasma cells in the bone marrow. Identification of a monoclonal immuno-globulin in the plasma cells by the immunoperoxidase method or immunofluorescence is useful for differentiating multiple myeloma from reactive plasmacytosis and also for recognizing myeloma cells that have an unusual morphologic appearance.

Minimal criteria for the diagnosis of multiple myeloma include the presence of at least 10% abnormal plasma cells in the bone marrow or histologic proof of an ex-tramedullary plasmacytoma, the usual clinical features of multiple myeloma, and at least one of the following abnormalities: a monoclonal protein in the serum (usually >3 g/dL), monoclonal protein in the urine, or osteolytic lesions. Connective tissue diseases, chronic infections, metastatic carcinoma, lymphoma, and leukemia may simulate some of the characteristics of myeloma and should be excluded in the differential diagnosis unless other features make the diagnosis of multiple myeloma clear.

Monoclonal gammopathy of undetermined significance (MGUS). Patients with multiple myeloma must be differentiated from those with MGUS (or benign monoclonal gammopathy). The latter condition is characterized by a monoclonal protein level less than 3 g/dl in the serum, less than 10% plasma cells in the bone marrow, no anemia or osteolytic bone lesions, normal serum albumin, no or small amounts of monoclonal protein in the urine, and no evidence of progression. Patients with MGUS should be observed indefinitely and not be given therapy.

Smoldering multiple myeloma (SMM): Not all patients who fulfill the criteria for the diagnosis of multiple myeloma should be treated. Patients with SMM also should not be given therapy. In contrast to patients with MGUS, patients with SMM have a monoclonal protein value more than 3 g per deciliter in the serum or more than 10% atypical plasma cells in the bone marrow. In addition, patients with SMM frequently have a small amount of monoclonal protein in the urine and a reduction of uninvolved immunoglobulins in the serum. Anemia, renal insufficiency, and skeletal lesions do not develop, however, and the patient's condition remains stable. Patients should not be treated unless laboratory abnormalities progress or symptoms of myeloma develop.

A plasma cell labeling index (PCLI) in which a monoclonal antibody to 5-bromo-2-deoxyuridine is used is helpful for differentiating patients with MGUS or SMM from those with multiple myeloma. Patients whose plasma cells have a high labeling index (≥1%) most likely have or soon will develop symptomatic multiple myeloma.

Disease progression: Patients should not be treated unless progression occurs. The most dependable means of differentiating a benign from a malignant course is the serial measurement of the monoclonal protein. Serum protein electrophoresis or quantitation of immunoglobulins is satisfactory for follow-up, but it is necessary to adhere to one method or the other. Clinically overt disease develops during follow-up of most patients who fulfill the criteria for the diagnosis of multiple myeloma. Because myeloma is not curable and therapy entails cost and morbidity, treatment should be delayed until evidence of progression develops, the patient becomes symptomatic, or treatment is needed to prevent imminent complications.

A clinical staging system based on a combination of findings that correlated with the myeloma cell mass has been used frequently:

- **Stage I.** Patients with low-cell mass (stage I) have all the following characteristics: hemoglobin more than 10 g per deciliter, normal serum calcium, serum IgG less than 5 g per deciliter, or IgA less than 3 g per deciliter, Bence Jones proteinuria less than 4 g daily, and no generalized lytic lesions.
- **Stage II.** Patients whose cell mass is between the limits specified for stage I and stage III are designated as having stage II disease.

- **Stage III.** Patients with high-cell mass (stage III) have at least one of the following: hemoglobin less than 8.5 g per deciliter, serum calcium more than 12 mg per deciliter, IgG more than 7 g per deciliter, IgA more than 5 g per deciliter, Bence Jones proteinuria more than 12 g daily, or advanced lytic bone lesions.

- Patients subclassified according to their serum creatinine values as A (< 2 mg/dL) or B (≥2 mg/dL).

Prognosis
The duration of survival of patients with multiple myeloma ranges from a few months to many years; the median is 3 years. The plasma cell labeling index, β_2-microglobulin (β_2-M) level, C-reactive protein (CRP) value, plasmablastic morphology, age, and levels of thymidine kinase, serum albumin, and soluble interleukin-6 receptor (sIL-6R) are all significant prognostic univariate factors. In our studies, multivariate analysis showed that the plasma cell labeling index, β_2-M level, and plasmablastic morphology are the most important prognostic variables. The median survival of patients with a low plasma cell labeling index and low β_2-M level was 6 years after starting chemotherapy.

Treatment
Although most patients who fulfill the diagnostic criteria for multiple myeloma have symptomatic disease at diagnosis and require therapy, some are asymptomatic and should not be treated. All symptoms, physical findings, and laboratory data must be considered before therapy is started. An increasing level of the monoclonal protein in the serum or urine suggests that therapy will be needed in the near future, whereas immediate treatment is indicated if significant anemia, hypercalcemia, renal insufficiency, lytic bone lesions, or extramedullary plasmacytomas develop. If there is doubt about beginning treatment, it is best to reevaluate the patient in 2 or 3 months and delay therapy until progressive disease is evident.

Systemic therapy is the preferred initial approach for overt symptomatic multiple myeloma. In most patients, analgesics in combination with systemic therapy can control the pain. This management is preferred over the use of local radiation because pain frequently occurs at another site, and radiation may further reduce the bone marrow reserve. Palliative radiation should be limited to patients who have disabling pain from a well-defined focal process or a localized tumor.

If the patient is younger than 70 years, the physician should discuss the possibility of autologous peripheral blood stem cell transplantation with the patient. The hematopoietic stem cells should be collected before the patient is exposed to alkylating agents. Chemotherapy is the preferred initial treatment for symptomatic multiple myeloma in patients older than 70 years or in younger patients in whom transplantation is not feasible.

Peripheral blood stem cells are preferable to bone marrow for transplantation because engraftment is more rapid, and there may be less contamination of the infused cells with tumor cells. The absolute number of CD34+ cells per kilogram of recipient weight is the most reliable and practical method for determining the adequacy of a stem cell product. Autologous peripheral stem cell transplantation is applicable for more than half of patients with multiple myeloma. Two major shortcomings are that (a) eradication of myeloma from the patient does not occur even with large doses of chemotherapy or total body radiation or both and (b) autologous peripheral blood stem cells are contaminated by myeloma cells or their precursors. Fortunately, mortality from autologous transplantation is 1% to 2% if patients are appropriately selected.

Most physicians initially treat the patient with vincristine, doxorubicin (Adriamycin), and dexamethasone (VAD) for 3 to 4 months to reduce the number of tumor cells in the bone marrow and peripheral blood. Dexamethasone with or without thalidomide is being evaluated for initial therapy. Peripheral stem cells then are collected after high-dose cyclophosphamide and granulocyte colony-stimulating factor (G-CSF). One then can proceed with the transplantation, for which the patient is given high-dose chemotherapy or total-body radiation or both followed by infusion of peripheral blood stem cells. The other choice is to treat the patient with alkylating agents after stem cell collection until a plateau is reached and then give the patient α_2-IFN or no therapy until early relapse. At that time, the patient is given high-dose melphalan or total-body radiation or both and the previously collected peripheral blood stem cells are infused. There is no difference in the median survival of patients receiving an autologous stem cell transplant after recovery from stem cell collection and that of patients treated with chemotherapy followed by autologous stem cell transplant at the time of relapse.

In a randomized trial by the French Myeloma Group comparing high-dose chemotherapy and autologous bone marrow transplantation with conventional combination chemotherapy, the 5-year event-free survival (28% vs. 10%) and overall survival (52% vs. 12%) favored the transplant group. The median duration of survival was 42 months in the chemotherapy group and 57 months in the transplant group.

There is controversy concerning the need for a double (tandem) stem cell transplant. In a randomized trial, there was no difference in event-free or overall survival between double and single autologous stem cell transplants at 2-year evaluation. In a subsequent evaluation, patients with a low β_2-microglobulin value at diagnosis appeared to have better results with the double transplantation.

The preparative regimen for autologous stem cell transplantation must be improved because it is the likely source of relapse in most patients. Most physicians now use melphalan (200 mg/m^2) as the preparative regimen rather than melphalan plus total-body irradiation because there is no survival advantage with total-body radiation and toxicity is less. Holmium-166 and samarium-153 plus melphalan are being explored as new preparative regimens.

Melphalan and prednisone: The oral administration of melphalan (Alkeran) (0.15 mg/kg daily for 7 days) and prednisone (20 mg three times a day for the same 7 days) every 6 weeks is a satisfactory regimen and produces objective response in 50% to 60% of patients. Leukocyte (neutrophil) and platelet counts must be determined at 3-week intervals, and the dosage of melphalan should be altered to achieve modest cytopenia at midcycle because absorption of melphalan is variable.

Many combinations of chemotherapeutic agents have been used because of the obvious shortcomings of melphalan and prednisone. Multivariate analysis comparing melphalan and prednisone with a variety of combinations of chemotherapeutic agents revealed higher response rates with combination chemotherapy, but there was no significant difference in overall survival. In addition, there was no evidence that high-risk patients benefited from combination chemotherapy.

Chemotherapy should be continued until the patient is in a plateau state or for a year. Continued therapy with alkylating agents may lead to the development of a myelodysplastic syndrome or acute leukemia. α_2-IFN has been used to prolong the response state. In a multivariate analysis, a modest survival benefit and a 6-month prolongation of the response state occurred with α_2-IFN on maintenance. In most cases, α_2-IFN is not used during maintenance because of its inconvenience, side effects, cost, and modest benefit. Chemotherapy must be reinstituted when relapse occurs. Although most patients again respond to the initial chemotherapy regimen, the duration and quality of response are usually inferior to those shown initially.

Allogeneic bone marrow transplantation: The major advantage is that the graft contains no tumor cells. Fewer than 10% of patients with multiple myeloma are eligible because of their age, lack of an human leukocyte antigen (HLA)-matched sibling donor, or inadequate renal, pulmonary, or cardiac function. In addition, the mortality rate is at least 25%. In an effort to reduce the mortality rate, a "mini-allo" (nonmyeloablative) transplant with a preparative regimen of fludarabine and melphalan may result in lower mortality. Depletion of T cells from the infusion of stem cells decreases the incidence of graft-versus-host disease and thus transplant-associated mortality is reduced, but relapse may be more frequent. If a patient has relapse after allogeneic transplantation, infusion of donor lymphocytes results in benefit in about half the patients. Currently, a conventional allogeneic transplant is not recommended because of its high mortality rate and lack of cure.

Therapy for Resistant Disease

All patients with multiple myeloma who have a response to chemotherapy eventually will have a relapse if they do not die of their disease or an unrelated cause. In addition, more than one third of patients treated initially with chemotherapy will not obtain an objective response.

Chemotherapy: The highest response rates reported for patients with multiple myeloma that is resistant to alkylating agents have been with vincristine, doxorubicin (Adriamycin), and dexamethasone (VAD). About 60% of patients respond if relapse occurs when chemotherapy is not being given, but approximately 40% respond if relapse occurs while they are receiving alkylating agents. Vincristine and doxorubicin are given in a 4-day continuous infusion (days 1–4) along with dexamethasone, 40 mg daily on days 1 through 4, 9 through 12, and 17 through 20. The cycle is repeated every 28 days. Most of the activity of VAD is from dexamethasone. A major shortcoming of VAD is that vincristine and doxorubicin (Adriamycin) must be given by a central venous catheter. Significant steroid toxicity is manifested by infections, gastrointestinal bleeding, and steroid myopathy. In addition, the median duration of response is less than 1 year. Dexamethasone can be given without vincristine and doxorubicin (Adriamycin) because it accounts for 80% of the benefit from VAD. We often use methylprednisolone, 2 g administered intravenously three times weekly for a minimum of 4 weeks. In the event of a response, we reduce the frequency to twice weekly and then to once weekly for maintenance. We find fewer side effects from methylprednisolone than dexamethasone.

Thalidomide produces benefit in approximately 30% of patients with previously treated progressive multiple myeloma. It is given in an initial dosage of 200 mg daily and gradually increased in 200-mg increments to a maximum of 800 mg daily. Constipation, weakness or fatigue, sleepiness, and peripheral neuropathy are undesirable side effects. Use of thalidomide in conjunction with dexamethasone is being explored. In most patients, response occurs within 6 weeks after beginning therapy and with only 400 mg of thalidomide daily.

Therapy with VBAP, a combination of vincristine (2 mg), carmustine (BCNU, 30 mg), doxorubicin (Adriamycin, 30 mg), administered intravenously on day 1, and prednisone (60 mg daily) for 5 days every 3 to 4 weeks has produced some benefit in approximately 30% of patients. The dosage of BCNU and doxorubicin should be increased in subsequent cycles if tolerated. Interferon produces objective improvement in approximately 10% of patients with refractory myeloma. Cyclophosphamide, 600 mg/m^2 given intravenously daily for 4 days, plus prednisone followed by granulocyte-macrophage colony-stimulating factor (GM-CSF) has been useful for refractory, aggressive myeloma but is quite toxic.

Management of Complications

Hypercalcemia, which occurs initially in one fifth of patients with multiple myeloma, must be suspected if the patient has anorexia, nausea, vomiting, polyuria, increased constipation, weakness, confusion, stupor, or coma. Treatment is urgent because renal insufficiency commonly develops. Hydration, preferably with isotonic saline, is essential. In addition, prednisone in an initial dosage of 25 mg four times daily should be given, but the dosage must be reduced and the use of the agent discontinued as soon as possible. If these measures fail, pamidronate disodium (Aredia) or etidronate disodium (didronel) is effective. Because prolonged bed rest often contributes to hypercalcemia, patients with myeloma should be encouraged to be as active as possible. Allopurinol is necessary if **hyperuricemia** is present.

Dehydration, infection, nonsteroidal antiinflammatory agents, and radiographic contrast media may contribute to **acute renal failure.** Patients with acute renal failure should be treated promptly with fluid and electrolyte correction and then hemodialysis if necessary. VAD should be given to reduce the tumor mass as quickly as possible. Plasmapheresis may be helpful for acute renal failure, but patients with irreversible renal changes are unlikely to benefit. Maintenance of a high urine output (3 L every 24 hours) is important for preventing renal failure in patients with Bence Jones proteinuria.

Anemia occurs in almost all patients during the course of multiple myeloma. Erythropoietin improves the hemoglobin level and quality of life in about 60% of patients. Side effects are negligible, and the major disadvantage is cost. The serum erythropoietin concentration is the most important factor predicting response, but some patients with normal levels will respond to the agent.

The prompt and appropriate treatment of **bacterial infections** is important. Pneumococcal and influenza immunizations should be given to all patients despite the suboptimal antibody response that occurs. Prophylactic daily oral penicillin may benefit patients with recurrent pneumococcal infections. Intravenously administered gamma globulin can be used for patients with recurrent infections, but it is inconvenient and very expensive. Because many infections occur in the first 2 months after institution of chemotherapy, the prophylactic use of daily oral trimethoprim-sulfamethoxazole is helpful.

As previously stated, patients should be as active as possible because confinement to bed increases **demineralization of the skeleton.** Trauma must be avoided because even mild stress may result in multiple fractures. Fixation of long-bone fractures or impending fractures with an intramedullary rod and methyl methacrylate has given excellent results. Bisphosphonates are specific inhibitors of osteoclastic activity and reduce the number of patients with pathologic fractures and the number of skeletal lesions that need surgical or radiation intervention for progressive skeletal disease. Improved quality of life and a lesser requirement for analgesics also is associated with bisphosphonate therapy. In addition, bisphosphonates may have an antitumor effect. Patients with multiple myeloma who have lytic lesions or osteopenia should be given pamidronate (90 mg intravenously over 2 hours every 4 weeks). The pamidronate should be continued indefinitely. The drug is well tolerated, but cost is a factor.

The symptoms of **hyperviscosity** may include oronasal bleeding, blurred vision, neurologic symptoms, and congestive heart failure. Most patients have symptoms when the relative serum viscosity reaches 6 to 7 centipoises (normal, < 1.8), but the relationship between serum viscosity and clinical manifestations is not precise. Although vigorous plasmapheresis with a cell separator relieves the symptoms of hyperviscosity, treatment with alkylating agents is necessary for long-term benefit.

If **spinal cord compression** is suspected clinically, magnetic resonance imaging or computed tomography is essential. Radiation therapy in a dose of approximately 3,000 cGy is beneficial. Dexamethasone should be administered daily during radiation therapy to reduce edema.

Emotional Support
All patients with multiple myeloma need substantial continuing emotional support. The physician's approach must be positive in emphasizing the potential benefits of therapy. It is reassuring for patients to know that some patients survive for 10 years or longer. It is vital that the physician caring for patients with multiple myeloma has the interest and capacity to deal with an incurable disease over the space of years with assurance, sympathy, and resourcefulness.

Variant Forms of Myeloma
Smoldering Multiple Myeloma
The diagnosis of SMM depends on the presence of a monoclonal protein level of more than 3 g per deciliter in the serum or more than 10% atypical plasma cells in the bone marrow but no anemia, renal insufficiency, or skeletal lesions. Often a small amount of monoclonal protein is found in the urine, and the uninvolved immunoglobulins are reduced in the serum. Clusters or aggregates of plasma cells often are seen on the bone marrow biopsy specimen. The plasma cell labeling index is low. It is important to recognize these patients because they should not be treated unless progression occurs. In some patients, symptomatic multiple myeloma does not develop for years.

Plasma Cell Leukemia
Patients with plasma cell leukemia have more than 20% plasma cells in the peripheral blood and an absolute plasma cell content of at least 2,000 per microliter. Plasma cell leukemia may be classified as *primary* when it is diagnosed in the leukemic phase or as *secondary* when there is leukemic transformation of a previously diagnosed multiple myeloma. Approximately 60% of patients with plasma cell leukemia have primary plasma cell leukemia. Patients with primary plasma cell leukemia are younger and have a greater incidence of hepatosplenomegaly and lymphadenopathy, a higher platelet count, fewer lytic bone lesions, a smaller serum monoclonal protein peak, and longer survival than do patients with secondary plasma cell leukemia.

Treatment of plasma cell leukemia is unsatisfactory. VAD is the preferred treatment, and if the patient responds, an autologous stem cell transplantation should be considered. Unfortunately, the survival is still short. Secondary plasma cell leukemia, which occurs in 1% to 2% of patients with myeloma, rarely responds to chemotherapy because patients already have received therapy agents and are resistant to them.

Nonsecretory Myeloma

Patients with nonsecretory myeloma have no monoclonal protein in either the serum or the urine, and this condition occurs in about 2% of patients with multiple myeloma. For certainty of diagnosis, a monoclonal protein should be identified in the plasma cells by immunoperoxidase or immunofluorescence methods. In some cases, there is no evidence of a monoclonal protein within the plasma cells, suggesting that no such protein is synthesized. The more carefully the serum and urine are examined for evidence of a monoclonal protein, the fewer cases of nonsecretory myeloma will be found. Treatment for nonsecretory myeloma is the same as that for multiple myeloma. Less renal involvement is seen and survival is longer than in typical myeloma.

Immunoglobulin D Myeloma

Immunoglobulin D myeloma differs enough from IgG and IgA myelomas to warrant discussion as a separate entity. The monoclonal protein spike is smaller, and Bence Jones proteinuria of the λ type is more common. Extramedullary plasmacytomas, plasma cell leukemia, and amyloidosis are more frequent in IgD myeloma. Treatment is the same as that for multiple myeloma. Survival is generally believed to be shorter than with other types, but IgD myeloma is often not diagnosed until later in its course. We have seen several patients with IgD myeloma who survived more than 5 years.

Osteosclerotic Myeloma

The acronym POEMS (polyneuropathy, organomegaly, endocrinopathy, M protein, skin changes) describes the complete syndrome. The major clinical feature in osteosclerotic myeloma is a chronic inflammatory demyelinating polyneuropathy with predominantly motor disability. Single or multiple osteosclerotic bone lesions are characteristic. In contrast to multiple myeloma, the hemoglobin level is usually normal, and erythrocytosis occurs in some patients. Thrombocytosis is common. The bone marrow aspirate usually contains less than 5% plasma cells, whereas hypercalcemia and renal insufficiency rarely occur. Most patients have a λ-monoclonal protein. The protein level of cerebrospinal fluid is high, and slow motor nerve conduction velocities are found. Hepatosplenomegaly, hyperpigmentation, gynecomastia, edema, digital clubbing, hypertrichosis, atrophic testes, and impotence may occur. The diagnosis is confirmed by biopsy of an osteosclerotic lesion.

Radiation of solitary osteosclerotic lesions decreases the neuropathy in most patients. If the patient has widespread osteosclerotic lesions, an autologous stem cell transplantation should be considered. Chemotherapy is usually less effective. Patients can survive for many years, and death rarely is due to multiple myeloma.

Solitary Plasmacytoma (Solitary Myeloma) of Bone

The **diagnosis** of solitary plasmacytoma is based on histologic evidence that the tumor consists of plasma cells identical to those in multiple myeloma. In addition, complete skeletal radiographs must show no other lesions of myeloma, the bone marrow aspirate must contain no evidence of multiple myeloma, and immunofixation of the serum and concentrated urine usually shows no monoclonal protein. Some exceptions to the last-mentioned criterion occur, but therapy for the solitary lesions should result in disappearance of the monoclonal protein. Treatment consists of tumoricidal radiation (40–50 Gy). The most uncertain criterion for the diagnosis of solitary plasmacytoma of bone is the duration of observation necessary before one can be certain that the disease will not become generalized. Overt multiple myeloma develops in approximately 55% of patients during 10 years of follow-up, whereas new solitary bone lesions or local recurrences occur in about 10%. About 50% of patients with solitary plasmacytoma of bone survive 10 years. There is no convincing evidence that adjuvant chemotherapy influences the incidence of conversion to multiple myeloma. Progression of myeloma occurs within 3 years in two thirds of those patients who have progression.

Extramedullary Plasmacytoma
This plasma cell tumor arises outside the bone marrow. The upper respiratory tract, including the nasal cavity and sinuses, nasopharynx, and larynx, is the most frequent location of lesions. Epistaxis, rhinorrhea, and nasal obstruction are the most frequent symptoms. Solitary extramedullary plasmacytomas can occur in virtually any organ, however, and spread locally or develop into multiple myeloma. There is a predominance of IgA monoclonal protein. The diagnosis is made on the basis of finding a plasma cell tumor in an extramedullary site and the absence of multiple myeloma on the basis of bone marrow, radiography, and appropriate studies of blood and urine. Treatment consists of tumoricidal radiation and is often curative. Extramedullary plasmacytoma develops into overt multiple myeloma in about 15% of patients, in contrast to solitary plasmacytoma of bone.

Waldenström Macroglobulinemia (Primary Macroglobulinemia)
This malignant lymphoplasma cell proliferative disorder produces a monoclonal IgM protein. The condition bears similarities to multiple myeloma, lymphoma, and chronic lymphocytic leukemia. The lymphoid cells express CD19, CD20, and CD22 on their surface membrane. CD5 is expressed in about 15% of patients, whereas CD10 and CD23 expressions are absent.

Epidemiology and Etiology
The incidence is 5.1 per million per year, and approximately 1,400 cases occur in the United States each year. Although the cause of Waldenström macroglobulinemia is unknown, the disease may be more frequent in certain families. Studies of relatives of patients with macroglobulinemia reveal an increased frequency of IgM monoclonal proteins and quantitative immunoglobulin abnormalities.

Clinical Features
Macroglobulinemia has a predilection for older men, and the onset is usually insidious. Weakness, fatigue, and bleeding (especially oozing from the oronasal region or gastrointestinal tract) are common presenting symptoms. Blurring or other impairment of vision may occur. In contrast to multiple myeloma, bone pain is rare. In addition to bleeding and blurred vision, there may be hyperviscosity, which can produce dizziness, headache, vertigo, nystagmus, paresthesias, somnolence, and coma. Fever, night sweats, and weight loss also may occur. Pallor, splenomegaly, hepatomegaly, and peripheral lymphadenopathy are the most frequent physical findings. Retinal lesions, including hemorrhages, exudates, and venous congestion with vascular segmentation ("sausage" formation), may be impressive.
  Peripheral neuropathy may be the initial symptom and usually involves both sensory and motor functions. Sudden deafness, progressive spinal muscular atrophy, and multifocal leukoencephalopathy all have been noted. Pulmonary involvement is manifested by diffuse pulmonary infiltrates, isolated masses, or pleural effusion. Renal failure rarely occurs. The skin may be infiltrated by plasmacytoid lymphocytes or deposits of IgM. Systemic amyloidosis has been found in Waldenström macroglobulinemia.

Laboratory Features
Almost all patients have a normocytic, normochromic anemia. Occasionally, there is Coombs'-positive hemolytic anemia. Hemoglobin and hematocrit values are often spuriously reduced because of the increased plasma volume. A tall, narrow peak or dense band of gamma mobility constituting the IgM monoclonal protein is seen on the electrophoretic pattern; 75% are κ. The reduction in uninvolved immunoglobulins is less striking than in multiple myeloma. The urine contains a monoclonal light chain in 70% to 80% of cases. Rouleau formation is striking, and erythrocyte sedimentation is greatly increased. Mild lymphocytosis or monocytosis is not uncommon. The serum creatinine level is almost always normal. The bone marrow aspirate is usually hypocellular, but biopsy specimens are hypercellular and infiltrated with lymphoid and plasma cells. The lymphocytes tend to be small, are often basophilic, and resemble plasma cells. The number of plasma cells is greater than normal. The number of mast cells is increased, and this finding helps differentiate macroglobulinemia from myeloma or lymphoma.

Differential Diagnosis
The combination of typical symptoms and physical findings, more than 3 g per deciliter of IgM monoclonal protein, and lymphoplasma cell infiltration of the bone marrow provides the diagnosis of Waldenström macroglobulinemia. Patients with a malignant lymphoproliferative process manifested by an increase in lymphocytes and plasmacytoid lymphocytes in the bone marrow, anemia, constitutional symptoms requiring therapy, and a serum M spike of less than 3 g per deciliter should be classified as having Waldenström macroglobulinemia. They have the same survival as those with classic Waldenström macroglobulinemia. The major problems in the differential diagnosis center around the distinction from multiple myeloma, chronic lymphocytic leukemia, lymphoma, and MGUS of the IgM type. An IgM monoclonal protein concentration of less than 1 g per deciliter, an absence of anemia and organomegaly, mild lymphocytosis of the bone marrow, and absence of clinical symptoms are suggestive of MGUS rather than macroglobulinemia. The patient must be observed carefully, however, because in some instances of apparently benign monoclonal gammopathy, Waldenström macroglobulinemia subsequently develops.

Treatment
Therapy should be withheld until the patient has constitutional symptoms such as weakness, fatigue, night sweats, weight loss, features of hyperviscosity, anemia, significant hepatosplenomegaly, or lymphadenopathy. Chlorambucil, in an initial daily dose of 6 to 8 mg, produces objective benefit in 70% of patients. The dosage must be altered depending on the leukocyte and platelet counts, which should be determined every 2 weeks. Chlorambucil also may be given on an intermittent schedule in combination with prednisone. Cyclophosphamide or combinations of alkylating agents such as the M-2 protocol (VBMCP) have been beneficial. Chemotherapy should be discontinued when the patient has reached a plateau state.

Cladribine (2-chlorodeoxyadenosine) (2CDA) and fludarabine have produced impressive responses in macroglobulinemia. These agents are more effective for previously untreated patients than those resistant to alkylating agents. No prospective trials have compared conventional chemotherapy such as chlorambucil with 2CDA or fludarabine. Rituximab (Rituxan), an anti-CD20 monoclonal antibody, produces a response in approximately half of refractory patients. Plasmapheresis is effective for the management of symptomatic hyperviscosity. The use of a cell separator alleviates the symptoms quickly. The median survival of patients with Waldenström macroglobulinemia is approximately 5 years after diagnosis.

Heavy-chain Diseases
The heavy-chain diseases (HCDs) are lymphoplasma cell proliferative disorders characterized by the production of a monoclonal protein consisting of an incomplete heavy chain devoid of light chains. There are three major types: γ, α, and μ.

Gamma Heavy-chain Disease
Diagnosis: This lymphoplasma cell proliferative syndrome produces a monoclonal γ heavy chain in the serum or urine (or both). In all instances, the abnormal protein consists of a monoclonal γ chain with significant amino acid deletions, including deletion of the CH1 domain and a portion of the VH1 constant (C) region. The median age at diagnosis is approximately 60 years, although the condition has been noted in persons younger than 20 years. Patients with γ-HCD usually present with a lymphoma-like illness, but the clinical findings are diverse and range from an aggressive lymphoproliferative process to an asymptomatic state. Weakness, fatigue, and fever are common, but other features, including parotid swelling, severe soreness of the tongue, nodular infiltration of the skin, extranodal non-Hodgkin lymphoma, autoimmune hemolytic anemia, idiopathic thrombocytopenic purpura, rapid enlargement of the thyroid gland, neutropenia from hypersplenism, and an atypical lymphoproliferative process, have all been recognized. Hepatosplenomegaly is present in about 60% of patients. The histopathologic findings are nonspecific and usually include generalized or localized malignant lymphoma, myeloma, or macroglobulinemias, but there may be no evidence of a lymphoplasmacytic proliferative process. Anemia occurs in about 80% of patients.

The serum protein electrophoretic pattern is variable and often does not suggest a monoclonal gammopathy. It may appear as a broad-based increase of gamma globulin or a discrete localized band. The urinary heavy-chain protein concentration ranges from traces to 20 g in 24 hours, but more than half of patients excrete less than 1 g in that time. Bence Jones proteinuria is not found. Osteolytic lesions are rare.

Treatment is not indicated for the asymptomatic patient. Many different drugs have been used, including nitrogen mustard, melphalan, cyclophosphamide, prednisone, vincristine, vinblastine, procarbazine, azathioprine, chlorambucil, and doxorubicin. Radiotherapy also has been tried. The results have been inconsistent and generally disappointing in that responses often are incomplete or brief. On the basis of experience, we recommend a trial of cyclophosphamide, vincristine, and prednisone for patients with symptomatic γ-HCD and evidence of a progressive lymphoplasma cell proliferative process. If there is no response to this regimen, doxorubicin should be added. The median duration of survival is 1 year.

Alpha Heavy-chain Disease
α-Heavy-chain disease is the most common type and is characterized by the presence of a monoclonal α chain with extensive internal deletions encompassing the VH region and the entire first constant domain.

Diagnosis: Most patients with α-HCD are from the Mediterranean area and have involvement of the digestive tract with severe malabsorption, loss of weight, diarrhea, and steatorrhea. The term *immunoproliferative small intestinal disease* (IPSID) is restricted to patients with small intestinal lesions that have the same pathologic pattern as that of α-HCD, but these patients do not synthesize α-heavy chains. Infrequently, the respiratory tract is involved. Patients in their second or third decade of life are affected most often, and 60% of patients are men. Poor hygiene and low socioeconomic status are important risk factors. The serum protein electrophoretic pattern is normal in half the cases; in the remainder, an unimpressive broad band may appear in the $α_2$- or β-regions. Bence Jones proteinuria does not occur. The bone marrow is normal. The small bowel is infiltrated with mature plasma cells or lymphoplasmacytic cells, and in later stages, it has the appearance of an immunoblastic lymphoma. The mesenteric lymph nodes are usually affected, but liver, spleen, and peripheral lymph node involvement is uncommon. The stomach and colon may be affected. The diagnosis depends on the recognition of a monoclonal α-heavy chain that is not associated with a light chain.

Treatment: Most often α-HCD is progressive and fatal, and yet remissions have been recorded with the use of melphalan or cyclophosphamide and prednisone and, surprisingly, antibiotics. Patients with superficial lesions limited to the bowel and the mesenteric lymph nodes should be treated initially with oral antibiotics. Any documented parasites should be eradicated. If patients do not respond or if more advanced disease is present initially, they should be treated with cyclophosphamide, doxorubicin (Adriamycin), vincristine, and prednisone (CHOP). The complete remission rate is about 50%, with two thirds of patients surviving at 3 years.

Mu Heavy-chain Disease
μ-Heavy-chain disease is characterized by a monoclonal μ-heavy chain in which the VH domain is absent. Other deletions also may occur. In μ-HCD, chronic lymphocytic leukemia or a lymphoma-like pattern is most common. A stable, asymptomatic state also has been noted. The clinical spectrum of μ-HCD should broaden, as it has in γ-HCD. Serum electrophoresis usually reveals hypogammaglobulinemia; a localized peak or band occurs in 40% of cases. Bence Jones proteinuria has been found in two thirds of patients. The presence of vacuolated plasma cells in the bone marrow aids in the diagnosis. Demonstration of a monoclonal μ-heavy chain in the serum is necessary for diagnosis. Treatment with corticosteroids and alkylating agents is beneficial. The median survival is about 2 years.

Amyloidosis
Amyloid (a substance that is homogeneous and amorphous under the light microscope) stains pink with hematoxylin-eosin and metachromatically with methyl violet or crystal violet. When amyloid tissue is present, Congo red produces an apple-green birefringence

under polarized light. The amorphous, hyaline-like appearance of amyloid is misleading because it is a fibrillar protein. Electron microscopy, the most specific diagnostic method, reveals that amyloid consists of rigid, linear, nonbranching, aggregated fibrils that are hollow, 7.5 to 10.0 nm wide, and of indefinite length.

All amyloid fibrils are arranged in an antiparallel or cross-β pleated sheet formation and appear the same with Congo-red staining and on electron microscopy. Amyloid fibrils are insoluble and generally resist proteolytic digestion. The deposition of amyloid fibrils destroys and replaces normal tissue. The fibrils are composed of various proteins, depending on the type of amyloid, and include monoclonal light chains (κ or λ) in primary amyloidosis, protein A in secondary amyloidosis, transthyretin (TTR) (prealbumin) in hereditary or senile amyloidosis, β_2-microglobulin (β_2-M) in dialysis-associated amyloidosis, β protein in Alzheimer disease, and gelsolin, cystatin C, apolipoprotein A1, procalcitonin, atrial natriuretic factor, islet amyloid polypeptide, scrapie protein, and γ-heavy chains.

Classification
No truly satisfactory classification of amyloidosis exists. The classification provided in Table 4 is based on what is currently known about the biochemistry of the amyloid fibril.

Pathogenesis
1. **Primary amyloidosis:** The fibrils of primary amyloidosis (AL) consist of the variable or constant (or both) portions of a monoclonal immunoglobulin light chain. AL can be divided into two categories–AL and AL with multiple myeloma—on the basis of the appearance and number of plasma cells in the bone marrow, the amount of monoclonal protein in the serum and urine, and the presence or absence of skeletal lesions. The presence or absence of multiple myeloma is often difficult to determine, however, and is artificial because both categories represent a plasma cell proliferative process. The mechanism for deposition of monoclonal light-chain fragments as amyloid is not clear.

2. **Secondary amyloidosis:** The fibrils of secondary amyloidosis (AA) consist of protein A, a nonimmunoglobulin. Protein A has a molecular weight of 8,500 and consists of 76 amino acids. Protein AA is derived from protein SAA (serum amyloid A), which is produced by the liver. Deposition of protein AA is associated with a chronic inflammatory process, malignancy, or a wide variety of other conditions. The catabolism of amyloid fibrils is undoubtedly an important factor in pathogenesis. Monocytes from patients with AA fail to degrade protein SAA, whereas monocytes from normal subjects do, suggesting that monocyte dysfunction may contribute to the development of AA. Elastase-type proteases in the monocyte have been implicated in the degradation of protein SAA.

Diagnosis
The diagnosis of amyloidosis requires the demonstration, by appropriate staining procedures, of amyloid deposits in the tissue. Congo red produces an apple-green birefringence when amyloid tissue is viewed under polarized light and is the most widely accepted stain. Identification of the type of protein component in the amyloid fibril is most reliably accomplished by specific antisera to the proteins. We have seen several specimens in which the staining of tissue with Congo red or the metachromatic stains was negative, and yet electron microscopy revealed typical amyloid fibrils. Thus, in some situations, electron microscopy may be necessary for the diagnosis.

Primary Amyloidosis (AL)
Clinical features: The possibility of AL must be considered in any patient who has a monoclonal protein in the serum or urine and refractory congestive heart failure, nephrotic syndrome, sensorimotor peripheral neuropathy, carpal tunnel syndrome, orthostatic hypotension, or steatorrhea. Any patient older than 40 years who has unexplained nephrotic syndrome or renal insufficiency should have electrophoresis and immunofixation of the serum and urine.

The incidence of AL is 0.9 per 100,000 per year. AL is found more often in men (66%) than in women. The median age at diagnosis is about 65 years, and 98% of the patients are 40 years old or older.

Table 4. Classification of amyloidosis

Amyloid type	Classification	Protein precursor	Protein type or variant
AL	Primary: no evidence of preceding or coexisting disease, except multiple myeloma	κ, λ (i.e., λ$_{VI}$)	Aκ, Aλ (i.e., Aλ$_{VI}$)
AA	Secondary: coexistence with other conditions such as rheumatoid arthritis or chronic infection, familial Mediterranean fever (FMF), Muckle-Wells syndrome	SAA	—
AL	Localized: involvement of a single organ without evidence of systemic involvement (e.g., urinary bladder, urethra, ureter, tracheobronchial)	κ, λ	Aκ, Aλ
ATTR (AF)	Familial amyloid polyneuropathy (FAP) (Portuguese, Swedish, and Japanese)	Transthyretin (prealbumin)	Met 30
	FAP II (Indiana/Swiss, German)	Transthyretin (prealbumin)	SER 84
	Appalachian	Transthyretin (prealbumin)	Ala 60
AApoA1	FAP III (Iowa, Van Allen)	ApoA1	Arg 26
Aβ$_2$-M	Associated with chronic dialysis	β$_2$-Microglobulin	—

AA, secondary amyloidosis; AL, primary amyloidosis; APO, apolipoprotein; SER, serine.
From Husby G, et al. The 1990 guidelines for nomenclature and classification of amyloid and amyloidosis. In: Natvig JB, Forre O, Husby G, et al, eds. *Amyloid and amyloidosis 1990*, 6th International Symposium on Amyloidosis. Oslo, Norway, 1990. Dordrecht, The Netherlands: Kluwer Academic Publishers, 1990: 7–11, with permission.

Weakness and fatigue are the most frequent symptoms. Loss of weight may be striking; many patients lose more than 22.7 kg (50 lb). Dyspnea, pedal edema, paresthesias, light-headedness, syncope, and periorbital purpura may occur. Jaw claudication occurs in about 10% of patients, and approximately half of these also have arm or calf claudication on the basis of occlusion of small vessels by amyloid. Changes in the voice are not uncommon.

Hepatomegaly occurs in one fourth of patients, but splenomegaly is found in less than 5%. Macroglossia, present in 10% of patients, may be prominent. Purpura is common and often involves the neck and face, particularly the upper eyelids. Gross bleeding may occur. Ankle edema is common and usually results from congestive heart failure or the nephrotic syndrome.

At diagnosis, one fourth of patients have the nephrotic syndrome, one fifth have the carpal tunnel syndrome, one sixth have congestive heart failure, and about 15% have peripheral neuropathy. The presence of one of these syndromes and a monoclonal protein in the serum or urine is highly suggestive evidence of amyloidosis, and appropriate diagnostic studies must be done.

Laboratory features: Initially, anemia is not a prominent feature in AL. When present, anemia is usually due to multiple myeloma, renal insufficiency, or gastrointestinal bleeding. Thrombocytosis is present in 10% of patients. Abnormality of liver function tests is common, but hepatic insufficiency is uncommon. The serum protein electrophoretic pattern shows a modest-sized localized band or spike (median, 1.4 g/dL) in only 45% of patients, whereas approximately one fourth have hypogammaglobulinemia; therefore, electrophoresis is unsatisfactory for screening a monoclonal protein or for the diagnosis of AL. Immunofixation of the serum increases the detection of a monoclonal protein to about two thirds of patients. Almost one fourth of patients have a free monoclonal light chain in the serum (Bence Jones proteinemia). Light chains of the λ type (65%) are more common than κ light chains (35%), in contrast to multiple myeloma, in which the ratio is reversed. Electrophoresis of the urine shows an albumin peak in three-fourths of patients. Immunofixation reveals a monoclonal light chain in 70% of patients. The serum or urine contains a monoclonal protein in 90% of patients with AL and represents the single most helpful screening method. A monoclonal protein is not seen in secondary, senile, familial, or localized amyloidosis. Modest plasmacytosis of the bone marrow is common, and one half of patients have greater than 5% plasma cells, whereas one fifth have more than 20%. Lytic bone lesions are rare in AL without myeloma.

Cardiac and circulatory involvement: Congestive heart failure is present initially in one sixth of patients and develops during the course of the disease in an additional 5% to 10%. Electrocardiography shows low voltage or loss of anterior septal forces, findings mimicking those of myocardial infarction. The results of echocardiography are abnormal in two thirds of patients at diagnosis. The major features are increased thickness of the ventricular walls, abnormal myocardial texture, atrial enlargement, valvular thickening and regurgitation, pericardial effusion, and abnormal diastolic function. Ultimately, reduced systolic ventricular function occurs. Amyloid may infiltrate the conduction system and produce the sick sinus syndrome or atrioventricular block. Angina pectoris and myocardial infarction may result from deposits of amyloid in the coronary arteries. Constrictive pericarditis may be difficult to differentiate from the restrictive cardiomyopathy of cardiac amyloidosis.

Renal involvement: Proteinuria is present initially in more than 80% of patients, whereas renal insufficiency is found in nearly half of patients at diagnosis. A nephrotic syndrome is present initially in one fourth of patients. Although it is believed that the kidneys are enlarged in amyloidosis, normal-sized or small and contracted kidneys may be present. Gross hematuria is rare in AL. The adult Fanconi syndrome, renal vein thrombosis, and priapism all have been reported.

Other organ involvement: Although microscopic evidence of respiratory tract involvement is common, AL rarely produces pulmonary symptoms. Microscopic involvement of the gastrointestinal tract is common, but it frequently is asymptomatic. Pseudo-obstruction or diarrhea may result from extensive infiltration by amyloid, but more frequently it represents neurologic dysfunction from involvement of the autonomic nervous system. Steatorrhea occurs in up to 5% of patients. Striking hepatomegaly may be present, but abnormalities of hepatic function are generally modest. Intrahepatic cholestasis with jaundice is an ominous finding, and death usually occurs within a few weeks. Spontaneous splenic rupture resulting in hypovolemic shock has been the presenting feature of AL in several instances.

Peripheral neuropathy occurs in about 15% of patients. It is usually distal, symmetric, and progressive. Dysesthetic numbness is more frequent than paresthesias. Usually, the lower extremities are more often involved than the upper extremities.

Involvement of the skin by systemic amyloidosis may take the form of petechiae, ecchymoses, papules, plaques, nodules, tumors, bullous lesions, alopecia, and thickening of the skin (resembling scleroderma). Bleeding may be a major manifestation. In addition to the well-known deficiency of factor X, we have found deficiency of the vitamin K–dependent clotting factors (factor IX) and, to a lesser extent, factors VII and II, increased antithrombin activity, increased fibrinolysis, and intravascular coagulation.

The **diagnosis** of AL amyloidosis depends on the demonstration of amyloid deposits in tissues. The possibility of AL must be considered in every patient who has a monoclonal protein in the serum or urine and who also has nephrotic syndrome, congestive heart failure, sensorimotor peripheral neuropathy, carpal tunnel syndrome, giant he-patomegaly, or idiopathic malabsorption. In 98% of patients, there is a monoclonal protein in the serum or urine, or there is a monoclonal proliferation of plasma cells in the bone marrow. The initial diagnostic procedure in AL should be biopsy of the bone marrow because it is easy to perform, carries little risk, and provides an estimate of the degree of plasmacytosis, which is helpful in identifying patients with frank multiple myeloma. The bone marrow biopsy is positive for AL in 55% of patients. Biopsy of subcutaneous fat is positive in 70% to 80% of patients, but one must be alert for the possibility of both false-positive and false-negative results. If the bone marrow and subcutaneous fat are normal, one should proceed to a rectal biopsy, which is positive in 70% of patients. To be adequate, the biopsy specimen must contain submucosa because submucosa and the vessels that it contains are involved more frequently than the mucosa. If these tissues are negative, tissue must be obtained from an involved organ. Renal biopsy specimens have a higher incidence of positive findings, but the procedure is more difficult and costly than the taking of bone marrow biopsy, subcutaneous fat, or rectal specimens. The incidence of hematuria is not greater than that after renal biopsy in nonamyloid patients. Liver biopsy frequently discloses AL. The procedure occasionally results in bleeding, however; in rare instances, the liver has ruptured. Tissue obtained at carpal tunnel decompression always be should be stained for amyloid because it is positive in more than 90% of patients with AL. Biopsy of the small intestine is often positive. In patients with peripheral neuropathy, the sural nerve is an excellent source of biopsy material; however, this is appropriate only if the peripheral neuropathy is severe, because taking a biopsy specimen results in loss of local sensation. Endomyocardial biopsy is useful and carries little risk. Iodine 123-labeled human serum amyloid P component is useful for detecting the extent of amyloid deposition, but it is not readily available. The increased uptake of ^{99m}Tc-pyrophosphate is not a reliable diagnostic approach.

Prognosis: The median duration of survival for patients with AL seen within 30 days of diagnosis is 13 months. Survival mainly depends on the associated syndrome. The median survival of patients with AL presenting with congestive heart failure is 4 to 6 months. It is more than 2 years when peripheral neuropathy is the major presentation, however (Fig. 7).

The use of a proportional-hazards model in a stepwise multivariate fashion to evaluate the risk factors in 168 cases of AL revealed that congestive heart failure, presence of urine light chain, hepatomegaly, and degree of weight loss were the major factors adversely affecting survival during the first year of diagnosis. Increased serum creatinine levels and the presence of multiple myeloma, orthostatic hypotension, and monoclonal serum protein were the most important variables adversely affecting survival for patients surviving 1 year. Cardiac involvement is the cause of death in about one half of patients.

Treatment of AL is not satisfactory. Because the amyloid fibrils consist of the variable portions of monoclonal immunoglobulin light chains and are synthesized by plasma cells, it is reasonable to attempt treatment with alkylating agents known to be effective against plasma cell proliferative processes. Colchicine inhibits the deposition of casein-induced amyloid in mice and is effective for controlling recurrent attacks of abdominal pain and the amyloidosis (AA) associated with familial Mediterranean fever.

In a prospective randomized study of 220 patients conducted at Mayo Clinic, patients were randomized to receive (a) colchicine, melphalan, and prednisone; (b) melphalan and prednisone; or (c) colchicine alone. Patients were stratified according to their major clinical manifestation, age, and sex. Measurement of response included improvement in renal function, as demonstrated by a 50% decrease in the 24-hour urine protein excretion in the absence of progressive renal insufficiency; a reduction in the size of the liver by at least 2 cm, and a 50% decrease in serum alkaline phosphatase; disappearance of serum monoclonal protein or a reduction of more than 50%; disappearance of urinary monoclonal protein or a decrease of more than 50%; an increase of at least 1 g per deciliter in serum albumin if the initial value was 3 g per deciliter or lower; and improvement in the echocardiogram with a 2-mm reduction in the thickness of the interventricular septum or an increase of 20 percentage points in the ejection fraction. The median duration of survival was 8.5 months for the colchicine-treated group, 18 months for the melphalan and prednisone group, and 17 months for the melphalan, prednisone,

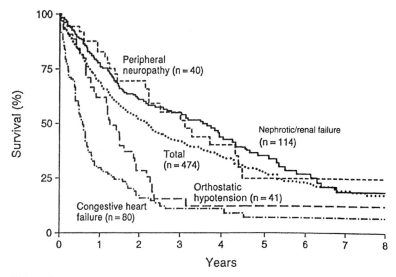

FIG. 7. Survival in primary amyloidosis, by syndrome, arranged hierarchically.

and colchicine group (p <0.001). In patients who had a reduction in serum or urine monoclonal protein at 12 months, the overall duration of survival was 50 months, whereas among those without a reduction at 12 months, the overall duration of survival was 36 months (p = 0.03). This finding indicates that response to chemotherapy affects survival. Thirty-four patients (15%) survived for 5 years or longer.

In an effort to determine whether more intensive combination chemotherapy was beneficial, 101 patients were randomized to either melphalan and prednisone or a combination of vincristine, BCNU, melphalan, cyclophosphamide, and prednisone (VBMCP). The latter combination did not result in a higher response rate or longer survival than use of melphalan and prednisone. In addition, treatment with alkylating agents may be associated with myelodysplastic syndrome or acute leukemia.

High-dose dexamethasone produces some benefit in 15% to 20% of patients. Vitamin E and α_2-IFN have not been beneficial. The use of 4'-iodo-4'-deoxydoxorubicin, which has an affinity for amyloid deposits, may aid in their dissolution.

Encouraging results have been reported with high-dose intravenous melphalan (200 mg/m²), followed by autologous peripheral stem cell rescue. Improvement in hepatic, gastrointestinal, neurologic, renal, or cardiac involvement has been reported along with decreased proteinuria and stable or improved performance status. The monoclonal protein in the serum and urine and the number of bone marrow plasma cells usually decrease. Because of the short follow-up, the impact of this treatment approach on response duration and survival is to be determined. Selection of patients for autologous stem cell transplantation plays a significant role in morbidity and survival. In a group of Mayo Clinic patients who met eligibility criteria for an autologous stem cell transplantation, the survival with conventional chemotherapy was 3.5 years. Thus, selection of patients plays a major role in survival.

The **nephrotic syndrome** should be managed with salt restriction and diuretics as needed. Furosemide is usually satisfactory, but occasionally, the addition of metolazone is helpful. Albumin infusions have only transient benefit and are not useful for long-term treatment of edema. If symptomatic azotemia develops, chronic renal dialysis is necessary. Either hemodialysis or peritoneal dialysis is effective; peritonitis may occur with peritoneal dialysis, whereas hypotension may lead to difficulties in hemodialysis. Death usually results from cardiac amyloid rather than from complications of dialysis.

Patients with **congestive heart failure** also must be treated with salt restriction and diuretics such as furosemide. Digitalis must be used with care and reserved for control of supraventricular tachycardia. Patients with AL are unusually sensitive to this drug, and heart block and arrhythmias are common. Ambulatory electrocardiographic monitoring is useful because the placement of a pacemaker for heart block or the use of antiarrhythmic agents may be life-saving. Cardiac transplantation may be considered for patients younger than 60 years who have severe amyloid cardiomyopathy and no evidence of renal involvement, multiple myeloma, or other symptomatic organ impairment.

Treatment of orthostatic hypotension is difficult. Patients should be instructed to rise slowly and sit on the edge of the bed for a few minutes before assuming an upright position. The use of elastic stockings or leotards may help. Fludrocortisone (Florinef) often is associated with increased fluid retention. Midodrine or L-threo-3, 4-dihydroxyphenylserine may be useful. Orthostatic hypotension and autonomic-induced diarrhea may be benefited by octreotide.

Sensorimotor neuropathy does not benefit from alkylating agent therapy. In most patients, the neurologic symptoms continue to progress. Dysesthesias are replaced by numbness. Analgesics may be needed. In some patients, amitriptyline and fluphenazine are useful. Codeine is helpful for controlling the discomfort from dysesthesias, and the long-term risk of habituation and tolerance is minimal. Macroglossia may produce obstructive sleep apnea and may be helped by nasal continuous positive airway pressure. In some instances, a permanent tracheostomy may be needed. Resection of the tongue is not advised because of bleeding. Patients with intestinal pseudo-obstruction must not be treated surgically because resection does not relieve the obstructive symptoms and complications are common. Bleeding or perforation of the gastrointestinal tract may occur.

Secondary Amyloidosis (AA)

Diagnosis: AA is associated with an inflammatory process, malignancy, or a wide variety of other conditions. Rheumatoid arthritis or its variants—ankylosing spondylitis, juvenile rheumatoid arthritis, psoriatic arthritis, and Reiter syndrome—are the most common causes. Infections associated with paraplegia or cystic fibrosis, bronchiectasis, osteomyelitis, tuberculosis, or lepromatous leprosy also may produce AA. Long-standing inflammatory bowel disease is a well-recognized cause. Hypernephroma, Hodgkin disease, and lymphoma also may be associated with secondary amyloidosis. In 90% of patients with AA, nephrotic syndrome or renal failure is the major manifestation. The gastrointestinal tract and thyroid also may be involved. In contrast to AL, the heart is rarely compromised.

Treatment of AA depends on the underlying disease. Response has occurred after appropriate treatment of osteomyelitis, pulmonary tuberculosis, and other infections. The therapy for rheumatoid arthritis with methotrexate, chlorambucil, or cyclophosphamide may reduce the inflammatory response and decrease the amyloidosis. Renal transplantation may be helpful. Dimethyl sulfoxide (DMSO) may help some patients who have amyloidosis due to rheumatoid arthritis. Colchicine is effective for the treatment of acute episodes of abdominal pain and fever from familial Mediterranean fever and reduces the possibility of amyloidosis.

Localized Amyloidosis

Localized amyloidosis is limited to the involved organ and does not become systemic. Such amyloidosis most commonly involves the lungs, urinary bladder, ureter, urethra, skin, synovia, and tendons. Although the amyloid fibrils consist of κ or λ light chains, no monoclonal protein is present in the serum or urine. The amyloidosis never becomes systemic, and treatment is unnecessary unless it causes local symptoms:

1. **Lung:** Amyloidosis localized to the lung can be classified as tracheobronchial, single or multiple nodular, or diffuse interstitial. In the tracheobronchial form, mucosal amyloid deposits occur and may produce cough, dyspnea, wheezing, and hemoptysis. Solitary amyloid nodules, which may be single or multiple, are confused with carcinoma of the lung. Amyloid may be confined to the larynx or adjacent structures.

2. **Bladder:** Localized amyloidosis of the bladder has been noted in more than 100 patients. Gross hematuria is the most frequent symptom. On cystoscopic study, localized tumefactive deposits of amyloid often are confused with carcinoma. For life-threatening

hematuria, conservative fulguration or surgical resection is indicated. Local instillation of DMSO may be helpful.

3. **Ureter:** Amyloid has been found localized in the ureter in more than 30 patients. A patient may have flank discomfort or gross hematuria. All patients have evidence of ureteral obstruction with hydronephrosis, and the preoperative diagnosis is usually ureteral carcinoma. Occasionally, bilateral ureteral amyloid may occur and produce anuria. Surgical alleviation of the obstruction is necessary.

4. **Urethra:** Amyloid has been localized to the urethra in more than 20 patients. The usual symptom is stricture associated with intermittent hematuria or a bloody urethral discharge. Conservative resection of the amyloid deposits is indicated.

Dialysis-associated Amyloidosis
Amyloidosis is seen with both hemodialysis and peritoneal dialysis. Amyloid deposits may be found in the synovia and tendons of patients with carpal tunnel syndrome who have received long-term hemodialysis. The amyloid consists of β_2-microglobulin, a protein homologous to the light-chain component of the class I HLA. Areas of cystic radiolucency are common. Renal transplantation often leads to dramatic improvement in joint symptoms. When it is performed early, it is the most effective preventive measure. Although amyloid deposits occur in visceral organs, they are of little or no clinical consequence.

Familial Amyloidosis
Familial amyloidosis can be classified most easily as neuropathic, nephropathic, cardiopathic, or miscellaneous. All forms except familial Mediterranean fever have autosomal dominant inheritance. This topic is not discussed here because it is not associated with a monoclonal gammopathy.

Monoclonal Gammopathy of Undetermined Significance (MGUS) (or Benign Monoclonal Gammopathy)

Patients with MGUS have a monoclonal protein in the serum without evidence of myeloma, macroglobulinemia, amyloidosis, or related diseases. The frequency is approximately 3% of persons older than 70 years. At Mayo Clinic, of the patients with monoclonal proteins, 65% have MGUS, 13% have multiple myeloma, and 11% have AL.

Characteristic features include the following:

1. The monoclonal protein value in serum is less than 3 g per deciliter.
2. Either no Bence Jones proteinuria is present, or small amounts are present.
3. Bone marrow aspirate contains less than 10% plasma cells.
4. Anemia is not present.
5. Renal function is normal.
6. Hypercalcemia is absent.
7. Osteolytic lesions are not present (unless caused by other diseases).
8. No progressive increase of the monoclonal protein or development of a plasma lymphoproliferative process occurs during long-term follow-up.

Differential Diagnosis
The differentiation of a "benign" monoclonal gammopathy from myeloma or macroglobulinemia is difficult at the time that the monoclonal protein is detected. Help in this differentiation may be derived from the following:

1. More than 3 g per deciliter of monoclonal protein usually indicates overt myeloma or macroglobulinemia, but some exceptions (e.g., smoldering myeloma) do exist.
2. Levels of immunoglobulin classes not associated with the monoclonal protein (normal polyclonal or background immunoglobulins) are reduced in most patients with myeloma, but a reduction also occurs in more than one third of patients with MGUS.
3. The association of significant Bence Jones proteinuria with a serum monoclonal protein usually indicates a neoplastic process.
4. More than 10% of plasma cells in the bone marrow is usually indicative of myeloma, but in some patients with more pronounced plasmacytosis, the disease has remained stable for long periods.

5. The atypical morphologic changes of the plasma cells in multiple myeloma also may appear in MGUS and smoldering myeloma.
6. The presence of osteolytic lesions is suggestive of multiple myeloma, but metastatic carcinoma also may produce lytic lesions.
7. β_2-Microglobulin levels, although increased in multiple myeloma, are not helpful for differentiating MGUS from low-grade or smoldering multiple myeloma.
8. Monoclonal plasma cells can be detected in the peripheral blood of 80% of patients with active multiple myeloma, but patients with MGUS or smoldering multiple myeloma have very few or no circulating plasma cells.
9. Patients with MGUS or smoldering myeloma have a low plasma cell labeling index. A series of 241 patients with a serum monoclonal protein but no evidence of multiple myeloma, macroglobulinemia, amyloidosis, or lymphoma (benign monoclonal gammopathy) were followed for more than 20 years. The patients were classified as follows:
   - **Group 1:** Patients alive and without increase in serum monoclonal protein during follow-up (benign) (10%).
   - **Group 2:** Patients with a monoclonal protein level of more than 3 g per deciliter who did not require therapy (11%).
   - **Group 3:** Patients who died of unrelated causes (53%).
   - **Group 4:** Patients in whom myeloma, macroglobulinemia, amyloidosis, or related diseases developed (26%).

The initial values of hemoglobin, quantity, and type of the serum monoclonal protein, levels of normal immunoglobulins, and the number of plasma cells in the bone marrow did not differ substantially between those whose condition progressed and those who remained stable. Analysis of age, sex, presence of organomegaly, presence of small amounts of monoclonal light chain in the urine, serum albumin, and IgG subclass did not initially help differentiate patients with benign monoclonal gammopathy from those in whom various diseases developed.

Multiple myeloma, macroglobulinemia, amyloidosis, or a malignant lymphoproliferative process developed in 63 patients (actuarial rate is 16% at 10 years, 33% at 20 years, and 40% at 25 years). Forty-three (68%) of the 63 patients developed multiple myeloma. The intervals from recognition of the monoclonal gammopathy to diagnosis of multiple myeloma ranged from 2 to 29 years (median, 10 years). Median survival after the diagnosis of multiple myeloma was 33 months.

Waldenström macroglobulinemia occurred in seven patients 4 to 20 years (median, 8.5 years) after recognition of an IgM monoclonal protein. These patients had serum levels of IgM κ monoclonal protein that ranged from 3.1 to 8.5 g per deciliter during the course of the disease. All patients had anemia, and their bone marrow aspirates and biopsy or autopsy specimens showed increased numbers of lymphocytes and plasma cells.

Systemic amyloidosis was found in eight patients 6 to 19 years (median, 9 years) after the recognition of a serum monoclonal protein. Histologic evidence of amyloidosis was present at autopsy in three patients, on renal biopsy in two, on lymph node biopsy in one, on rectal biopsy in one, and as an incidental finding at the time of operation for carcinoma of the colon in one patient.

A malignant lymphoproliferative process developed in five other patients 6 to 22 years (median, 10.5 years) after detection of the monoclonal protein: malignant lymphoma in three patients, chronic lymphocytic leukemia in one, and a malignant lymphoproliferative process in one.

Although MGUS frequently exists without other abnormalities, certain diseases are associated with it, as would be expected in an older population. Therefore, studies of such a relationship must include a control group to determine whether the association is merely a coincidence. Monoclonal proteins have been noted in lymphoma, leukemia, and a wide variety of hematologic conditions.

The clinician must periodically reexamine patients who have an apparently benign monoclonal gammopathy to determine whether the disorder is benign or is the initial manifestation of multiple myeloma, systemic amyloidosis, macroglobulinemia, or another malignant lymphoproliferative disorder. Patients with MGUS should not be treated.

Biclonal Gammopathies

Biclonal gammopathies occur in 8% to 9% of patients with monoclonal gammopathy. IgG and IgA are the most frequent combinations, followed by IgG and IgM monoclonal immunoglobulins. The clinical findings are similar to those of monoclonal gammopathies. In two thirds of patients, the biclonal gammopathies are of undetermined significance. The remainder have multiple myeloma, amyloidosis, macroglobulinemia, or other lymphoproliferative disorders. In many cases, the serum protein electrophoretic pattern shows only a single band, and the biclonal gammopathy is unrecognized until immunofixation is performed. More than 20 patients with triclonal gammopathy have been reported.

Idiopathic Bence Jones Proteinuria

Although Bence Jones proteinuria is most frequently associated with multiple myeloma, primary amyloidosis, Waldenström macroglobulinemia, or other malignant lymphoproliferative disorders, it may be benign. Small amounts of monoclonal light chains (Bence Jones proteinuria) are not uncommon. Most patients who excrete more than 1 g of Bence Jones protein in 24 hours and have no evidence of malignant plasma cell proliferation eventually develop multiple myeloma or amyloidosis. This may not occur for up to 20 years, however. Therefore, patients with such idiopathic Bence Jones proteinuria should be observed indefinitely.

Acknowledgment

Supported in part by CA62242 from the National Institutes of Health.

Suggested Readings

Alexanian R, et al. Primary dexamethasone treatment of multiple myeloma. *Blood* 1992;80:887.

Alexiou C, et al. Extramedullary plasmacytoma: tumor occurrence and therapeutic concepts. *Cancer* 1999;85:2305.

Attal M., et al. A prospective, randomized trial of autologous bone marrow transplantation and chemotherapy in multiple myeloma: Intergroupe Français du Myelome. *N Engl J Med* 1996;335:91.

Baldini L, et al. Role of different hematologic variables in defining the risk of malignant transformation in monoclonal gammopathy. *Blood* 1996;87:912.

Barlogie B, et al. Total therapy with tandem transplants for newly diagnosed multiple myeloma. *Blood* 1999;93:55.

Ben-Ayed F, et al. Treatment of alpha chain disease: results of a prospective study in 21 Tunisian patients by the Tunisian-French Intestinal Lymphoma Study Group. *Cancer* 1989;63:1251.

Berenson JR, et al. Efficacy of pamidronate in reducing skeletal events in patients with advanced multiple myeloma: Myeloma Aredia Study Group. *N Engl J Med* 1996;334:488.

Berenson JR, et al. Long-term pamidronate treatment of advanced multiple myeloma patients reduces skeletal events: Myeloma Aredia Study Group. *J Clin Oncol* 1998;16:593.

Bladé J, Kyle RA. Monoclonal gammopathies of undetermined significance. In: Malpas JS, Bergsagel DE, Kyle RA, et al., eds. *Myeloma: biology and management,* 2nd ed. Oxford: Oxford University Press, 1998:513–544.

Bladé J, Kyle RA. Nonsecretory myeloma, immunoglobulin D myeloma, and plasma cell leukemia. *Hematol Oncol Clin North Am* 1999;13:1259.

Buxbaum JN, et al. Monoclonal immunoglobulin deposition disease; light chain and light and heavy chain deposition diseases and their relation to light chain amyloidosis: clinical features, immunopathology, and molecular analysis. *Ann Intern Med* 1990;112:455.

Cohen HJ, et al. Racial differences in the prevalence of monoclonal gammopathy in a community-based sample of the elderly. *Am J Med* 1998;104:439.

Comenzo RL, et al. Intermediate-dose intravenous melphalan and blood stem cells mobilized with sequential GM+G-CSF or G-CSF alone to treat AL (amyloid light chain) amyloidosis. *Br J Haematol* 1999;104:553.

Comenzo RL, et al. Dose-intensive melphalan with blood stem-cell support for the treatment of AL (amyloid light-chain) amyloidosis: survival and responses in 25 patients. *Blood* 1998;91:3662.

Dimopoulos MA, et al. Treatment of Waldenström macroglobulinemia with 2-chlorodeoxyadenosine. *Ann Intern Med* 1993;118:195.

Dimopoulos MA, et al. Waldenström's macroglobulinemia: clinical features, complications, and management. *J Clin Oncol* 2000;18:214.

Durie BG, Salmon SE. A clinical staging system for multiple myeloma: correlation of measured myeloma cell mass with presenting clinical features, response to treatment, and survival. *Cancer* 1975;36:842.

Falk RH, Comenzo RL, Skinner M. The systemic amyloidoses. *N Engl J Med* 1997;337:898.

Fermand JP, et al. Gamma heavy chain "disease": heterogeneity of the clinicopathologic features: report of 16 cases and review of the literature. *Medicine (Baltimore)* 1989;68:321.

Fermand JP, et al. High-dose therapy and autologous peripheral blood stem cell transplantation in multiple myeloma: up-front or rescue treatment? Results of a multicenter sequential randomized clinical trial. *Blood* 1998;92:3131.

Frassica DA, et al. Solitary plasmacytoma of bone: Mayo Clinic experience. *Int J Radiat Oncol Biol Phys* 1989;16:43

Gahrton G, Bjorkstrand B. High-dose treatment of multiple myeloma. *Crit Rev Oncol Hematol* 1999;30:173.

Gahrton G, et al. Prognostic factors in allogeneic bone marrow transplantation for multiple myeloma. *J Clin Oncol* 1995;13:1312.

Garcia-Sanz R, et al. Primary plasma cell leukemia: clinical, immunophenotypic, DNA ploidy, and cytogenetic characteristics. *Blood* 1999;93:1032.

Gertz MA, Kyle RA. Secondary systemic amyloidosis: response and survival in 64 patients. *Medicine (Baltimore)* 1991;70:246.

Gertz MA, Kyle RA, Thibodeau SN. Familial amyloidosis: a study of 52 North American-born patients examined during a 30-year period. *Mayo Clin Proc* 1992; 67:428.

Gregory WM, Richards MA, Malpas JS. Combination chemotherapy versus melphalan and prednisolone in the treatment of multiple myeloma: an overview of published trials. *J Clin Oncol* 1992;10:334.

Greipp PR, et al. Plasmablastic morphology—an independent prognostic factor with clinical and laboratory correlates: Eastern Cooperative Oncology Group (ECOG) myeloma trial E9486 report by the ECOG Myeloma Laboratory Group. *Blood* 1998;91:2501.

Greipp PR, et al. Plasma cell labeling index and beta 2-microglobulin predict survival independent of thymidine kinase and C-reactive protein in multiple myeloma. *Blood* 1993;81:3382.

Hallek M, Bergsagel PL, Anderson KC. Multiple myeloma: increasing evidence for a multistep transformation process. *Blood* 1998;91:3.

Hartmann A, et al. Fifteen years' experience with renal transplantation in systemic amyloidosis. *Transpl Int* 1992;5:15.

Husby G, et al. The 1990 guidelines for nomenclature and classification of amyloid and amyloidosis. In: Natvig JB, Forre O, Husby G, et al., eds. *Amyloid and amyloidosis 1990.* Dordrecht, The Netherlands: Kluwer Academic Publishers, 1990:7–11.

Kyle RA. "Benign" monoclonal gammopathy—after 20 to 35 years of follow-up. *Mayo Clin Proc* 1993;68:26.

Kyle RA. High-dose therapy in multiple myeloma and primary amyloidosis: an overview. *Semin Oncol* 1999;26:74.

Kyle RA. Multiple myeloma: review of 869 cases. *Mayo Clin Proc* 1975;50:29.

Kyle RA. The role of bisphosphonates in multiple myeloma [Editorial]. *Ann Intern Med* 2000;132:734.

Kyle RA. Sequence of testing for monoclonal gammopathies. *Arch Pathol Lab Med* 1999;123:114.

Kyle RA, Garton JP. The spectrum of IgM monoclonal gammopathy in 430 cases. *Mayo Clin Proc* 1987;62:719.

Kyle RA, Gertz MA. Primary systemic amyloidosis: clinical and laboratory features in 474 cases. *Semin Hematol* 1995;32:45.

Kyle RA, Gertz MA. Systemic amyloidosis. *Crit Rev Oncol Hematol* 1990;10:49.

Kyle RA, et al. A trial of three regimens for primary amyloidosis: colchicine alone, melphalan and prednisone, and melphalan, prednisone, and colchicine. *N Engl J Med* 1997;336:1202.

Kyle RA, Greipp PR. "Idiopathic" Bence Jones proteinuria: long-term follow-up in seven patients. *N Engl J Med* 1982;306:564.

Kyle RA, Greipp PR. Smoldering multiple myeloma. *N Engl J Med* 1980;302:1347.

Kyle RA, Greipp PR, Banks PM. The diverse picture of gamma heavy-chain disease: report of seven cases and review of literature. *Mayo Clin Proc* 1981;56:439.

Kyle RA, et al. Waldenström's macroglobulinaemia: a prospective study comparing daily with intermittent oral chlorambucil. *Br J Haematol* 2000;108:737.

Kyle RA, Greipp PR, O'Fallon WM. Primary systemic amyloidosis: multivariate analysis for prognostic factors in 168 cases. *Blood* 1986;68:220.

Kyle RA, et al. Clinical indications and applications of electrophoresis and immunofixation. In: Rose NR, ed., *Manual of clinical laboratory immunology,* 6th ed. Washington, D.C.: American Society for Microbiology (*in press*).

Kyle RA, Rajkumar SV. Monoclonal gammopathies of undetermined significance. *Hematol Oncol Clin North Am* 1999;13:1181.

Kyle RA, Robinson RA, Katzmann JA. The clinical aspects of biclonal gammopathies: review of 57 cases. *Am J Med* 1981;71:999.

Laurencet FM, et al. Cladribine with cyclophosphamide and prednisone in the management of low-grade lymphoproliferative malignancies. *Br J Cancer* 1999;79:1215.

Liebross RH, et al. Solitary bone plasmacytoma: outcome and prognostic factors following radiotherapy. *Int J Radiat Oncol Biol Phys* 1998;41:1063.

Myeloma Trialists' Collaborative Group. Combination chemotherapy versus melphalan plus prednisone as treatment for multiple myeloma: an overview of 6,633 patients from 27 randomized trials. *J Clin Oncol* 1998;16:3832.

Noel P, Kyle RA. Plasma cell leukemia: an evaluation of response to therapy. *Am J Med* 1987;83:1062.

Rambaud JC, et al. Immunoproliferative small intestinal disease (IPSID): relationships with alpha-chain disease and "Mediterranean" lymphomas. *Springer Semin Immunopathol* 1990;12:239.

Singhal S, et al. Antitumor activity of thalidomide in refractory multiple myeloma. *N Engl J Med* 1999;341:1565.

Soesan M, et al. Extramedullary plasmacytoma: clinical behaviour and response to treatment. *Ann Oncol* 1992;3:51.

Wahner-Roedler DL, Kyle RA. Heavy-chain diseases. In: Malpas JS, Bergsagel DE, Kyle RA, et al., eds. *Myeloma: biology and management,* 2nd ed. New York: Oxford University Press, 1998:604–638.

Wahner-Roedler DL, Kyle RA. Mu-heavy chain disease: presentation as a benign monoclonal gammopathy. *Am J Hematol* 1992;40:56.

Waldenström JG. POEMS: a multifactorial syndrome [Editorial]. *Haematologica* 1992;77:197.

Witzig TE, et al. Peripheral blood monoclonal plasma cells as a predictor of survival in patients with multiple myeloma. *Blood* 1996;88:780.

14. BENIGN LYMPHOCYTE DISORDERS

Neil E. Kay

Benign lymphocyte disorders (BLDs) are clinical syndromes that result from either qualitative (functional) or quantitative abnormalities in lymphocyte subsets. In general, lymphocytes in BLD do not show any biologic features typically seen in malignant lymphocyte and can be characterized as polyclonal. With increasing sophistication of molecular techniques, however, it is possible to detect clonal B- or T-cell populations in some BLDs. There is little reason to believe that these clonal populations are truly malignant, but further studies of the natural history of patients with BLD in relation to the presence of these clonal populations will be of interest.

There is an increasing sophistication for both the characterization of the exact nature of the lymphocyte subsets and their function. Many of these advances have made their way into the routine clinical evaluation of patients with BLD and will be discussed herein. The lymphocyte subsets discussed in this chapter include the B-cell, T-cell subsets, and natural killer (NK) cells. The latter cell is also commonly referred to as the *large granular lymphocyte* (LGL).

Ontogeny and Function

During fetal life, the mesenchyme quickly differentiates into a recognizable lymphopoietic system. There is detectable immunoglobulin (Ig) synthesis and a cellular proliferative response to plant mitogen by 11 to 12 weeks of gestation. These parameters reflect two major lymphocyte functions: humoral (B-lymphocyte) and cellular (T-lymphocyte) immunity. Lymphoid stem cells develop from precursor cells and differentiate into T, B, or NK cells, depending on the organs or tissues to which the stem cells traffic.

B-cell Maturation

A pluripotent lymphoid stem cell that resides in the fetal liver first and then in bone marrow (the major production site) differentiates into a lymphopoietic progenitor (Fig. 1). These pluripotential stem cells (CD34+) appear on the yolk sac at 2.5 to 3 weeks of gestational age and migrate to the fetal liver by 5 weeks. They later migrate to the bone marrow (to the bone marrow of the clavicles by 8 weeks of embryonic life and to the long bones by 10 weeks, where they remain throughout life). By an as yet incompletely understood set of interactions, presumably involving cytokines and interaction with stromal cells, this cell differentiates into a B cell through an orderly process (Fig. 1).

Most recently, the combined assessment of recombinase activating gene (*RAG*) and surface membrane antigens as defined by cluster differentiating (CD) monoclonal antibodies has permitted detailed studies of B-cell maturation, which can be divided into antigen-independent and antigen-dependent phases. The antigen-independent phase has been defined based on both immunoglobulin gene rearrangement patterns and the

---

FIG. 1. Human B-cell development. There are several recognizable stages in human B-cell development that are based on nuclear, cytoplasmic, and membrane features. The numbers in boxes indicate the CD antigens that have been used to define B-cell subsets as they mature. The various nuclear enzymes, recombinase activating gene (*RAG*), and terminal deoxynucleotidyl transferase (TdT) needed for immunoglobulin (Ig) rearrangements are indicated in the nucleus of the developing B-cell subsets. Finally, the increasingly functional nature of Ig rearrangements in B cells are depicted in order as D to J rearrangements (DJ$_H$), V to D to J rearrangements (VDJ$_H$), V to J kappa (VJ$_k$), and surface Ig as μ-κ/λ κ/λ. Stromal cells are depicted below the B cells and should be providing critical cytokines or other secreted molecules and surface interactions that are important for survival and differentiation of the human B cells.

Human B-cell development

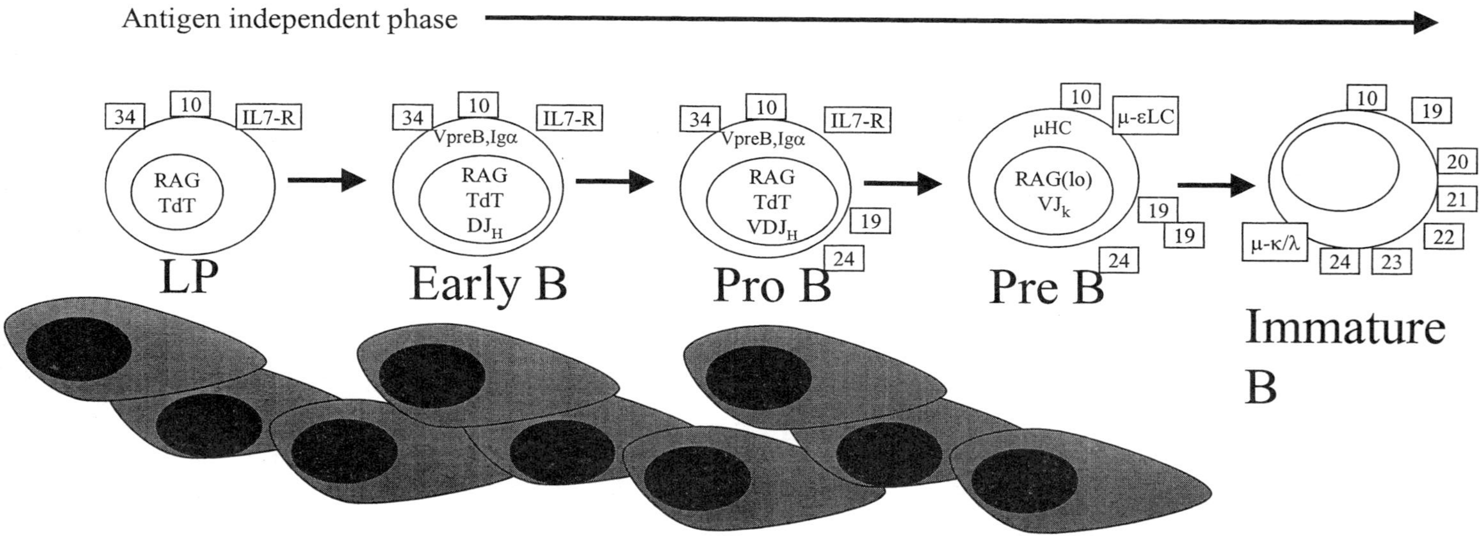

Antigen independent phase →

LP

34	10	IL7-R

RAG
TdT

Early B

34	10	IL7-R

VpreB,Igα

RAG
TdT
DJ_H

19

Pro B

34	10	IL7-R

VpreB,Igα

RAG
TdT
VDJ_H

19
24

Pre B

10	μ-εLC

μHC

RAG(lo)
VJ_k

19
19
24

Immature B

10	19
20	
21	
22	
23	
24	

μ-κ/λ

surface proteins expressed by the B cells (Fig. 1). The antigen-independent phase involves maturation of pro-B cell to pre-B cell and finally to the immature B cell.

During maturation of the B cell, a series of DNA rearrangements of immunoglobulin heavy-chain genes (driven by a recombinase activating gene) and light-chain genes results in the production of membrane-bound and secreted immunoglobulin molecules. As the pre-B cell matures, it acquires the surface expression of immunoglobulin M (IgM) after μ-chain gene and then κ or λ gene rearrangements. Mature B cells coexpress surface IgM and IgD after heavy-chain messenger RNA splicing. All these maturation events are antigen independent. At approximately 2 to 3 months of fetal life, B cells that express surface immunoglobulin (SIg) and are Fc receptor positive are present in the spleen. At birth, cord blood B cells represent about 15% to 20% of the cord blood lymphocytes, whereas 50% to 75% of human fetal spleen B cells and 90% of human cord B cells are CD5+ (1). In adult blood, 15% to 20% of lymphocytes are B cells, with SIg patterns of approximately 9% IgM, 6% IgD, 3% IgG, and 2% IgA. Approximately 15% are κ-chain positive and 7% λ-chain positive, which is evidence that these cells represent a polyclonal population. The spleen and lymph nodes are composed of about 25% to 40% B cells. The typical adult B cell coexpresses CD19+, CD20+, and CD21+; a small percentage of B cells are CD5+. The mature B cells are primarily responsible for production and secretion of functional immunoglobulin molecules.

T-lymphocyte Maturation
Blood-borne T-cell precursors from the fetal liver begin to colonize the thymic mesenchyme at 8 weeks' gestation. Under thymic influence, precursor cells differentiate toward fully mature, functional T lymphocytes. The thymic cortex is the site of most of human T-cell lymphopoiesis. As maturation proceeds, the T cells migrate to the thymic medulla, where they become immunocompetent and acquire or lose certain surface antigens (Fig. 2). The thymus is crucial for T-cell development and until recently was believed to decline with age. Recent information, however, suggests that thymic tissue may be present, albeit much smaller, even in centenarians. T-cell development in the thymus requires that genes coding for the T-cell receptor (TCR) undergo gene rearrangement. The TCR gene rearrangement involves the process of splicing noncontiguous DNA regions called V (*variable*), D (*diversity*), and J (*joining*) regions together. Random combinations of these diverse VDJ segments account for most of the diversity of TCR and the ability of the mature T-cell system to recognize millions of unique antigens. TCR rearrangement requires at least the *RAG1* and *RAG2* genes. TCRs, in conjunction with gene products of the major histocompatibility complex, recognize and bind antigen. The antigen specificity of T cells is maintained by the TCR, which consists of a two-chain heterodimer (γ and β chains) in physical association with CD3 (trimolecular complex of γ, δ, and ζ). Most T cells in the blood express the α, β TCR, but a minority of T cells express a γ, δ heterodimer. The TCR γδ+ cells may be a separate, distinct lineage; they are more dominant in the gut, intraepithelium, and vaginal mucosa; and they may be needed for first-line defense against pathogens.

Analysis of T-cell surface antigens in the thymus has revealed a complex, sequential change in membrane antigens that reflects the stage of maturation and functional capacity of thymic T cells. With expression of the TCR, the T cells undergo a process of selection. A positive selection for T cells will occur if the TCR has a low affinity for major histocompatibility complex (MHC) antigens on cortical thymic epithelial cells. This results in either CD4+ T cells (self–class II HLA restricted) or CD8+ T cells [self–class 1 human leukocyte antigen (HLA) restricted]. A negative selection will result if the TCR expressing T cells interact with self-peptides presented by dendritic cells. That interaction may result in programmed cell death or apoptosis of T cells with high affinity for self-antigens. The mature T cells of the thymus migrate to the peripheral blood and usually represent 70% to 85% of the blood lymphocytes. In addition, competent T cells leave the thymus to populate the thymic-dependent areas of spleen, nodes, tonsils, and Peyer's patches. Surface phenotype analysis of T-lymphocyte populations has provided evidence that each lymphocyte containing organ and blood has a characteristic distribution of T-lymphocyte populations. T cells have their heaviest concentrations in node paracortical areas, periarteriolar areas in the spleen, and the lymph of the thoracic duct.

Stages in Human T-cell Development

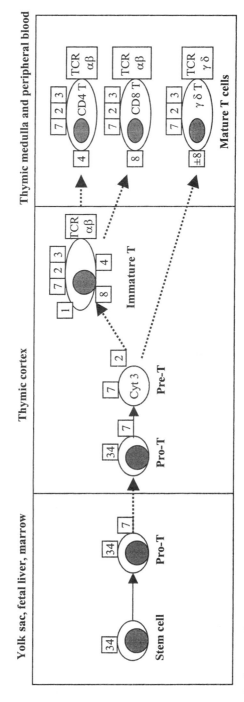

FIG. 2. Stages in human T-cell development. This schema illustrates human T-cell maturation from stem cell to mature T cell subsets. Note the different organs in which T-cell maturation occurs, with the sequential alteration in membrane antigens (boxes) and eventual expression of mature T-cell receptor (TCRαβ) for either CD4+ or CD8+ T cells. The other mature T cell is the γδ cell. This cell is found in a minor population in blood but also in mucosal environments. CYT3 indicates the presence of cytoplasmic CD3 protein.

Natural Killer Development

Natural killer (NK) function has been detected in human fetal liver at around 10 weeks of gestation. NK cells have been found in marrow and thymus but do not require thymic tissue for development. NK cells are believed to migrate from marrow to enter the blood pool and the spleen with few NK cells in lymph nodes.

Surface expression of CD56+ and CD16+ (FCγR111) is present on 90% to 100% of all NK cells; lesser levels of CD57 (50% to 60%), CD7, and CD2 are present. These cells also possess membrane receptors for CR2 (C3d), EBV, and Fc receptors for IgG.

NK cells constitute 5% to 10% of the normal human blood lymphocyte population. They are characterized morphologically as LGLs with slightly indented nuclei and large azurophilic granules.

Lymphocyte Function

T lymphocytes: Two distinct groups of T cells are distributed in the periphery: (a) CD4+, CD8- cells, which provide T cell–mediated help and (b) CD4-, CD8+ cells, which are responsible for T cell–mediated cytotoxicity and suppression.

CD4+T cells and even CD8+T cells are now subdivided into *naive* and *memory* subsets. Naive T cells migrate to T-cell areas of secondary lymphoid organs and, when exposed to antigen presented by dendritic cells, they are activated. These cells proliferate and generate effector cells that can migrate to B-cell areas or areas of inflammation. Some of the activated T cells persist as memory cells and with secondary challenge give rise to both a qualitative and quantitatively enhanced response.

Although this topic is controversial, the phenotype of naive and memory T cells can be used to discriminate between the two subsets. These markers include CD45 isoforms, but the CD45RO isoform can revert back to CD45RA. Other phenotypes that may be helpful in distinguishing naive T cells include the combination of CD45RA and CD62L or lack of CD95 antigen.

The CD4+T cell can be further subdivided into a T helper (Th2) versus T suppressor type (Th1) cell based on their cytokine synthesis profile. The former subset is capable of assisting B-cell immunoglobulin synthesis and production, whereas the latter is able to mediate antigen-specific induction of suppressor T-cell activity. Th1 cells may produce more interferon-gamma (IFN-γ) and interleukin-2 (IL-2), whereas Th2 cells produce IL-4, IL-5, IL-6, and IL-13.

Thus, the fully mature T-cell population is able to perform multiple functions, including T-cell–mediated cytotoxicity, T-cell help and suppression, production of cytokines (i.e., IL-2), proliferation in response to mitogen, and participation in graft-versus-host reactions.

B-cell function: The primary function of the B-cell pool is to generate diverse repertoire of immunoglobulin synthesizing and secreting cells called *plasma cells*. Each plasma cell produces and secretes only one of five immunoglobulin isotypes (i.e., IgG, IgM, IgA, IgD, or IgE) with one light-chain subtype.

The only complement-fixing isotypes are IgG and IgM, and these are the most important immunoglobulins for protection against infectious agents. IgM is found primarily to the intravascular compartment because of its large size, whereas IgG is present in all internal body fluids. IgA is the major protective immunoglobulin in the gastrointestinal, respiratory, and urogenital tracts where it is externally secreted. IgE, present in both internal and external body fluids, is used primarily for host defense against parasites and is the principal mediator of allergic reactions of the immediate type.

There are also immunoglobulin subclasses, including four subclasses of IgG (IgG1, IgG2, IgG3, and IgG4) and two subclasses of IgA (IgA1 and IgA2). For example, IgG1 and IgG3 have enhanced complement-fixing activity. Finally, there is evidence that the human B cell can function as an antigen presenting cell (APC).

Natural killer function: These cells are responsible for antibody-dependent cellular cytotoxicity (ADCC) and spontaneous cytotoxicity or natural killing. This latter function is critical for host response to viral infections and may be important in controlling malignant cell growth. If the NK cell population is exposed to IL-2, these cells are capable of becoming lymphokine activated killer (LAK) cells. Although it is unclear what the *in vivo* correlate of the LAK cell may be, the LAK cell has enhanced *in vitro* functional killing capacities for tumor cells.

Natural killer T cells: This cell is a minor cell population in the blood (<0.01%), but it is an important subset because these cells may be immunoregulatory cells (2). They can kill tumor cells but have an apparent role in preventing development of autoimmune disorders. They express the TCR of an α, β type and also NK markers such as NK1.1. TCR on NK T cells recognize glycolipids associated with the monomorphic-like, MHC-like CD1 molecule. These T cells have a limited TCR repertoire compared with other mature T cells.

Interleukins
Interleukins (ILs) (See Chapter 1) are proteins or glycoproteins, mostly with molecular weights in the range of 15,000 to 40,000 and are a family of molecules with pleiotropic cell regulatory functions. This pleiotropism results from the expression on multiple cell types of receptors for the same interleukin. Interleukins (meaning "between leukocytes") are hormone-like polypeptides that induce changes in metabolism, cell division, and gene activity. Cells have membrane receptors that recognize individual ILs; the cell–IL interaction generates signal transduction events that allow cell-cell communication or behavioral changes.

Most ILs act as paracrine or autocrine drivers for cells of the immune system. ILs can be subdivided into the following: (a) immunoregulatory ILs involved in the activation, growth, and differentiation of lymphocytes and monocytes, for example, IL-2, IL-4; (b) proinflammatory ILs that are produced mostly by mononuclear phagocytes in response to infectious agents, for example, IL-1, tumor necrosis factor (TNF)-α, and the chemokine family of inflammatory cytokines, that is, IL-8, monocyte chemotactic protein (MCP)-1, MCP-2, MCP-3, and macrophage inflammatory protein (MIP)-1; and (c) ILs that regulate immature leukocyte growth and differentiation, for example, IL-3, IL-7, and granulocyte–macrophage colony-stimulating factor (GM-CSF).

A partial list of ILs that interact with immune cells include IL-1, IL-2, IL-3, IL-4, IL-5, IL-6, IL-7, IL-8, IL-10, IL-12, IL-15, IL-18, IFN-α, IFN-β, IFN-γ, tumor growth factor (TGF)-β, TNF-α, and TNF-β. With increasing biologic information about these Ils, they are being tested for use in the treatment of human disease, particularly in the field of immunotherapy for malignancies.

General workup for lymphocyte disorders is usually done for patients suspected of immunoincompetence. Typical process comprises taking a complete history (especially family history), physical, and blood work. Most of this can be done at minimal expense and includes a complete blood count, erythrocyte sedimentation rate, absolute lymphocyte count, serum protein electrophoresis, and skin tests. Additional screening tests to help further define the nature of the abnormality are listed in Table 1. The usual clinical clue is the presence of repeated infections. It is unusual, however, for patients

Table 1. Initial screening tests for evaluation of a patient (pediatric or adult) with potential abnormalities in the immune system

Function	Test
Lymphocyte pool	CBC with differential, include microscopic morphologic assessment
Lymphocyte subsets	Flow cytometry to detect CD4, CD8 levels, CD4/CD8 ratios, and numbers of B and NK cells
B cell	Quantitative and qualitative serum protein electrophoresis isohemagglutinins. Antibody titers to; tetanus, diphtheria, *H. influenza,* pneumococci, rubella
T cell	Total lymphocyte count, skin tests (i.e., candida), mitogen response (to PHA, Con A, PWM)
NK cell	NK assay, ADCC assay

ADDC, antibody-dependent cell-mediated cytotoxicity; CBC, complete blood count; Con A, concanavalin A; NK, natural killer (cell); PHA, phytohemagglutinin; PWM, pokeweed mitogen.

with recurrent infections to have an identifiable immunodeficiency disorder. The most important clinical aspect is sufficient clinical concern by the physician that results in efforts to make a true diagnosis of immunodeficiency prior to significant clinical damage. For children, an immunodeficiency workup should start if there is chronic or recurrent infections at unusual sites, with unusual pathogens (e.g., *Serratia marcescens, Aspergillus*), or systemic infections. In adults, the same clinical findings may indicate a secondary immunodeficiency such as acquired immunodeficiency syndrome (AIDS), or it may be seen in association with immunosuppressive therapies. For both groups of patients, however, a detailed history, in particular a detailed family history, can be most informative. After that, a physical examination followed by selected screening tests based on the clinical suspicion should be obtained.

Lymphocyte Population: Quantitative and Qualitative Assessment
Measurements usually are performed most exclusively on blood cell populations, but lymphoid cells in bone marrow and nodes may be used to help characterize the lymphoid populations. The combined use of morphology and monoclonal antibodies specific for membrane markers (i.e., surface Ig for B cells) has permitted a more detailed and relevant quantitative measurement of human peripheral blood lymphocyte populations (Table 2).

Routine laboratory tests can be very helpful in enhancing the clinical suspicion or diagnosis of most immunodeficiencies (Table 1). Age-related differences are also important in the assessment of the lymphocyte levels (Table 2). B-cell function is assessed by measurement of isohemagglutinins, which are predominantly IgM antibodies to blood group polysaccharide antigens A and B. To assess IgG antibodies, antibodies to diphtheria or tetanus toxoid should be measured both before and after toxoid booster. IgA deficiency is best delineated by the quantification of serum IgA because IgA is typically very low or absent. Protein electrophoresis and IgG subclass assays are very helpful in assessment of B-cell function.

Skin testing, especially with a *Candida* skin test, is the best evaluation of T-cell function. A positive skin test (10 mm of erythema and induration) excludes most primary T-cell defects.

More laboratory tests are appropriate if your clinical impression suggests significant risk of immunodeficiency despite a normal routine laboratory evaluation. This could include specific lymphocyte function tests such as phagocytosis, proliferation to other antigens, cytotoxicity assays, and production of Ig.

Human Disease
The remaining discussion deals only with "benign" lymphocyte disorders. (See Chapter 12 for information on malignant lymphoproliferative diseases.) Benign lymphocyte disorders are still capable of inducing significant clinical symptoms in many patients. In general, benign lymphocyte disorders can be subclassified into *primary* (i.e., congenital immunodeficiency) and *secondary* (i.e., postviral, therapy-related) categories. Further classification of the latter category according to whether the disorders result in lympho-

Table 2. Normal lymphocyte counts (ranges) in humans from birth to adulthood[a]

	Cord blood	0–1 yr	1–6 yr	7–17 yr	18–70 yr
WBCs	10–15	6.4–11	6.8–10.0	4.7–7.3	4.6–7.1
Lymphocytes	4.2–6.9	2.7–5.4	2.9–5.1	2.0–2.7	1.6–2.4
T cells	2.4–3.7	1.7–3.6	1.8–3.0	1.4–2.0	1.1–1.7
CD4+ T cells	1.5–2.4	1.7–2.8	1.0–1.8	0.7–1.1	0.7–1.1
CD8+ T cells	1.2–2.0	0.8–1.2	0.8–1.5	0.6–0.9	0.5–0.9
B cells	0.7–1.5	0.5–1.5	0.7–1.3	0.3–0.5	0.2–0.4
NK cells	0.8–1.8	0.3–0.7	0.2–0.6	0.2–0.3	0.2–0.4

NK, natural killer (cells); WBC, white blood cells.
[a] Absolute counts are expressed in 10^3 cells/μL.

cytosis or lymphocytopenia is useful. In addition, the "physiologic" impairment of human immune lymphocytes noted in newborn infants must be considered.

Neonatal Lymphocytes: Physiologic Dysfunction
B-cell Function
Fetal and neonatal B lymphocytes are deficient in their ability to produce and secrete normal amounts of diverse Ig isotypes (1). IgM, normal at birth, is acquired transplacentally during the last trimester, but newborns will have deficiencies in some specific IgM antibodies to gram-negative organisms. IgM levels rise quickly around 1 week after birth. Maternally acquired IgG is usually sufficient for resistance to gram-positive organisms. Significant IgG production is reached at 3 to 6 months of life, with adult levels reached at 6 to 8 years. Serum IgA is poorly produced in the newborn, and adult levels are achieved only over the first decade. The physiologic hypogammaglobulinemia of infancy is most pronounced in premature infants, and even in full-term infants, the total Ig level is lowest around 4 to 6 months after birth.

T-lymphocyte Function
Many T-lymphocyte functions are present at adult levels early in gestation, including antigen recognition and binding, cell-mediated lympholysis, and mitogen-induced proliferation. The higher blood lymphocyte counts at birth give normal infants higher T cells than adults. In general, there is a predominance of naive T cells over memory type cells for the first few years of life. Because newborns may have unrecognized T-cell defects, it is prudent to irradiate blood products if they are to be given to newborns.

"Activated" T Lymphocytes
Normal, healthy newborns have blood T-lymphocyte membrane expression of certain activation antigens that are not noted in adults. For example, adult T cells express CD38 (activation antigen) on 5% of all cells, whereas in neonates, 85% of cord T cells express CD38. In addition, Tal, a late activation antigen, is noted on 30% of cord T cells and fewer than 15% of adult T cells. The appearance of these "activation" antigens on large numbers of cord T cells suggests that neonatal T cells are being activated or induced in an undefined manner.

"Activated" B Lymphocytes
Enriched cord B cells, most of which are CD5⁺, have increased expression of either immature B-cell antigens or bright-staining of other B-cell antigens (3). These findings may indicate "activated" B cells or an immature cell population.

Natural Killer Lymphocytes
NK activity is present at birth but is less than that in adult blood. This function will rise to adult levels and may gradually diminish in old age.

Lymphoid Organs
Lymphoid tissue is well developed and fully replete with normal histology at birth. The thymus is large but enlarges further over the first year of life. By puberty, the thymus is at its maximum size and thereafter involutes to a remnant size. Although this topic is controversial, it is now thought that thymic function, albeit low level, may be present even in more aged humans.

Lymphocytic Disorders
Lymphocytosis
Lymphocytosis is an absolute increase in circulating lymphocytes and is defined as a lymphocyte count in excess of 5.0×0^9 per liter. Typically, there is no associated change in lymphocyte functional capacity. As the normal lymphocyte count alters with age (Table 1), a lymphocytosis is detected when blood lymphocyte counts are consistently above the upper limit range for the different age groups as outlined in Table 2.

Etiologic Agents Associated with Lymphocytosis
In **acute infectious lymphocytosis,** the **clinical features** are as follows: Onset is accompanied by varying degrees of constitutional symptoms. There is a marked increase

in lymphocyte count, with the mean count varying from 20 to 30×10^9 per liter. No other hematologic abnormalities are evident. Usually, there is no hepatosplenomegaly, and no long-term sequelae are apparent. Affected persons are usually young, but this condition may be seen in young adults, and outbreaks frequently occur in epidemic form. The outcome is usually recovery to normal health.

The **laboratory features of acute infectious lymphocytosis** are the following: Lymphocytosis persists for 3 to 7 weeks and consists mostly of normal mature lymphocytes; the average peak value is 34.0×10^9 per liter. Occasional striking eosinophilia has been seen with the lymphocytosis. Acute infectious lymphocytosis usually is diagnosed because it occurs in epidemics; most viral cultures [i.e., EBV and cytomegalovirus (CMV)] are negative. To rule out a malignant disorder, the use of tissue biopsy or, more often, flow cytometry on the peripheral blood lymphocytes to evaluate for a malignant B- or T-cell clone is very helpful.

Treatment: The disease is self-limited and does not require therapy.

Infectious mononucleosis (IM): The **clinical features** of infectious mononucleosis (IM) are the following: IM is likely by infection with the EBV. Often subclinical in young children (<10 years), a primary infection results in the mononucleosis syndrome in young adults. Prominent features of EBV infection are acute pharyngitis; markedly enlarged tonsils; thick, white palatal exudate; and a petechial rash on the palate. In addition, lymphadenopathy parallels the pharyngitis. Other prominent features are fatigue, chills, sweats, and fever. Both hepatomegaly and splenomegaly are prominent. Rupture of the spleen is rare but has been reported.

Laboratory features of IM are as follows: Atypical lymphocytes in the blood are a dramatic finding on blood smear contrasting with acute infectious lymphocytosis. The diagnostic laboratory feature is the positive heterophil antibody test. Hemolytic anemia with anti-i antibody can be present, and the platelet count is usually lowered. Cold agglutinins, antinuclear factor antibody, and rheumatoid factor are sometimes present. Antibody to horse red cells that is not absorbed by the guinea pig kidney is almost always diagnostic for IM.

Treatment of IM: IM is self-limiting, and usually no therapy is indicated. Glucocorticoid therapy (prednisone) has been used to manage the direct antiglobulin-positive hemolytic anemia.

Cytomegalovirus (CMV): The clinical features of cytomegalovirus (CMV) are as follows: CMV is a syndrome that resembles IM. Approximately 8% of cases of IM may be caused by CMV. Spontaneous CMV is characterized by high fever and persistent, profound fatigue. Organomegaly may be prominent but is unusual. Posttransfusion CMV is typically milder. The disease also may be transmitted by transplant allografts with CMV infection, which after allograft transplantation is the most common infection in the posttransplant period. The incubation period is about 1 month (range, 30–60 days). A lymphocytosis greater than 10.0×10^9 per liter with atypical lymphocytes is common. In CMV, the symptoms may last longer than in EBV mononucleosis. Possible clinical complications include myocarditis, Guillain–Barré syndrome, pneumonia, hemolytic anemia, and splenomegaly with infarction. Other agents that may cause a mononucleosis syndrome include human immunodeficiency virus (HIV) I, herpes simplex II, rubella virus, and adenovirus.

Laboratory features of CMV are as follows: CMV is an IM-like disease with a negative heterophil test. There may also be signs of chemical hepatitis and cholestasis. Detection of antibody titers and culture of the virus from urine and blood are possible. Persons with circulating antibodies to CMV are not always protected from a second CMV infection. One should be very suspicious of CMV if a mononucleosis syndrome occurs in an immunosuppressed patient. Serologic determination of CMV is most helpful when both IgG and IgM virus-specific antibodies are measured but usually only in normal hosts. Finally, polymerase chain reaction (PCR) has been used successfully to detect viremia and plasma CMV/DNA. Quantifying PCR results have defined a threshold of viral burden that is associated with a high likelihood of development of invasive disease.

Treatment of CMV: No specific therapy is indicated in the normal host; if therapy is needed in immunocompromised patients, two agents (i.e., ganciclovir and foscarnet) have been shown to be virostatic *in vitro* and *in vivo*. Clinical trials have documented efficacy with these drugs in treating invasive CMV disease in both transplant and AIDS patients.

***Bordetella pertussis* and toxoplasmosis:** The typical clinical picture of childhood pertussis is characterized by large increases in peripheral lymphocyte counts. The total lymphocyte count may be up to 60×10^9 per liter, whereas the typical ranges are from 20 to 30×10^9 per liter. Toxoplasmosis can be seen in both neonates and adults. In the adult, this disease may present as IM with a negative heterophil test. Absolute lymphocytosis is not common, however, whereas relative lymphocytosis without atypical lymphocytes is usual.

Other viral and infectious diseases: In postviral infection (i.e., mumps, chickenpox, roseola, infectious hepatitis, and respiratory infections), immediate lymphopenia develops followed a few days later by lymphocytosis. Usually, the more severe the disease, the more dramatic the modulation of the lymphocyte blood values. Lymphocyte morphology may resemble that seen in IM syndromes. T lymphocytes, often of the suppressor phenotype (CD8+), usually constitute the increase in blood lymphocytes. Other miscellaneous infectious causes include measles, varicella, hepatitis, coxsackievirus, adenovirus, human immunodeficiency virus-1 (HIV-1, often with acute lymphadenopathy), toxoplasmosis, brucellosis, tuberculosis, typhoid fever, and secondary syphilis.

Miscellaneous causes: Numerous inflammatory or immune complex-related illnesses may be associated with lymphocytosis, including Crohn disease, ulcerative colitis, serum sickness, vasculitis, and drug hypersensitivity. In addition, a relative increase in circulating lymphocytes may be seen in a minority of patients with thyrotoxicosis or Addison disease.

Lymphocytopenia occurs when the peripheral blood lymphocyte counts fall consistently below the lower limits of the absolute lymphocyte ranges. Lymphocytopenia is a peripheral blood lymphocyte count below 1.5×10^9 per liter; severe lymphocytopenia is considered to be less than 0.7×10^9 per liter. Lymphocytopenia can result from abnormalities in (a) lymphocyte production, (b) lymphocyte traffic, and (c) lymphocyte loss and destruction. The most common well-understood mechanisms for lymphocyte reduction include chemotherapy or bone marrow and blood irradiation. Removal of stem cells and destruction of lymphocytes are the main factors in these cases. Mechanisms are diverse and sometimes unknown. Clinical presentations for patients with lymphocytopenia are not specific, but the workup should include evaluation of the nature of the remaining blood lymphocytes and estimation of immune function as listed in Table 1. Treatment depends on the specific disease and may include transplantation of allogeneic bone marrow, fetal liver, or thymic epithelial cells or even the use of gene therapy.

Etiologic Agents Associated with Lymphocytopenia

1. Decreased lymphocyte production
   - Inherited Ig diseases (i.e., ataxia–telangiectasia, Wiskott–Aldrich syndrome, and combined immunodeficiency diseases)
   - Advanced malignancy
   - Stage III to IV Hodgkin disease
   - Aplastic anemia
2. Increased lymphocyte destruction
   - Treatment related (i.e., chemotherapy and irradiation)
   - Excess corticosteroid (i.e., stress and Cushing syndrome)
3. Increased gastrointestinal lymphatic loss
   - Thoracic duct drainage or intestinal lymphectasia
   - Impaired gut lymphatic drainage (i.e., obstruction due to tumor infiltration and Whipple disease)
   - Severe right-sided heart failure
4. Miscellaneous causes
   - Renal failure
   - Myasthenia gravis
   - Systemic lupus erythematosus (SLE)
   - Miliary tuberculosis
   - AIDS: HIV may not often be associated with lymphocytopenia, but it infects the helper (CD4+) subset of T lymphocytes and destroys them resulting in a marked

decline in the absolute numbers of helper (CD4+) T cells in the peripheral circulation. This decrease may be a combination of decreased production and accelerated destruction of lymphocytes. A blood CD4 cell count of less than 500 per microliter frequently is associated with a poor clinical prognosis and frequent opportunistic infections for these patients.

Assessment of T-cell repertoire post chemotherapy: The kinetics and nature of T-cell reconstitution post chemotherapy is becoming more well-defined based on the use of phenotype analysis, which allows for determination of whether cells are naive or memory type T cells and the use of methods to determine T-cell repertoire. Thus, the presence of CD4 and CD8 T cells that possess either CD45RA (naive type) or CD45RO (memory type) cells can tell us much about the type of immunity that patients have post chemotherapy.

In the normal immunocompetent adult, the total number of CD4+ and CD8+ T peripheral lymphocytes with subpopulations of naive and memory cells is quite constant and likely is maintained by separate homeostatic regulators. This helps to ensure that the host can recognize new pathogens and respond vigorously to previously encountered pathogens. The administration of intensive cytotoxic chemoradiotherapy to patients with malignancy depletes peripheral T cells and challenges these homeostatic mechanisms, leading to defects in their immunologic status.

The reconstitution of CD4+ T-cell numbers after intensive chemotherapy is inversely related to age, with pediatric patients more rapidly recovering their total CD4+ T cells, including the CD45RA subset. This is likely to result from increased thymic activity, in which it is frequent to see thymic enlargement on chest films. The thymus undergoes involution in adolescence, however, and in older patients, the recovery of CD4+ T cells is slow and often quantitatively incomplete (Fig. 3). In adults, most CD4+ cells express the memory cell marker CD45RO, suggesting expansion of residual peripheral T cells that survived cytotoxic chemotherapy.

Surprisingly, recovery of CD8+ T cell numbers after intensive chemotherapy is more rapid than CD4+ T cell recovery and unrelated to age in adults and young children. However, the early recovering CD8+ T cells are mostly CD45RO+ and CD28- 57+ cells. These probably are terminally differentiated cells with limited remaining replication capacity and also are found in increased numbers in elderly patients. By contrast, naive CD8+ T-cell recovery requires a thymic contribution and parallels the recovery of naive CD4+ T cells.

A major effort is needed to reconstitute T-cell immunity after intensive chemoradiotherapy, particularly in adults. This is currently being explored by using a variety of approaches, including adoptive transfer of antigen-specific lymphocytes or expansion of autologous lymphocytes by *in vitro* manipulations. The most exciting future for a complete T-cell reconstitution is likely to come from the use of agents that help to regenerate thymic tissue in aging humans.

Immunodeficiency Diseases
There are now at least 70 inherited (primary) immunodeficiency diseases. More frequently, the exact molecular etiology or pathophysiology is being described for these diseases with obvious implications for therapy. The usual clinical presentation is increased susceptibility to infection. Immunodeficiency disorders also may be characterized by increased incidence of malignancies (especially leukemia and lymphoma). The clinical spectrum of immunodeficiency varies from the transient hypogammaglobulinemia of infants to severe congenital or inherited disorders that manifest at different times during human life (3).

1. **Classification:** The primary immunodeficiencies are classified according to the specific immune system defect. Antibody (B-cell) immunodeficiencies are most common and represent about half of all primary immunodeficiencies. Cellular (T-cell) immunodeficiencies constitute about 40% of the remainder. In cellular immunodeficiency diseases, 75% have associated Ig deficiencies and are designated as *combined immunodeficiencies.* Other immunodeficiencies include phagocytic (neutrophil/monocyte) or complement deficiency diseases; these will not be discussed here.

2. **Diagnosis:** Laboratory tests that assist in the diagnosis of immunodeficiency diseases are summarized in Table 1.

Transient hypogammaglobulinemia of infancy (THI) (see also section entitled **Neonatal Lymphocytes: Physiologic Dysfunction**):

1. **Clinical features:** At birth, the normal infant's serum contains little IgA, IgD, IgE, and IgM; but neonatal serum IgG is at a level comparable to normal serum. After birth, the levels of serum antibodies diminish with the decline of maternal-derived antibodies and are lowest at 3 to 4 months of age; they then rise as an infant's own IgG production gradually increases. In some infants, the development of Ig synthesis is delayed (i.e., transient hypogammaglobulinemia beyond 6 months of age and is termed THI) and occurs equally in males and female infants. Whereas this Ig defect is present (up to 18–30 months of age), infants may have increased susceptibility to infections of the skin, central nervous system (CNS), and respiratory tract. By the latter part of their first year, these infants usually can synthesize antibodies to blood type A and B

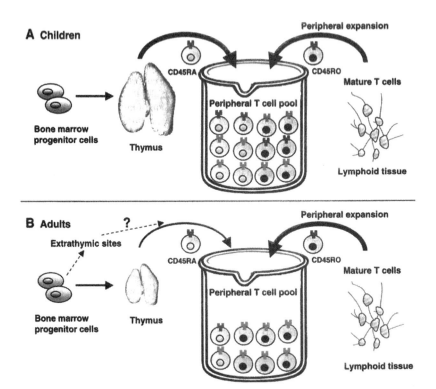

FIG. 3. T cells recovery from chemotherapy for children versus adults. Most lymphocytes are destroyed by cytotoxic chemotherapy. Recovery in children **A:** results from expansion of mature memory T cells (CD45RO) in the periphery and production of naive T cells (CD45RA) in the thymus, leading to restoration of normal T-cell numbers and a diverse repertoire. Because of the thymic involution in adults **B:** the production of naive T cells is reduced, resulting in a prolonged immunodeficient state characterized by reduced T-cell numbers and a restricted repertoire. (From Greenberg PD, Riddell SR. Deficient cellular immunity—finding and fixing the defects. *Science* 1999;285,546, with permission.).

and to tetanus toxoids. This condition is more likely an extreme variation on the normal maturation of the immune system.

2. **Laboratory features:** Serum Ig isotype is measured at serial intervals to monitor changes. B and T lymphocytes are present at normal levels and T-lymphocyte function is normal. Unlike inherited immunodeficiencies, patients with THI synthesize antibodies to human type A and B erythrocytes, diphtheria, and tetanus toxoids normally by 6 to 11 months of age, even before Ig concentrations normalize.

3. **Pathophysiology** is not precisely known; however, maturation of lymphoid tissue is delayed, and there are almost no germinal centers and few plasma cells in the nodes of these infants.

4. **Treatment:** Use of appropriate antibiotics for specific infections may be appropriate, but prophylactic use of immune serum globulin is not usually indicated.

Primary B-cell Deficiencies
X-linked agammaglobulinemia (Bruton's agammaglobulinemia):

1. **Clinical features.** X-linked agammaglobulinemia, the first immunodeficiency described, is a complex disorder with defects in regulatory genes (X chromosome) that perturb the structural Ig genes on several autosomal chromosomes. Because infants are born with adequate IgG (i.e., maternal transfer), infants with this disease do not manifest clinical problems until late in the first year of life. There is an unusual susceptibility to pyogenic organisms (i.e., *Haemophilus influenzae,* pneumococci, and streptococci). The infections are frequent and severe, and recurrences with the same organism are common. Typical sites of infection are sinus, lung, ear, skin, CNS, and blood. Recurrent infections may lead to bronchiectasis and pulmonary insufficiency. Gastrointestinal infection with *Giardia lamblia* is common. Some infants may have a syndrome that resembles rheumatoid arthritis. A fatal syndrome sometimes noted late in the disease course is characterized by neurologic involvement and dermatomyositis. There is normal resistance to most viruses, fungi, and gram-negative organisms; however, fatal infection with CNS infection by echovirus has occurred in several patients, and paralysis following administration of polio vaccine also has been noted.

2. **Laboratory features:** Diagnosis is made by serum immunoelectrophoresis and measurement of serum levels of all Ig classes. IgG is usually less than 100 mg per microliter, and any IgA, IgM, IgD, or IgE is almost undetectable. No B cells are detectable by surface membrane phenotype, whereas blood T-cell numbers and function are usually normal. Prenatal diagnosis can be made by restriction fragment length polymorphism (RFLP) of the *Btk* gene in affected male fetuses.

3. **Pathophysiology:** The abnormal gene for X-linked agammaglobulinemia is present on the proximal portion of the long arm of the X chromosome (Xq 21.3 to 22). This gene encodes for B-cell protein kinase (designated Bruton tyrosine kinase, Btk). Btk is a src-related tyrosine kinase molecule; it is involved in signal transduction and probably plays an important role in B-cell differentiation. The absence or mutation of this gene results in a total lack of B cells in lymph nodes. Although pre-B cells are detectable in normal numbers in bone marrow, apparently they are unable to mature into normal B cells. There is hypoplasia of lymph nodes, an absence of germinal centers, and few plasma cells.

4. **Treatment** revolves around the use of monthly administration of gamma globulin to maintain relatively normal levels of serum IgG (i.e., 400 mg/μL). The use of antibiotics and regular administration of antibodies are the only effective treatments for B cell disorders. Intravenous globulin preparations (4,5) are now recommended at a dosage of 100 to 200 mg per kilogram a month with higher doses sometimes necessary to achieve adequate serum levels. Most commercial preparations are isolated from normal plasma by the Cohn's alcohol fractionation method. To adjust the intravenous dose of Ig for each patient, it is best to measure serum IgG just before each infusion. On occasion, higher doses of intravenous globulin are needed for acute, severe bacterial infections. The use of intrathecal administration of immunoglobulin for CNS echovirus can be a life-saving maneuver.

Common variable immunodeficiency with predominant antibody deficiency:

1. **Clinical features:** This hypogammaglobulinemia does not appear to be genetically transmitted; however, recent work suggests that there may be gene defects on chromosome 6 that can account for this malady. Family clusters are rarely noted, and both sexes are affected equally, but female morbidity is greater. This disease occurs in first-degree relatives of patients with selective IgA deficiency. The onset is usually after puberty and typically is characterized by depressed Ig levels. The IgG level is less than 250 mg per microliter, and concentrations of all other Ig molecules are also low. T cell–mediated functions are frequently abnormal, and patients have frequent, chronic infections that typically involve the sinuses and respiratory tract. The association between this immunodeficiency disorder and autoimmune diseases that resemble rheumatoid arthritis, SLE, and pernicious anemia is high. Other associated disorders include gastrointestinal malabsorption, which may involve *G. lamblia,* chronic lung disease, and massive enlargement of the lymph nodes and spleen. There is a striking increase in the incidence of lymphoma in female patients who survive to more than 50 years of age.

2. **Pathophysiology:** This syndrome may have multiple causes. Genetic factors combined with exposure to environmental factors, including drugs (e.g., sulfasalazine, gold, penicillamine, phenytoin) could result in full expression of this disease.

3. **Laboratory features:** Serum Ig levels are severely depressed in young male or female subjects following onset of puberty. The number of blood B cells is normal, but these cells do not differentiate into plasma cells. T cell–mediated functions are frequently abnormal. Because there is a familial relationship to serum IgA deficiency, serum IgA levels of patient or family members may be helpful.

4. **Treatment:** (a) Replacement of immunoglobulin as described above in **Treatment**; and (b) timely, aggressive use of antibiotics during acute infections.

X-linked lymphoproliferative disease (Duncan disease):

1. **Clinical features:** This inherited, recessive disease results from a suboptimal reaction to EBV infection. Patients are typically healthy until around 5 years of age and later develop IM. Mortality is high: Approximately 70% of these patients may die of EBV-induced B-cell proliferation with extensive liver damage. They are unable to mount an effective antibody response to the EBV nuclear antigen. Survivors often have more extensive immune defects of their B-, T-, and NK-cell systems along with hypogammaglobulinemia and can develop B-cell lymphomas.

2. **Laboratory features:** Serum electrophoresis reveals low levels of serum Ig. Cellular dysfunction includes defective antibody-dependent cell–mediated cytotoxicity for EBV-infected cells and low NK cell activity. In addition, T-cell responses to EBV are impaired. Cytogenetics studies have indicated a defective gene on the X chromosome at the Xq25 region. The specific gene is called *SAP*, and it encodes for a signal lymphocyte-activated protein (SLAM) that helps prevent the lymphoproliferation of EBV in infected humans.

Specific Immunoglobulin Deficiencies
These disorders are relatively common, with approximately 1 in 200 hospital patients exhibiting an individual Ig deficiency. These patients may be relatively healthy but can present with bacterial infections that do require immunoglobulin replacement.

Lack of serum IgA:

1. **Clinical features:** This is the most frequently recognized immunodeficiency disorder, with a potential incidence of at least 1 in 333 persons (3). IgA deficiency often is associated with clinical sequelae, especially in the gut, lungs, and urogenital tracts. In addition, patients may have steatorrhea and nontropical sprue, but affected persons do not have an increased propensity for viral infections. Transfusion reactions, some anaphylactic, have occurred in this group of patients. This condition may be noted in families, but an inheritance pattern is not obvious. Patients have an increased incidence of

autoimmune diseases and malignancy, and some patients can develop common variable immunodeficiency (see preceding discussion).

2. **Pathophysiology:** These patients lack IgA-producing cells in the lamina propria of the intestinal tract. Their cell-mediated immune system is normal.

3. **Laboratory features:** Quantitative electrophoresis demonstrates an isolated absence of serum IgA and usually secretory IgA. Occasionally, secretory IgA is absent with normal serum IgA. Circulating anti-IgA antibodies may be detected in about half of the patients, and the incidence of autoantibodies is high. Patients have normal values of B cells and serum Ig, but IgG subclass deficiency and monoclonal IgM has been reported.

4. **Treatment:** There is no treatment except to avoid transfusions where possible to decrease the incidence of serum transfusion reaction. Only red blood cells from an IgA-deficient donor should be transfused and blood products with IgA or anti-IgA antibodies (i.e., intravenous immune serum globulin products) should be avoided. Extensive washing (200-mL volumes) of healthy donor red cells are the infusion product of choice when transfusion is absolutely necessary. Sometimes the IgA deficiency will remit spontaneously with removal of prescribed phenytoin (Dilantin).

IgG subclass deficiency:

1. **Diagnosis:** These patients have recurrent pyogenic (*H influenzae* and pneumococci) infections, particularly involving the respiratory tract. Serum qualitative and quantitative Ig analysis may reveal decreased IgG1, IgG2, IgG3, or various subclass combinations (6). A selective IgG2 deficiency may predispose an affected patient to recurrent infection and a progressive immunodeficiency, and most patients with IgG2 deficiency also have low IgA levels. Alternatively, this disorder may occur without a clinical diagnosis of immunodeficiency. The inheritance pattern of IgG subclass deficiency is not clear.

2. **Treatment** consists of serum immune globulin replacement through intravenous administration. Appropriate antibiotics may also be useful.

κ-chain deficiency:

1. **Clinical features:** κ-Chain deficiency is an unusual, complex disorder in which kappa-type serum Ig is completely or virtually absent. One patient had concomitant cystic fibrosis and diabetes mellitus.

2. **Pathophysiology:** Familial incidence has been documented. The disorder probably results from the failure of B cells to produce κ chains, but no exact mechanism or genetic defect has been determined.

3. **Laboratory features:** Serum electrophoresis does not detect IgM or IgG with kappa-light chains, but it does show Ig with λ-light chains. Associated serum IgA deficiency may also be evident.

4. **Treatment:** No therapy is indicated except for treatment of clinical complications associated with the disease. If IgA deficiency accompanies the κ-chain deficiency, avoidance of blood transfusions is warranted.

Combined B- and T-cell Defects
Severe combined immunodeficiency (SCID):

1. **Clinical features:** These patients are infected early (often before 6 months of age) and experience recurrent, severe infections that ultimately result in death before the age of 2 years. The most prominent sites of infection are the colon and lung; these infections result in chronic watery diarrhea and pulmonic abscesses. Other prominent clinical features include oral moniliasis, susceptibility to viral infections, disseminated viremia with vaccinations, and extreme wasting. These children are incapable of graft rejection and may develop graft-versus-host disease from maternal cells that cross the placenta or from transfused blood products.

2. **Pathophysiology:** There are two genetic modes of inheritance: autosomal recessive and X-linked. These two patterns result in an overall male-to-female ratio of 3:1. The thymus is tiny, it fails to descend normally, and it lacks a distinct cortical and medullary anatomy. The bone marrow and lymph nodes show severe deficiency in lymphoid elements or germinal contents, respectively. The X-linked recessive type is more common (1:100,000 births), approximately half of all SCID cases, and the gene defect is in the Xq 13-21.1 region. Patients with X-linked SCID have defects in the gene encoding for the γ chain common to many cytokines (IL-2, IL-4, IL-15) and in TCR-chain V-D-J rearrangements. The absence of TCR rearrangements may explain the lack of mature, functional T cells in this disorder, whereas defects in the common g chain for important cytokines may explain the severe immunodeficiency. The major defect appears to be the inability of stem cells to mature into functioning B and T cells.

3. **Autosomal recessive:** About one half of patients with the autosomal recessive type have a concomitant deficiency of adenosine deaminase (ADA). (Additional features of ADA are described subsequently.) In addition, some patients with SCID-like disease have purine nucleoside phosphorylase deficiency (see PNP features to follow). Genes with mutations implicated in this form of SCID include ADA deficiency, IL-7 receptor α chain, and *RAG1/RAG2* deficiency.

4. **Laboratory features:** Frequently, there is leukopenia because of low lymphocyte counts. ADA patients have the lowest lymphocyte blood counts, with no phenotypically mature T cells, but they may contain "immature" T cells. Affected infants lack sufficient numbers of NK/T cells, significant B- and T-cell function, or both. An inability to produce specific antibody (despite normal or increased numbers of B cells) or to develop cell-mediated immunity is uniform. Thus, serum Ig levels are very low, and skin grafts are accepted without rejection. Some patients may retain NK function.

5. **Treatment:** At present, SCID is uniformly fatal by 2 years of age unless bone marrow transplantation (BMT) or ADA replacement is successful. Most SCID cases can be cured with HLA-identical or T-cell–depleted haploidentical BMT procedures.

Wiskott–Aldrich syndrome:

1. **Clinical features:** The characteristic triad is eczema, thrombocytopenia with purpura, and recurrent infections or malignant lymphoma. This disease is usually fatal by age 10; death is usually due to overwhelming infection or hemorrhage. Abnormal bleeding is a frequent initial sign with prolonged bleeding after circumcision. Patients with a platelet count of less than 10,000 per microliter are at high risk for bleeding. Pneumococci or other bacteria with polysaccharide capsule cause serious infections; the usual sites for infection are the ear, lung, CNS, or blood. Subsequent infection agents include the herpes virus or *Pneumocystis carinii*. Patients may have autoimmunity and are also at risk for malignancy (EBV induced).

2. **Pathophysiology:** Wiskott–Aldrich syndrome is an X-linked disorder that results primarily in progressive diminution in cell-mediated immunity. The defective gene is on Xp11.22-11.23, which encodes a cytoplasmic protein found in lymphocytes and megakaryocytes. It has been designated the *Wiskott–Aldrich protein* (WASP), and it binds to the rac and rho family of guanosine triphosphatases. There appears to be a role for WASP in modulating the assembly of actin filaments, with subsequent interference in downstream tyrosine kinase signaling.

3. **Laboratory features:** T-lymphocyte function is decreased in most *in vitro* proliferative assays. Skin test results usually show subnormal responses. Serum electrophoresis often shows normal or slightly elevated IgA, IgE, and IgG but low IgM. Serum isohemagglutinins are absent, and the numbers of circulating T cells (CD3⁺) are reduced. Defective humoral responses to polysaccharide antigens are consistently found. Bone marrow biopsy reveals normal levels of megakaryocytes, but the circulating platelets are small and have defective function.

4. **Treatment:** BMT is the only method that has successfully changed the course of the disease.

Combined immunodeficiency (CID):

1. **Clinical presentation:** CID is distinguished from SCID by having low but not absent T-cell function. The clinical presentation is similar to SCID: failure to thrive, recurrent pulmonary infections, chronic diarrhea, skin infections, and severe varicella as infants. They live longer than SCID patients but still can die early in life.

2. **Laboratory:** Patients often have neutropenia and eosinophilia with normal Ig levels. The IgA is low, but IgE levels can be very high. Plasma cells can be found in various tissues of these patients, but the paracortical tissues are depleted of lymphocytes and T cells have deficient responses to mitogens and other antigens.

3. **Pathophysiology:** There are multiple genetic causes of CID; the most well characterized is purine nucleoside phosphorylase gene mutations located on the long arm of chromosome 14 (14q13.1).

Hyperimmunoglobulinemia E syndrome:

1. **Clinical features:** Affected persons suffer from recurrent staphylococcal abscesses that may involve the skin, joints, and respiratory tract. They present with a characteristic clinical facial appearance and a pruritic dermatitis; the syndrome appears in infancy. The genetic inheritance is probably autosomal dominant with incomplete penetration.

2. **Laboratory features:** Eosinophilia is common, and serum IgE levels are markedly elevated. Most other serum Ig levels are normal, but IgD may also be elevated. Abnormal neutrophil chemotaxis has been reported; however, there is poor concordance between that defect and clinical disease in persons who have elevated serum IgE levels. Defective humoral responses and cell-mediated response to neoantigens contrast with normal proliferative response to mitogen. Quantitative values for T cells are normal, but memory T cells (CD45RO+) apparently are decreased.

3. **Treatment:** The primary effective mode of therapy is chronic administration of antibiotics (penicillinase resistant). The use of antifungal agents is sometimes necessary. Intravenous Ig is also beneficial if the patient's other serum Ig values are low.

Ataxia–telangiectasia:

1. **Clinical features:** A progressive neurologic dysfunction (ataxia) becomes evident early when the patient begins to walk. Patients also develop choreoathetosis, myoclonic jerks, nystagmus, and difficulty with voluntary eye movements. Between the ages of 2 and 8 years, dilated venules (telangiectasia) occur on the bulbar conjunctiva, and these appear later in other exposed sites (i.e., ear, and flexor folds of arms). Other skin abnormalities include premature hair graying, skin atrophy, vitiligo, and café au lait spots. In addition, endocrine abnormalities are frequent, with more than half of affected persons having glucose intolerance with hyperinsulinemia and hyperglyceridemia. Growth retardation usually occurs. Girls often have delayed or absent development of secondary sexual features, and boys may have hypogonadism. Infections are common in most patients, and the respiratory system is frequently affected (>80% of all patients). In some patients, bronchiectasis may result and respiratory failure may occur as a terminal event. Children with this disorder have a marked increased incidence of hematologic neoplasms (leukemia and non-Hodgkin lymphoma), and most develop before age 15.

2. **Pathophysiology:** This autosomal recessive disorder affects both the humoral and cellular immune response. The abnormal gene is on the long arm of chromosome 11(11q22-23) with the gene product a DNA-dependent protein kinase. Lymphocytes from affected persons show a high frequency of spontaneous chromosome abnormalities (typically chromosomes 7 and 14) and have defective DNA repair pathways. In addition, these lymphocytes show an increased susceptibility to chromosome breakage from irradiation.

3. **Laboratory features:** Patients with ataxia–telangiectasia have defects in both cellular and hormonal immune systems. Selective deficiency of IgA is most common

(50%–80% of affected persons). IgE, IgG, or IgG2 serum levels also may be low. The serum IgM may be the low molecular (7S) variant rather than the 19S form. Patients may have low antibody titers to specific antigens, and their T-cell response to mitogens is usually decreased.

4. **Treatment** to date is restricted to therapy of the clinical complications (i.e., infections, and lymphoma).

Bare lymphocyte syndrome (BLS): There are two general categories of this disorder: one with lymphocytes lacking class I antigens and the other with a lack of MHC class II.

1. **Clinical presentation:** Persons with MHC class I antigen deficiency are rare and usually not so sick. These children also present later than do the MHC class II–deficient children. These latter patients are infants, usually of North African ancestry. They present with diarrhea (cryptosporidiosis) and later develop bacterial pneumonia, oral candidiasis, septicaemiae, *Pneumocystis* pneumonia, and high susceptibility to viral infections. Most patients are not able to survive past 3 years of age.

2. **Pathophysiology:** Patients with BLS have a form of combined immunodeficiency that is not quite as severe as SCID. BLS is characterized by an absence or decreased expression of HLAs and the absence of β_2-microglobulin on lymphocytes. In this heterogeneous disorder, some patients have defective expression of HLA class I but not HLA class II antigen, whereas other patients have decreased membrane expression of HLA class II antigen and partial abnormalities in HLA class I expression. The inheritance pattern is autosomal recessive. The genetic defect responsible for MHC class I deficiency may be mutations in TAP a protein needed for transport. In MHC class II deficiency, three gene defects have been noted; promoter region on 1q, promoter region on 13q, and a gene on 16p13 that encodes a protein that binds to the promoter region of MHC class II.

3. **Laboratory features:** Serum IgG and IgA levels are low with very poor antibody response to antigenic challenge. Lymphopenia, with abnormal T-cell function by both *in vitro* tests and skin test responses is evident. Pathology of the lymph nodes and thymus reveals severe hypoplasia. Low numbers of CD4 cells are seen with elevated or normal numbers of CD8 cells. No MHC class II antigens are detectable on B cells, and in the MHC class I deficiency no MHC I antigens are found on any cells.

Omenn syndrome:

1. **Pathophysiology:** Omenn syndrome is CID accompanied by hypereosinophilia. It is an autosomal recessively disease characterized by mutations in the recombinase activating genes *RAG1* and *RAG2*.

2. **Clinical:** This fatal condition is characterized by extreme susceptibility to infection, with T-cell infiltration of skin, intestines, liver, and spleen. Often an exfoliative erythroderma, lymphadenopathy, hepatosplenomegaly, and severe diarrhea are present.

3. **Laboratory:** Infants have a persistent leukocytosis, marked eosinophilia, elevated serum IgE, and low IgG, IgA, and IgM. These persons have low or absent blood B cells and elevated numbers of T cells that are dysfunctional because of restricted heterogeneity of their T-cell repertoire.

Primary T-cell Diseases
Congenital thymic hypoplasia (DiGeorge syndrome):

1. **Clinical features:** Congenital thymic aplasia (complete DiGeorge) presents in infancy as neonatal tetany and hypocalcemia. Facial abnormalities (i.e., hypertelorism, nasal clefts, low-set pinnae) are characteristic, and cardiac anomalies such as tetralogy of Fallot are usually present. These infants develop recurrent infections from viral, bacterial, or fungal sources, which are fatal for some patients. This last feature is not too dissimilar from that seen in SCID patients. The degree of hypoplasia in both thyroid and parathyroid tissue varies; variable hypoplasia patients (partial DiGeorge) fare much better.

2. **Pathophysiology:** This disorder is caused by failure of the third and fourth pharyngeal pouch endoderm to generate thymic tissue during embryogenesis. The absence of parathyroid tissue results in tetany and hypocalcemia. There is no obvious hereditary or familial inheritance pattern. Recently, deletions in the 22q11.1 region have been found in most patients, but no candidate genes have yet been identified.

3. **Laboratory features** include lymphopenia (suppressor cells CD8+ decreased more than helper CD4+ cells), normal Ig levels, and abnormally decreased response to antigen (i.e., *Candida,* streptokinase) skin testing. In general, *in vitro* T-cell function is decreased.

4. **Treatment:** Transplants of fetal thymic tissue and unfractionated HLA-identical marrow transplantation can reverse most of the lymphocyte qualitative and quantitative abnormalities characteristic of this disease.

X-Linked Immunodeficiency with Hyper-IgM (Hyper-IgM syndrome):

1. **Clinical features:** X-linked immunodeficiency with hyper-IgM, or hyper-IgM syndrome, is characterized by very low serum concentrations of IgG and IgA with a normal or, more frequently, a markedly elevated concentration of polyclonal IgM. This is a common Ig deficiency that appears in either a hereditary or acquired form. Affected males become symptomatic during the first 2 years of life with recurrent pyogenic infections, including otitis media, sinusitis, pneumonia, and tonsillitis. In contrast to patients with Bruton, the frequent presence of lymphoid hyperplasia often leads away from a diagnosis of immunodeficiency. Many patients suffer from complications such as cytopenias (i.e., thrombocytopenia, cyclic neutropenia, aplastic or hemolytic anemia) and renal disease.

2. **Pathophysiology:** The abnormal gene is on Xq26, and the gene product (CD154) is the ligand for CD40 receptor on B cells, which is upregulated on normal, activated T cells. The B cells of affected persons respond normally to IL-4 and anti-CD40. The T cells in some patients have a genetic defect in the CD40 ligand, with defective expression of CD40L on the membrane (7). This membrane glycoprotein is a critical antigen that is necessary for efficient T cell–mediated help for B-cell Ig synthesis and isotype switching. Mutations in CD154 on activated T cells from male subjects with X-linked hyper-IgM result in an inability to signal B cells to undergo isotype switching with the production of only IgM.

3. **Laboratory features:** Serum electrophoresis reveals decreased to absent levels of IgG and IgA, with IgM levels from 100 to 1,000 mg per microliter. On occasion, patients have increased levels of serum IgD. Plasma cells and lymphocytoid plasma cells in blood and nodes are increased. B cells with surface IgM or IgD are present in normal numbers. Mutations in CD154 gene can be used to detect carriers of X-linked hyper-IgM and can be used to make a prenatal diagnosis of this condition. The caveat is that mutations in CD154 are not the only cause of the hyper-IgM syndrome; some patients having an intrinsic defect in B-cell isotype switching that is not associated with that protein.

4. **Treatment** involves immune serum globulin replacement as reviewed previously.

Miscellaneous T-cell diseases: Two other diseases have primary T-cell defects that have been characterized as having specific chromosomal or molecular defects. These are T-cell cytokine production defects and abnormal expression of the TCR–CD3 complex:

1. **T-cell cytokine production defects.** Two main defects of cytokine production are now described. One is a selective inability to produce IL-2. The IL-2 gene was present in two patients, but no IL-2 message or protein could be detected; other T-cell cytokines were produced normally. As infants, these two patients had severe recurrent infections as infants. A second cytokine defect was described in a female infant patient who presented with failure to thrive and severe recurrent infections. This infant had defective transcription of several lymphokine genes (IL-2, IL-3, IL-4, and IL-5). The mechanism

could be via abnormal binding of nuclear factor of activated T cells (NFAT-1) to response elements in IL-2 and IL-4 enhancers. There was some response to IL-2 infusions.

2. **T-cell activation defects.** These diseases are featured by peripheral blood T cells that appear phenotypically normal but fail to proliferate or produce cytokines in response to stimulation with mitogens, antigens, or other signals delivered to the T-cell antigen receptor (TCR). The mechanism for this may be related to defective signal transduction from the TCR to intracellular metabolic pathways (8). These patients behave clinically like other T-cell–deficient patients. Indeed, some severe T-cell activation defects may resemble SCID disease.

Enzyme Deficiency in Immunodeficiency Disease
Several enzymes important in nucleoside/nucleotide metabolism have restricted distributions in human lymphocyte populations. Two enzymes, adenosine deaminase (ADA) and purine nucleoside phosphorylase (PNP), are present in T cells but bear a reciprocal relationship to each other. ADA is highest in the thymus and decreases as T-cell maturation proceeds. PNP activity increases as T cells mature. PNP and ADA are ubiquitous in human tissues, but peripheral blood elements contain the highest PNP enzyme activity. Deficiency of these two enzymes leads to unique, clinically significant immunodeficiency in humans.

Adenosine deaminase deficiency:

1. **Clinical features:** The disease usually manifests by 3 months of age. Variation in clinical presentation within affected families may be widespread. Some children have body deformities involving the ribs, iliac regions, and vertebrae; they are subject to recurrent chronic infections with viral, fungal, protozoal, and bacterial organisms. These infections are usually fatal, and a failure-to-thrive syndrome is often associated with this deficiency.

2. **Pathophysiology:** The structural gene encoding adenosine deaminase is on chromosome 20. Intracellular accumulation of lymphotoxic metabolites [i.e., deoxyadenosine triphosphate (deoxy-ATP), deoxyadenosine diphosphate (deoxy-ADP), 21-deoxyadenosine] ultimately results in a SCID. Adenosine and deoxyadenosine inactivate S-adenosylhomocysteine hydrolase, which results in high intracellular levels of S-adenosyl homocysteine (9). The latter substance is a potent inhibitor of cellular methylation and seems to enhance T-cell apoptosis.

3. **Laboratory features:** Severe lymphopenia and abnormalities in both T-cell and B-cell–dependent aspects of the immune system occur in most patients (90%). ADA-deficient patients usually have a much more profound lymphopenia than do infants with other SCID disease (mean absolute lymphocyte counts <500/μL). Erythrocyte ADA deficiency and elevated levels of deoxy-ATP and deoxy-ADP are also present. There are also large amounts of adenosine and deoxyadenosine in the plasma.

4. **Treatment:** These patients can be cured by HLA-identical or haploidentical T-cell–depleted BMT without the need for pretransplant or posttransplant chemotherapy. Enzyme replacement therapy should not be initiated if bone marrow transplantation is contemplated because it could generate graft-rejection capability. In the past, transfusions with irradiated erythrocytes from normal, healthy subjects was the only option resulting in a transient, partial reconstitution of the immunodeficiency.

Purine nucleoside phosphorylase deficiency:

1. **Clinical features:** In brief, children show signs and symptoms of immunodeficiency between 3 and 18 months of age, but if the deficiency of PNP is incomplete, the disease may not appear until 4 to 6 years of age. Initially, T-cell function appears normal, but advancing disease usually occurs secondary to declining T-cell function. Children become increasingly susceptible to viral infections, especially varicella, and often do not survive viral illness. Occasional autoimmune disease supervenes, leading to an additional array of clinical problems. Many patients have neurologic symptoms,

including mental retardation. Posttransfusion graft-versus-host disease also has been documented. In contrast to ADA deficiency, serum and urinary uric acid usually are markedly deficient, and there are no characteristic physical or skeletal abnormalities associated with this syndrome.

2. **Pathophysiology:** Point mutations are identified in the PNP gene on chromosome 14q13.1. This disease is inherited, probably as an autosomal recessive trait, but the genetic inheritance pattern is unclear.

3. **Laboratory features:** T-cell functional assays generally show markedly decreased function of T cells. Lymphopenia is common, and the thymus is severely hypocellular. Humoral immunity is preserved, but autoantibody production often is exaggerated. Serum and urine uric acid levels are very low. Specific diagnosis requires the *in vitro* assay of enzyme levels or purine metabolites.

4. **Treatment:** Transfusion with irradiated erythrocytes from normal, healthy persons may be of some help, but BMT has been the only successful form of therapy.

Miscellaneous Lymphocyte Disorders

Large granular lymphocytes (LGL) proliferations: There are two major types of LGL type proliferations. One is known as T-LGL; these proliferations are CD57$^+$ CD3$^+$ CD8$^+$ CD2$^+$. The other is known as NK-LGL; these proliferations are CD56$^+$ CD3$^-$ CD8$^-$ CD2$^+$(10).

1. **Clinical features:** Patients with T-LGL often have neutropenia, rheumatoid arthritis, and autoantibodies. These patients tend to have clonal proliferations as shown by TCR gene rearrangements, and the usual finding is neutropenia with an otherwise indolent clinical course. Males and females are approximately equally affected. Infections may be recurrent but are seldom debilitating. About one half of patients will have splenomegaly, and clinical progression is typically slow. NK-LGL leukemias are observed in younger patients and run an aggressive course. The typical clinical presentation is hepatosplenomegaly and involvement of the gastrointestinal system with ascites. The course of the disease is acute and often fatal within 1 to 2 months after diagnosis.

2. **Laboratory features** include obvious evidence of a peripheral blood expansion of LGL. Monoclonal antibody phenotyping reveals a CD3$^+$ CD16$^-$ in the majority cell population. In 15% of patients, the LGL have a CD3$^-$, CD16$^+$ (NK-like) phenotype.

3. **Treatment:** The long-term consequences of the T-LGL disease is not clear but appears to be relatively benign. Some patients benefit from therapy with corticosteroids or immunosuppressive–cytotoxic drugs. Splenectomy usually is not recommended for patients with this disease.

Leucocyte adhesion deficiency (LAD) is also frequently called CD11–CD18 deficiency.

1. **Clinical features** include delayed separation of the umbilical cord, gingivitis, recurrent otitis media, skin infections, pneumonia, perianal abscesses, and poor wound healing. Mortality results from severe bacterial or fungal infections. Risk for viral infections or malignancies is not increased.

2. **Pathophysiology:** There are two types, designated LAD-1 and LAD-2. An abnormal beta chain (CD18) used by three adhesion molecules is responsible for LAD-1 (11). Mutations in the CD16 gene on chromosome 21 q22.3 have been documented. This chain is used by CD11a (LFA-1), CD11b (MAC-1), and CD11c (p150, 95); each of these adhesion molecules has an α chain that is not expressed because of the abnormal β chain. In LAD-2, the cells are deficient in sialyl-Lewis X, a carbohydrate ligand for selectins (12).

3. **Laboratory features:** Although these patients have dysfunctional neutrophils, many lymphocyte functions are very impaired because of defects related to CD11-type adhesion molecules. Lymphocytes are not able to interact with other immune cells in an effective manner. The lack of CD11 also results in abnormal phagocytic cell adherence, chemotaxis, and reduced respiratory metabolic activity.

References
1. Wilson M. Immunology of the fetus and newborn: lymphocyte phenotype and function. *Clin Immunol Allergy* 1986;5:271.
2. van der Vliet HJJ, et al. Human natural killer T cells acquire a memory-activated phenotype before birth. *Blood* 2000;95:2440–2442.
3. Tosato G, et al. B cell differentiation and immunoregulatory T cell function in human cord blood lymphocytes. *J Clin Invest* 1980;66:383.
4. Ochs HD, et al. Comparison of high- and low-dose intravenous immunoglobulin therapy in patients with primary immunodeficiency diseases. *Am J Med* 1984;76:78.
5. Buckley RH, Schiff RI. The use of intravenous immune globulin in immunodeficiency diseases. *N Engl J Med* 1991;325:110.
6. Aucouturier P, et al. Frequency of selective IgG subclass deficiency: a reappraisal. *Clin Immunol Immunopathol* 1992;63:289.
7. Korthauër U, et al. Defective expression of T-cell CD40 ligand causes X-linked immunodeficiency with hyper IgM. *Nature* 1993;361:539.
8. Arnaiz-Villena A, et al. Human T-cell activation deficiencies. *Immunol. Today* 1992;13:259.
9. Fox IH, Kelley WN. The role of adenosine and 2-deoxyadenosine in mammalian cells. *Annu Rev Biochem* 47:655, 1978.
10. Zambello R, et al. Phenotypic diversity of natural killer (NK) populations in patients with NK-type lymphoproliferative disease of granular lymphocytes. *Blood* 1993;81:2381.
11. Buckley RH. Immunodeficiency diseases. *JAMA* 1992;268:2797.
12. Phillips ML, et al. Neutrophil adhesion in leucocyte adhesion deficiency syndrome. *J Clin Invest* 1995;96:2898–2906.

Suggested Readings
Allen RC, Armitage RJ, Conley ME, et al. CD40 ligand gene defects responsible for X-linked hyper IgM syndrome. *Science* 1993;259:990.
Buckley RH. Breakthroughs in the understanding and therapy of primary immunodeficiency. *Pediatr Clin North Am* 1994;41:665.
Buckley RH, Schiff RI. The use of intravenous immune globulin in immunodeficiency diseases. *N Engl J Med* 1991;325:110.
Buckley RH, Schiff RI, Schiff SE, et al. Human severe combined immunodeficiency (SCID): genetic, phenotypic and functional diversity in 108 infants. *J Pediatr* 1997; 130:378.
Buckley RH, Schiff SE, Schiff RI, et al. Hematopoietic stem-cell transplantation for the treatment of severe combined immunodeficiency. *N Engl J Med* 1999;340:508.
Comans-Bitter WM, de Groot R, van den Beemd R, et al. Immunophenotyping of blood lymphocytes in childhood. *J Pediatr* 1997;30:388.
Dalal I, Reid B, Nisbet-Brown E, et al. The outcome of patients with hypogammaglobulinemia in infancy and early childhood. *J Pediatr* 1998;133:144.
Fischer A, Malissen B. Natural and engineered disorders of lymphocyte development. *Science* 1998;280:237.
Greenberg PD, Riddell SR. Deficient cellular immunity—finding and fixing the defects. *Science* 1999;285:546.
Grimbacher B, Holland SM, Gallin JI, et al. Hyper-IgE syndrome with recurrent infections—an autosomal dominant multisystem disorder. *N Engl J Med* 1999; 340:692.
Kara CJ, Glimcher LH. *In vivo* footprinting of MHC class II genes: bare promoters n the bare lymphocyte syndrome. *Science* 1991;252:709.
Kingreen D, Siegert W. Chronic lymphatic leukemias of T and NK cell type. *Leukemia* 1997;11:46.
Lamy T, Loughran TP. Current concepts: large granular lymphocyte leukemia. *Blood Rev* 1999;13:230.
Lopez M, Fleisher T, deShazo RD. Use and interpretation of diagnostic immunologic laboratory tests. *JAMA* 1992;268:2970.
Markert ML. Purine nucleoside phosphorylase deficiency. *Immunodefic Rev* 1991;3:45.

Rijkers GT, Scharenberg JGM, VanDongen JJM, et al. Abnormal signal transduction in a patient with severe combined immunodeficiency disease. *Pediatr Res* 1991;29:306.

Rosenstein Y, et al. CD43, a molecule defective in Wiskott-Aldrich syndrome, binds ICAM-1. *Nature* 1991;354:233.

Sharfe N, Dadi HK, Shahar M, et al. Human immune disorder arising from mutation of the alpha chain of the interleukin-2 receptor. *Proc Natl Acad Sci U S A* 1997;94: 3168.

Spickett GP, Webster ADB, Farrant J. Cellular abnormalities in common variable immunodeficiency. *Immunodefic Rev* 1990;2:199.

Weinberg K, Parkman R. Severe combined immunodeficiency due to a specified defect in the production of interleukin-2. *N Engl J Med* 1990;322:1718.

Winton EF, et al. Spontaneous regression of a monoclonal proliferation of large granular lymphocytes associated with reversal of anemia and neutropenia. *Blood* 1986; 67:1427.

15. MALIGNANT LYMPHOMAS

Hodgkin Disease

William R. Friedenberg

Hodgkin disease (HD) is a disorder that was originally described in 1832 by Sir Thomas Hodgkin, who proposed that this malignancy originated in the lymphatic system. In the past 30 years, HD has become a model for the development of techniques permitting the cure of cancer. Despite the fact that the etiology and pathogenesis of HD are unknown, new insights have allowed more accurate diagnosis, appropriate staging, and effective treatment with a multidisciplinary approach. The clinician who first evaluates the patient must take responsibility for obtaining the tissue for diagnosis and for initiating appropriate staging, so that potentially curative treatment can be given to patients.

Epidemiology, Etiology, and Pathogenesis

Hodgkin disease is less common than non-Hodgkin lymphoma (NHL). It occurs in males more commonly than females, and in approximately 20,000 patients each year in the United States. The incidence of HD is bimodal in terms of age distribution, with the largest peak occurring in the late twenties and a gradual increase in incidence with age over 45 years.

Although the etiology of HD is unknown, epidemiologic data suggest that viral factors, especially Epstein–Barr virus (EBV) and perhaps human immunodeficiency virus (HIV), which interact with the environment, may play a causal role. Reports of clustering of cases and multiple cases of HD in a single household are frequent. There is a small increase in incidence in patients who have had infectious mononucleosis. In addition, some patients with HD have high titers of antibodies against the viral capsid antigen of EBV, and multiple studies have detected EBV in 20% to 80% of tumor specimens. HD appears to occur with increased incidence in patients with HIV infection, although not as frequently as NHL.

Although the t(14;18) translocation and the bcl-2 protein (produced by the *bcl*-2 oncogene) have been described in up to 32% of patients with HD, recent studies suggest that these abnormalities are present in the benign tissues that are reacting to the underlying HD cells in the majority of cases. Neither EBV nor HIV appears to be the direct cause of HD, and it seems likely that other environmental factors in conjunction with genetic predisposition play a significant role in the pathogenesis of the disease.

Pathology

Diagnosis

The **diagnosis** of HD depends on finding multinucleated Reed–Sternberg (RS) cells or their variants in the appropriate background of benign reactive cells consisting of lymphocytes, histiocytes, neutrophils, plasma cells, and fibroblasts. Fine needle aspiration (FNA) is inadequate for initial diagnosis. Open biopsy is preferred, and core biopsies may be adequate in exceptional cases (see the discussion of **Biopsy** in the section on **Diagnosis**). The most commonly used system, the Rye classification system (Table 1), divides the disease into four subtypes, all of which contain the RS cell but with a somewhat different background. Recent investigations found that these subtypes are not independent prognostic factors if appropriate treatment is given. RS cells or their variants are usually large cells with two or more nuclei, each with a prominent nucleolus that sometimes gives it an "owl's eyes" appearance. **Nodular sclerosis** is the most common subtype, and mixed-cellularity HD is the second most frequent, except in patients with the acquired immunodeficiency syndrome (AIDS), in whom mixed-cellularity HD is most common.

1. **Lymphocyte-predominant HD** is usually characterized by limited disease (stage I or II) in the neck; involvement of the mediastinum or hilar lymph nodes is unlikely. Recent studies documented that the nodular subtype of lymphocyte-predominant

Table 1. Histologic classification of Hodgkin disease

1. Lymphocyte predominance
2. Nodular sclerosis
3. Mixed cellularity
4. Lymphocyte depletion[a]

[a] The importance of subdividing lymphocyte depletion into (1) diffuse fibrosis and (2) reticular types, as originally proposed by Lukes, has been emphasized by Rosen *J Clin Oncol* 1986;4:275. From Lukes RJ. Report of the committee on Hodgkin's disease staging classification. *Cancer Res* 1971;31:1755, with permission.

HD is more closely related to a B-cell–indolent NHL and has a tendency to relapse after many years and yet retain the ability to respond to multiple treatments. This subtype of HD is frequently associated with a conversion to a diffuse, large-cell NHL and probably represents a "transformation" rather than a separate and distinct malignancy.

2. **Nodular sclerosis HD** is frequently associated with a mediastinal mass and hilar lymphadenopathy in addition to disease in the neck.

3. Constitutional symptoms and advanced disease are more common in **mixed-cellularity HD** and **lymphocyte-depleted HD.**

4. To establish the diagnosis, it is necessary to find RS cells, which is usually easier in lymph nodes than in the bone marrow, which may have the appropriate background but lack the typical RS cells.

5. In rare cases, typical-appearing RS cells may be found in benign illnesses, NHL, and carcinoma. The pathologist must be able to distinguish HD from NHL, in particular, Ki-1–positive large-cell anaplastic lymphomas and T-cell lymphomas, which may mimic lymphocyte-depleted HD.

The RS Cell
The RS cell is accepted as the neoplastic cell in HD, but the origin of this cell is controversial. Cell-culturing techniques and analysis of individual cells by immunophenotyping, gene rearrangement, and cytogenetic studies have shown a variety of antigens expressed on the surface of the RS cell, including CD30 (Ki-1), CD25 (interleukin-2 receptor), human leukocyte antigen DR locus (HLA-DR), and CD71 (transferrin receptor). The immunophenotype of the RS cell varies with the histological subtype of HD, in some cases having granulocyte markers (Leu-M-1), whereas T- or B-cell markers may predominate in others.

Diagnosis
Presentation
Most patients present with superficial lymphadenopathy, with cervical nodes being most common. Only 4% of the patients have disease limited to below the diaphragm. The lymph nodes are usually nontender and firm or rubbery; occasionally, the size varies spontaneously. Rarely, patients present with immune-mediated thrombocytopenia or autoimmune hemolytic anemia. Renal failure is uncommon, but it may be associated with bilateral obstruction of the ureters because of enlarged retroperitoneal lymph nodes. Infrequently, patients may present with the nephrotic syndrome as a paraneoplastic manifestation of HD.

Constitutional Symptoms
1. Fever (>38°C) and drenching night sweats requiring a change in bed clothes or a weight loss of more than 10% of usual weight occur in approximately 40% of patients and are associated with a poor prognosis.

2. Pruritus and alcohol-induced pain in areas of disease involvement are uncommon and not consistently associated with a poor prognosis. The pruritus may be intense and not localized to any particular portion of the body. The pain with alcohol usually comes on within a few minutes of ingestion and may occur in any area affected by the disease.

3. Constitutional symptoms occur more commonly in older patients and indicate advanced disease and poor histology. Fatigue and weakness are frequent but nonspecific.

Contiguous Spread
Hodgkin disease appears to spread contiguously from one group of lymph nodes to another. The disease usually begins in the neck and spreads to adjacent lymph nodes, with occasional spread to nonlymphoid structures (e.g., the mediastinum into the lung). In patients with left supraclavicular involvement, the disease may spread to the upper abdomen and skip the mediastinum.

The spleen or splenic hilar lymph nodes may be the only site of involvement below the diaphragm, and such involvement is not necessarily an indicator of widespread hematogenous dissemination. Visceral dissemination, including the liver, without splenic involvement, is rare. Spread to the periaortic or pelvic lymph nodes (stage III-2) implies more advanced disease (hematogenous dissemination) and frequently is associated with visceral involvement. Splenomegaly, as determined by either physical examination or by imaging techniques, may be reactive and not associated with pathologic involvement. Enlarged spleens that are pathologically affected by HD are more likely to be associated with liver involvement.

Laboratory Tests
1. **Abnormalities in the peripheral blood** are common and include anemia, neutrophilia, eosinophilia, monocytosis, lymphocytopenia, and thrombocytosis or thrombocytopenia. Lymphocytopenia may be a manifestation of replacement of normal lymph node structures with either advanced disease or HIV infection. Immunophenotyping the peripheral blood may show a deficiency of T cells; lymphocyte transformation may be decreased, and skin tests may demonstrate anergy.

2. **Liver function tests** may be abnormal, with a cholestatic pattern either secondary to a reactive phenomenon with noncaseating granulomas or attributable to liver involvement with HD. The LDH may be elevated because of the tumor itself or because of any organ involvement.

3. The erythrocyte sedimentation rate (ESR), serum ferritin, and copper levels may be elevated on a reactive basis. β_2-Microglobulin is frequently elevated in patients with advanced disease, similar to patients with NHL.

Abnormalities in T-cell Function
Abnormalities in T-cell function with deficiencies in cell-mediated immunity are frequent. The severity of the defect is proportional to the stage of disease. Because patients usually have normal immunoglobulins, they typically do not have bacterial infections; they may, however, present with viral infections, such as herpes zoster (shingles), pulmonary fungal infection, or cryptococcal meningitis. Because AIDS is associated with an increased incidence of HD, patients may present with one of the infections associated with HIV infection and found to have HD.

Thromboembolic Disease
Patients who develop a deep venous thrombosis or pulmonary embolism (not associated with a well-recognized risk for thromboembolic disease) have an increased incidence of malignancies, including HD and NHL.

Biopsy
The diagnosis of HD should be established by obtaining an adequate open biopsy. FNA is usually not sufficient to establish an accurate initial diagnosis of any kind of lymphoma but may be acceptable in some circumstances to confirm relapsing disease. Core biopsies may suffice in exceptional circumstances, for example, patients with severe cardiopulmonary disease who are unable to tolerate a general anesthesia and the risks of surgery required to obtain tissue.

Staging
Staging is the process of defining the extent of disease. The extent of disease has a direct relationship to prognosis and treatment. Clinical staging (CS) involves the history,

physical examination, laboratory data, and imaging techniques, whereas pathologic staging (PS) refers to the extent of disease following exploratory laparotomy and splenectomy.

Classification

The original staging classification adopted by the Ann Arbor Conference in 1971 was modified by the Cotswald Conference in 1989 (Table 2). Staging is important before initiating treatment for two reasons: (a) HD is thought to spread by contiguous rather than early hematogenous dissemination and (b) the staging of patients appears to have an excellent correlation with survival. The initial staging was designed to distinguish patients who might benefit from radiotherapy (*limited disease*) from those who require chemotherapy (*advanced disease*). Stages I through III represent increasingly disseminated lymphadenopathy with or without extra nodal spread by contiguous involvement (E). The spleen (S) is considered a specialized lymph node. Stage IV represents disseminated disease with visceral involvement (i.e., lung, liver, bone marrow). All patients are subclassified as A or B, depending on the absence (A) or presence (B) of an unexplained fever (>38°C), drenching night sweats or weight loss (>10% of usual body weight in the previous 6 months). The Cotswald Conference added the designation of bulky disease (X) for patients who had mediastinal widening greater than one third of the diameter of the chest on radiograph or any tumor mass with a maximum single dimension of more than 10 cm. In addition, the number of anatomic regions involved is now part of the general staging (e.g., II-3). The stage III patients have been subdivided into two groups, depending on the involvement of splenic hilar, celiac, or portal nodes (III-1) as opposed to the periaortic, iliac, or mesenteric nodes (III-2). Patients with HD, especially those with bulky disease, frequently have residual abnormalities after treatment, and the Cotswald staging system recommends that these

Table 2. Hodgkin disease staging classification

Stage I—Involvement of a single lymph node region (I) or of a single extralymphatic organ or site (I_E).

Stage II—Involvement of 2 or more lymph node regions on the same side of the diaphragm (II) or localized involvement of extralymphatic organ or site and of 1 or more lymph node regions on the same side of diaphragm (II_E). The number of anatomic sites should be indicated by a subscript (e.g., II_4).

Stage III—Involvement of lymph node regions on both sides of the diaphragm (III), which may also be accompanied by localized involvement of extralymphatic organ or site (III_E) or by involvement of the spleen (III_S) or both (III_{SE}), involvement of splenic, hilar, celiac, or portal nodes (III_1), or involvement of periaortic iliac or mesenteric nodes (III_2).

Stage IV—Diffuse or disseminated involvement of 1 or more extralymphatic organs or tissues with or without associated lymph node enlargement. Involvement of liver or bone marrow is always considered stage IV.
　　Each stage is further subdivided into various categories:
　　A—Absence of systemic symptoms
　　B—Presence of systemic symptoms: unexplained fever (>38°C); night sweats;
　　　　>10% weight loss in previous 6 months
　　E—Involvement of an extranodal site by local extension from a nodal site
　　X—Bulky disease: mediastinal widening greater than one third the diameter of
　　　　the chest at the T6–7 level, or >10 cm in any single dimension
　　CR_U—Unconfirmed or uncertain complete remission in patients with residual
　　　　masses
　　CS—Clinical stage
　　PS—Pathological stage (laparotomy)

From Lister TA, et al. Report of the committee convened to discuss the evaluation and staging of patients with Hodgkin's disease: Costwald meeting. *J Clin Oncol* 1989; 7:1630, with permission.

patients be designated CR (U), representing unconfirmed or uncertain complete remission (CR).

Recommended Staging Procedures
1. **History:** The history should determine whether the patient has constitutional (B) symptoms and the presence or absence of pruritus. Following ingestion of alcohol, occasional patients have pain in sites of disease involvement with HD. Although present in only 2% of patients with HD, this response may be a very specific symptom of involvement in a specific area.
2. **Physical examination** (Table 3)
3. **Blood studies:** The usual hematologic tests, including a white blood cell (WBC) count and differential, may be useful because of frequently encountered leukocytosis and occasional eosinophilia. The ESR, although nonspecific, may be helpful in following the patient's response to treatment and may be an indication of relapse following treatment.
4. **Imaging studies:** Computed tomography (CT) scans of the chest, abdomen, and pelvis should be performed along with a plain chest film. Lymphangiography can detect

Table 3. Staging procedures for patients with biopsy-proven Hodgkin disease

Procedures to be used in all patients	
History	Detailed with specific inquiry regarding presence or absence of systemic symptoms (e.g., fever, night sweats, weight loss), including pruritus and pain with alcohol
Physical examination	Detailed examination of Waldeyer's ring, all peripheral lymph node chains, liver, and spleen and search for body tenderness
Blood studies	ESR, CBC, liver function tests, serum creatinine, uric acid, LDH, calcium
Imaging studies	Chest roentgengram; CT scan of chest, abdomen, and pelvis; bipedal lymphangiogram if CT scan negative below diaphragm; bone scan and roentgenogram of appropriate area if patient has bone pain or tenderness. A Gallium scan may support involvement in equivocally positive areas on other tests. MRI may be useful for questionable areas of bone involvement.
Procedures to used in selected patients	
Bone marrow biopsy	Iliac crest needle biopsy for patients with anemia, systemic symptoms, or stage III disease; also may be appropriate for stage IV (e.g., liver, lung) to serve as a guide for evaluation of complete response following therapy
Liver biopsy	Should be performed in selected patients either by peritoneoscopy or by laparotomy when indicated
Laparotomy	Should be performed only when results will substantially change therapeutic plan; strong indication is for situations when irradiation alone will be the preferred therapy; not indicated for patients who will receive multidrug chemotherapy regardless of findings at laparotomy

CBC, complete blood cell count; CT, computed tomography; ESR, erythrocyte sedimentation rate; MRI, magnetic resonance imaging
From Rosenberg SA, et al. Report of the committee of Hodgkin disease staging procedures. *Cancer Res* 1971;31:1862, and Lister TA, et al. Report of the committee convened to discuss. The evaluation and staging of patients with Hodgkin's disease: Cotswald meeting. *J Clin Oncol* 1989;7:1630, with permission.

abnormalities in architecture as well as size and is thus more sensitive in determining periaortic lymph node disease. CT scanning can visualize areas rarely or never seen on lymphangiography (celiac, splenic, portal, mesenteric nodes). Lymph nodes are assumed to be normal if they are less than 1.5 cm in cross-sectional diameter. If the CT scan is negative and the proposed treatment plan involves using extended-field radiation therapy and not total nodal irradiation (TNI) or chemotherapy, consideration should be given to obtaining a lymphangiogram. If, however, lymphangiograms are not done frequently at the treating institution, they may not be worth doing. A bone marrow should be done in patients with anemia, leukopenia, or thrombocytopenia, B symptoms, and at least stage III disease on preliminary evaluation. Bone scanning, gallium scanning, positron emission tomography (PET) scanning, and magnetic resonance imaging (MRI) may be helpful based on the preliminary staging evaluation.

Staging Laparotomy
A staging laparotomy should be performed only if the evaluating physicians believe the results of the procedure would significantly influence the treatment. Patients who appear to be in **stage I or II** without constitutional symptoms, and are therefore candidates for curative radiation therapy, may need laparotomy if the philosophy at the treating institution does not include chemotherapy. About one third of the patients with clinically diagnosed early stage disease are placed in a higher stage after laparotomy (50% of patients with B symptoms and 25% without B symptoms). The decision regarding the need for laparotomy should be multidisciplinary; the radiation oncologist and the hematologist or medical oncologist must agree on the proposed treatment, and the surgeon needs to have a reasonable rationale for performing the operation.

Most institutions have abandoned laparotomy for clinical **stage III patients,** because most of these patients will receive chemotherapy with or without radiation therapy. In patients with **stage I and II HD with B symptoms,** some institutions give only radiation therapy if the laparotomy is negative for advanced disease, but if the planned treatment involves combining radiation therapy with chemotherapy, laparotomy is not indicated.

Another controversy regarding laparotomy is the **role of splenectomy.** If the spleen is enlarged and the presumptive plan is to treat with radiation therapy for early stage III disease, then many radiation therapists believe that the spleen should be removed to avoid excessive damage to the left lung and kidney. If the spleen can be irradiated because it is of normal size, then the question of whether the liver is involved should be evaluated by CT scan and other techniques. In addition to the slight increase in risk of overwhelming sepsis in splenectomized patients, there is an increased risk of acute leukemia.

Although **staging laparotomy** for HD is very safe (operative mortality <0.5%), patients who have an extremely low incidence of intraabdominal involvement, such as young women with either lymphocyte predominance histology with isolated lymph nodes high in the neck and epitrochlear area or patients with isolated mediastinal disease of nodular sclerosis type can be treated with mantle irradiation therapy without exploratory laparotomy or extended-field radiation. A laparotomy is necessary for patients with stage IIB and IIIA HD in treating institutions that plan only radiation therapy if the laparotomy is negative. If chemotherapy is to be used with or without radiation therapy, however, exploratory laparotomy is unnecessary.

Treatment
Controversies persist regarding the management of HD because treatment for both early and advanced disease has become so successful that comparing therapeutic regimens without randomized controlled studies of large treatment groups has become difficult. Successful treatment strategies have evolved at many institutions in the United States and Europe and continue to evolve as new data on treatment programs emerge. In most centers, patients with early stage HD (stages I through IIA–E) are treated with radiation therapy, whereas patients with advanced disease (stages IIB through IV) are treated with combination chemotherapy. Patients who have constitutional symptoms (B) or who are at intermediate stages may be treated with chemotherapy, radiation therapy, or combined-modality treatment, depending on the institution.

Early Stage Hodgkin Disease

Early studies using radiation therapy were designed to cure patients in whom all disease could be covered by radiation fields. The development of the linear accelerator allowed higher doses and larger fields. The simultaneous development of more accurate staging with imaging studies lymphangiogram and laparotomy made treatment more accurate and less toxic. Early studies by Peters at the Princess Margaret Hospital showed that radiation therapy could cure HD and sterilize sites of involvement by the administration of sufficient doses. Randomized clinical trials were performed to evaluate limited radiation therapy versus more extensive treatment.

Radiation therapy: Patients who are considered to have early stage disease are those with stages I and II without bulky disease or B symptoms. These patients usually are treated with high-dose irradiation of between 3,600 and 4,400 cGy to contiguous regions of lymphoid tissue; all major sites of lymphoid tissue above the diaphragm are encompassed in a *mantle field* (Fig. 1). Below the diaphragm, the periaortic and splenic nodes or spleen constitute the *spade field,* and the *inverted Y field* extends the periaortic and splenic field to include the iliac, hypogastric, and inguinal nodes. Patients usually are treated with the mantle field first. Following several weeks of rest, they are given "extended-field radiation," or TNI, which includes the combination of mantle and inverted Y fields, to encompass the periaortic nodes and splenic pedicle. Several clinical trials have demonstrated an improvement in freedom from progression or disease-free survival with extended-field as opposed to involved-field treatment. When pathologic staging is used, the differences in overall survival have been less obvious because of potential salvage with combination chemotherapy if and when patients have a relapse. In Europe, many patients are not pathologically staged, and the size of the irradiation fields are somewhat less than what is standard in the United States. This treatment philosophy limits early toxicity, but it increases the need for salvage chemotherapy and the possibility of late side effects, including acute myelogenous leukemia (AML).

Prognostic indicators: A mediastinal mass greater than one third of the chest diameter on chest radiograph, age greater than 40 years, B symptoms, extranodal disease, more than three lymph node sites, an ESR over 30, male sex, and histologic features of mixed cellularity or lymphocyte depletion all have been determined to be important prognostic indicators in predicting relapses after radiotherapy. In addition, the treatment outcome appears to be related to the experience of the radiation oncologist's experience.

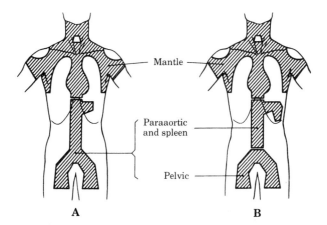

FIG. 1. Diagrammatic representation of irradiation fields used in the treatment of Hodgkin disease. **A:** Mantle and inverted Y fields. **B:** Mantle, paraaortic/splenic, and pelvic fields. (From Kaplan HS. *Hodgkin's disease,* 2nd ed. Cambridge, MA: Harvard University Press, 1980:376, with permission.).

The risk of HD below the diaphragm is very low (<10%) in the following patients: women with stage IA lymphocyte predominant disease above the level of the clavicles, epitrochlear disease, and women with nodular sclerosis limited to the mediastinum. These patients can be effectively treated with radiation therapy without the extended field approved and without staging laparotomy. In other patients with stage IA and IIA HD, if laparotomy is omitted in the evaluation process or radiation therapy is limited, the risk of relapse is increased. Chemotherapy to salvage these patients has been so successful that overall survival has not been seriously affected. If laparotomy is omitted in stage I or stage II disease, it may be necessary that the patient and physician accept the increased risk of sequential radiation therapy followed by chemotherapy.

Combined-modality treatment using chemotherapy and radiation therapy has been used instead of more extensive radiation therapy (e.g., TNI) in early stage disease. Three studies showed that brief chemotherapy with ABVD (Adriamycin, bleomycin, vinblastine, and dacarbazine; two to four cycles) followed by irradiation for early stage HD provides highly effective treatment with minimal infertility, cardiopulmonary toxicity, or second malignancies. This strategy appears to be the most effective and least toxic treatment for most patients with early stage disease who have some poor prognostic features.

Massive mediastinal involvement: Different criteria have been used to determine whether mediastinal involvement is massive. The Cotswald Conference recommends that a mass with a maximal horizontal width on a standing chest radiograph of more than one third of the chest diameter at the T6–7 level should be considered massive. A study using CT scan measurements compared with plain chest films showed no improvement. The mediastinum is involved in more than 50% of patients with HD. If the involvement is small and localized with no evidence of HD outside the mediastinum, the prognosis is excellent even with involved-field radiation therapy. Between 50% and 74% of patients with stage II massive mediastinal HD treated with total nodal radiotherapy will relapse. Most relapses occur above the diaphragm in the lung, chest wall, pleura, or thoracic extranodal sites. This relapse rate is excessive; therefore, combined-modality therapy is recommended. Usually, chemotherapy is administered first to shrink the mediastinal mass and allow radiation therapy to be given to a smaller port with less potential toxicity to the adjacent tissues (i.e., lung and heart).

Chemotherapy with MOPP, MOPP alternated with ABVD, the hybrid regimen, or ABVD alone combined with radiotherapy have been used (Tables 4 and 5). The combination of radiation therapy and ABVD alone appears to be less likely to cause myelodysplasia, acute nonlymphoblastic leukemia (ANLL), and infertility, although the incidence of cardiopulmonary toxicity is increased. Alternative combinations and numbers of cycles of chemotherapy are being investigated.

Chemotherapy alone: Biti et al. compared chemotherapy alone, using MOPP, with extended-field radiotherapy. All patients were laparotomy staged to be early stage disease and randomized to receive mantle-field radiation followed by periaortic irradiation or six cycles of MOPP chemotherapy. All patients in the radiation therapy group and 40 of 44 in the chemotherapy group achieved complete remission. The overall survival was greater in the radiation therapy group (93%) compared with the chemotherapy group (56%; $p < 0.001$). In patients with pathologically staged I and IIA HD with good prognostic features, chemotherapy alone does not appear to be as efficacious as radiation therapy or combined-modality treatment.

Constitutional symptoms: At most institutions, if patients with B symptoms do not undergo exploratory laparotomy, they receive chemotherapy with or without radiation therapy. In a large study combining the data of pathologically stage IB and IIB patients, those with night sweats with no other B symptoms had a prognosis similar to patients with pathologically stage IA and IIA disease when treated with radiation therapy alone. Although total lymphoid irradiation or extended-field treatment has been used by these institutions, the rate of relapse following irradiation alone is high. Patients with B symptoms are similar to others with poor prognostic features and may be salvaged by combination chemotherapy if the decision is made to treat with radiation therapy alone.

(text continues on page 309)

Table 4. Chemotherapy regimens for Hodgkin disease

Regimen	Drugs	Dosage (mg/m²)	Route	Treatment schedule (days)	Cycle length (days)	Duration	Reference
Induction therapy							
MOPP	Mechlorethamine	6	i.v.	1 and 8	28	6 mo minimum (2 cycles beyond complete remission)	35
	Vincristine	1.4	i.v.	1 and 8			
	Procarbazine	100	p.o.	1–14			
	Prednisone	40	p.o.	1–14[a]			
MOPP/ABVD MOPP	As above, alternating every cycle with ABVD				28	12 mo minimum	5
ABVD	Doxorubicin	25	i.v.	1 and 15	28		
	Bleomycin	10	i.v.	1 and 15			
	Vinblastine	6	i.v.	1 and 15			
	Dacarbazine (DTIC)	375	i.v.	1 and 15			
BCVPP	Carmustine (BCNU)	100	i.v.	1	28	6 mo minimum	1
	Cyclophosphamide	600	i.v.	1			
	Vinblastine	5	i.v.	1			
	Procarbazine	50	p.o.	2–10			
	Procarbazine	100	p.o.	1–10			
	Prednisone	60	p.o.	1			
MOP/BAP	Mechlorethamine	6	i.v.	1	28	10–14 mo	28
	Doxorubicin	30	i.v.	8			
	Vincristine	1.4[b]	i.v.	1 and 8			
	Bleomycin	2	i.v.	1 and 8			
	Procarbazine	100	p.o.	2–7 and 9–12			
	Prednisone	40	p.o.	2–7 and 9–12[c]			

continued

Table 4. (continued).

Regimen	Drugs	Dosage (mg/m²)	Route	Treatment schedule (days)	Cycle length (days)	Duration	Reference
MOPP/ABV	Mechlorethamine	6	i.v.	1	28	6–12 mo	29
	Vincristine	1.4[b]	i.v.	1			
	Procarbazine	100	p.o.	1–7			
	Prednisone	40	p.o.	1–14			
	Doxorubicin	35	i.v.	8			
	Bleomycin	10	i.v.	8			
	Vinblastine	6	i.v.	8			
MVPP	Mechlorethamine	6	i.v.	1 and 8	28	6 mo	44
	Vinblastine	6	i.v.	1 and 8			
	Procarbazine	100	p.o.	1–15			
	Prednisone	40[d]	p.o.	1–5			
ChlVPP	Chlorambucil	6	p.o.	1 and 8	28	6 mo (2 cycles beyond complete remission)	41
	Vinblastine	6	i.v.	1 and 8			
	Procarbazine	100	p.o.	1–14			
	Prednisone	40	p.o.	1–14[a]			
Salvage therapy							
ABVD	As above						6, 7, 16, 17, 33, 46
B-CAVe							23
	Lomustine (CCNU)	100	p.o.	1	42	6 mo minimum cycles beyond complete remission	23
	Doxorubicin	60	i.v.	1			
	Vinblastine	5	i.v.	1			
	Bleomycin	5	i.v.	1, 28, and 35			

Regimen	Drug	Dose	Route	Days	Cycle	Comments	Ref
ABDIC	Doxorubicin	45	i.v.	1	28	Continued until 450 mg/m^2 doxorubicin given +1–3 cycles minus doxorubicin	45
	Bleomycin	5	i.v.	1 and 5			
	Dacarbazine (DTIC)	200	i.v.	1–5			
	Lomustine (CCNU)	50	p.o.	1			
	Prednisone	40	p.o.	1–5			
MOPP	As above			1 and 8	28	6 mo minimum 2 cycles beyond complete remission	34
CVPP/ABOS					28	Cycles are alternated between CVPP and ABOS + 12 cycles	47
CVPP	CCNU	75	p.o.	1			
	Vinblastine	4	i.v.	1 and 8			
	Procarbazine	100	p.o.	1–14			
	Prednisone	40[e]	p.o.	1–14			
ABOS	Doxorubicin	50	i.v.	1	28	See above	47
	Bleomycin	5	i.v.	1 and 8			
	Vincristine	1.4[b]	i.v.	1 and 8			
	Streptozotocin	1500	i.v.	1 and 8			

i.v., intravenously; p.o., orally.

[a] Cycles 1 and 4 only.
[b] Maximum dose 2.0 mg.
[c] Cycles 1, 4, 7, and 10 only.
[d] 40 mg total dose.
[e] Courses 1, 3, and 5.

Table 5. Survival of patients with Hodgkin disease following therapy

Stage	Therapy	Disease-free survival (%)		Overall survival (%)		References
		5 yr	10 yr	5 yr	10 yr	
IA, IIA	Radiation	80–85	75–85	95–97	95–95	3, 11, 12, 25, 30, 31, 36
IIB	Radiation	70–75	65–70	85–90	75–85	13, 25, 30
IIIA	Radiation	66	64	86	63	24
IIIA	Radiation + chemotherapy	74–88	86–90	70–88	92–94	4, 14, 26, 37
IIIA	Chemotherapy	—	90	90 (7 yr)	90–94	14, 32, 35
III$_1$A	Radiation	63	65	91	73–85	21, 37, 43
III$_2$A	Radiation	32	10	56	44	21, 37, 43
III$_2$A	Radiation + chemotherapy	76	80	84	66	21, 37, 43
IIIA, B;IVA,B	Chemotherapy					18
	MOPP	45–55	54	55–67	40–50	1, 4, 9, 35
	BCVPP	64	—	67	—	1
	MOPP/ABVD	73	73 (8 yr)	—	76 (8 yr)	4, 5
	MOP-BAP	—	—	60	—	28
	MOPP/ABV	75	—	84	—	10

Advanced Disease

Combination chemotherapy is the treatment of choice for patients with advanced disease (Tables 4 and 5). Combination chemotherapy for advanced HD was the first example of a chemotherapy program consisting of multiple agents, all of which had shown significant individual success in treating HD. These drugs were combined to avoid overlapping toxicity and successfully eradicated all disease. The first four drugs that were combined to form the MOPP regimen were mechlorethamine (nitrogen mustard), vincristine (Oncovin), procarbazine, and prednisone. Eighty-four percent of patients in this original study achieved complete remission; 54% were disease free at 15 years. Relapses beyond four years were very few, and none occurred after 11 years. Similar programs of combination chemotherapy consisting of four different drugs induced CR in 70% to 90% of patients. One third eventually relapsed, resulting in cure of 50% to 65% of all patients with advanced disease (Table 4). It is apparent that a variety of different agents is crucial to the success of each regimen, minimizing the toxicity of each agent and maximizing dose intensity.

Nadir blood counts are necessary to monitor treatment and avoid excessive myelosuppression. In patients who have hypersplenism or bone marrow involvement, reductions in the doses of myelosuppressive drugs should not be made during the initial cycles of therapy because of the potential compromise of effectiveness of the regimen.

The usual plan is to administer four cycles of the combination chemotherapy and repeat the staging procedures that were positive before treatment was instituted. Following the sixth cycle, the previously positive tests are repeated (restaging). If the studies are completely normal or residual abnormalities persist and are unchanged after the last two cycles, treatment should be discontinued on the assumption that whatever residual abnormalities are present may result from fibrosis rather than residual tumor. Gallium scans or PET scans may provide useful information regarding residual disease. If a response continues between cycles four and six, two additional cycles of treatment beyond the planned six treatments are given until there is either stability of disease or disappearance of all previously visible residual disease.

Growth factors have been used to maintain the schedule and maximize dose intensity by decreasing myelotoxicity and hastening marrow recovery.

Maintenance chemotherapy has been attempted without showing any signs of improving overall survival and with the possible increased risk of secondary acute myeloid leukemia or myelodysplasia.

In some studies, **radiotherapy** is given to either limited areas of bulky disease or to broader fields. Although adding radiation therapy increased the complete remission rate and FFP, it does not improve overall survival. Patients who have advanced disease and massive mediastinal involvement do have high relapse rates, particularly in the lung, and may benefit from the addition of radiation therapy.

To increase the complete remission, failure-free survival (FFS), and overall survival, several presumably non–cross-resistant combination chemotherapy regimens were put together to try to improve the results achieved by MOPP (Tables 4 and 6). In an effort to avoid drug resistance, as postulated by the Golde-Coldman hypothesis, seven or eight drugs were combined to try to avoid overlapping toxicity and improve efficacy. Canellos showed that ABVD was better than MOPP and equivalent to MOPP/ABVD. A comparison of the hybrid regimen MOPP/ABV with ABVD showed that ABVD was less toxic.

A consensus has emerged that ABVD (Diehl V, et al.) is the best chemotherapy currently available for advanced-stage HD. A German regimen using escalated BEACOPP plus irradiation and the abbreviated 12-week chemotherapy regimen (Stanford V) are under investigation.

The *optimal choice* for an individual patient depends not only on the efficacy of the treatment regimen but also on the possible early and late toxicity associated with the treatment. Although some regimens have been reported to be less emetogenic than others, the recent use of more effective agents, such as ondansetron and granisetron, minimizes the concern for this toxicity. Both ondansetron and granisetron have proven so effective in preventing vomiting that this side effect is no longer relevant. Myelotoxicity is a major side effect of chemotherapy and is worse with MOPP and its variants.

Late toxicities include infertility, pulmonary and cardiac dysfunction, and second malignancies, especially acute leukemia and severe myelodysplasia. These effects are

Table 6. Selected controlled trials comparing combination chemotherapy regimens in advanced Hodgkin's disease [17, 46]

Regimen	CR (%)	RFS (%)	PFS (%)	OS (%)	Comment	References
LOPP	57	32	—	66	RT was given to residual masses	22
vs		p < 0.001 (5 yr)		p < 0.05 (5 yr)		
LOPP/EVAP	64	47		75		
MOPP	57	61	43	57	RT was given to nodes >5 cm originally, or residual masses	42
vs		p = 0.42 (6 yr)	p = 0.13 (6 yr)	p = 0.13 (6 yr)		
MOPP/ABVD	59	69	60	65		
BCVPP	73	56	47	68	Combining the 2 BCVPP arms produced statistically significant results	19
vs	} 69		} 48	} 65		
BCVPP+RT	67	61	49	63		
MOPP/ABVD	80	61	61	75 p ≠ 0.005	MOPP/ABVD and ABVD were superior to MOPP and equivalent to each other when both were combined in the analysis	8
vs						
MOPP	67	—	50	66		
ABVD	82	—	61	73		20
vs	} p ≠ 0.006 (5 yr)		} p ≠ 0.02 (5 yr)	} p ≠ 0.28 (5 yr)		
MOPP/ABVD	83	—	65	75		
MOPP/ABV	81	—	80	90	The hybrid regimen was superior with a median follow-up of 22 mo	
vs						
MOPP/ABVD	76	—	67	85		
MOPP+RT	80.7	77.2	62.8	67.9	ABVD+RT improved survival, decreased gonadal dysfunction and acute leukemia, without increased cardio-pulmonary toxicity	40
vs	p = 0.02	p = 0.06	p < 0.02	p = 0/03		
ABVD+RT	92.4	87.7	80.8	77.4		
MOPP/ABV	85	75	—	84	The two treatments were equivalent with a median follow-up of 60 mo	10
vs						
MOPP/ABVD	82	70	—	84		

CR, complete remission; OS, overall survival; PFS, progression-free survival; RFS, relapse-free survival; RT, radiation therapy.

dose related; MOPP variants with high doses of alkylating agents or procarbazine increase the rate of infertility, acute leukemia and myelodysplasia, and solid tumors.

The risk of acute leukemia with MOPP alone within the first 10 years is approximately 2% and increases with the addition of radiation therapy, maintenance chemotherapy, or the inclusion of a nitrosourea in a MOPP variant. The seven- and eight-drug regimens (MOPP/ABVD and MOPP/ABV hybrid) reduce the total dose of the MOPP drugs by 50% and the rate of infertility by approximately 50%.

The addition of radiation therapy to aggressive combination chemotherapy regimens has not demonstrated an overall survival advantage; thus, most institutions no longer advocate "adjuvant" radiation therapy except for bulky mediastinal disease.

The risk of acute leukemia with either the Stanford VBM or ABVD protocol with or without radiation therapy is nearly zero. The exact risk of late cardiac and pulmonary toxicity with ABVD alone with or without radiation therapy has not been completely assessed beyond 5 to 7 years. It appears likely, however, that late fatal pulmonary and cardiac disease with regimens containing Adriamycin and bleomycin will be similar to the risk of leukemia/myelodysplasia after alkylating agent–containing regimens.

Salvage Treatment

The length of first CR has a dramatic impact on the subsequent response to salvage treatment and the duration of that response. Patients who have a relapse within 1 year are considered resistant to the original regimen because responses to this same regimen are low (about 30%) and not durable. Patients who remain in remission for more than 1 year have a greater chance of achieving a second CR (about 95%), and the second remissions are more likely to be durable.

In the initial National Cancer Institute experience, patients who relapsed after MOPP and who again achieved a second remission with MOPP had a relapse-free survival at 10 years of 45%, but only 24% lived for more than 11 years because of the development of second malignancies and treatment-related complications. Only 11% of patients who were retreated with MOPP after early relapse survived 10 years. Patients who had a relapse after treatment with ABVD have had a similar experience. For patients who were initially managed with radiation alone, systemic chemotherapy is the treatment of choice. Patients who relapse locally at the margin of a previously irradiated field may be salvaged by isolated radiation therapy to that site.

The addition of radiation therapy to chemotherapy for patients who relapse with disseminated disease has not been shown to improve survival. Conventional-dose salvage chemotherapy in patients who relapse after a seven- or eight-drug regimen within 1-year of the original combination chemotherapy regimen or who are more than 30 years of age are very unlikely to live beyond ten years (<11%) without stem cell transplant.

Stem cell rescue using autologous bone marrow, peripheral stem cells or allogeneic bone marrow transplantation (BMT) with high-dose chemotherapy or radiation therapy has been used as potentially curative treatment for relapsing patients (Table 7). Patients who have continued sensitivity to chemotherapy, a limited number of prior treatments, and good performance status are more likely to do well with stem cell rescue. Patients who have never achieved a CR or who have a relapse early following CR still can be salvaged by this approach, whereas standard salvage chemotherapy is unlikely to produce long-term survival. In a review of eight series consisting of 268 patients who received stem cell transplants, the CR rate was 59%, with a 61% relapse-free rate at 3 years. Patients with good prognostic features do better than those with poor indicators (Hasenclever D, et al.).

In patients treated with autologous stem cells derived from the bone marrow or peripheral blood, early mortality is less than 10%, whereas with allogeneic BMT, the risk of graft-versus-host disease increases morbidity and mortality. Allogeneic transplantation is limited to patients who have a good HLA match, either from a related or unrelated donor, and who are less than 50 to 55 years of age.

Stem cell transplants from autologous bone marrow or peripheral blood may be used in patients up to age 60 or 65 years. Because many of these patients have had radiation therapy, high dose regimens such as CBV (cyclophosphamide, BCNU, and etoposide) and BEAM (BCNU, etoposide, cytarabine, and melphalan) have been developed without total body irradiation.

Table 7. Autologous bone marrow transplantation

No. of patients	Conditioning regimen	CR (%)	PFS (%)	OS (%)	Reference
58	Cytoxan Carmustine Etoposide ± Cisplatin (CBV ± P)	—	64 at median follow-up of 2.3 yr	72	39
73	Etoposide Melphalan RT	75	38.6 at 4 yr	—	15
30	CBV	50	37	—	27
26	Cytoxan TBI ± involved field RT	50	27	38	38

CR, complete remission; OS, overall survival; PFS, progression free survival; RT, radiation therapy; TBI, total body irradiation.

The use of growth factors [granulocyte colony-stimulating factor (G-CSF), granulocyte-macrophage–colony-stimulating factor (GM-CSF)] as adjuvant to high-dose therapy with stem cell rescue has decreased the duration of neutropenia and length of hospital stay and appears to be cost effective.

Randomized controlled studies have not been done to compare conventional salvage chemotherapy with high-dose chemotherapy with stem cell rescue. Selected patients for whom chemotherapy induction has failed, who have a short initial remission, or have had multiple relapses but remain sensitive to treatment and have a good performance status have an excellent chance of being salvaged by stem cell transplant. Peripheral stem cells appear superior to unstimulated bone marrow because of more rapid engraftment and better neutrophil and platelet recovery, an absence of general anesthesia, and ability to be collected.

Toxicity
As discussed previously, the choice of treatment for HD at its various stages has been so successful that the selection depends significantly on the acute and chronic toxicity associated with the modality chosen. Individual patients may choose one treatment modality over another, depending on their concerns. The duration of treatment and the geographic availability of radiation therapy may determine which modality the patient chooses. The long-term effects on the quality of life, including infertility, are predominant in the minds of some patients.

Radiation Therapy
Mantle irradiation: Acute toxicity frequently includes stomatitis with a decrease in taste and appetite associated with weight loss. Superimposed thrush is sometimes seen. Although acute cardiopulmonary toxicity is uncommon, long-term toxicity is frequent. Radiation pneumonitis of mild degree occurs in most patients, and pulmonary fibrosis in the apical and perimediastinal areas is usually evident on routine chest radiographs 6 months or longer following treatment. An asymptomatic pericardial effusion may occur, but symptomatic constrictive pericarditis is rare (1%).

One study showed mediastinal radiation to be the most consistent factor in the reduction of pulmonary function more than 36 months following treatment (32%). The addition of bleomycin increased the risk to 37%, and bleomycin alone reduced long-term pulmonary function in only 19% of patients.

When VBM chemotherapy was given to a group of 30 patients who also received involved-field radiotherapy to the mediastinum, 14 of 30 patients had significant symptoms (cough and dyspnea) associated with impairment of pulmonary function. Although myocardial fibrosis and coronary artery disease are known complications of radiation and may be increased by the addition of doxorubicin, the true incidence of these complications is not yet known.

Thyroid irradiation: Hypothyroidism (increased thyroid-stimulating hormone, or TSH) is a frequent complication following mantle irradiation, and patients should be monitored indefinitely. At least 25% of patients develop clinical hypothyroidism within 6 years following treatment, and an additional 40% show signs of early disease with an elevated TSH and normal thyroxine (T4) levels.

Pelvic irradiation: When irradiation is given below the diaphragm, irradiation of the periaortic nodes without the complete inverted Y field is associated with nausea and vomiting but avoids severe myelosuppression (leukopenia and thrombocytopenia) requiring the interruption of therapy to allow time for marrow recovery.

Infertility is frequent, with 70% of menstruating females becoming amenorrheic. This can be avoided by the use of oophoropexy, in which the ovaries are moved to the midline at the time of laparotomy to avoid the radiation fields. The permanent induction of menopause occurs more frequently in older patients, whereas menses return in approximately 60% of patients, more commonly in younger patients. Oligospermia is frequent in men, although the testicles are not in the radiation field. Some recovery may occur following completion of therapy, but fertility remains low.

Second malignancy: The incidence of nonhematologic second malignancies varies between 7% and 9%. Sarcomas, lung cancer, thyroid cancer, malignant melanoma, basal cell carcinoma, and breast cancer occur in radiation fields, with a slow increase beyond 10 years. Patients who develop breast cancer after radiation therapy for HD more frequently have bilateral disease, with more frequent involvement of the medial half of the breast. AML does not appear to be increased by radiation alone. Because of the increased risk of breast cancer, screening of these patients has been recommended, although the role of mammography in premenopausal women remains controversial. Unlike AML, in which the risk of leukemia falls dramatically after 10 years following chemotherapy, the risk of solid tumors increases beyond 15 years.

Chemotherapy

The type and severity of toxicity depend on the exact regimen used. **Acute toxicities** include the following:

1. **Nausea and vomiting** associated with emetogenic chemotherapy have been dramatically reduced by new agents such as ondansetron and granisetron.
2. **Malaise, anorexia, fatigue, and weakness** are common, especially during periods of myelosuppression, when patients may be severely leukopenic.
3. In patients treated with vincristine, **peripheral neuropathy** is common; severe weakness, constipation, ileus, or bladder retention occur infrequently; the dose of vincristine should be limited to 2 mg per injection.
4. Doxorubicin is associated with **cardiomyopathy,** and the incidence increases significantly with accumulative doses above 400 mg/m^2.
5. Bleomycin is frequently associated with **fever** with the first dose, but severe acute pulmonary toxicity and respiratory failure rarely occur.
6. The use of growth factors to prevent neutropenia may prevent some infections, but serious **infectious complications** (e.g., cryptococcal meningitis, pneumonia) are still a major concern with chemotherapy.
7. **Thrombocytopenia** may occur, but seldom does it contribute to bleeding or require platelet transfusions.
8. **Anemia** may require red cell transfusions and can be decreased by the use of erythropoietin.

Long-term toxicity includes the following:

1. Patients who receive vincristine for prolonged periods have an increased incidence of **peripheral neuropathy.**

2. **Gonadal dysfunction** is more frequent and more common in adult males who receive MOPP. Irreversible azoospermia occurred in at least 80% of patients; sperm banking has allowed successful fertilization, but azoospermia is frequent even before treatment.
3. Although transient **amenorrhea** occurs in at least 50% of women, ovarian function recovers more often, especially in younger women who are not approaching menopause.
4. ABVD and other nonalkylating agent–containing regimens may completely avoid the induction of infertility in patients treated with multiple cycles of chemotherapy.

See the discussion of optimal treatment choices in the section entitled **Advanced Disease** and the discussion of mantle irradiation in the section entitled **Toxicity** for more information concerning toxicities associated with various treatment regimens.

Second malignancy includes the following:

The most serious long-term toxicity of chemotherapy is second malignancy, especially myelodysplasia AML. The risk of AML for patients treated with MOPP is approximately 5% to 7%, with most cases occurring between 4 and 7 years. The risk is significantly lower after 10 years. The combined use of alkylating agents plus irradiation increases the incidence only slightly, suggesting that the chemotherapy in combined modality therapy regimens is primarily responsible for the leukemogenic effect. Regimens that contain alkylating agents, especially mechlorethamine, have the highest incidence of AML. Protocols such as ABVD that do not contain alkylating agents have less leukemogenic potential even when combined with radiation therapy. When alkylating agent–based chemotherapy is given as salvage therapy after prior radiation therapy, the leukemogenic effect may be greater. The risk of NHL also appears to be increased in patients treated with combined-modality therapy as well as those treated with chemotherapy or radiation alone.

Splenectomy
Patients with HD who undergo splenectomy are at increased risk of developing severe and sometimes fatal bacteremia due to encapsulated organisms (e.g., *Streptococcus pneumoniae, Haemophilus influenzae*). Although this condition is rare in adults, it may be partially prevented by the use of pneumococcal vaccine. Patients with HD, even when immunized before splenectomy, do not respond as well to immunization as otherwise normal adults do, however. Prophylactic daily penicillin as is given in children who have had splenectomy may be useful in preventing this complication.

The incidence of AML is also greater in those patients who have had splenectomies.

Psychosocial Adaptation
Survivors of advanced HD are at increased risk for developing problems with psychosocial adaptation. Problems are more frequent in patients who have a lower income (< $15,000/year) or who develop gonadal dysfunction. As a consequence of having had HD, survivors frequently are denied life and health insurance, have sexual problems (37%), and suffer from conditioned nausea when reminded of chemotherapy (39%). The majority of patients are cured with current therapies, and new efforts are under way to investigate treatments that minimize long-term physical and psychological side effects.

Suggested Readings
Ahmed T, Lake DE, Beer M, et al. Single and double autotransplants for relapsing/refractory Hodgkin's disease: results of two consecutive trials. *Bone Marrow Transplant* 1997;19:449.

Anderson JE, Litzow MR, Appelbaum FR, et al. Allogeneic, syngeneic, and autologous marrow transplantation for Hodgkin's disease: the 21-year Seattle experience. *J Clin Oncol* 1993;11:2342.

Andre M, Henry-Amar M, Pico J-L, et al. Comparison of high-dose therapy and autologous stem-cell transplantation with conventional therapy for Hodgkin's disease induction failure: a case–control study. *J Clin Oncol* 1999;17:222.

Bakemeier RF, et al. BCVPP chemotherapy for advanced Hodgkin's disease. Evidence for greater duration of complete remission, greater survival and less toxicity than with a MOPP regimen: results of the Eastern Cooperative Oncology Group study. *Ann Intern Med* 1984;101:447.

Bartlett NL, Rosenberg SA, Hoppe RT, et al. Brief chemotherapy, Stanford V, and adjuvant radiotherapy for bulky or advanced-stage Hodgkin's disease: a preliminary report. *J Clin Oncol* 1995;13:1080.

Bierman PJ, Anderson JR, Freeman MB, et al. High-dose chemotherapy followed by autologous hematopoietic rescue for Hodgkin's disease patients following first relapse after chemotherapy. *Ann Oncol* 1996;7:151.

Bierman PJ, Vose JM, Armitage JO. Autologous transplantation for Hodgkin's disease: Coming of age? *Blood* 1994;83:1161.

Biti GP, et al. Extended-field radiotherapy is superior to MOPP chemotherapy for the treatment of pathologic stage I–IIA Hodgkin's disease: eight-year update of an Italian prospective randomized study. *J Clin Oncol* 1992;10:378.

Bonadonna G, Santoro A. Clinical evolution and treatment of Hodgkin's disease. In: Wiernik PH, et al. eds. *Neoplastic diseases of the blood.* New York: Churchill Livingstone, 1985:789–826.

Bonadonna G, Valagussa P, Santoro A. Alternating non-cross resistant combination chemotherapy or MOPP in stage IV Hodgkin's disease. *Ann Intern Med* 1986;104:739.

Bonfante V, Santoro A, Viviani S, et al. Outcome of patients with Hodgkin's disease failing after primary MOPP-ABVD. *J Clin Oncol* 1997;5:528.

Buzaid AC, Lippman SM, Miller TP. Salvage therapy of advanced Hodgkin's disease: critical appraisal of curative potential. *Am J Med* 1987;83:523.

Canellos GP. The second chance for advanced Hodgkin's disease [Editorial]. *J Clin Oncol* 1992;10:175.

Canellos GP, et al. Chemotherapy of advanced Hodgkin's disease with MOPP, ABVD, or MOPP alternating with ABVD. *N Engl J Med* 1992;327:1478.

Coltman CA Jr. Chemotherapy of advanced Hodgkin's disease. *Semin Oncol* 1980;7:155.

Connors JM, Klimo P, Adams G, et al. Treatment of advanced Hodgkin's disease with chemotherapy-comparison of MOPP/ABV hybrid regimen with alternating courses of MOPP and ABVD: a report from the National Cancer Institute of Canada clinical trials group. *J Clin Oncol* 1997;15:1638.

Connors JM, et al. MOPP/ABV hybrid versus alternating MOPP/ABVD for advanced Hodgkin's disease. *Proc Am Soc Clin Oncol* 1992;11:317.

Cornbleet MA, et al. Pathologic stages IA and IIA Hodgkin's disease: results of treatment with radiotherapy alone (1968–1980). *J Clin Oncol* 1985;3:758.

Cosset JM, et al. The EORTC trials for limited stage Hodgkin's disease. *Eur J Cancer Clin Oncol* 1992;28A:1847.

Crnkovich MJ, Hoppe RT, Rosenberg SA. Stage IIB Hodgkin's disease: the Stanford experience. *J Clin Oncol* 1986;4:472.

Crowther D, et al. A randomized study comparing chemotherapy alone with chemotherapy followed by radiotherapy in patients with pathologically staged IIIA Hodgkin's disease. *J Clin Oncol* 1984;2:892.

Crump M, et al. High-dose etoposide and melphalan, and autologous bone marrow transplantation for patients with advanced Hodgkin's disease: importance of disease status at transplant. *J Clin Oncol* 1993;11:704.

Desch CE, et al. The optimal timing of autologous bone marrow transplantation in Hodgkin's disease patients after a chemotherapy relapse. *J Clin Oncol* 1992;10:200.

DeVita VT Jr, Hubbard SM. Hodgkin's disease. *N Engl J Med* 1993;328:560.

Diehl V, Franklin J, Hasenclever D, et al. BEACOPP, a new dose-escalated and accelerated regimen, is at least as effective as COPP/ABVD in patients with advanced-stage Hodgkin's lymphoma: interim report from a trial of the German Hodgkin's Lymphoma Study Group. *J Clin Oncol* 1998;16:3810.

Diehl V, Sieber M, Ruffer U, et al. BEACOPP: an intensified chemotherapy regimen in advanced Hodgkin's disease: the German Hodgkin's Lymphoma Study Group. *Ann Oncol* 1997;8:143–148.

Duggan D, Petroni G, Johnson J, et al. MOPP/ABV versus ABVD for advanced Hodgkin's disease. *Proc Am Soc Clin Oncol* 1997;16:13a(abst 43).

Friedenberg WR, et al. Improved survival in the treatment of advanced Hodgkin's disease at a nonuniversity institution (1970–1979). *Cancer* 1986;57:12.

Glick J, et al. Improved survival with MOPP–ABVD compared to BCVPP ± radiotherapy (RT) for advanced Hodgkin's disease: 6-year ECOG results. *Blood* 1990; 76:351A.

Glick J, et al. A randomized phase III trial of MOPP-ABV hybrid vs. sequential MOPP-ABVD in advanced Hodgkin's disease: preliminary results of the intergroup trial. *Proc Am Soc Clin Oncol* 1991;10:271.

Golomb HM, et al. Importance of substaging of stage III Hodgkin's disease. *Semin Oncol*. 1980;7:136.

Hancock BW, et al. LOPP alternating with EVAP is superior to LOPP alone in the initial treatment of advanced Hodgkin's disease: results of a British National Lymphoma Investigation Trial. *J Clin Oncol* 1992;10:1252.

Harker WG, Kushlan P, Rosenberg SA. Combination chemotherapy for advanced Hodgkin's disease after failure of MOPP: ABVD and B-CAVe. *Ann Intern Med* 1984; 101:440.

Hasenclever D, Diehl V. A prognostic score for advanced Hodgkin's disease: International Prognostic Factors Project on Advanced Hodgkin's Disease. *N Engl J Med* 1998;339:1506.

Hoppe RT. Radiation therapy in the treatment of Hodgkin's disease. *Semin Oncol* 1980;2:144.

Hoppe RT, et al. The management of stage I–II Hodgkin's disease with irradiation alone or combined modality therapy: the Stanford experience. *Blood* 1982;59:455.

Horning SJ, Hoppe RT, Rosenberg SA. The Stanford Hodgkin's Disease Trials 1968–1984: results of combined modality therapy in PSI, II, and III. In: Jones SE, Salmon SE, eds. *Adjuvant therapy of cancer IV*. Orlando: Grune and Stratton, 1984:633.

Horning SJ, Rosenberg SA, Hoppe RT. Brief chemotherapy (Stanford V) and adjuvant radiotherapy for bulky or advanced Hodgkin's disease: an update. *Ann Oncol* 1996; 7(Suppl 4):105.

Horning SJ, Chaeo NJ, Negrin RS, et al. High-dose therapy and autologous hematopoietic progenitor cell transplantation for recurrent or refractory Hodgkin's disease: analysis of the Stanford University results and prognostic indices. *Blood* 1997;89:801.

Horning SJ, Hoppe RT, Mason J, et al. Stanford-Kaiser Permanente GI study for clinical stage I to IIA Hodgkin's disease: subtotal lymphoid irradiation versus vinblastine methotrexate, and bleomycin chemotherapy and regional irradiation. *J Clin Oncol* 1997;5:1736.

Horning SJ, Williams J, Bartlett N, et al. Assessment of the Stanford V regimen and consolidative radiotherapy for bulky and advanced Hodgkin's Disease: Eastern Cooperative Oncology Group Pilot Study E1492. *J Clin Oncol* 2000;18:972.

Jagannath S, et al. High-dose cyclophosphamide, carmustine, and etoposide and autologous bone marrow transplantation for relapsed Hodgkin's disease. *Ann Intern Med*. 1986;104:163.

Johnston LJ, Horning SJ. Autologous hematopoietic cell transplantation in Hodgkin's disease. *Biol Blood Marrow Transplant* 2000;6:289.

Jones SE, et al. Comparison of Adriamycin-containing chemotherapy (MOP-BAP) with MOPP-bleomycin in the management of advanced Hodgkin's disease: a Southwest Oncology Group Study. *Cancer* 1983;51:1339.

Josting A, Katay I, Reuffer U, et al. Favorable outcome of patients with relapsed or refractory Hodgkin's disease treated with high-dose chemotherapy and stem cell rescue at the time of maximal response to conventional salvage therapy (Dex-BEAM). *Ann Oncol* 1998;9:289.

Klasa RJ, Connors JM, Fairey R, et al. Treatment of early stage Hodgkin's disease: Improved outcome with brief chemotherapy and radiotherapy without staging laparotomy. *Ann Oncol* 1996;7(Suppl 3):21 (abst 67).

Klimo P, Connors JM. MOPP/ABV hybrid program: combination chemotherapy based on early introduction of seven effective drugs for advanced Hodgkin's disease. *J Clin Oncol*. 1985;3:1174.

Lazarus HM, Rowlings PA, Zhang MJ, et al. Autotransplants for Hodgkin's disease in patients never achieving remission: a report from the Autologous Blood and Marrow Treatment Registry. *J Clin Oncol* 1999;7:534.

Leslie NT, Mauch PM, Hellman S. Stage IA to IIB supradiaphragmatic Hodgkin's disease: long-term survival and relapse frequency. *Cancer* 1985;55:2072.

Levitt SH, et al. The role of radiation therapy in Hodgkin's disease: experience and controversy. The 54th Annual Janeway Lecture: 1989. *Cancer* 1992;70:693.

Lister TA, et al. The treatment of stage IIIA Hodgkin's disease. *J Clin Oncol* 1983;1:745.

Lohri A, et al. Outcome of treatment of first relapse of Hodgkin's disease after primary chemotherapy: identification of risk factors from the British Columbia experience 1970 to 1988. *Blood* 1991;77:2292.

Longo DL, et al. Conventional-dose salvage combination chemotherapy in patients relapsing with Hodgkin's disease after combination chemotherapy: the low probability for cure. *J Clin Oncol* 1992;10:210.

Longo DL, et al. Twenty years of MOPP therapy for Hodgkin's disease. *J Clin Oncol* 1986;4:1295.

Mauch P, et al. Stage III Hodgkin's disease: Improved survival with combined modality therapy as compared with radiation therapy alone. *J Clin Oncol* 1985;3:1166.

Mauch PM. Controversies in the management of early stage Hodgkin's disease. *Blood* 1994;83:318.

Mauch PM, Canellos GP, Shulman LN, et al. Mantle irradiation alone for selected patients with laparotomy-staged IA to IIA Hodgkin's disease: preliminary results of a prospective trial. *J Clin Oncol* 1995;3:947.

Milpied N, Fielding AK, Pearce RM, et al. Allogeneic bone marrow transplant is not better than autologous transplant for patients with relapsed Hodgkin's disease. European Group for Blood and Bone Marrow Transplantation. *J Clin Oncol* 1996; 14:1291.

Phillips GL, et al. Treatment of progressive Hodgkin's disease with intensive chemoradiotherapy and autologous bone marrow transplantation. *Blood* 1989;73:2086.

Reece DE, et al. Intensive therapy with cyclophosphamide, carmustine, etoposide ± cisplatin, and autologous bone marrow transplantation for Hodgkin's disease in first relapse after combination chemotherapy. *Blood* 1994;83:1193.

Santoro A, et al. Long-term results of combined chemotherapy—radiotherapy approach in Hodgkin's disease: superiority of ABVD plus radiotherapy versus MOPP plus radiotherapy. *J Clin Oncol* 1987;5:27.

Santoro A, Bonfante V, Viviani S, et al. Subtotal nodal (STNI) vs. involved field (IFRT) irradiation after 4 cycles of ABVD in early stage Hodgkin's disease (HD). *Proc Am Soc Clin Oncol* 1996;15:415(abst 67).

Selby P, et al. ChlVPP combination chemotherapy for Hodgkin's disease: long-term results. *Br J Cancer* 1990;62:279.

Somers R, et al. A randomized study in stage IIIB and IV Hodgkin's disease comparing eight courses of MOPP versus an alternation of MOPP with ABVD: a European Organization for Research and Treatment of Cancer Lymphoma Cooperative Group and Groupe Pierre- et- Marie-Curie Controlled Clinical Trial. *J Clin Oncol* 1994;2:279.

Specht L, Gray RG, Clarke MJ, et al. Influence of more extensive radiotherapy and adjuvant chemotherapy on long-term outcome of early-stage Hodgkin's disease: a meta-analysis of 23 randomized trials involving 3,888 patients. International Hodgkin's Disease Collaborative Group. *J Clin Oncol* 1998;6:830.

Stein RS, et al. Anatomical substages of stage III—A Hodgkin's disease: a collaborative study. *Ann Intern Med* 1980;92:159.

Sutcliffe SB, et al. MVPP chemotherapy regimen for advanced Hodgkin's disease. *BMJ* 1978;1:679.

Sweetenham JW, Taghipour G, Milligan D, et al. High-dose therapy and autologous stem cell rescue for patients with Hodgkin's disease in first relapse after chemotherapy: results from EBMT. Lymphoma Working Party of the European Group for Blood and Marrow Transplantation. *Bone Marrow Transplant* 1997;20:745.

Tannir N, et al. Long-term follow up with ABDIC salvage chemotherapy of MOPP-resistant Hodgkin's disease. *J Clin Oncol* 1983;1:432.

Tesch H, Sieber M, Ruffer JU, et al. 2 cycles of ABVD plus radiotherapy is more effective than radiotherapy alone in early stage Hodgkin's disease—interim analysis of the HD7 trial of the GHSG (abstr 2001). *Blood* 1999;485a.

Urba WJ, Longo DL. Hodgkin's disease. *N Engl J Med* 1992;326:678.

Vinciguerra V, et al. Alternating cycles of combination chemotherapy for patients with recurrent Hodgkin's disease following radiotherapy: a prospective randomized study by the Cancer and Leukemia Group B. *J Clin Oncol* 1986;4:838.

Viviani S, Bonadonna G, Santoro A, et al. Alternating versus hybrid MOPP and ABVD combinations in advanced Hodgkin's disease: ten-year results. *J Clin Oncol* 1996;14: 1421.

Wheeler C, Eickhoff C, Elias A, et al. High-dose cyclophosphamide, carmustine, and etoposide with autologous transplantation in Hodgkin's disease: a prognostic model for treatment outcomes. *Biol Blood Marrow Transplant* 1997;3:98.

Non-Hodgkin Lymphomas

Leo I. Gordon

This section reviews the pathogenesis and biology of non-Hodgkin lymphomas (NHLs). An attempt has been made to highlight important aspects of pathology, molecular biology, cytogenetics, and epidemiology, but the focus is on relevant clinical features to provide a framework with which to approach these complex diseases.

Pathogenesis
History
Most NHLs are neoplasms of B-lymphocyte origin with characteristic cell membrane surface markers. These surface markers can be identified by various techniques that utilize fresh, frozen, or paraffin-embedded tissue. These techniques have improved our accuracy in distinguishing lymphomas from epithelial malignancies. Most patient samples should be available for surface marker analysis. In difficult cases, frozen tissue should be available for molecular analysis using Southern blotting or polymerase chain reaction (PCR) techniques to identify the characteristic immunoglobulin heavy-chain gene rearrangement.

Cytogenetics and Oncogenes
Manolov and Manolova (1), who described the presence of an abnormally long chromosome 14 in the malignant cells of patients with Burkitt lymphoma, were the first to demonstrate chromosome abnormalities in NHL. Zech et al. (2) later found that this abnormal chromosome (chromosome 14) was part of a translocation of genetic material from chromosome 8, such that t(8;14) of (q24;q32). Two additional variations, t(8;22) and t(2;8), have since been discovered. All of these involve 8q24. Of major interest and importance were the observations by Erikson et al. (3) that the breakpoints on chromosome 14 directly involved the immunoglobulin heavy-chain locus on chromosome 14 and that the immunoglobulin light-chain (lambda and kappa) loci also are interrupted by the translocations in the Burkitt variants (8;22) and t(2;8). Of even greater interest was the observation that c-*myc*, the human homolog of the v-*myc* oncogene (which is present in avian myelomatosis virus, a retrovirus capable of inducing B-cell lymphoma in children) is mapped at 8q24 and is translocated to the region of the immunoglobulin heavy-chain on chromosome 14. In the indolent lymphomas, chromosomal abnormalities are found in 10% to 30% of cases and commonly involve chromosomes 8, 14, 9, 22, 18, and 11. The oncogenes *bcl*-1 and *bcl*-2 are found on chromosomes 11 and 18, respectively. Recently, *bcl*-6 was identified as an important prognostic feature in patients with diffuse large-cell lymphoma. Some of these oncogenes can become deregulated when translocated near the immunoglobulin gene at 14q32. Translocations are the most common abnormality in NHL, but deletions may also occur. For example, mutations of the tumor suppressor gene *p53* were described in NHL by Gaidano et al. (4). Table 8 lists some of the common chromosome abnormalities in NHL.

Table 8. Associations between nonrandom chromosomal aberrations
and histologic subgroups of non-Hodgkin lymphoma

Histologic subgroup	Chromosomal abnormality		
	Numerical	Structural	Break
A. SL	+3, +12	del11q	14q22–24, 14q
B. FSC	—	t(14;18), del(6q), i(6p) or t(6p)	1p22, 6p, 14q, 18q
C. FM	+8, +3/3q[a]	t(14;18), del(2q)	2p, 10q23–25, 18q
D. FL	+7	t(14;18)	7p, 13q, 14q, 17q21–25, 18q
E. Mantle cell	—	t(11;14), del(8p), del(20q)	2p13, 12q23
F. DM	+3, +5, +7, +14	—	9p, 11p, 19p
G. DL	+X, +4, +7, −8, +9, −13, +12, +21	del(6q)	1p22, 1q, 2q, 3q21, 4q, 6q, 7q, 9q, 13q, 14q, 18q
H. IBL	+X, +3, +5, +7	del(3p), del(5q), del(q)	5p, 5q, 13q, 16q, 19p
I. LBL	—	—	14q11–13, 9q32–34
J. SNC	—	—	8q, 11q23, 14q

SL, small lymphocytic; FSC, follicular small cleaved; FM, follicular mixed; FL, follicular large;
DM, diffuse mixed; DL, diffuse large; IBL, immunoblastic; LBL, lymphoblastic; SNC, small non-cleaved.
[a] Trisomy 3 or structural changes of 3q.
Adapted from Mrozek K, Bloomfield CD. Cytogenetics of indolent lymphomas. *Semin Oncol* 1993;
20:47, with permission.

Viruses
Viruses, including retroviruses such as human t-cell leukemia virus type 1 (HTLV-1),
linked with a rare type of T-cell lymphoma–leukemia syndrome prevalent in certain
regions of Japan, the Caribbean, and the southeastern United States, have been associated with NHL. Liebowitz (5) reviewed the association of the Epstein–Barr virus
(EBV) and lymphoma, and it is clear that immunomodulation may result in tumor
shrinkage. We now accept this form of immunomodulation as the first intervention in
most patients with posttransplant lymphoproliferative disorders (PTLDs). Hepatitis
C virus also was more prevalent in patients with lymphoma, but no cause and effect
relation can be established yet (6).

Epidemiology
Approximately 56,000 new cases of NHL were diagnosed in the United States in 1999,
and more than 19,000 deaths are attributed to NHL (7). The incidence of this disorder
is increasing at an annual rate of 4% for men and 3% for women, which makes NHL
the most rapidly increasing cancer, with the exceptions of lung cancer in women and
malignant melanoma. The reasons for this increase are unclear, but possible expla-
nations include nutritional factors and exposure to viruses and radiation. The increased
incidence of NHL among farmers led to theories that pesticides may play a role, but
other factors, such as exposure to animal viruses, solvents, fuels, and dust, may be involved. For example, there is an increased incidence of both follicular and diffuse NHL
in association with benzene exposure, a highly volatile organic solvent frequently used
in industry.
    The increased incidence of NHL in patients infected with the human immunodefi-
ciency virus (HIV) is well documented. In a case–control study, Levine et al. (8) found

that of 294 lymphoma cases and 181 control cases, high-grade lymphoma was diagnosed in 82% of HIV-positive cases and in 40% of the HIV-negative cases.

Pathology

The numerous classification schemes for NHLs indicate some of confusion about the understanding of these diseases. In the past, the most widely used classification scheme was the Rappaport classification, but the Working Formulation and, more recently, the Revised European American Lymphoma Classification (REAL) (9) and the Kiel classification are now supplanting the Rappaport classification in large clinical trials and in everyday use. All systems attempt to correlate clinical behavior with histopathology; they are summarized in Table 9. Although this can be done by classifying the malignant lymphomas into low-grade and high-grade groups based on morphology alone, it seems likely that other biologic features, such as oncogene expression and characteristics such as ploidy or cell-cycle kinetics, may be better predictors of clinical behavior. Newer technologies, such as gene array analysis, will likely lead to major changes in NHL classification. Table 10 divides NHL into indolent and aggressive disease based on histologic features.

Clinical Features

Most patients with NHL present with peripheral adenopathy. This is especially true in the indolent lymphomas, and most patients with indolent lymphomas also have bone marrow involvement. Patients with more aggressive B-cell lymphomas (diffuse large cell and small noncleaved) present with large abdominal or mediastinal masses. Patients with lymphoblastic lymphoma (T-cell lymphoma) often present with a mediastinal mass and central nervous system (CNS) or bone marrow involvement. Waldeyer's ring is involved in 15% to 30% of patients with NHL, and the incidence of gastrointestinal tract involvement is higher in this group of patients.

The bone marrow is affected in about 50% of patients; it is not unusual to see small cells involving the marrow in a paratrabecular arrangement with larger cells in the lymph nodes. Some investigators believe this discordant histologic presentation has a different natural history than either purely small-cell or large-cell lymphoma. Marrow involvement with large cells is thought to predict CNS involvement, and some clinicians routinely use CNS prophylactic therapy in this setting. In the United States, Burkitt's lymphoma (small noncleaved cell) often presents with large abdominal or pelvic masses, whereas in Africa, it frequently presents with massive head and neck tumors that involve the jaw and facial bones. NHL tends to spread in centrifugal fashion, skipping anatomic compartments, unlike Hodgkin disease (HD), which more often spreads centripetally from one lymph node region to the next in a more predictable anatomic progression.

Laboratory Features

Patients with low-grade (small-cell or nodular small-cell types) lymphoma may have peripheral blood involvement that may be evident on the peripheral blood smear as immature lymphocytes with cleft nuclei (buttock cells). If sensitive immunologic (flow cytometry) or molecular (gene rearrangement) techniques are used, peripheral blood or bone marrow involvement is more common; however, the clinical significance of blood or marrow involvement documented by molecular or immunologic techniques has not yet been determined.

The most important laboratory parameter, especially in aggressive NHL, is the lactate dehydrogenase (LDH) level. Numerous studies have found LDH to be an important predictor of outcome in NHL. β_2-microglobulin levels also may be an important predictor of outcome, although different patterns of β_2-microglobulin levels have been described by Rodriguez et al. (10). The serum uric acid level may be elevated when the tumor burden is high.

Liver function abnormalities that suggest liver involvement may be present, but an elevated bilirubin may also be caused by the presence of extrahepatic disease with biliary tract obstruction. This presentation may mimic pancreatic cancer, which is why patients with pancreatic masses with biliary tract obstruction must never be assumed to have "incurable" malignancies based on radiographic criteria alone, without tissue confirmation. Occasionally, these "incurable" tumors, in fact, may be curable large-cell lymphomas. Elevations in serum creatinine may reflect either direct renal involve-

Table 9. Comparison of Kiel classification, Revised European–American Lymphoma (REAL) classification, International Working Formulation, and Rappaport classification

Kiel classification	REAL classification	International Working Formulation	Rappaport classification
B-lymphoblastic	Precursor B-lymphoblastic lymphoma/leukemia	Lymphoblastic (high grade)	
B-lymphocytic, CLL B-lymphocytic prolymphocytic leukemia	B-cell chronic lymphocytic leukemia/prolymphocytic leukemia/small lymphocytic lymphoma	Small lymphocytic, consistent with CLL Small lymphocytic, plasmacytoid	Diffuse well differentiated
Lymphoplasmacytoid immunocytoma	Lymphoplasmacytoid lymphoma		
Lymphoplasmacytic immunocytoma	Mantle-cell lymphoma	Small lymphocytic, plasmacytoid Diffuse, mixed small and large cell Small lymphocytic	Diffuse mixed lymphocytic histiocytic
Centrocytic Centroblastic, centrocytoid subtype		Diffuse, small cleaved cell Follicular, small cleaved cell Diffuse, mixed small and large cell Diffuse, large cleaved cell	
Centroblastic-centrocytic, follicular	Follicular center lymphoma, follicular Grade I Grade II Grade III	Follicular, predominantly small cleaved-cell Follicular, mixed small and large cell Follicular, predominantly large cell	Nodular poorly differentiated lymphocytic Nodular mixed lymphocytic histiocytic Nodular histiocytic
Centroblastic-centrocytic, diffuse	Follicular center lymphoma, diffuse, small cell (provisional)	Diffuse, small cleaved cell Diffuse, mixed small and large cell	Diffuse poorly differentiated lymphocytic

continued

Table 9. (*continued*).

Kiel classification	REAL classification	International Working Formulation	Rappaport classification
—	Extranodal marginal zone B-cell lymphoma (low-grade B-cell lymphoma of MALT type)	Small lymphocytic Diffuse, small cleaved cell Diffuse, mixed small and large cell	Diffuse mixed lymphocytic histiocytic
Monocytoid, including marginal zone immunocytoma	Nodal marginal zone B-cell lymphoma (provisional)	Small lymphocytic Diffuse, small cleaved cell Diffuse, mixed small and large cell unclassifiable	
—	Splenic marginal zone B-cell lymphoma [provisional]	Small lymphocytic diffuse small cleaved cell	
Hairy-cell leukemia	Hairy-cell leukemia		
Plasmacytic	Plasmacytoma/myeloma	Extramedullary plasmacytoma	
Centroblastic (monomorphic, polymorphic, and multi-lobated subtypes)	Diffuse large B-cell lymphoma	Diffuse, large cell; large cell immunoblastic	Diffuse histiocytic, diffuse lymphoblastic
B-immunoblastic			
B-large cell anaplastic (Ki-1)		Diffuse, mixed small and large cell	
—	Primary mediastinal large B-cell lymphoma	Diffuse, large cell; large cell immunoblastic	Diffuse histiocytic, diffuse lymphoblastic
Burkitt's lymphoma	Burkitt lymphoma	Small noncleaved cell, Burkitt	Diffuse undifferentiated
—	High-grade B-cell lymphoma	Small noncleaved cell, non-Burkitt	
Some cases of centroblastic and immunoblastic	Burkitt-like [provisional]	Diffuse, large cell, large cell immunoblastic	

CLL, chronic lymphocytic leukemia.

Table 10. A clinical classification of non-Hodgkin lymphomas for therapeutic purposes

Indolent
    Small lymphocytic
    Follicular, predominantly small cleaved cell
    Follicular, mixed small cleaved and large cell
    Diffuse, small cleaved cell

Aggressive
    Follicular, predominantly large cell
    Diffuse, mixed small and large cell
    Diffuse, large cell
    Diffuse, large cell immunoblastic
        Small, noncleaved cell

Lymphoblastic

Burkitt lymphoma

Adapted from Rosenberg SA. Current concepts in cancer: non-Hodgkin's lymphoma. *N Eng J Med* 1979;301:924–928, and Jaffe ES. Relationship of classification to biologic behavior of non-Hodgkin's lymphomas. *Semin Oncol* 1986;13:3–9, with permission.

ment by lymphoma or ureteral obstruction. This should be easy to differentiate on computed tomography (CT) scan.

Diagnosis

The diagnosis of NHL requires adequate tissue and an experienced hematopathologist. Most often, it is necessary to perform biopsies of peripheral lymph nodes rather than rely on needle aspirates because the architecture of the tissue is important to the classification of NHL. Some patients, however, present with large abdominal or mediastinal masses without peripheral adenopathy. In these instances, attempts could be made to obtain tissue by CT or ultrasound-guided Tru-Cut needle biopsies. If only aspirates can be obtained, it is possible to diagnose NHL by using newer immunologic and molecular techniques, but every attempt should be made to obtain adequate tissue for a histologic diagnosis.

Occasionally, the histology of a lymph node biopsy will reveal only an undifferentiated malignancy, and differentiation between an epithelial tumor and a lymphoid tumor is impossible by histologic criteria alone. In such instances, immunologic analysis by flow cytometry or immunohistochemistry and molecular analysis for immunoglobulin gene rearrangement can be very useful and clinically important. It is critical that the clinician review all pathology material with the hematopathologist because the clinical presentation may influence the pathologic diagnosis in difficult cases.

Staging

At present, the Ann Arbor staging system is used for clinical and pathologic staging. Unfortunately, this has not proved as useful in NHL as it has been in HD because stage alone is not as predictive of outcome.

Problems may result because NHL does not spread by orderly, anatomic pathways but rather in more unpredictable fashion. In addition, other prognostic factors such as tumor bulk (measured as serum LDH level or size of dominant mass), performance status, number of extranodal sites, and age are important predictors of outcome. The Ann Arbor staging system is listed in Table 11.

Shipp et al. (11) published a retrospective experience involving more than 3,000 patients with diffuse aggressive lymphomas. The investigators identified five risk factors that predicted outcome in a hazards model. The resulting International Index (Table 12) now can be used as a staging system in patients with diffuse aggressive lymphoma.

Some of the staging studies that are useful in NHL are listed in Table 13. Although the diagnostic tests listed are similar to those used in HD, some differences are apparent. For example, lymphangiograms have limited usefulness in NHL because most

Table 11. Ann Arbor staging classification for non-Hodgkin lymphoma

Stage I—Involvement of a single lymph node region or a single extralymphatic organ or site

Stage II—Involvement of 2 or more lymph node regions on the same side of the diaphragm

Stage III—Involvement of lymph node regions on both sides of the diaphragm

Stage IV—Diffuse or disseminated involvement of one or more extralymphatic organs

nodal disease is bulky enough to be seen easily on CT scans. Evaluation of response to treatment was reviewed by Cheson et al. (12), and response criteria were established.

Treatment

The treatment of NHL is quite variable, depending on the histology (indolent versus aggressive), the age of the patient, and the philosophy of the physician and the patient.

Indolent NHL

This disease often occurs in elderly, asymptomatic patients. The median survival is 4 to 6 years, but some patients may live for more than 20 years with slowly growing or waxing and waning disease. Although the introduction of aggressive chemotherapy and radiation regimens (short of bone marrow transplant) resulted in more rapid remissions and perhaps a higher incidence of remission, it has not had significant impact on overall survival. For this reason, some investigators have advocated a "watch and wait" approach, often deferring treatment until symptoms dictate.

When treatment is given, single alkylating agents such as chlorambucil or cyclophosphamide are often used. Data from Smalley (13) suggested that the addition of interferon may have advantages, but this treatment has not yet become standard, and some investigators have suggested that the "aggressive" chemotherapy regimens were not aggressive enough and that new studies of novel chemotherapy regimens are warranted.

Newer studies using purine analogues such as fludarabine (14) and 2-chlorodeoxy-adenosine (2-CDA) (15) are under way in patients with indolent NHL, and these results may change the way these patients are treated [reviewed by Cheson and colleagues (12, 16)]. Some clinicians advocate very aggressive therapy, including high-dose chemoradiation followed by autologous bone marrow or peripheral stem cell transplantation; studies to test these ideas have been reported.

In elderly or frail patients, "no treatment" or single-agent alkylators seems to be an excellent approach. In young, vigorous patients with a disease that will likely result in death within 4 to 6 years, a "no treatment" approach often is not acceptable.

Monoclonal antibodies have been developed for treatment of NHL. Rituxan, an immunoglobulin G (IgG)-"chimeric" antibody directed against the CD20 antigen present in most B-cell lymphomas, has been approved by the U.S. Food and Drug

Table 12. International Index (prognostic factors in diffuse aggressive lymphoma)[a]

Age ($\leq$60 or >60 yr)
Stage (I/II or III/IV)
Number of extranodal sites (0, 1, or >1)
Performance status (0, 1 or 2, 3, 4)
LDH ($\leq$nl or >nl)

LDH, lactate dehydrogenase; nl, normal.
[a] For each factor, the left-hand side of parentheses carries a better prognosis.
Adapted from Shipp M. A predictive model for aggressive lymphoma: the international NHL prognostic factors project. *N Engl J Med* 1993;329:987, with permission.

Table 13. Staging procedures in non-Hodgkin lymphoma (NHL)

Procedures to be used in all patients
History
Physical examination
Imaging studies
CT scan of chest, abdomen, pelvis
Chest radiograph
Bilateral bone marrow biopsies
Procedures to be used in selected patients
Gallium scan or PET scan[a]
GI tract endoscopy[b]
MRI[c]
Lymphangiogram[d]

CT, computed tomography; GI, gastrointestinal; MRI, magnetic resonance imaging; PET, positron emission tomography
[a] May be an early marker of recurrence in aggressive NHL and may help determine response in patients with "bulky" disease.
[b] Use when Waldeyer's ring involvement is present.
[c] May detect bone marrow involvement.
[d] May be useful in some institutions.

Administration (FDA), and some clinical trials have suggested that it can be used in combination with chemotherapy (17). The exact place for monoclonal antibody therapy in NHL is still unclear but is the subject of ongoing investigation. Although most patients with indolent NHL have advanced disease, there are some who, after careful clinical staging, have limited stage I disease. For these patients, local radiation may result in 10-year disease-free survival of 50% to 60%.

Anti-CD20 antibodies linked to radionuclide, such as I^{131} and Y^{90}, have been used with promising early results in patients with low-grade lymphomas. Some commonly used chemotherapy regimens for indolent lymphomas are listed in Table 14.

Aggressive NHL
Most aggressive lymphomas fall into the Working Formulation designation F through H, and the following discussion concerns this group of patients. Although these patients have more aggressive disease and are likely to die quickly if untreated, aggressive chemotherapy may result in complete remissions in 50% to 85% of patients, with half of these free of disease and likely cured (25%–45%).

Several years ago, investigators were interested in the use of very intensive (second- and third-generation) regimens and suggested that the cure rates were higher for patients treated in this fashion. Phase 3 randomized clinical trials demonstrated, however, that there were no significant differences in survival when a "first-generation" regimen (CHOP: cyclophosphamide, hydroxydaunorubicin, Oncovin, and prednisone) was compared with a "second-generation" regimen (m-BACOD: moderate-dose methotrexate, bleomycin, Adriamycin, cyclophosphamide, Oncovin, and dexamethasone) (18–20). Figure 2 shows the lack of survival differences between the two regimens. In another study comparing first- through third-generation chemotherapy, no differences were found between four chemotherapy regimens (21). The results are shown in Figure 3. These studies suggest that the standard chemotherapy regimen for diffuse aggressive lymphomas (Working Formulation F–H) is CHOP. Newer, more aggressive treatments probably appeared more effective because of patient selection in small, non-randomized studies.

It appears that inherent prognostic factors (such as those outlined in the International Index criteria) are more predictive of outcome than the choice of chemotherapy. Other prognostic factors may also be important; β_2-microglobulin levels, serum LDH levels, proliferation markers such as Ki-67, and molecular markers such as *bcl*-6 may help

Table 14. Selected chemotherapy regimens for treatment of indolent non-Hodgkin lymphoma

Regimen	Drugs	Dosage mg/day	Dosage mg/m²	Route	Treatment schedule (days)	Cycle length (days)	Duration	References
Single oral alkylating agent	Cyclophosphamide or chlorambucil	100[a] 4–6[a]		p.o. p.o.	Daily Daily	— —	[b] [b]	Rosenberg (1985) Ezdinli et al. (1985)
CP	Cyclophosphamide Prednisone		600 100	i.v. p.o.	1 and 8 1–5	28	[b]	Ezdinli et al. (1985)
CVP	Cyclophosphamide Vincristine Prednisone		400 1.4[c] 100	p.o. i.v. p.o.	1–5 1 1–5	21	[b]	Gallagher et al. (1985)
C-MOPP	Cyclophosphamide Vincristine Procarbazine Prednisone		650 1.4 100 40	i.v. i.v. p.o. p.o.	1 and 8 1 and 8 1–14 1–14	28	[b]	Fisher et al. (1977)
BCVP	Carmustine Cyclophosphamide Vincristine Prednisone		60 1,000 1.2[c] 100	i.v. i.v. i.v. p.o.	1 1 1 1.15	21	[b]	Ezdinli et al. (1985)
Rituxan	Rituxan		375	i.v.	Weekly × 4	28		

i.v., intravenously; p.o., orally.
[a] Initial total dose (mg/day); reduce for maintenance.
[b] Treatment continued until complete remission or stable partial remission attained.
[c] Maximum dose 2.0 mg.

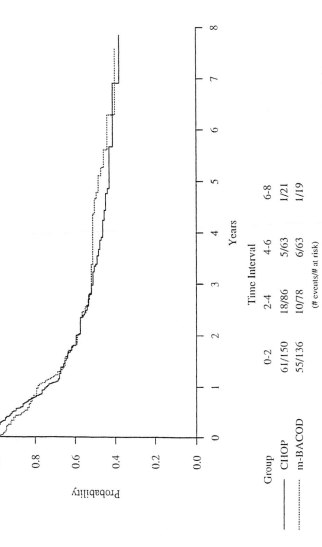

Group	0-2	2-4	4-6	6-8
CHOP	61/150	18/86	5/63	1/21
m-BACOD	55/136	10/78	6/63	1/19

Time Interval

(# events/# at risk)

FIG. 2. Kaplan–Meier plot of 286 patients randomized between CHOP (*solid line*) and m-BACOD (*dotted line*) chemotherapy. The ratio of the number of events to the number of patients at risk is shown for each yearly interval. Median follow-up was 3–5 years. CHOP, cyclophosphamide, doxorubicin, vincristine, and prednisone; m-BACOD, methotrexate bleomycin, doxorubicin, cyclophosphamide, vincristine, and dexamethasone.

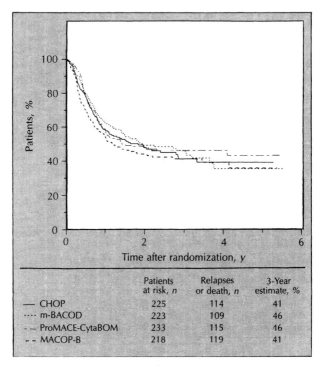

	Patients at risk, n	Relapses or death, n	3-Year estimate, %
— CHOP	225	114	41
···· m-BACOD	223	109	46
– – ProMACE-CytaBOM	233	115	46
– – MACOP-B	218	119	41

FIG. 3. Time to treatment failure according to treatment group ($p = 0.35$). CHOP, cyclophosphamide, doxorubicin, vincristine, and prednisone; m-BACOD, methotrexate, bleomycin, doxorubicin, cyclophosphamide, vincristine, and dexamethasone; ProMACE-CytaBOM, prednisone, methotrexate, doxorubicin, cyclophosphamide, etoposide, cytarabine, bleomycin, vincristine, and methotrexate; MACOP-B, methotrexate, doxorubicin, cyclophosphamide, vincristine, prednisone, and bleomycin. (From Fisher RI, et al. Comparison of a standard regimen (CHOP) with three intensive chemotherapy regimens for advanced non-Hodgkin lymphoma. *N Engl J Med* 1993;328:1002, with permission).

predict outcome and delineate groups of patients appropriate for more aggressive and less aggressive therapy.

For patients with Working Formulation designation J (Table 8) (diffuse, undifferentiated non-Burkitt or Burkitt lymphoma, i.e., small, noncleaved cell), aggressive chemotherapy, including high-dose alkylating agents and CNS prophylaxis is warranted. Patients with lymphoblastic lymphoma (Working Formulation designation I) are frequently treated as though they have acute lymphoblastic leukemia because they often have bone marrow, peripheral blood, and CNS involvement.

The commonly used chemotherapy regimens for aggressive NHL are summarized in Table 15. The role for radiation therapy in aggressive NHL is controversial, and as yet no data show that the eventual outcome (measured as survival) is affected by the addition of radiation. Some studies indicate that recurrences tend to be in sites of previous involvement so that radiation to sites of bulky disease should be considered.

For patients with Ann Arbor stage I or II diffuse aggressive lymphoma, limited chemotherapy (e.g., three cycles of CHOP), followed by involved-field radiation, has resulted in improved disease-free survival compared with eight cycles of CHOP without radiation (22). We will await longer follow-up to see if these data hold true.

(*text continues on page 332*)

Table 15. Selected chemotherapy regimens for treatment of aggressive non-Hodgkin lymphoma

Regimen	Drugs	Dosage (mg/m²)	Route	Treatment schedule (days)	Cycle length (days)	Duration	Reference
1st Generation							
CHOP	Cyclophosphamide	750	i.v	1	21	6 mo	Gordon (1992) (18)
	Doxorubicin	50	i.v	1			
	Vincristine	1.4[a]	i.v	1			
	Prednisone	100[d,g]	p.o.	1–5			
BACOP	Cyclophosphamide	650	i.v.	1 and 8	28	6 mo or 2 cycles following remission	Fisher (1997) (20)
	Doxorubicin	25	i.v.	1 and 8			
	Vincristine	1.4	i.v.	1 and 8			
	Bleomycin	5	i.v.	15 and 22			
	Prednisone	60	p.o.	15–29			
COMLA	Cyclophosphamide	1,500	i.v.	1	85	8 mo	Gaynor (1985)
	Vincristine	1.4[a]	i.v.	1, 8, and 15			
	Methotrexate	120	i.v.	22, 29, 36, 43, 50, 57, 64, and 71			
	Leucovorin	25	p.o.	q64 X 4, 24 h after each dose of methotrexate			
	Cytosine arabinoside	300	i.v.	22, 29, 36, 43, 50, 57, 64, and 71			
CPOB	Cyclophosphamide	1,000	i.v.	1	21	6 mo	Johnson et al. (1983)
	Prednisone	100	p.o.	1–5			
	Vincristine	1.2[a]	i.v.	15			
	Bleomycin	10	i.v.	15			
2nd Generation							
m-BACOD	Cyclophosphamide	600	i.v.	1	21	7 mo	Gordon (1992) (18)
	Doxorubicin	45	i.v.	1			

continued

Table 15. (continued).

Regimen	Drugs	Dosage (mg/m²)	Route	Treatment schedule (days)	Cycle length (days)	Duration	Reference
	Vincristine	1.0	i.v.	1			
	Bleomycin	4.0	i.v	1			
	Dexamethasone	6.0	p.o.	1–5			
	Methotrexate	200	i.v.	8 and 15			
	Leucovorin	10	p.o.	q6h × 8, 24 h after methotrexate			
ProMACE-MOPP							
ProMACE	Cyclophosphamide	650	i.v.	1 and 8	28	6–9 months[b]	Longo et al. (1991)
	Doxorubicin	25	i.v.	1 and 8			
	Etoposide	120	i.v.	1 and 8			
	Prednisone	60	p.o.	1–14			
	Methotrexate	1,500	i.v.	14			
	Leucovorin	50	i.v.	q6h × 5[c], 24 h after methotrexate			
MOPP (see Table 4)							
3rd Generation							
MACOP-B	Cyclophosphamide	350	i.v.	1, 22, 36, 50, 64, and 78	Treatment weekly	12 wk	Fisher (1993) (21)
	Doxorubicin	50	i.v.	1, 22, 36, 50, 64, and 78			
	Vincristine	1.4[a]	i.v.	15, 29, 43, 57, 71, and 85			
	Bleomycin	10	i.v.	29, 57, and 85			
	Methotrexate	400	i.v.	15, 43, and 71			
	Leucovorin	15[c]	p.o.	q6h × 6, 24 h after methotrexate			
	Prednisone	75[d]	p.o.	Daily for 10 wk, taper weeks 11 and 12			

Regimen	Drug	Dose	Route	Day	Reference
ProMACE-CytaBOM	Cotrimoxazole	2 tablets	p.o.	b.i.d.	Fisher (1993) (21)
	Cyclophosphamide	650	i.v.	1	
	Doxorubicin	25	i.v.	1	
	Etoposide	120	i.v.	1	
	Prednisone	60	p.o.	1–15	
	Cytarabine	300	i.v.	8	
	Bleomycin	5	i.v.	8	
	Vincristine	1.4	i.v.	8	
	Methotrexate	120	i.v.	8	
	Leucovorin	25[f]	p.o.	q6h × 4, 24 h after methotrexate	
200% ProMACE-CytaBOM	Doxorubicin	50	i.v.	1	Gordon (1999) (19)
	Etoposide	240[d]	i.v.	1	
	Prednisone	60[d]	p.o.	1–15	
	Cytarabine	600	i.v.	8	
	Bleomycin	5	i.v.	8	
	Vincristine	1.4 (cap 2 mg)	i.v.	8	
	Methotrexate	120	i.v.	8	
	Leucovorin	25[e]		q6h × 4, 24 h after methotrexate	
	G-CSF	5 µg/kg		9–19	
	Bactrim DS[f]	M, W, F			
	Ketoconazole[g]				
	Fluconazole				

b.i.d., twice daily; G-CSF, granulocyte colony-stimulating factor; i.m, intramuscularly; i.v., intravenously; PCP, *Pneumocystis carinii* pneumonia; p.o., orally; q6h, every 6 hours.

[a] Maximum dose 2.0 mg.
[b] Treatment induction with ProMACE, consolidation with MOPP, and late intensification with ProMACE [see Longo et al. (1991)].
[c] Leucovorin continued until methotrexate level <5 and 10^{-7}M.
[d] mg/m²/day
[e] mg/dose
[f] Consider PCP prophylaxis in regions which are immunosuppressive
[g] Some trials use 100 mg/day rather than 100 mg/m²/day.

Special Clinical Syndromes

1. **CNS lymphoma (23):** Primary CNS lymphoma continues to carry a poor prognosis; only a few patients are alive 2 to 4 years after diagnosis. This is true both in the acquired immunodeficiency syndrome (AIDS)-related lymphomas and in non-AIDS lymphomas. More recently, combined-modality radiation and systemic and intrathecal chemotherapy regimens have reportedly improved response rates. The CNS may become involved in patients who present with aggressive NHL, usually at the time of relapse elsewhere. Risk factors for CNS disease (which may be parenchymal or involve the brain or cerebrospinal fluid) include histology (Burkitt, undifferentiated, non-Burkitt, and lymphoblastic); bone marrow involvement with large cells; testicular presentation; bulky sinus or head and neck lymphoma; and epidural lymphoma.

2. **Gastric lymphoma (24):** Patients who have primary gastric lymphoma may present with symptoms similar to a peptic ulcer or gastritis, with pain and anorexia, or with a gastrointestinal bleed. The diagnosis is frequently made at the time of exploratory surgery, and a total or partial gastrectomy is performed. Most often, the NHL pathology is of the aggressive type, with large-cell or mixed-cell lymphoma being most common. The diagnosis can be difficult to make by endoscopy because the malignant cells are often submucosal or on the stomach wall (like linitis plastica). Nonhealing gastric "ulcers" or "gastritis" may prove on follow-up to be lymphoma. Although the literature advocating gastrectomy as the primary therapy for gastric lymphoma is abundant, more recent studies investigated the possibility of using chemotherapy and radiation in place of surgery, thus saving patients the potential morbidity of a gastric resection. This idea remains controversial. Some patients are found to have small cells involving gastric mucosa and surrounding glands and have been referred to as *mucosa-associated lymphomas* or MALT lymphomas. These patients often have a protracted indolent course. It is interesting that several reports of association of these MALT lymphomas with *Helicobacter pylori* have appeared, and treatment with antibiotics and Pepto-Bismol results in complete regression (25). The molecular pathology of these tumors was reviewed (26,27) and raises consideration of the role of *H. pylori* in the etiology of this lymphoma.

3. **Testicular lymphoma (29,30):** This diagnosis should be suspected in any man with a testicular mass. A testicular mass in a young man is usually testicular cancer, but in men over 45 or 50 years of age, the diagnosis of lymphoma is more common. Most often, these patients have aggressive histologic features, and frequently, they also have bone marrow or CNS disease. Treatment is dictated by the histologic appearance of the mass, but aggressive histology calls for aggressive chemotherapy (CHOP), CNS prophylaxis, and prophylactic irradiation to the normal testicle.

4. **Ki anaplastic large cell lymphoma (29):** Primary Ki-1 (CD-30) anaplastic large-cell lymphoma is now recognized as a distinct clinicopathologic entity. The histopathology is distinctive and is characterized by large cells that most often express T-cell markers. The cells stains with CD-30 using immunoperoxidase techniques. A specific chromosomal translocation, t(2;5)(p23;q35), now has been described. This translocation encodes for a fusion protein, the anaplastic lymphoma kinase (ALK), which results from fusion of the *ALK* and *NPM* genes. From the pathologist's viewpoint, the differential diagnosis is most often HD. Unfortunately, the clinician can offer little help because the clinical presentation resembles both HD and NHL. In young children, where this entity was first described, the skin is often involved, and the course is thought to be indolent. In adults, however, the disease appears to be like other large-cell lymphomas and generally is treated like diffuse, large-cell lymphoma. Durable complete responses to Adriamycin-based chemotherapy regimens are seen if the lymphoma is localized to skin and nodal tissue. Patients with the t(2;5) tend to have better outcome, and recently, a subgroup t(2;5) lymphomas that encode for ALK variants other than ALK-NPM has been described (30). Adults who are ALK negative do poorly.

Dose Intensity

The important studies by Hyrniuk and colleagues (31,32) and Skipper (33) suggested that received dose intensity was important in cancer chemotherapy in general and in lymphoma treatment in particular. A given dose of cytotoxic chemotherapy is able to kill a certain fraction of tumor cells, and some drugs have a dose–response curve in some tumors. Thus, it is logical that higher dose intensity should result in more complete responses and more cures. Most of the retrospective data in lymphoma trials support this conclusion (34,35), and newer dose intensive regimens have been designed (19). In a recent Eastern Cooperative Oncology Group (ECOG) trial, however, a retrospective review of dose intensity data did not clearly show that delivered higher-dose chemotherapy had any relationship to outcome (18). Apparently factors such as toxicity of the drugs result in dosage reductions, which makes retrospective comparisons difficult. A prospective, randomized trial of dose intensity will need to be conducted to answer this question more completely.

Salvage Therapy

Although some progress has been made in treatment of the aggressive lymphomas, most patients have a relapse and require some regimen of second-line or salvage therapy. Most series report some responses in these patients, but there are few complete responses; of these responses, few are lasting (36,37). Combinations, including the platinum derivatives (cis-platinum or carboplatinum), Ara-C, VP-16, ifosfamide, and mitoxantrone have been used with modest success, but these regimens do not result in cures. Trials with radiolabeled monoclonal antibodies or ricin-linked antibodies are in progress; preliminary results suggest significant activity (38,39). Autologous bone marrow transplantation or peripheral stem cell transplantation has been used following high-dose chemotherapy or chemoradiotherapy. Some durable complete responses have been obtained using these methods, most often in patients with tumors that are still responsive to conventional therapy (40). Patients with resistant disease probably should not undergo transplantation with currently available regimens (see Chapter 19).

References

1. Manolov G, Manolova V. Marker band in one chromosome 14 from Burkitt lymphomas. *Nature* 1972;237:33.
2. Zech L, et al. Characteristic chromosomal abnormalities in biopsies and lymphoid cell lines from patients with Burkitt and non-Burkitt lymphomas. *Int J Cancer* 1976;7:47.
3. Erikson J, et al. Translocation of immunoglobulin VH genes in Burkitt lymphoma. *Proc Natl Acad Sci U S A* 1982;79:5611.
4. Gaidano G, et al. p53 mutations in human lymphoid malignancies: association with Burkitt lymphoma and chronic lymphocytic leukemia. *Proc Natl Acad Sci U S A* 1991;88:5413.
5. Liebowitz D. Epstein-Barr virus and a cellular signaling pathway in lymphomas from immunosuppressed patients. *N Engl J Med* 1998;338:1413.
6. Zuckerman E, Zuckerman T, Levine AN, et al. Hepatitis C virus infection in patients with B-cell non-Hodgkin's lymphoma. *Ann Intern Med* 1997;27:423.
7. McKean-Cowdin R, Feigelson HS, Ross PK, et al. Declining cancer rates in the 1990s. *J Clin Oncol* 2000;18:2258.
8. Levine AM, et al. Epidemiological and biological study of AIDS-related lymphoma in the county of Los Angeles: preliminary results. *Cancer Res* 1992;52(Suppl): 54842S.
9. Harris NL, Jaffee ES, Stein H, et al. A revised European-American classification of lymphoid neoplasms: a proposal from the International Lymphoma Study Group. *Blood* 1994;4:1361.
10. Rodriguez J, Pugh WC, Romaguera JE, et al. Primary mediastinal large cell lymphoma is characterized by an inverted pattern of large tumoral mass and low B-2 immunoglobulin levels in serum and frequently elevated levels of LDH. *Ann Oncol* 1999;5:847.
11. Shipp M, et al. A predictive model for aggressive lymphoma: the international NHL prognostic factors project. *N Engl J Med* 1993;329:987.
12. Cheson BD, Horning SJ, Coiffier B, et al. Report of an international workshop to standardize response criteria for non-Hodgkin's lymphomas. *J Clin Oncol* 1999; 17:1244.
13. Smalley RV, et al. Interferon combined with cytotoxic chemotherapy for patients with non-Hodgkin's lymphomas. *N Engl J Med* 1992;327:1336.

14. Luzzarino M, Orlandi E, Mantillo M, et al. Fludarabine, cyclophosphamide and dexamethasone (FluCyD) combination is effective in pre-treated low-grade non-Hodgkin's lymphoma. *Ann Oncol* 1999;10:59.

15. Kong LR, Huang CF, Hakimian D, et al. Long term follow-up and late complications of 2-chlorodeoxyadenosine in previously treated, advanced, indolent non-Hodgkin's lymphoma. *Cancer* 1998;82:957.

16. Cheson BD. New antimetabolites in the treatment of human malignancies. *Semin Oncol* 1992;19:695.

17. Czuczman MS, Grilo-Lopez AJ, White CA, et al. Treatment of patients with low grade B-cell lymphoma with the continuation of chimeric anti-CD20 monoclonal antibody and CHOP chemotherapy. *J Clin Oncol* 1999;17:268.

18. Gordon LI, et al. Comparison of a second generation combination chemotherapeutic regimen (CHOP) with a standard regimen (m-BACOD) for advanced diffuse non-Hodgkin's lymphoma. *N Engl J Med* 1992;327:1342.

19. Gordon LI, et al. A phase II trial of 200% ProMACE-CytaBOM in patients with previously untreated aggressive lymphomas: analysis of response, toxicity and dose intensity. *Blood* 1999;94:3307.

20. Fisher RI, et al. Prognostic factors for advanced diffuse histiocytic lymphoma following treatment with combination chemotherapy. *Am J Med* 1977;63:177.

21. Fisher RI, et al. Comparison of a standard regimen (CHOP) with three intensive chemotherapy regimens for advanced non-Hodgkin's lymphoma. *N Engl J Med* 1993;328:1002.

22. Miller TD, Dahlberg S, Cassady JR, et al. Chemotherapy alone compared with chemotherapy plus radiotherapy for localized intermediate and high-grade non-Hodgkin's lymphoma. *N Engl J Med* 1998;339:21.

23. DeAngelis L. Primary CNS lymphoma. *PPO update, principles and practice of oncology* vol 11. Philadelphia: JB Lippincott, 1992.

24. Frazie RL, Robert J. Gastric lymphoma treatment. Medical vs Surgical (A review). *Surg Clin North Am* 1992;72:423.

25. Witherspoon AC, et al. Regression of primary low-grade B-cell gastric lymphoma of mucosa associated lymphoid tissue after eradication of *Helicobacter pylori*. *Lancet* 1993;342:575.

26. Zucca E, Bertoni F, Roggero E, et al. Molecular analysis of the progression from *Helicobacter pylori*-associated chronic gastritis to mucosa-associated lymphoid tissue lymphoma of the stomach. *N Engl J Med*. 1998;338:804.

27. Zucca E, Bertoni F, Roggero E, Cavalli F. The gastric marginal zone B-cell lymphoma of MALT type. *Blood* 2000;96:410.

28. Nomura N, et al. Malignant lymphoma of the testis: histological and immunological studies of 28 cases. *J Urol* 1989;14116:1368.

29. Shulman LN, et al. Primary Ki-1 anaplastic large-cell lymphoma in adults: clinical characteristics and therapeutic outcome. *J Clin Oncol* 1993;11:937.

30. Falini B, Pulford K, Pucciarini A, et al. Lymphomas expressing ALK fusion protein(s) other than NPM-ALK. *Blood* 1999;94:3509.

31. Hryniuk W, Bush H. The importance of dose intensity chemotherapy of metastatic breast cancer. *J Clin Oncol* 1984;2:1281.

32. Hryniuk W, Goodyear M. The calculation of received dose intensity. *J Clin Oncol* 1990;8:1935.

33. Skipper HE. Dose intensity vs total dose of chemotherapy: an experimental basis. In: DeVita VT Jr, Hellman S, Rosenberg SA, eds. *Important advances in oncology 1990*. Philadelphia: JB Lippincott, 1990:43.

34. Kwak LW, et al. Prognostic significance of actual dose-intensity in diffuse large cell lymphoma: Results of a tree-structured survival analysis. *J Clin Oncol* 1990;8:963.

35. Meyer RM, Hryniuk W, Goodyear M. The role of dose-intensity in determining outcome in intermediate grade non-Hodgkin's lymphoma. *J Clin Oncol* 1991;9:339.

36. Cabanillas F, Velasquez WS, Hagemeister FB. Clinical, biologic and histologic features of late relapses in diffuse large cell lymphoma. *Blood* 1992;79:1024.

37. Haim N, et al. Salvage therapy for non-Hodgkin's lymphoma with a combination of dexamethasone, etoposide, ifosfamide and cisplatin. *Cancer Chemother Pharmacol* 1992;30:243.

38. Kaminski MS, et al. Imaging, dosimetry and radioimmunotherapy with iodine 131-labeled anti-CD37 antibody in B-cell lymphoma. *J Clin Oncol* 1992;10:1696.
39. Kaminski MS, Zasadny KR, Francis IR, et al. Iodine-131-anti-B1 radioimmunotherapy for B-cell lymphoma. *J Clin Oncol* 1996;14:1974.
40. Vose JM, et al. Long-term sequelae of autologous bone marrow or peripheral stem cell transplantation for lymphoid malignancies. *Cancer* 1992;69:784.

Suggested Readings

Cohen JI. Epstein-Barr virus infection. *N Engl J Med* 2000;343:481.
Ezdinli EZ, et al. Moderate versus aggressive chemotherapy of nodular lymphoma. *J Clin Oncol* 1985;3:769.
Freedman AS, Neuberg D, Mauch P, et al. Long-term follow-up of autologous bone marrow transplantation in patients with relapsed follicular lymphoma. *Blood* 1999; 94:3325.
Gallagher CJ, et al. Follicular lymphoma: prognostic factors for response and survival. *J Clin Oncol* 1986;4:1470.
Gaynor ER, et al. Treatment of diffuse histiocytic lymphoma with COMLA: a 10-year experience in a single institution. *J Clin Oncol* 1985;3:1596.
Grossbard ML, Nadler LM. Monoclonal antibody therapy for indolent lymphomas. *Semin Oncol* 1993;20(Suppl 5):118.
Johnson GS, et al. Sequential cyclophosphamide-prednisone and vincristine-bleomycin (CPOB): an effective, schedule-dependent treatment for advanced diffuse histiocytic lymphoma. *Cancer* 1983;52:1133.
Longo DL, et al. Superiority of ProMACE-CytaBOM over ProMACE MOPP in the treatment of advanced diffuse aggressive lymphoma: results of a prospective randomized trial. *J Clin Oncol* 1991;9:25.
Malignant lymphomas. In: Rappaport H. *Tumors of the hematopoietic system: atlas of tumor pathology.* Section 3, Fascicle 8. Washington, DC: Armed Forces Institute of Pathology, 1966:91.
National Cancer Institute. The non-Hodgkin's lymphoma classification project. National Cancer Institute–sponsored study and description of a working formulation for clinical usage. *Cancer* 1982;49:2112.
Rosenberg SA. The low grade non-Hodgkin's lymphomas: challenges and opportunities. *J Clin Oncol* 1985;3:299.
Witzig T, White CA, Wiseman G, et al. Phase I/II trial of IDEC-Y2B8 radioimmunotherapy for treatment of relapsed or refractory CD20 (+) B-cell non-Hodgkin's lymphoma. *J Clin Oncol* 1999;17:3793.

Cutaneous T-cell Lymphomas

Joseph J. Mazza

The definitive recognition of neoplasms of human T cells was not possible until advances in immunology enabled the characterization of subclasses of human lymphocytes. The precise immunologic categorization of T-cell neoplasms is an ongoing process that is far from complete, and its eventual therapeutic and prognostic implications are uncertain. It appears that many of the molecules on cell surfaces that are recognized as immunologic markers function as receptors or processors of chemical signals that the cell receives from outside. As the functions of individual surface-marker molecules are characterized, their identification on cell surfaces of individual neoplasms may open up new, potent, and highly specific biologic therapies. It should be a source of satisfaction to the clinician that the major varieties of T-cell neoplasms (Table 16) were identified principally on clinical grounds, with some help from conventional histopathology, long before modern immunologic techniques were available. Thus, the syndrome of male sex,

Table 16. European Organization for Research and Treatment of
Cancer (EORTC) classification for primary cutaneous lymphomas

Primary CTCL	Primary CBCL
Indolent	Indolent
MF	Follicle center cell lymphoma
MF + follicular mucinosis	
Pagetoid reticulosis	Immunocytoma (marginal zone B-cell lymphoma)
Large cell CTCL, CD30+	
Anaplastic	
Immunoblastic	
Pleomorphic	Intermediate
Lymphomatoid papulosis	Large B-cell lymphoma of the leg
Aggressive	
SS	
Large cell CTCL, CD30	
Immunoblastic	
Pleomorphic	
Provisional	Provisional
Granulomatous slack skin	Intravascular large B-cell lymphoma
CTCL, pleomorphic small/ medium-sized	Plasmacytoma
Subcutaneous panniculitis-like T-cell lymphoma	

CBCL, cutaneous B-cell lymphoma; CTCL, cutaneous T-cell lymphoma; MF, mycosis fungoides; SS, Sézary syndrome.
From Willemze R, et al. EORTC classification for primary cutaneous lymphomas: a proposal from the Cutaneous Lymphoma Study Group of the European Organization for Research and Treatment of Cancer. *Blood* 90:354, 1997; with permission.

mediastinal tumor in the location of the thymus, hyperleukocytosis, early central nervous system (CNS) involvement, and short survival was well recognized as an adverse variant of acute lymphocytic leukemia long before the concept of T and B lymphocytes was formulated. The cutaneous T-cell lymphomas (CTCLs) were characterized many years ago on clinical grounds, and it was appreciated that there were morphologic resemblances to other lymphomas but important differences in biologic behavior.

With the discovery of the human T-lymphotropic viruses (HTLVs), there has been a major upsurge of interest in T-cell neoplasias. The HTLV-1 virus appears likely to be at least a contributory, or perhaps the definitive, cause of adult T-cell lymphoma/leukemia (ATL), a subacute malignant disease that is endemic in parts of Japan and the Caribbean. The rare T-cell variant of hairy-cell leukemia (T-HCL) has an association with HTLV-2, whereas HTLV-3, now termed *the human immunodeficiency virus* (HIV), is infamous as the etiologic agent of the acquired immune deficiency syndrome (AIDS). A study of T-cell lymphomas other than mycosis fungoides (MF) showed a 49% incidence of disease confined to the skin, diverse cytologic and immunologic features, and a lack of correlation between clinical, morphologic, and immunologic features. Table 16 emphasizes the complexity of this group of entities that present as neoplastic disease involving the skin.

Primary cutaneous lymphomas can be divided into primary CTCLs and primary B-cell lymphomas. This classification is based on a combination of clinical, histologic, immunohistochemical, and genetic criteria. It does not incorporate the terms *low-grade* and *high-grade,* which refer primarily to cell size and have no clinical significance in primary cutaneous lymphomas. Distinction in this classification is based on the clinical behavior of the specific type of cutaneous lymphoma, that is, indolent, intermediate, or aggressive. Thus, the situation with respect to CTCLs has become much more complex, and careful analysis of the various cell types that make up these lymphomas using currently available molecular testing is imperative to make a more accurate diagnosis. It is hoped that this will allow for better, more effective treatment.

History and Nomenclature

Mycosis fungoides (MF) was first described in 1806 by the great French dermatologist Alibert, who named it much later in 1832. The name, an interlingual hybrid, is also somewhat redundant: *mycosis* is Greek for fungus and *fungoides,* is of Latin origin, signifies mushroom-like. It recognizes the mushroom-like tumors that sometimes are observed in the very advanced stages of the disease; they are rarely seen today. Three clinical variants of MF were recognized:

1. The **classic,** or **Alibert-Bazin form,** which evolves from a dermatitis or patch stage into a plaque stage and then a tumor stage
2. The rarer **d'emblee form,** in which the disease begins with tumor formation
3. The **erythrodermic form,** without plaques or tumors, which may precede, occur with, or follow the diagnosis of MF.

In 1946, Sézary described four patients who presented with generalized severe erythroderma (*l'homme rouge*) and skin lesions of lymphoma. Characteristic large cells with convoluted or even encephaloid nuclei were present in the skin and peripheral blood; the total leukocyte count was frequently elevated. Morphologic studies by light and electron microscopy and studies of cell-surface markers suggest that Sézary syndrome is closely related to MF and may be considered a variant. The late progression of both conditions tends to be similar.

More recently, several T-cell variants of chronic lymphocytic leukemia (T-CLL) have been described. The cells may bear surface markers characteristic of helper cells (CD4) or suppressor cells (CD8) or express both markers simultaneously. The condition may progress in a subacute or chronic fashion. Comparison of T-CLL, Sézary syndrome, and MF (Table 17) suggests a gradation from a disease that is predominantly leukemic (T-CLL) to one that predominantly affects the skin (MF), with Sézary syndrome having intermediate characteristics. The boundary lines are not sharply defined but may reflect quantitative differences in the homing patterns of various subtypes of T cells.

Incidence

The age-adjusted incidence of CTCL in the United States is 4.2 per million per year; thus, about 1,000 new cases are diagnosed each year. MF is the most frequently occurring of the CTCLs, but it is still an uncommon disease. Sézary syndrome constitutes approximately 5% of CTCL, with 40 new cases diagnosed annually (see section the entitled **Pathogenesis** for further discussion of Sézary syndrome). The peak incidence of diag-

Table 17. Comparison of T-cell chronic lymphocytic leukemia (T-CLL), Sézary syndrome (SS), and mycosis fungoides (MF)

Disease	T-CLL	SS	MF
Skin	±	+ +	+ + +
Blood	+ + +	+ +	±[a]
Marrow	+ + +	+ +	−[b]
Lymph nodes	+	±	−[b]
Spleen	+ +	+	−[b]
Light microscopy	±[c]	+	+
Electron microscopy	+	+	+
T-markers	+	+	+

[a] Many cases (+) when closely scrutinized.
[b] In early stages of disease.
[c] T-helper cells (convoluted) are recognizable; T-suppressor variant may not be recognized.

nosis of MF is between the ages of 30 and 70 years. Approximately 60% of patients with MF are men. No racial predilection has been demonstrated. Like many diseases whose diagnosis may be difficult, MF is likely to be more frequent in a factitious manner among populations who receive a high standard of medical care.

Etiology

The cause of MF is unknown. Epidemiologic studies suggest that exposure to chemicals and drugs, possibly on a background of chronic skin disorders, may predispose to the disease, but no agent has been clearly identified. Many patients with MF have a history of chronic dermatitis extending back 20 years or longer before the diagnosis of MF. The chronic immune stimulation of the dermatitis may promote the eventual onset of a T-cell neoplasm. Although human retroviruses are intimately involved in the onset of other T-cell disorders, they have not been shown to play a role in MF or Sézary syndrome.

Pathogenesis

The cell of origin of MF is undoubtedly a T cell, and marker studies show the phenotype of a helper cell (CD4+). Helper cell activity has been demonstrated *in vitro*.

Patients with MF show both enhanced delayed hypersensitivity reactions and elevated levels of immunoglobulins, suggesting increased helper cell activity *in vivo*. True neoplasia is shown by the demonstration of cellular monoclonality and also cytogenetic abnormalities. An apparently nonneoplastic counterpart of the MF cell occurs in normal individuals and is seen forming an infiltrate in some chronic benign inflammatory dermatoses, including lichen planus. It has been postulated but not proven that chronic antigenic stimulation of normal T cells occasionally may result in neoplastic transformation and the development of MF over time. The characteristic distribution of MF cells, showing epidermotropism and a tendency to avoid the bone marrow, is not different from that of normal T cells.

Diagnosis

The diagnosis of MF may be difficult or impossible in the early stages of the disease, particularly if only classic morphologic evaluation by histopathology is used. Many patients have a history of 5 to 10 years of nonspecific dermatitis. Numerous periodic skin biopsies may be necessary before the diagnosis is established. Many patients have had a series of dermatologic diagnoses attached to their disease before MF is proved. In many cases, one of these earlier diagnoses may have been correct, and MF then follows another chronic skin disease.

The **differential diagnosis of MF** includes the following:

1. Psoriasiform dermatitis
2. Tinea corporis
3. Neurodermatitis
4. Seborrheic dermatitis
5. Parapsoriasis
6. Other obscure and polysyllabic chronic dermatoses
7. Primary cancers of the skin, including small-cell cancer
8. Other lymphomas, including those of B-cell origin, which occasionally produce a picture resembling MF (Table 16)

Biopsy

Definitive diagnosis is by biopsy, with demonstration of characteristic MF cells infiltrating the dermis and epidermis. In the early stage of MF, the epidermal and dermal infiltrate may be nonspecific, and it may be impossible to diagnose the disease with confidence or to distinguish it from **lymphomatoid papulomatosis.** When MF cells are arranged in small groups with a surrounding clear space, the appearance is that of a Pautrier microabscess in the epidermis, which is virtually pathognomonic of MF.

Electron Microscopy

Sometimes electron microscopy helps make the diagnosis by demonstrating MF cells with highly convoluted nuclei (Fig. 4). Electron microscopy usually shows MF cells in nodes that are only dermatopathic by light microscopy.

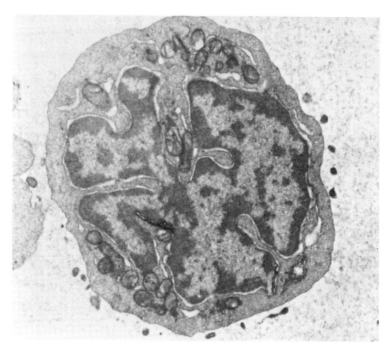

FIG. 4. Electron micrograph of a Sézary cell from the peripheral blood of a patient with T-cell lymphocytic leukemia and skin infiltrates. Note the deep convolutions that make the nucleus genuinely cerebriform and the peripheral concentration of electron-dense chromatin around the nuclear membrane. (Original magnification × 30,000).

Enlarged Lymph Nodes
Enlarged lymph nodes from patients with MF may show a nonspecific "dermatopathic lymphadenopathy" or frank involvement with MF. The belief that overt involvement by MF carries a worse prognosis than dermatopathic changes alone has been challenged.

Immunophenotyping
Using a panel of commercially available monoclonal antibodies, it is now possible to differentiate the monoclonal (*neoplastic*) T-cell infiltrate from a polyclonal (*inflammatory*) process. The neoplastic cells of MF usually have a helper phenotype (CD4+) and express pan T-cell markers (CD2, CD3, and CD5). The cells are frequently CD7– and CD62L–.

Molecular Genetic Techniques
Molecular genetic techniques, usually involving studies of the rearrangement of the T-cell receptor gene, may be used to prove monoclonality and hence the neoplastic nature of a cutaneous lymphoid infiltrate. Gene studies show consistent rearrangement of the T-cell receptor β (TCR-β)-chain gene.

Dermatopathology
The diagnosis of MF should be made or verified by an experienced dermatopathologist, especially since treatment frequently involves radiation and cytotoxic drugs. These modalities should be used only rarely in the management of nonneoplastic disorders. When doubt exists, these potentially harmful therapies should be held in reserve.

Clinical Forms and Progression
The usual course is one of inexorable, but sometimes very slow, progression from one stage of the disease to the next, followed by progression beyond the skin. Most patients

follow the classic Alibert–Bazin pattern of a three-stage disease, with one very important exception. Elderly patients with indolent MF may succumb to intercurrent unrelated disease without ever developing the more advanced, and serious, stages of cutaneous lymphoma. It follows that aggressive treatment for MF usually is inappropriate in such patients.

Initial Patch Stage or Early Phase
A clinically and histologically nonspecific dermatitis with erythematous patches and frequent scaling is evident. The patches are usually on the trunk but may occur anywhere on the body; they may be small and of little significance or extensive and a source of major symptoms. Pruritus varies from none to severe. This stage frequently lasts 2 to 5 years but may persist as long as 30 years (Tables 18 and 19).

Second or Plaque Stage
Infiltrating plaques of cutaneous lymphoma, frequently appearing annular, are present. Spontaneous waxing and waning of the plaques is not uncommon. Occasionally, the disease appears to oscillate between cutaneous and blood involvement. Periods of leukocytosis with many circulating MF cells and minor skin involvement alternate with phases of multiple large plaques and a paucity of MF cells in the blood.

Third or Tumor Stage
1. Multiple nodules that involve the skin and subcutaneous tissues are apparent.
2. Tumors are pink or red, usually soft, and frequently lobulated.
3. Pruritus is less in this stage, but the tumors are likely to ulcerate, become infected, and as a result become very tender.
4. Lymphadenopathy in the area of an ulcerated, infected tumor is difficult to evaluate, because it may represent involvement by lymphoma or simply lymphadenitis in response to infection.
5. Painful tumors may occur on the tongue or other parts of the oral mucous membranes.

If the patient is so unfortunate as to survive for a prolonged period in the tumor stage, the eventual clinical picture may be pitiful, with painful, infected, weeping ulcers involving 50% or more of the body surface. Complications at this stage include hypoalbuminemia, cachexia, and episodes of bacteremia arising from the skin lesions. Substantial

Table 18. TNMB classification for mycosis fungoides

Classification	Description
T (skin)	
T1	Limited patch/plaque (<10% of total skin surface)
T2	Generalized patch/plaque (≥10% of total skin surface)
T3	Tumors
T4	Generalized erythroderma
N (nodes)	
N0	Lymph nodes clinically uninvolved
N1	Lymph nodes enlarged, histologically uninvolved (includes "reactive" and "dermatopathic" nodes)
N2	Lymph nodes clinically uninvolved, histologically involved
N3	Lymph nodes enlarged and histologically involved
M (viscera)	
M0	No visceral involvement
M1	Visceral involvement
B (blood)	
B0	No circulating atypical (Sézary) cells (<5% of total lymphocytes)
B1	Circulating atypical (Sézary) cells (≥5% of total lymphocytes)

From Kim YH, et al. Prognostic factors in erythrodermic mycosis fungoides and the Sézary syndrome. *Arch Dermatol* 1995;131:1003, with permission.

Table 19. Clinical staging system for mycosis fungoides

Clinical stages	TNM classification[a]
IA	T1, N0, M0
IB	T2, N0, M0
IIA	T1–2, N1, M0
IIB	T3, N0–1, M0
IIIA	T4, N0, M0
IIIB	T4, N1, M0
IVA	T1–4, N2–3, M0
IVB	T1–4, N0–3, M1

[a] The "B" classification does not alter clinical stage.
From Kim YH, et al. Prognostic factors in erythrodermic mycosis fungoides and the Sézary syndrome. *Arch Dermatol* 1995; 131:1003, with permission.

amounts of narcotic analgesics may be required, particularly for dressing changes. Death is a merciful release from severe suffering.

Staging

Several staging systems have been proposed for MF and related diseases, and no system is universally accepted. Tables 18 and 19 represent the currently available and used classification and staging of MF. In a theoretical sense, the staging is artificial because MF appears to be a systemic disease from the outset, with a traffic in neoplastic cells between the skin, the blood, and other organs. The staging system simply reflects *overt* involvement but appears to be clinically valid because life expectancy decreases with increasing stage (Tables 18 and 19). The stages of MF broadly represent the bulk of disease that is present and also the increasingly invasive and replicative proclivities of the MF cells. There is no evidence that the stage of disease has the important implications for therapy as is the case, for example, in Hodgkin disease. As a result, staging laparotomy has not won a place in the management of MF, although it has contributed to the understanding of the disease.

Prognosis

From Tables 18 and 19, it is apparent that the prognosis varies quite widely within the lower stages (0–I) and becomes poorer, with a narrower range of variation, in the higher stages. The outlook is particularly poor when major visceral involvement is present. As yet, no good evidence shows that therapy alters the median survival of patients with high-stage MF, but preliminary evidence in some studies indicates that aggressive treatment in the early stages of MF may eradicate the disease or suppress it for prolonged periods. Other studies have failed to show such an advantage. The occurrence of a favorable response to treatment does not appear to influence the duration of life, but it can significantly improve its quality. The major **prognostic variables** in MF are as follows:

1. Stage of disease
2. Extent or bulk of disease within a stage
3. The tempo of disease progression in the individual patient
4. The age of the patient
5. The presence or absence of other diseases that significantly affect life expectancy
6. Immunophenotype of the malignant lymphocytes (CD30+ versus CD30−)

Similar variables apply to chronic lymphocytic leukemia and to low-grade non-Hodgkin lymphomas of B-cell origin.

Extracutaneous Manifestations

The extracutaneous manifestations of MF are numerous (Table 20). Although the classic progression from skin to lymph nodes to blood is the most frequent evolution, virtually any organ or system may become involved, as in other lymphomas and in the

Table 20. Extracutaneous manifestations of T-cell cutaneous lymphomas

System	Manifestation
Pulmonary	Nodules Infiltrates Pleural effusion Mediastinal or hilar lymphadenopathy
Skeletal	Osteolytic lesions Osteoporosis Arthritis
Ocular	Intraocular: retina, choroid, optic nerve Extraocular: cornea, conjunctiva, lid, orbit
Oral	Tumors and ulcers on lips, tongue, larynx
Nervous system	Intracerebral: tumor, hemorrhage, progressive multifocal leukoencephalopathy Meningeal infiltration Peripheral neuropathy
Gastrointestinal	Diarrhea Ascites Hemorrhage
Cardiac	Congestive failure; arrhythmias
Renal	Progressive renal failure
Hematologic	Eosinophilia, monocytosis Monoclonal paraprotein, cryoglobulinemia Leukemic phase of mycosis fungoides Marrow invasion (uncommon even as terminal event)
Subcutaneous tissue, viscera	Tumors (nondermatotrophic mycosis fungoides)

Note: An extensive bibliography of these relatively rare manifestations can be found in Carney DM, Bunn PA. Manifestations of cutaneous T-cell lymphoma. *J Dermatol Surg Oncol* 1980;6:369, (192 references).

leukemias. Carney and Bunn described these manifestations and included an excellent bibliography.

Pulmonary infiltrates may cause a major clinical problem in determining their etiology, particularly when they arise in a patient who has received cytotoxic drugs and adrenal corticosteroids, and pose the question, Is this opportunistic infection or pulmonary fibrosis a result of cytotoxic agents or aggressive MF? Both might be signs of advancing MF, which is sometimes accompanied by eosinophilia, or the findings might indicate a pulmonary fungal infection. A transbronchial lung biopsy may show infiltration with MF cells and no evidence of infection. The infiltrates and the eosinophilia usually respond to intensive cytotoxic drug therapy.

Orbital or ocular involvement by MF is important because of the disability it may cause. A patient who develops exophthalmic ophthalmoplegia of sudden onset due to retrobulbar MF may respond at once to urgent radiotherapy with resolution of all clinical signs. Delay in diagnosis probably would result in long-term visual impairment. Involvement of the retina, vitreous, or lens of the eye is a rare but serious problem that responds to irradiation. It is important to note that, in such cases, the probability of coexisting involvement of the brain and meninges is high. Such involvement should be sought by magnetic resonance imaging and lumbar puncture for cerebrospinal fluid cytology and immunophenotyping.

Oral lesions of MF are rarely missed because they tend to be highly symptomatic. In a patient with known MF, it is seldom necessary to biopsy such lesions to prove their identity. Prompt treatment with radiation produces excellent relief and spares the patient unnecessary surgery. **Nondermatotropic lesions** of MF may occur in the oral cavity (e.g., as masses within the substance of the tongue). These lesions respond to irradiation, but not surprisingly, problems of radiation-induced mucositis may occur.

Central nervous system involvement by MF can be diagnosed by immunophenotyping the cells in the cerebrospinal fluid. As mentioned, it occurs more frequently in patients with involvement of the eye or the orbit.

1. **Meningeal** involvement by MF produces a clinical picture resembling meningeal leukemia.
2. **Direct cerebral** involvement is rare but life threatening.
3. **Progressive multifocal leukoencephalopathy** is extremely rare but tends to be overdiagnosed in MF as in other lymphomas. The diagnosis is seldom confirmed.

Nondermatotropic Mycosis Fungoides
Nondermatotropic mycosis frequently is a source of diagnostic problems. Some patients develop large masses in the subcutaneous tissues, orbit, retroperitoneum, or other sites that may be obvious clinically or visualized on computed tomography (CT) scans. These masses bear no relation to cutaneous tumors or plaques and frequently are unrelated to major lymph node groups. Biopsy discloses sheets of MF cells without recognizable lymph node structures. Apparently, these neoplastic T-cells have lost their normal homing characteristics and no longer have a predilection for the skin and subcutis. This manifestation of MF is readily diagnosed by the physician who is familiar with it.

Non-Hodgkin Lymphomas and Hodgkin Disease
Non-Hodgkin lymphomas and Hodgkin disease may develop in patients with MF but should be diagnosed only after careful review of biopsy material by an expert pathologist. Atypical appearances of MF may be misdiagnosed as a new disease.

Finally, it should be noted that the incidence of extracutaneous manifestations of MF is much higher in autopsy series than it is in clinical series. This reflects the fact that autopsy is a more than usually aggressive investigation and usually is performed in a patient with MF that was extremely advanced unless the cause of death was unrelated. Clinical studies are important for making clinical judgments (e.g., frequency of clinically significant meningeal involvement), whereas autopsy studies provide more information about the biology of the disease (e.g., involvement of the bone marrow is not uncommon at autopsy but rarely constitutes a clinical problem).

Management of the Patient
Initial Evaluation
In any patient with neoplastic disease, the initial evaluation includes the assembly of data on all other coexisting illnesses and inquiry about psychosocial factors that are relevant to the care of the patient. Thus, it is imperative to take a complete history of the patient's past and present illnesses and to carry out a comprehensive medical examination.

Assessment of the Cutaneous Lymphoma.
Table 21 lists the data required for assessment of MF and other cutaneous lymphomas.

1. **The history and physical examination,** as usual, are the most cost-effective steps. A history of very slow evolution and the finding of very limited disease indicate a good prognosis, particularly in an elderly patient, in whom the prognosis of the lymphoma may exceed the life expectancy of the patient.
2. Review of the histopathology is important because the more noxious forms of therapy are contraindicated if the diagnosis of neoplasia is in doubt.
3. The extent of further investigation is determined both by the results of initial laboratory tests and by the overall clinical picture.
4. Younger patients and those with systemic symptoms merit more extensive evaluation. In patients with cutaneous tumors or lymphadenopathy, investigations for the presence of visceral disease (e.g., abdominal CT scans) are more likely to yield positive results.

Table 21. Initial evaluation of a patient with mycosis fungoides (MF)

Basic
  History
  Physical examination
    Special attention to skin and lymph nodes
    Baseline clinical photographs are desirable
  Investigations
    Review of pathology, rebiopsy if indicated
    Complete blood count
    Examination of buffy-coat films for MF cells
    Biochemical profile
    Serum electrophoresis
    Chest radiograph
Special
  Enumeration of peripheral blood lymphocyte subpopulations
  Immunophenotyping of buffy coat cells and biopsy specimens
  Electron-microscopic studies of buffy-coat cells
Extensive disease suspected
  Biopsy of suspicious lymph nodes
  Abdominal CT scan
  Bone marrow aspiration and biopsy
  Pointers suspicious of extensive disease include lymphadenopathy, organomegaly,
    abnormal chest radiograph. MF cells in peripheral blood, severe systemic
    symptoms, neurologic, or ophthalmologic findings
Other
  Many other tests are required occasionally, on the basis of abnormal findings from
    the original investigation, e.g., cranial or chest CT, transbronchial lung biopsy,
    liver biopsy, lumbar puncture; they are not part of the routine evaluation of the
    usual case.

CT, computed tomography.

5. As in other diseases, an investigation should be done only if its results will significantly affect the physician's course of action.

The **treatment** of MF and other CTCLs has not evolved in the same manner as that of other malignant lymphomas, in part because these conditions are usually diagnosed and then managed by dermatologists. Until recently, hematologist–oncologists were rarely consulted until patients developed advanced, resistant disease, frequently with extensive visceral involvement. Undoubtedly, another reason is that most patients do very well, sometimes for many years, with simple treatments that are purely palliative but nonetheless effective. The usual modern approach to malignant disease—aggressive staging and intensive therapy with curative intent—has frequently been thought inappropriate for a condition that may run a very indolent course with minimal therapy. Although this view is generally correct for the elderly patient with multiple medical problems, a different approach is required for younger, otherwise healthy patients who in the long run are at high risk of death from MF if it is not treated effectively. Programs that treat MF from the outset as the systemic disease it is and that aim at cure through intensive therapy represent a logical approach to the disease. These programs must, however, be regarded as investigational because there is no certain evidence that cure can be effected or even that survival can be enhanced by such treatment. Table 22 summarizes current therapeutic approaches to MF.

Early Stages
Particularly when the diagnosis of MF is not established beyond question, radiotherapy or the use of cytotoxic drugs is not recommended. These mutagenic and carcinogenic treatments should not be used in the absence of a firm diagnosis of malignant disease.

Table 22. Treatment of cutaneous T-cell lymphomas[a]

Stage	Treatment
Dermatitis stage	Topical steroids Bland ointments Topical and oral antipruritic agents Psoralens with ultraviolet A (PUVA): photo-chemotherapy and photopheresis techniques Radiation and chemotherapy are not recommended at this stage, particularly when the diagnosis of a neoplastic disease has not been firmly established
Cutaneous plaques or tumors	Topical nitrogen mustard Topical carmustine (BCNU) Superficial radiotherapy, preferably electron beam
Spread beyond the skin to nodes and viscera	Single-agent chemotherapy (e.g., methotrexate) Multiple-agent chemotherapy (e.g., CHOP, CHOPE, CHOP-Bleo)
Localized extracutaneous lesions (e.g., orbit, eye, meninges, brain bone)	Megavoltage radiotherapy

Newer and investigational therapies	Leukapheresis
	Retinoids
	Immunotherapy
	  Biologic response modifiers
	  Antithymocyte globulin
	  Monoclonal antibodies
	  Cyclosporine
	  Thymopentin
	Bone marrow transplantation
	  Allogeneic
	  Autologous
	Newer chemotherapeutic agents
	  Pentostatin
	  Fludarabine
	  Cladribine

[a] The recommendations primarily concern mycosis fungoides, about which experience is most extensive.

Topical and Oral Agents

Topical corticosteroids, bland ointments, and topical and oral antipruritic agents are all of some value. Some patients obtain significant relief from the administration of systemic corticosteroids (e.g., prednisone), but such treatment rarely produces long remissions. The manifestations of MF reappear when prednisone is discontinued, or they may recur during prednisone therapy, indicating the acquisition of resistance to the drug. The toxic effects of corticosteroid therapy, particularly in older patients who have multiple medical problems, mean that corticosteroids should be used carefully in a chronic condition like MF.

Photochemotherapy

Photochemotherapy with methoxsalen followed by ultraviolet light in the "A" range (PUVA) can be beneficial in early disease and can be used before MF is unequivocally diagnosed because it is not a highly carcinogenic form of therapy. PUVA therapy may cause mild nausea, generalized pruritus, or sunburn-like changes, and it may provoke secondary cutaneous malignancies, particularly when given over prolonged periods or in combination with other therapies.

More Advanced Stages
When the diagnosis of MF is not in doubt or is in more advanced stages, the mainstays of treatment are topical nitrogen mustard and superficial radiotherapy. More recently, extracorporeal ultraviolet irradiation of the neoplastic lymphocytes, a process termed *photophoresis* has been added to the list of available treatments.

Traditionally, **nitrogen mustard** is applied every day as an aqueous solution to local lesions of MF. The solution is unstable and must be made up by the patient at home, which limits its usefulness. A formulation of nitrogen mustard in petrolatum may be superior to the aqueous solution and has the advantage that it is stable and can be prepared by the pharmacist, which eliminates potential errors when the patient prepares an aqueous solution at home. More intensive treatment with whole-body application of nitrogen mustard has been reported to produce lengthy complete remissions of MF, but this has not been widely confirmed, and the method is used infrequently. It occasionally may be curative, but this has not been proved.

The **mode of action** of nitrogen mustard in MF may be twofold. In addition to the usual cytotoxic action of the alkylating agent, the induction of cutaneous hypersensitivity may also be beneficial in securing resolution of MF lesions. The general practice, however, is to attempt to avoid hypersensitivity reactions because the resultant pruritus may become sufficiently severe as to preclude the further use of topical nitrogen mustard. If this occurs, patients may be successfully desensitized with the use of very dilute solutions of nitrogen mustard. Carmustine (BCNU) also may be used as an alternative to nitrogen mustard. Results tend to be poor when MF is very extensive or in the tumor stage. Long-term use of topical nitrogen mustard may be associated with an increased risk of squamous cell and basal cell skin cancers.

Superficial radiotherapy: In the past, low-voltage x-rays (grenz rays) were used, but the preferred modern treatment is with electrons (β rays) from strontium-90 or from a linear accelerator. Because the skin penetration of electrons is limited (1 cm for each 2 MV), bone marrow suppression is seldom a problem. Bulky skin tumors may be undertreated because of this low penetration, and traditional radiographs of 50 to 100 kV may be used in such cases.

Electron beam therapy: The aggressive and early use of whole-body electrons has been reported to bring about lengthy remissions and possibly cure. This approach merits further study. Whole-body electron beam therapy requires a powerful linear accelerator and a relatively large treatment room, so that the patient can be placed sufficiently far from the accelerator to permit a whole-body field. For these technical reasons, whole-body electron beam therapy is not available everywhere.

The **adverse effects of electron beam therapy** are substantial. They include acute radiodermatitis (72%) associated with erythema, hair loss, and occasional blistering and skin breakdown that may be slow to heal. Chronic complications include a decreased ability to sweat (*hypohidrosis*) because of the loss of sweat glands (84%) and reduced lacrimation (62%). Whether electron beam therapy is superior to either topical nitrogen mustard or PUVA is unclear. Electron beam therapy often is reserved for patients who fail to respond to another approach because it may be more expensive and toxic.

Photophoresis: Attempts have been made to treat MF by **leukapheresis,** the physical removal of leukocytes from the blood by a cell centrifuge. This treatment was based on the knowledge that MF cells circulate in the blood and that in some patients there appears to be a two-way commerce between the blood and the skin. Cycles of leukocytosis and improved skin lesions alternate with phases when MF cells are less numerous in the blood and skin lesions are larger. Although repeated leukapheresis removed MF cells and produced clinical improvement in some patients, the technique is labor intensive and therefore costly and the improvement is temporary. Leukapheresis is of scientific interest as a treatment for MF but is of little practical importance and is not widely practiced.

More recently, animal experiments showed that if peripheral blood lymphocytes were removed by leukapheresis, treated in ways that rendered them antigenic, and then *returned* to the host animal, the host then mounted an immune reaction against cell clones whose representatives were present in sufficiently large numbers. An abnormal clone could be reduced more effectively by this technique than by simple leukapheresis. That is, returning the altered cells to the animal had effects that exceeded those of physical removal and discarding the cells. This technique then was applied to human MF.

In normal human blood, the lymphocyte population is made up of scores or hundreds of separate clones, each with only a few representatives circulating in the blood at any one time. If altered antigenically, none of these clones would have sufficient cells present to elicit a major immune response. In patients with MF, circulating MF cells at times constitute a relatively large monoclonal population that, if antigenically altered, is sufficient to trigger an immune reaction.

In **clinical photophoresis,** the patient ingests a dose of 8-methoxypsoralen (8-MOP), a photoactivatable drug. Exposure to ultraviolet light activates 8-MOP and enables it to bind to DNA. The patient then undergoes leukapheresis (i.e., the leukocytes are separated from the blood by cell centrifuge in an extracorporeal circuit). The erythrocytes and plasma then are returned to the patient, and the harvested leukocytes are passed through a chamber illuminated by ultraviolet light to activate the 8-MOP, which then combines with the cellular DNA. The irradiated cells are returned to the patient. Leukapheresis is an essential step in the process; exposing *whole* blood to ultraviolet light would be ineffective because the semiopaque erythrocytes would prevent effective irradiation of the leukocytes. The process resembles PUVA treatment, except that the irradiation is carried out extracorporeally rather than in the skin. The cutaneous side effects of PUVA treatment are, of course, avoided. Photophoresis treatments are carried out on two consecutive days once a month. Typically, responses are gradual, and 6 months may elapse before significant improvement of skin lesions is seen.

The following are the **advantages** of photophoresis:

1. The treatment is relatively safe and nontoxic.
2. 8-MOP only exerts its cytotoxic activity when in its photoactivated form, *outside* the body.
3. Photophoresis can prove effective when resistance to topical therapies has developed.
4. Major remissions occur and may be very durable without maintenance therapy. This suggests that, in some patients at least, photophoresis makes possible the long-term control of MF by the patient's own immune system.

The following are the **drawbacks** of photophoresis:

1. Expense of the procedure
2. The long time required to bring about initial improvement
3. Unpredictable absorption of 8-MOP from the gastrointestinal tract, requiring the repeated measurement of blood levels. Eventually, this may be circumvented by the licensing of an 8-MOP preparation that can be directly added to the separated leukocytes in their collecting bag before their exposure to ultraviolet light.
4. Problems with venous access
5. Significantly less effectiveness in tumor stage and visceral stage disease

It follows that photophoresis is best used before MF has become too far advanced. Photophoresis is unsuitable for patients with severe symptoms that require rapid relief. Because of its immunologic basis, photophoresis would likely be relatively ineffective in patients who have had extensive exposure to immunosuppressive cytotoxic chemotherapy. The best results may be expected in patients with *minimal* MF in whom photophoresis theoretically could affect long-term suppression of the disease. It may be impractical, however, to subject patients with minimal MF to this costly and demanding therapy. Detailed accounts of experience with photophoresis are included in the **Suggested Readings.**

Chemotherapy
When MF has spread beyond the skin to the lymph nodes and viscera, chemotherapy is the treatment of choice. Careful studies of peripheral blood buffy-coat films, including electron microscopic examinations, frequently document the presence of MF cells

even in early stage disease. Thus, systemic chemotherapy may well be the most logical approach in newly diagnosed MF because the disease is already systemic. Although this aggressive approach may be the best way to treat the *disease,* in most instances it is not the best way to treat the *patient.* As a result, most current experience with chemotherapy in MF is with far-advanced disease. Thus, the results of chemotherapy may be biased toward an unpromising lack of efficacy.

1. Many single agents and multiple-drug regimens have been reported to elicit responses in patients with advanced MF. The CHOP regimen (cyclophosphamide, doxorubicin, vincristine, prednisone), with or without etoposide (CHOPE), or bleomycin (CHOP-Bleo) is effective in many patients.

2. Response duration and survival have usually been brief, which may reflect the selection of patients with advanced disease and poor performance status.

3. Weekly intermediate-dose methotrexate (200–500 mg by intravenous bolus injection) with leucovorin rescue by mouth is a simple, relatively nontoxic therapy that can be administered in the outpatient clinic and frequently produces good palliation.

4. Because of the small size of published series and a paucity of comparative studies, no regimen has been recognized as superior or has become generally accepted as the treatment of choice.

5. Much further research in the chemotherapy of CTCLs is needed. This should be conducted in patients of good performance status whose disease is not far advanced, so that the potential value of cytotoxic therapy is not obscured. Randomized studies that compare different regimens are necessary to determine efficacy of these treatment programs. These can be done only through a large cooperative group of institutions using specific protocols.

Biologic Response Modifiers
These modifiers are beginning to find a role in CTCLs.

1. **Interferon-α** (IFN-α) may be the most active single agent in refractory MF, with objective responses in 45% of patients. Early studies used high doses (50 million U/m^2 administered intramuscularly three times per week). All patients experienced typical side effects of interferon: malaise, anorexia, weight loss, and declining performance status. Later studies achieved similar response rates using much lower doses (5 million U/m^2, 3 times per week) with much less toxicity. Interferon has also been administered intralesionally with good effect.

2. Limited experience with **interferon γ** (IFN-γ) showed a response rate of 31%, with reversible side effects of fever, weight loss, mild neutropenia, and elevated liver function tests. Unlike conventional cytotoxic agents, the IFNs are not immunosuppressive. Theoretically, they can be combined with photophoresis without loss of the host-versus-tumor reaction that is thought to underlie the effectiveness of the latter treatment.

Localized Extracutaneous Lesions
Localized extracutaneous lesions of MF are best treated with megavoltage radiotherapy because responses are more rapid and dependable than those obtained with presently available chemotherapy. The prompt administration of radiation therapy is particularly desirable when the lesions are at critical sites, such as the orbit, eye, and cranial cavity.

Investigational Therapies
1. **Retinoids** are natural or synthetic analogs of vitamin A that have been used to treat many skin diseases. The use of 13-*cis*-retinoic acid, which has produced responses in extensive MF with plaques and tumors, is potentially promising. This substance has not yet been widely used, however. **Isotretinoin** (Accutane), 2 mg per kilogram of body weight daily administered orally, produced objective responses in 44% of patients; the median duration of response is 8 months. **Etretinate** (Tegison) has produced similar results. Both these agents are promising and merit further study. More recently, a new oral retinoid, bexarotene (Targretin) that is specific for the x-receptor (RXR) has demonstrated efficacy in all stages of CTCL and is currently available for clinical use.

2. **Immunotherapy: biologic response modifiers** [IFN-α, IFN-γ, interleukin-2 (IL-2)] may prove important in the control of neoplasms of T lymphocytes. As previously discussed, IFN has been used alone; it is also used as an adjunct to photophoresis in the treatment of MF with significant success. Thus far, the data remain insufficient to assess the role of interferon and other cytokines in the clinical management of MF.

Antithymocyte globulin (ATG), a crude xenogeneic antibody to T lymphocytes, has antitumor activity in MF, produces regression of skin lesions, but the effects are temporary because of modulation of the tumor cell antigens. Toxic effects, particularly allergic reactions and serum sickness, are significant.

Monoclonal antibody therapy with highly specific antibodies that do not damage normal T cells has greater potential value than the use of ATG, which reacts with normal cells as well as lymphoma cells. Murine monoclonal antibodies to the T-cell differentiation antigens (CD5, CD25, and CD52) have produced brief partial responses.

1. Monoclonal antibodies can be rendered more potent by the attachment of toxins (e.g., ricin A-chain) or radionuclides (e.g., yttrium-90, iodine 131) to the antibody molecule.

2. A recently developed unique fusion protein that combines the cytotoxic A chain and translocation B chain of diphtheria toxin with recombinant IL-2 (DAB$_{389}$IL-2), marketed as Ontak, has shown significant response rates in patients with MF–Sézary syndrome. Downregulation of antigen expression on the neoplastic T cells and the production of human antimouse antibodies that neutralize the monoclonal antibodies (so-called HAMA reaction) are two obstacles to this approach.

3. Current studies with B-cell lymphomas suggest that monoclonal antibodies may be most effective *after* major cytoreduction has been secured by other means, usually involving conventional cytotoxic chemotherapy. This requires further investigation for use in CTCLs.

4. Monoclonal antibodies labeled with radioactive iodine or indium (γ-emitters) can also be useful as imaging agents in patients with suspected visceral involvement by T-cell lymphoma.

Cyclosporine, an immunosuppressive agent that exerts its effects by acting on T lymphocytes, inhibits the growth of MF cells by suppressing IL-2 production. Cyclosporine suppressed the symptoms of MF for up to 2 years but had little objective effect on the skin lesions. Because of this problem and associated immunosuppressive and nephrotoxic effects, cyclosporine is indicated only in patients who are severely symptomatic and lack other treatment options.

Thymopentin, a synthetic pentapeptide with numerous immunologic effects, including the promotion of T-cell differentiation, produced objective responses in all four patients with MF who were treated. Increases in natural killer cells were noted, which might explain the antitumor effect.

Bone marrow transplantation (BMT): Many patients with MF are too old for *allogeneic* BMT. Because MF frequently does not involve the bone marrow, there may be considerable scope for high-dose chemotherapy coupled with *autologous* bone marrow transplantation (ABMT). In one pilot study of ABMT, five of six patients had a complete response, three for less than 100 days and two for more than a year. This treatment may be of value for patients with severe MF who are otherwise healthy and able to withstand the procedure.

New Chemotherapeutic Agents

Recently, three new antipurine drugs with activity in MF have been licensed for sale in the United States. Although none of these agents was actually licensed for the treatment of MF, a growing body of literature attests to their activity in this condition.

1. **Pentostatin** (2′-deoxycoformycin, dCF, Nipent) is a tight-binding inhibitor of adenosine deaminase, an enzyme important in the metabolism of lymphoid cells, and is extremely toxic to normal and neoplastic lymphocytes, both T and B cells. This agent is of little value in rapidly progressive disorders (e.g., acute lymphocytic leukemia) but is active in indolent lymphoid neoplasms, including hairy-cell leukemia, chronic lym-

phocytic leukemia, and CTCLs. Good partial remissions and occasional complete remissions have been documented in patients with refractory MF, which suggests that pentostatin may have a useful role in this disease. This agent should be considered for the treatment of patients with MF that is less advanced and refractory. Pentostatin has CNS, renal, and hepatic toxicities and is highly immunosuppressive, promoting severe opportunistic infections. Therefore, caution is required in its use, and it should be restricted to patients of good performance status.

2. **Fludarabine** (Fludara), another adenosine deaminase inhibitor, produced a 19% response rate in 31 patients with previously treated, extensive-stage MF. One complete response lasted more than 17 months. Thus, this important new drug is active in MF as well as chronic lymphocytic leukemia (for which it was licensed) and low-grade non-Hodgkin lymphomas. Fludarabine has major myelosuppressive activity and must be used with caution, particularly in patients who have received cytotoxic chemotherapy in the past.

3. **Cladribine** (2-chlorodeoxyadenosine, 2-CDA, Leustatin): This agent is a purine analog that is resistant to degradation by adenosine deaminase and is cytotoxic to normal and neoplastic lymphocytes. In 15 patients with CTCLs, three (20%) achieved complete remission and four (27%) had a partial remission. Additional studies have shown significant response rate in previously treated patients when treated with cladribine. Myelosuppression was the major toxicity encountered, and cladribine should be used with caution in heavily pretreated patients. Because this drug also has potent immunosuppressive activity, opportunistic infections may be a significant hazard.

Summary
The therapy of MF has been marred because it evolved in an era when palliation was the goal of treatment. Early cases of MF were managed by nononcologists, and medical oncologists were not involved until advanced, refractory disease had become established. The continuing use of local therapy for a systemic disease is a reflection of this less than optimal evolution. Fortunately, ongoing therapeutic research has been directed toward a cure for MF; the concept of early systemic therapy is winning acceptance just as it did years ago in the control of breast cancer. It must be stressed, however, that despite well-founded theoretical concepts, there is as yet no proof that early systemic chemotherapy or biologic therapy can substantially alter the natural history of MF. The production of such evidence is a task for the future.

Complications of Cutaneous T-Cell Lymphomas
Cutaneous
Pruritus, disfigurement, weeping skin lesions, and painful ulcers are almost universal in advanced MF and may make patients' lives miserable. In severe cases, serum loss causes hypoproteinemia.

Infection
Infection secondary to loss of dermal integrity is the most frequent major complication.

1. The most frequent infecting organism in an initial episode is *Staphylococcus aureus.*
2. In second episodes, particularly in hospitalized patients, **gram-negative organisms,** including *Pseudomonas aeruginosa,* become increasingly important.
3. **Venous access devices,** such as implanted ports and catheters are especially prone to become infected in patients with MF, presumably because the ecology of their skin flora is very abnormal; when possible, implanted venous access devices should be avoided in these patients.
4. **Bacteremic episodes** are not uncommon, particularly if patients have been made granulocytopenic by cytotoxic drug therapy.
5. Initial antibiotic therapy should always include good antistaphylococcal coverage.
6. In hospitalized patients, **vancomycin** is the best choice because it is active against methicillin-resistant *S. aureus* (MRSA) and also against *Staphylococcus epidermidis.*

Extracutaneous
Involvement of extracutaneous sites (Table 20) may produce a wide range of complications comparable to those produced when acute leukemia affects the same organs.

1. **Meningeal involvement** by MF may produce headache, vomiting, and visual disturbance.
2. **Gastrointestinal involvement** may lead to abdominal pain, melena, and bowel obstruction.
3. **Pulmonary involvement** may produce infiltrates on chest radiographs that can only be distinguished from infectious processes by invasive procedures—transbronchial biopsy or open lung biopsy.

Elderly Patients
Older patients with indolent MF frequently die of cardiac or cerebrovascular diseases, and the lymphoma may thus have no impact on their lifespan.

Younger Patients
Younger patients, defined as those younger than 65 years, are at much greater risk of dying from complications of the neoplastic disease. This is particularly true if their general health is good and their life expectancy longer.

Terminal Care
The terminal care situation arises when MF is believed to be resistant to both chemotherapy and radiotherapy. The efforts of the physician are then concentrated on the relief of symptoms with analgesics, antipruritics, sedatives, and antidepressant drugs. Currently available antipruritic agents are virtually worthless in many patients, and only narcotics and potent sedatives are of any value. In severely debilitated and profoundly uncomfortable patients, the decision eventually must be made as to the propriety of administering antimicrobial agents when life-threatening infection occurs.

As in all terminal illness, the precise details of management should reflect the wishes of the patient. The wishes of the physician and the family are important but must be subordinate to those of the patient. The issue of resuscitation should be discussed with the patient, and the signing of a Living Will should be encouraged to ensure that the patient's wishes are carried out.

Sézary Syndrome
Sézary syndrome is the leukemic variant in the spectrum of CTCLs; it is a distinct clinical entity associated with severe morbidity and mortality. Although much has been written about CTCL, the bulk of the patients described are sufferers from MF. Few articles specifically address the problems of prognosis and treatment in Sézary syndrome.

History
Although MF was described by Alibert in 1806, its erythrodermic variant was not reported until 1892 by Besnier and Hallopeau. In 1938, Sézary and Bouvrain described the clinical constellation of erythroderma, intense pruritus, lymphadenopathy, and mononuclear cells with hyperconvoluted cerebriform nuclei circulating in the peripheral blood. In 1961, Taswell and Winkelmann named this entity *Sézary syndrome*. In the early 1970s, immunologic studies showed that the circulating neoplastic cells were T lymphocytes.

Epidemiology
Sézary syndrome is uncommon, constituting approximately 5% of all cases of CTCL, or an annual incidence of 30 to 40 cases in the United States. Most patients are between 45 and 70 years of age at diagnosis. There is a 1.5:1 male predominance. In absolute numbers, more whites have Sézary syndrome than do African Americans, but the incidence is twice as high in African Americans.

Etiology
The cause of Sézary syndrome is unknown, but exposures to tobacco, air pollutants, pesticides, solvents, analgesics, radiation, and detergents have been cited. A causative role for retroviruses, specifically HTLV-1, has been suggested but not proved. The adult T-cell leukemia-lymphoma caused by HTLV-1 is a more aggressive disease than Sézary syndrome and has a poorer prognosis.

Clinical Features

In addition to generalized erythroderma, edema, and intense pruritus, which occur in all patients, the major clinical features include lymphadenopathy (57%), hepatomegaly (36%), alopecia (32%), onchodystrophy (32%), and keratoderma (29%). When keratoderma affects the palms and soles, extremely painful fissuring of the skin may be present.

Pathology

Histopathologically, Sézary syndrome often demonstrates dense infiltrates of atypical lymphocytes in the dermis. Epidermotropism, the infiltration of these atypical lymphocytes into the epidermis, can also be seen. The cells also form clusters within the epidermis that are referred to as *Pautrier microabscesses*. In the later stages of Sézary syndrome, epidermotropism may be lost, with resulting absence of Pautrier microabscesses. The peripheral blood shows abnormal lymphocytes with cerebriform nuclei, and the leukocyte count may be markedly elevated (20,000–100,000/L). The mechanism involved in the production of the pruritus and erythroderma is not known.

Treatment

Because of its rarity, no randomized, controlled trials have been carried out in Sézary syndrome. Few articles specifically address the treatment of Sézary syndrome: Most describe one or more patients with Sézary syndrome and a much larger number of patients with MF or other types of CTCL. As a result, the relative merits of the many treatment options that exist for Sézary syndrome are difficult to evaluate.

1. **Electron beam irradiation** causes improvement of skin lesions in more than two thirds of patients, but the duration of response is usually less than 7 months. There is no convincing evidence that this treatment improves the survival of patients with Sézary syndrome.

2. **Topical nitrogen mustard** leads to improvement of the skin in approximately 50% of patients, but it does not affect the systemic disease. Side effects include dermatitis, hyperpigmentation, telangiectasia, pruritus, urticaria, hypersensitivity reactions, and the development of cutaneous malignancies.

3. **Intravenous nitrogen mustard** produced cutaneous responses in 8 of 14 patients, but the duration of response was not stated.

4. **Topical corticosteroids** in the form of fluocinolone acetonide with occlusive dressings proved effective in a single study.

5. **Topical carmustine** produced four responses, two of which were complete, in nine patients with Sézary syndrome. The side effects were similar to those of topical nitrogen mustard.

6. **Systemic chlorambucil and prednisone** produced 9 complete and 14 partial remissions in 25 patients with Sézary syndrome. The remission duration was not stated, and there was no evidence of an effect on survival.

7. **Systemic methotrexate** produced seven complete and six partial responses in the skin lesions of 17 patients; a decline in circulating Sézary cell counts also occurred. Responses lasted for 9 to 63 months, and the 5-year survival in this series was a favorable 71%. Thus, methotrexate appears to be a useful agent in this disease.

8. **Multiple-drug chemotherapy regimens** are effective in Sézary syndrome, but all published series are small. CHOP produced four complete and three partial responses in seven patients, and the median duration of response and median survival were 24 and 184 weeks, respectively. COP-Bleo produced two complete and nine partial responses in 12 patients, with a median duration of 53 weeks and a median survival of 107 weeks. Apparently, chemotherapy with multiple drugs is active in Sézary syndrome, but the evidence needed to determine the regimen of choice or the effect, if any, on survival is insufficient.

9. **PUVA** produces responses of the skin in Sézary syndrome, but few of these are complete and the responses are brief. The blood picture is not improved; ultraviolet light cannot penetrate to the Sézary cells circulating in the blood. PUVA therapy for Sézary syndrome is not an effective primary treatment.

10. **Leukapheresis** results in improvement in both skin and leukocyte counts in Sézary syndrome, but the treatment is expensive and time consuming, and the re-

sponses are incomplete and transient. Leukapheresis is not an effective therapy for Sézary syndrome.

11. **Antithymocyte globulin and monoclonal antibodies** have been administered to a few patients with Sézary syndrome. No complete responses have been observed, and the partial responses have lasted for only a few weeks. Toxic effects include fever, chills, nausea, angioedema, serum sickness, and immunosuppression. In its present form, antibody therapy has no value in Sézary syndrome. Whether this treatment is more effective when administered after effective cytoreductive chemotherapy is yet to be determined.

12. **Retinoids** (isotretinoin and etretinate) appear to be less effective in Sézary syndrome than they are in MF. When these drugs are administered to some patients with Sézary syndrome, their skin disease worsens.

13. **Cyclosporine** has relieved pruritus and erythroderma in patients with Sézary syndrome, but responses were short-lived. There was no objective decrease in the cutaneous infiltrate or the peripheral Sézary cell count. Serious nephrotoxicity and hepatotoxicity negate the value of cyclosporine in Sézary syndrome.

14. **Interferon** has been used in only a few patients with Sézary syndrome. Two complete and five partial responses were reported in 13 patients, with response duration ranging from 3 to 36 months. Many patients required dose reduction because of side effects. The information is insufficient to determine the role of interferon in this disease.

15. **Photophoresis** appears to be highly active in patients with Sézary syndrome. Among 37 patients, 27 (73%) showed clinical improvement as measured by defined skin scores. Circulating Sézary cell counts were not reduced, which suggests that the impact on the disease process is relatively minor. Patients experienced relief of symptoms and a notable lack of toxicity was evident. Photophoresis should be considered as a front-line treatment option for Sézary syndrome.

16. **Pentostatin, fludarabine, and cladribine** all possess activity against CTCL cells. Because of the rarity of Sézary syndrome and the newness of these cytotoxic agents, there are insufficient data to evaluate their role, if any, in the management of Sézary syndrome.

Summary

Because of its rarity, which results in a lack of both precedent and experience, Sézary syndrome has been treated along the same lines as MF. Whether this is truly appropriate is not known. Reports of treatment of patients with Sézary syndrome have tended to be lost or incorporated in a patient population, most of whom suffered from MF. In the future, treatment and outcomes in patients with Sézary syndrome should be reported separately. Further evaluations of the role of photophoresis and the newer antipurine drugs should be made in Sézary syndrome so that the treatment of this lethal disease can be improved.

Suggested Readings

Carney DN, Bunn PA. Manifestations of cutaneous T-cell lymphoma. *J Dermatol Surg Oncol* 1980;6:369.

Colby TV, Burke JS, Hoppe RT. Lymph node biopsy in mycosis fungoides. *Cancer* 1981;47:351.

Fuks Z, Hoppe RT, Bagshwa MA. The role of total skin irradiation with electrons in the management of mycosis fungoides. *Bull Cancer (Paris)* 1977;64:291.

Girardi M, Edelson RL. Cutaneous T-cell lymphoma: pathogenesis and treatment. *Oncology* 2000;14:1061.

Heald PW, et al. Photophoresis. *Yale J Biol Med* 1989;62:565. (This is a compilation of nine articles devoted to photophoresis.)

Holloway KB, Flowers FP, Ramos-Caro F. Therapeutic alternatives in cutaneous T-cell lymphoma. *J Am Acad Dermatol* 1992;27:367.

Horning SJ, et al. Clinical and phenotype diversity of T-cell lymphomas. *Blood* 1986; 67:1578.

Kemme DJ, Bunn PA. State of the art therapy of mycosis fungoides and Sézary syndrome. *Oncology* 1992;6:31. (A valuable 12-page review with 80 references.)

Kessler JF, et al. Treatment of cutaneous T-cell lymphoma (mycosis fungoides) with 13-*cis*-retinoic acid. *Lancet* 1983;1:1345.

Klein E, Schwartz RA. Cancer of the skin. In: Holland JF, Frei E, eds. *Cancer medicine* Philadelphia: Lea and Febiger, 1982:2085.

Kong LR, Samuelson E, Rosen ST, et al. 2-chlorodeoxyadenosine in cutaneous T-cell lymphoproliferative disorders. *Leuk Lymphoma* 1997;26:89.

Kuzel T, Hurria A, Samuelson E, et al. Phase II trial of 2-chlorodeoxyadenosine for the treatment of cutaneous T-cell lymphoma. *Blood* 1996;87:306.

Kuzel T, et al. Pivotal phase III trial of two dose levels of $DAB_{389}IL$-2 (Ontak) for the treatment of mycosis fungoides. *Blood* 1997;90(Suppl 1):586a.

Levi JA, Wiernik PH. Management of mycosis fungoides—current status and future prospects. *Medicine* 1975;54:73.

Long JC, Mihm MC. Mycosis fungoides with extracutaneous dissemination: a distinct clinicopathologic entity. *Cancer* 1974;34:1745.

Magrath IT. Lymphocyte differentiation, an essential basis for the comprehension of lymphoid neoplasia. *J Natl Cancer Inst* 1981;67:501.

McDonald CJ, Bertino JR. Treatment of mycosis fungoides lymphoma: effectiveness of infusions of methotrexate followed by oral citrovorum factor. *Cancer Treat Rep* 62:1009, 1978;62:1009.

O' Brien S, Kurzrock R, Duvic M, et al. 2-chlorodeoxyadenosine therapy in patients with T-cell lymphoproliferative disorders. *Blood* 1994;84:733.

Redman JR, et al. Phase II trial of fludarabine phosphate in lymphoma: an effective new agent in low-grade lymphoma. *J Clin Oncol* 1992;10:790.

Roenigk HH. Photochemotherapy for mycosis fungoides: long-term follow up study. *Cancer Treat Rep* 1979;63:669.

Saleh MN, et al. Antitumor activity of $DAB_{389}IL$-2 fusion toxin in mycosis fungoides. *J Am Acad Dermatol* 1998;39:63.

Saven A., et al. 2-chlorodeoxyadenosine: an active agent in the treatment of cutaneous T cell lymphoma. *Blood* 1992;80:587.

Siegel RS, et al. Primary cutaneous T-cell lymphoma: review and current concepts. *J Clin Oncol* 2000;18:2908.

Spiers ASD, Ruckdeschel JC, Horton J. Effectiveness of pentostatin (2'-deoxyco-formycin) in refractory lymphoid neoplasms. *Scand J Haematol.* 1984;32:130.

Spiers ASD, et al. T-cell chronic lymphocytic leukaemia: anomalous cell markers, variable morphology and marked responsiveness to pentostatin (2'-deoxycoformycin). *Scand J Haematol* 1985;34:57.

Variakojis D, Rosas-Uribe A, Rappaport H. Mycosis fungoides: pathologic findings in staging laparotomies. *Cancer* 1974;33:1589.

Whitbeck EG, Spiers ASD, Hussain M. Mycosis fungoides: subcutaneous and visceral tumors, orbital involvement and ophthalmoplegia. *J Clin Oncol* 1983;1:270.

Wieselthier JS, Koh HK. Sézary syndrome: diagnosis, prognosis and critical review of treatment options. *J Am Acad Dermatol* 1990;22:381. (This is an extremely useful 21-page review with 172 references.)

Willemze R, et al. EORTC classification for primary cutaneous lymphomas: a proposal from the Cutaneous Lymphoma Study Group of the European Organization for Research and Treatment of Cancer. *Blood* 1997;90:354.

16. INITIATION AND CONTROL OF COAGULATION

Dennis A. Gastineau

Hemostasis is the maintenance of a normal state of fluid blood flow within the vascular system. In the normal state, the balance of coagulation favors the liquid or anticoagulated state. Normal flow may require transient development of a new piece of solid matter, a clot, through the **coagulation** mechanism, and subsequent dissolution of that clot through the **fibrinolysis** mechanism. Localization of the coagulation mechanism is controlled through an endogenous **anticoagulant** mechanism. The balance of all these is required for normal health, and the perturbation by any missing abnormal or consumed element may result in abnormal thrombosis or bleeding.

Coagulation Preview
A fibrin clot is the result of activation of the coagulation pathway(s) through a number of mechanisms. Although simplified versions of the coagulation pathways are helpful for learning the processes and the tests of the system, the interactions are actually numerous and complex (Fig. 1). It should be carefully and frequently remembered that our models are based on *in vitro* reactions and observations and that *in vivo* mechanisms are undoubtedly different at least in quantity and probably qualitatively as well. There is still value in understanding the models and mechanisms to help predict disease characteristics, diagnosis, and responses to therapy.

Coagulation Mechanism
Initiation of the coagulation mechanism may occur from a number of sources, but commonly, **tissue injury** results in a combination of **platelet activation** and initiation of tissue activation by increased exposure of **tissue factor.**

The initial generation of small amounts of enzyme **thrombin,** which cleaves fibrinogen to fibrin, results in positive feedback amplification by further activation of coagulation factors back "upstream" and generation of increasing amounts of thrombin. These reactions occur in coagulation complexes, which assemble on various surfaces (platelets, leukocytes, membrane fragments). These complexes help to localize the reaction and increase the rate of reaction by bringing together the enzyme and its substrate. During activation of platelets, phosphatidylserine is translocated from the inner layer of the membrane to the outer exposed platelet membrane layer. The assembly of these complexes increases the rate of reaction logarithmically. Therapeutic intervention often focuses on the interference with complex assembly, such as limiting calcium binding of proteins to the phospholipid membrane surface either by limiting calcium availability (citrate anticoagulation) or by preventing modification of the proteins to allow the calcium binding (warfarin anticoagulation to prevent carboxylation of glutamic acid residues).

Platelets must activate to form what is termed the *primary hemostatic plug.* Platelets activate with exposure to the subendothelium exposed in tissue trauma and adherence via von Willebrand factor (vWF) to collagen. Platelets then release the content of cytoplasmic granules, including adenosine diphosphate (ADP), which binds to specific receptors on nearby platelets, activating them in a cascade effect that results in a conglomeration of activated platelets, bridged to one another by fibrinogen binding to the glycoprotein IIb/IIIa receptor. Further activation occurs with the release of thromboxane A_2, which is generated from arachidonic acid in the platelet. Platelets are strongly inhibited by prostacyclin, also derived from arachidonic acid but produced in the endothelial cells. Thus, the balance between coagulation and fluid blood is maintained by balance of the arachidonic acid pathways. Platelets also release growth factors, which induce vascular proliferation, which promotes healing.

The coagulation system begins *in vitro* with the assembly of contact activation factors on a surface (factor XII on a surface, which then can activate factor XI). The generation of factor Xa (activated clotting factors are denoted by a lower case "a" after the

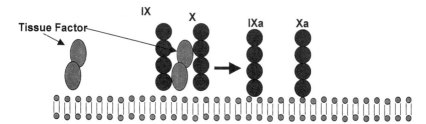

FIG. 1. Coagulation activation: tissue factor/factor VII complexes on phospholipid surfaces bind to activate factors IX and X, which become active serine proteases able to cleave substrates in their appropriate complexes on the phospholipid surface.

particular factor symbol) then activates factor IX to IXa. Factor IXa then can activate factor VIII, which circulates bound to vWF, an adhesion molecule key in the formation of the initial platelet plug. Factor VIIIa then functions as large template molecule bound to a negatively charged surface that has a binding site for IXa and also for factor X. This juxtaposition of IXa and X increases the rate of activation of X to Xa. Factor Xa then migrates over the membrane surface to factor Va, a molecule that has high homology to factor VIII and functions in the same way, bringing together factor Xa and its substrate, factor II (prothrombin). The factor Va, factor Xa, calcium, phospholipid complex is referred to as the *prothrombinase complex,* which then will cleave prothrombin (factor II) to IIa, which then will cleave fibrinogen to fibrin. The cleavage of fibrinogen to fibrin generates small fragments.

Along with contact activation, another pathway, traditionally referred to as the **extrinsic** pathway, is the primary *in vivo* coagulation activation pathway with tissue injury. Exposure of tissue factor on endothelial cell injury results in increased factor VII expression; activation of factor VII; and the assembly of a tissue factor VIIa complex on a phospholipid surface, which activates factor X. The activated factor X then migrates in a fashion analogous to its movement after activation by factor IX to the factor Va molecule to assemble the prothrombinase complex (Fig. 1).

The *in vivo* coagulation system does not follow the simple two-pathway model, but the need for the presence of adequate activity in both arms is explained by the model of initiation of coagulation through tissue factor and factor VII with a generation of a small amount of thrombin. This small amount of thrombin then activates factor VIII, additional factor VII, and factor IX. The intrinsic pathway provides necessary amplification of thrombin generation to generate adequate fibrin clot (Fig. 2). In normal coagulation,

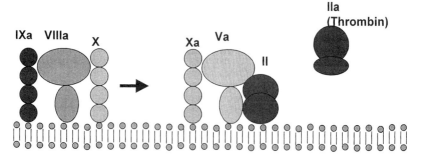

FIG. 2. Coagulation activation: Factor IXa is bound by factor VIIIa on a phospholipid surface in the presence of calcium, bringing it into proximity of factor X, and it cleaves factor X to Xa. Factor Xa then moves along the phospholipid surface to be bound by factor Va, which presents factor II to be cleaved to IIa (thrombin).

the intrinsic pathway cannot provide sufficient thrombin because of tissue pathway inhibitor (TFPI) activity. The maximum rate of thrombin formation occurs after the formation of fibrin, and the additional thrombin is necessary for additional fibrin formation and the activation of factor XIII and thrombin-activatable fibrinolysis inhibitor. Factor XIIIa is a transglutaminase (not a serine protease) that cross-links fibrin covalently. Thrombin-activatable fibrinolysis inhibitor cleaves lysines from fibrin, and these free lysines competitively prevent the binding of fibrinolytic enzymes to fibrin.

The rate of activity of the coagulation pathway is limited by an inhibitor that functions as a regulator of the rate of thrombin generation, TFPI. The TFPI inhibition of the pathway depends on the activation of factor X, and a complex of TFPI-Xa, which then inhibits the FVIIa-tissue factor complex.

This model provides an understanding of why hemophiliacs bleed despite having an intact extrinsic pathway. Inadequate levels of factor VIII (classic hemophilia or hemophilia A) or factor IX (Christmas disease or hemophilia B), or factor XI (hemophilia C) result in symptomatic bleeding. Factor XII and high-molecular-weight kininogen (HMWK) do not appear to participate to a significant degree in clot formation *in vivo*.

The concentrations of the coagulation proteins in plasma reflect their role in the coagulation reaction. The highest concentration is owned by fibrinogen (10 µmol/L). Factor VII (10 nmol/L) is outstripped by factors IX and X (100 nmol/L), and prothrombin has the highest concentration (2 µmol/L) after fibrinogen. Deficiencies of the various enzymes provide some clue to the potential for additional functions of these proteins; deficiency of tissue factor is embryonically lethal, and factor VII deficiency causes fatal bleeding at birth. Severe deficiencies of factor V and prothrombin are fatal, but factor VIII and IX deficiencies cause bleeding after birth.

Anticoagulation

The **limiting** of the clot is accomplished by two systems that depend on an intact endothelial cell surface. The antithrombin (previously called *antithrombin III*) system requires the presence of endogenous heparins on the endothelial surface. Antithrombin inhibits the coagulation mechanism by binding activated proteases 1:1. Most enzymes in the coagulation pathway can be inhibited by the serine protease inhibitor antithrombin. Free enzymes are inhibited most efficiently, whereas factors contained in the prothrombinase or tenase complexes are protected in part from inhibition.

The protein C system inhibits coagulation by cleaving the large template coenzyme proteins factors V and VIII. Cleavage of these proteins slows the rate of thrombin activation sufficiently to shut down the process. The system requires intact endothelial cells that have a receptor called *thrombomodulin*. In turn, thrombomodulin binds thrombin and changes its conformation and thereby its specificity from fibrinogen to cleaving protein C. Activated protein C (APC), in complex with protein S on the plasma membrane of intact endothelial cells, then can cleave factors V and VIII (Fig. 3). The inactivation of factor VIIIa is accelerated by protein S and factor C, the latter acting as an anticoagulant protein in this context. APC cannot cleave inactive factor VIII because of its being bound to vWF. APC, however, can cleave factor V bound on a membrane surface, which forms factor V, which can accelerate the activity of APC along with protein S. Factor V therefore actually has two activated forms: factor Va, which forms the tenase complex, and the active form after cleavage by APC, which accelerates the anticoagulant activity of that same enzyme. The common aspects of these systems are that intact endothelial cell surfaces are required and that the rate of the coagulation reaction is slowed to the point that new clot does not form.

Fibrinolysis

The control and remodeling of the thrombus are accomplished by cleavage of fibrin by plasmin, the precursors of which are contained within the fibrin clot. Plasmin will cleave fibrin and other coagulation proteins into many fragments, reducing their activity and concentration. Plasmin is activated from its precursor plasminogen through a number of pathways. Urokinase, located primarily in the urinary tract, has several active forms and cleaves plasminogen to plasmin. Tissue plasminogen activator is present in more tissues and binds to fibrin to come in contact with plasminogen. The activation of plasminogen by tissue plasminogen activator (t-PA) causes

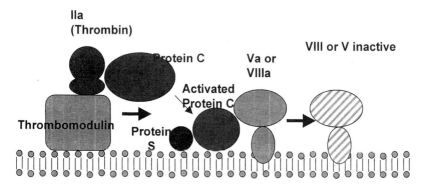

FIG. 3. Coagulation control: Thrombin is bound by thrombomodulin, which is present on intact endothelial cells. Thrombin's protease activity is not blocked, but the specificity is changed from fibrinogen to protein C. Activated protein C then can cleave and inactivate either factor VIIa or factor Va. The complexes formed by the binding proteins factors V and VIII then break apart, and the rate of coagulation shows.

localized fibrinolysis, restricted by the location of plasminogen, and removes fibrin, which is no longer necessary.

Plasminogen activator inhibitors (PAIs) prevent "premature" activation. Deficiency of these inhibitors can cause a clinical bleeding disorder similar to hemophilia. Plasmin that spills over into the general circulation is neutralized by several inhibitors, including α_2-antiplasmin. The fibrinolytic products produce an inhibitory effect in the coagulation assays by interfering with the protease activity of multiple clotting factors that play important roles in the generation of a clot.

Coagulation Proteins

Intrinsic Pathway: High-Molecular-Weight Kininogen
1. Molecule active in both modulation of vascular resistance and coagulation
2. Activation of factor XII
3. Deficiencies not well characterized
4. Can cause marked prolongation of activated partial thromboplastin time (APTT)

Factor XII
1. Deficiency is not associated with bleeding.
2. Marked prolongation of activated APTT: If APTT is greater than 55 seconds, think factor XII deficiency or lupus anticoagulant if no bleeding is present.
3. Does not require replacement.
4. Activator of factor XI *in vitro*
5. *In vivo* activity and importance of factor XI are unclear.

Factor XI
1. Autosomal inheritance
2. Critical for normal *in vivo* coagulation
3. There is great variation of bleeding for a given level of activity.
4. Intraarticular and muscle bleeding is typical.
5. Hemostasis usually occurs with levels greater than 30%.
6. Replacement is fresh frozen plasma (FFP).
7. Investigational concentrate has been used but is associated with a high rate of thrombosis and difficult to obtain.
8. Has been called hemophilia C

Factor IX
1. X-linked inheritance
2. Critical for normal *in vivo* coagulation

3. 1/10 as common as factor VIII deficiency
4. Intraarticular and muscle bleeding, spontaneous in severe disease
5. Clinically indistinguishable from factor VIII deficiency
6. Treatment is with recombinant factor IX.
7. Dose is 75 U per kilogram of body weight initially every 24 hours. Subsequent doses need lower dose (an apparent saturation effect).
8. Levels should be monitored.
9. Hemophilia B and Christmas disease are synonymous terms.

Factor VIII
1. X-linked inheritance
2. Intraarticular and muscle bleeding
3. Predictable bleeding based on level of activity:
   * Severe: less than 1% activity—spontaneous bleeding
   * Moderate: 1% to 5% activity—bleeding with moderate trauma
   * Mild: 6% to 35% activity—bleeding with significant trauma or surgery
4. Treatment is recombinant factor VIII.
5. Requires 75% to 100% activity for surgical hemostasis.
6. Prophylaxis to maintain level greater than 1% at all times
7. Dose is 50 U per kilogram of body weight for initial bolus, with continuous infusion of 4 U per kilogram per hour for maintenance of 100% activity, 2 U per kilogram per hour for 50% activity. Adjust according to factor levels; dose administered every 12 hours if not administered by continuous infusion.

Factor X
1. Rare congenital deficiency
2. Acquired deficiency associated with primary systemic amyloidosis
3. Replacement with FFP
4. Requires about 30% level of hemostasis

Factor V
1. Very rare congenital deficiency
2. Acquired deficiency in myeloproliferative disorders
3. Mucosal bleeding
4. Contained in platelets
5. Platelet transfusion is best therapy.

Factor II
1. Very rare congenital deficiency
2. Acquired deficiencies usually nutritional or related to warfarin (Coumadin)
3. FFP is best therapy.
4. Requires about 30% activity for hemostasis.

Factor VII
1. Extrinsic pathway
2. Congenital deficiencies unusual but not rare
3. Most do not bleed; level needed varies widely, but about 30% is usually enough (for single-factor deficiency); some patients have adequate hemostasis with lower levels.
4. FFP is the best replacement.

Tissue Factor Pathway Inhibitor
1. Regulator of the extrinsic pathway, yielding a maximal generation of thrombin, which alone is insufficient for hemostasis
2. TFPI deficiency has not been described and may be incompatible with life.
3. Inhibition of TFPI or manipulation to effect hemostasis has not been successful.

Common Screening Coagulation Tests
The APTT measures the coagulation factors from HMWK to fibrinogen, except factor VII and tissue factor. The limitations of the APTT are important to understand, and mild bleeding disorders, which are important in surgical bleeding risk, may be

undetected by an APTT. The precise threshold for each coagulation factor varies by brand and even by lot of partial thromboplastin reagent.

The prothrombin time (PT) measures factor VII through the prothrombinase complex and fibrinogen, but tissue factor is not well assayed by plasma-based tests available routinely. The PT is most valuable to screen for vitamin K deficiency and for oral anticoagulation effect (inducing vitamin K deficiency). The characteristics of thromboplastin are described by a relationship to a World Health Organization standard consisting of a logarithmic formula assigning a number called the International Sensitivity Index (ISI).

Tests for fibrinolysis include fibrin degradation products (FDPs), which may be derived from both fibrinogen and fibrin and from D-dimer assays, which measure crosslinked digested products of cross-linked fibrin (fibrin acted on by factor XIII). Some tests that are now rarely used include euglobulin clot lysis, which is intended to look for generalized fibrinolytic activity that should not be present in the usual remodeling of localized thrombus or hematoma.

Platelets
Quantitative Abnormalities
1. Having a platelet count less than 100,000 will prolong bleeding time.
2. Surgical hemostasis may be impaired.
3. Destruction may be increased.
   - Less bleeding with destructive processes compared with lack of production
   - Causes: hypersplenism, antibody-mediated extravascular destruction, platelet activation in disseminated intravascular coagulation (DIC), platelet activation in heparin-associated thrombocytopenia (HAT), or thrombotic thrombocytopenia (TTP).
   - Therapy: splenectomy, intravenous immunoglobulin, platelet transfusion in ITP can increase platelet count, platelet transfusion in HAT or TTP contraindicated except in life-threatening bleeding due to thrombosis risk.
   - Decreased production: greater bleeding compared with increased destruction group. Causes include megakaryocytic aplasia; aplastic anemia; leukemic replacement; myelophthisic (marrow replacement); and drug [idiosyncratic, dose-dependent (chemotherapy agents, nonchemotherapy)].
4. Treatment
   - Therapy of underlying cause
   - Recombinant thromboprotein (not yet available commercially): Effect is less dramatic than granulocyte macrophage–colony-stimulating factor (GM-CSF); it is not effective in transplant patients.
   - Stop drugs.

Qualitative Abnormalities
See Chapter 8.

Screening Testing
Bleeding time has been criticized extensively and is vulnerable to many operator and patient variables (age, cooperation, skin characteristics). It remains, however, the only broadly available screening for platelet function [and platelet adhesion molecule abnormalities such as von Willebrand disease (vWD)]. The bleeding time is sufficiently variable that it is unusual to obtain meaningful serial measurements in response to various interventions.

Approach to Bleeding Disorders
Personal History
History is the single most important tool in diagnosis of bleeding disorders and bleeding risk. The screening tests commonly available (PT, APTT) have sensitivities that cannot exclude clinically important deficiencies (most APTT reagents will have a normal clotting time with a 35% factor VIII level). A coagulation history should be obtained for any patient scheduled to undergo surgical procedures. The history of a mild bleeding disorder may be sufficiently subtle that the simple question "do you bleed normally?" is unlikely to discover the abnormality.

Personal history with specific questioning about bleeding with previous surgery, tooth extractions, and epistaxis. Specifically, inquiry should be made about tonsillectomy (patients do not always think of this as "surgery"). Very prolonged wound healing time or bleeding from an umbilical cord stump may suggest the extremely rare factor XIII deficiency preventing cross-linking and stabilization of the fibrin clot. Circumcisional bleeding may be the first indication of factor VIII deficiency (15% of cases are sporadic, new mutations). Ask about the patient having missed school or going to the nurse's office for epistaxis. Some patients compare themselves with other family members who may also have the same mild bleeding disorder and thus not realize they have abnormally frequent epistaxis. Menstrual bleeding patterns are important to obtain but have limited specificity.

Bruising may be nonspecific (> 25% of women will answer "yes" to the question "Do you bruise abnormally?"). Asking about the number of bruises typically present at any time (>3 is suggestive of an abnormality), the presence of pain and swelling in typical bruises (uncommon except with major trauma), or the presence of bruises on the trunk as opposed to the extremities will help to discriminate abnormal bruising.

The timing of bleeding after trauma or surgery can help guide investigation toward platelets or the plasma coagulation system. Immediate bleeding suggests platelet or severe protein abnormalities, whereas initial good hemostasis with bleeding 2 to 5 days later suggests a plasma protein deficiency.

Bleeding in joints (hemarthrosis) or deep-muscle bleeding is suggestive of a plasma protein disorder, whereas mucosal bleeding or extended bleeding from superficial cuts is suggestive of a platelet-related abnormality. Improvement of symptoms at adolescence is a common feature of some mild bleeding disorders, such as vWD. Determination of the duration of symptoms may help to determine whether this is acquired or indeed a congenital disorder. Significant recent-onset bleeding may be due to an inhibitor of coagulation factors.

Family History
A family history of at least two prior generations is important to confirm the presence of a familial pattern to the disorder. Disorders may be either sex-linked or autosomal and may "skip" generations in clinical penetrance (although it is important to recall that women may experience symptomatic X-linked disorders). Proceed with gentle prompting of all the same questions as in the personal history, but with the additional questions of whether any family member has ever died as a result of surgery (a sufficiently rare event that bleeding should be considered as a cause). Where there is a positive history, careful documentation of the entire pedigree with notation of the type of bleeding in each member should be done because some bleeding may be due to the hereditary disorder and other bleeding from acquired disorders. Analysis of the pattern of sex and age occurrences allows the probability of various disorders to be determined. History might **not** detect mild bleeding disorders that have been insufficiently challenged but may cause bleeding during major surgery.

Physical Examination
Examination of the skin may reveal evidence of connective tissue diseases (hyperelasticity), telangiectasias suggesting vascular disorders. Examination of the abdomen may reveal splenomegaly suggesting a systemic disorder. Examination of the joints is done to look for evidence of secondary joint changes resulting from intraarticular hemorrhage.

Approach to Bleeding Disorders
Disorders of Platelets and Vascular Diseases (Primary Hemostatic Plug)
See Chapter 8 for details. (For a discussion of vWD, see section entitled **Disorder of Platelet Adhesion Molecule** to follow.)

Coagulation Protein Abnormality Approach
Preliminary testing with the PT and the APTT may detect a prolonged clotting time. If a prolonged clotting time is found, the next step is to perform a 1:1 mix of normal plasma and patient plasma. If the repeat test with the mixture becomes normal, a protein deficiency is suggested. A 50% level of any single coagulation protein will support

a normal clotting time. If the test of the mixture remains prolonged, an inhibitor is suggested. Mild or moderate deficiencies of coagulation factors may have normal or only minimal prolonged coagulation times. If the tests are normal but the history is suggestive of a bleeding disorder, additional testing should be performed, including individual coagulation factor assays and platelet function testing.

Disorder of Platelet Adhesion Molecule
Disorders of platelets adhesion may be due to either intrinsic platelet receptor abnormalities or to abnormalities or deficiencies of the ligand molecules such as **vWF.** vWD was discovered through a careful family pedigree study of a family on the Åland Islands.
   The typical clinical features of vWD include mucosal bleeding, particularly epistaxis. Many have normal APTT values. Patients with severe vWD may have bleeding similar to hemophilia as a result of the concomitantly decreased factor VIII levels. Generally, no excessive bleeding at the time of delivery occurs as a result of the rise of vWF throughout pregnancy. vWF rises and reaches a peak at the beginning of the third trimester. If a normal value is present during the third trimester, no special preparation for delivery is needed. Postpartum bleeding may occur because of a rapid fall of vWF levels back to baseline over 3 to 5 days following delivery.
   Pathophysiology: Decreased or abnormal vWF, the ligand that binds to platelet glycoprotein Ib/IX. The classes of vWD are the following:

1. Type 1. Normal protein with decreased but detectable vWF activity; normal distribution of polymers
2. Type 2
   - Abnormal protein structure
   - Polymeric distribution is usually abnormal.
   - Unusual subtype of type 2 (Normandy) has abnormal factor VIII binding and looks like hemophilia A with markedly decreased factor VIII levels. Clue is the presence of affected males and females in the pedigree.
   - Type 2b molecules are hyperactive and cause increased platelet agglutination.
3. Type 3
   - Virtually absent vWF; polymers often invisible on electrophoresis.
   - Concomitantly decreased factor VIII levels (due to decreased half-life of factor VIII in absence of vWF)
   - May be sporadic; mechanism is not well understood. Not necessarily double heterozygote state.

Inherited Coagulation Factor Deficiencies
Classic **hemophilia A:**

1. Factor VIII deficiency
2. About 15% of cases are sporadic.
3. Multiple gene mutations
   - Most common gene abnormality is inversion of the large factor VIII gene, leading to early termination of an abnormal protein; it occurs in about 45% of cases.
   - Deletions, point mutations
   - No apparent difference in the development of inhibitors
4. Inhibitors to factor VIII develop in about 20% of patients after the first 50 treatments with exogenous factor VIII.
5. Clinical features vary with severity:
   - Severe (<1% activity): bleeding in joints and muscle with inconsequential activity; requires frequent replacement therapy.
   - Moderate (1%–5% activity): bleeding with moderate trauma.
   - Mild (6%–35% activity): bleeding with significant trauma; may not be diagnosed until late in life.
6. Bleeding sites: Bleeding into joints with a secondary inflammatory reaction is the most obvious expression of disease. The secondary inflammatory response induces neovascularization and new bone growth, which result in more frequent bleeding, leading to early osteoarthritis. Soft-tissue bleeding in deep muscle and retroperitoneal spaces can result in large decrease in hemoglobin and compartment syndromes.

Urinary tract bleeding can be problematic because therapy of the bleeding can result in the development of an obstructive clot. Central nervous system bleeding (which occurs almost exclusively in patients with severe disease) has high morbidity and mortality and requires treatment with a high index of suspicion.

7. Treatment of bleeding: The ideal treatment is actually prophylaxis. Prophylactic therapy of young children can be accomplished by three times weekly therapy with the goal of maintaining the trough factor VIII activity above 1%. The presence of a small amount of factor VIII activity changes the character of the disease dramatically. Prophylaxis has succeeded in preventing the development of hemophilic arthropathy through adolescence into early adulthood. Prophylaxis in adults may not be as important if the joints are reasonably normal because adults tend to be much less active and have fewer bleeding episodes. Replacement therapy with recombinant factor VIII may be administered at a dose of 50 U per kilogram of body weight to reach an activity of 100%. Continuous infusion with 4 U per kilogram per hour usually maintains a level of 100%, and 2 U per kilogram hourly for a level of 50%, sufficient for hemostasis 48 hours postoperatively. Intermittent therapy must be given every 12 hours. Rapid treatment with self-infusion provides the optimal reduction of morbidity and symptom duration for a bleeding episode. Treatment of bleeding in patients with antibodies (inhibitors) to factor VIII requires a high-dose factor VIII in low-titer inhibitors, or treatment that "bypasses" the inhibition. The approaches have either been to give clotting complex concentrates that contain small amounts of activated clotting factors or to overwhelm the extrinsic pathway by giving very large doses of recombinant factor VIIa, which overcomes the inhibition of TFPI and obviates the need for the intrinsic pathway amplification. The disadvantages of these approaches include risk of thrombosis, high cost, and the need to administer the drug frequently because of a short half-life.

Hemophilia B:

1. Factor IX deficiency
2. X-linked disorder 10% as common as hemophilia A
3. Symptomatically identical to factor VIII deficiency
4. The correlation of clinical severity with factor activity is less strong than in hemophilia A.
5. Treatment is with recombinant factor IX at an initial dose of 75 U per kilogram of body weight to reach 100% activity. The volume of distribution of factor IX is larger than that of factor VIII, but the volume of distribution decreases with subsequent doses, and the dose can almost always be reduced while following levels during replacement therapy.

Factor XI deficiency: Symptomatically, it is similar to hemophilia A and B, but bleeding is more variable with similar levels of factor XI activity. Treatment is with concentrate of FFP.

Factor II deficiency is a rare disorder. Replacement is with FFP, requiring 20% to 30% activity for adequate hemostasis.

Factor V deficiency is a rare disorder. Factor V is present on platelet membranes, and transfusion of platelet concentrates can reduce bleeding.

Factor XI deficiency most commonly presents as an acquired disorder associated with amyloidosis. FFP administration usually corrects the bleeding problem associated with deficiency.

Acquired Coagulation Disorders
Vitamin K deficiency:

1. Vitamin K is essential for the carboxylation of factors II, VII, IX, and X as well as proteins C and S in the natural anticoagulant system. In the absence or deficiency of vitamin K, abnormal coagulation molecules called PIVKAs (proteins induced by vitamin K absence) are produced, which have minimal coagulation activity because they cannot bind calcium and participate in the coagulation reaction.
2. **Causes** include inadequate vitamin K. Poor diet, usually from alcohol dependency or hospitalized patients receiving nutrition without vitamin K supplementation

(e.g., tube feedings or total parenteral nutrition, TPN). Impaired absorption of vitamin K is caused by the absence of bile salts resulting from bile duct obstruction or intestinal malabsorption resulting from sprue or inflammatory bowel disease. It is common in postsurgical patients who are taking nothing orally (NPO) and taking antibiotics over an extended period. Vitamin K antagonists such as warfarin or long-acting warfarin analogs sometimes are taken to obtain medical attention. Warfarin or brodifacoum are not detected by standard warfarin assay; specific assay for brodifacoum must be performed.

3. **Diagnosis** is done by measuring PT. Sometimes specific factor assays will uncover recent vitamin K replacement reflected by normal factor VII and depressed levels of the longer surviving factors II and X.

4. **Treatment:** Moderate prolongation of the PT may be treated with small doses (1 mg) of vitamin K if continued anticoagulation is desired; 5 mg of vitamin K administered subcutaneously daily for 3 days will differentiate vitamin K deficiency from liver failure.

Liver disease usually is associated with multiple factor deficiencies, including vitamin K–dependent factors but also factor V, fibrinogen, α_2-antiplasmin, plasminogen, protein C, and protein S. There is usually increased factor VIII in liver disease, most markedly with chronic liver disease.

1. **Diagnosis** is confirmed by abnormal or elevated liver enzymes or function tests. The APTT will be prolonged as well as the PT in severe cases, although the elevated factor VIII may mute the rise in the APTT. Elevated factor VIII suggests chronic liver disease. Elevated fibrinolytic products may be present in chronic liver disease and can be confused with DIC.

2. **Treatment:** Replacement therapy with FFP is the most common therapy because it replaces all plasma components. If fibrinogen is decreased, cryoprecipitate is most appropriate. Antifibrinolytic therapy must be used in rare instances, either tranexamic acid 20 mg per kilogram three times daily, or epsilonaminocaproic acid (EACA) 4 g every 4 hours administered orally or intravenously.

Disseminated intravascular coagulation (DIC) is a term used to describe a syndrome of coagulation activation to an abnormal degree resulting in generation of sufficient thrombin to overwhelm the physiologic thrombin inhibitors, including antithrombin and thrombomodulin. Thrombin activates the coagulation factors rapidly enough for their levels to fall, sometimes to levels that do not allow normal hemostasis to occur. The generation of fibrin also initiates fibrin and fibrinolysis, resulting in the overproduction of FDPs. The presence of fibrin strands can damage red blood cells, producing an abnormal blood smear with fragmented red cells, which are considered diagnostic of a microangiopathic hemolytic anemia.

Although DIC is not a disease itself, it is a condition brought on by some other process such as infection (endotoxins), trauma, cell necrosis, foreign substances (chemicals or hypotonic solutions), and foreign enzymes, such as snake venoms that activate the coagulation system by the overproduction or generation of thrombin.

Bleeding is the most commonly recognized clinical sign and usually is present in more than one site. Thrombotic events may be more subtle but can manifest as changes in mental status, renal failure, or other localized organ ischemia caused by small-vessel obstruction.

There is no single test that unequivocally identifies DIC. The presence of fibrinolysis products such as D-dimers, decreases of fibrinogen or platelets, and the prolongation of the PT reflecting reduced levels of circulating coagulation factors are common abnormalities accompanying this syndrome. The presence of fibrin monomers (soluble fibrin monomer complex, or SFMCs) is also usually detected. Protamine and ethanol precipitation tests may be helpful but are qualitative and more operator-dependent.

Therapy: If coagulation factors are decreased and the patient is bleeding, factor replacement with FFP (the plasma coagulation proteins), cryoprecipitate (concentrated fibrinogen), and platelets is indicated. **Never** treat just because abnormal test values are present. If thrombosis is occurring, anticoagulation, usually with heparin is appropriate. Antithrombin (AT) concentrates may be needed if AT levels are low. Heparin in the absence of thrombosis is rarely indicated and only if concerted efforts to replace the coagulation factors have failed. Accurate diagnosis and vigorous treatment of an underlying cause are necessary for successful outcome.

Fibrinolysis: Pure fibrinolysis or fibrinogenolysis is very rare, occurring in amyloidosis (the best documented setting), sometimes with liver disease (although the decreased clearance of fibrinolytic products in liver disease complicates this interpretation and rare malignancies where a specific fibrinogen cleaving activity or enzyme may be present. Diagnosis and differentiation from DIC can be difficult, but no evidence of decreases in coagulation factors other than fibrinogen, plasminogen, and α_2-antiplasmin should be present (Table 1). Treatment of fibrinolysis with inhibitors, tranexamic acid (1,500 mg three times daily. for the average adult), or EACA 4 g every 6 hours or 1 g per hour continuous infusion may be helpful in turning off the fibrinolytic process.

Factor X deficiency occurs in about 1% of patients with amyloidosis and appears to be caused by binding of the coagulation factor to the amyloid fibrils. It has been treated with splenectomy when the spleen is the dominant site of amyloid tissue.

Cardiopulmonary bypass induced disorders: Cardiopulmonary bypass for treatment of acute pulmonary toxicity is associated with an increased risk of bleeding. All patients have an acquired qualitative platelet defect that reverses in the first several hours after stopping bypass. The bleeding tendency can be treated with platelet transfusion. Partial activation causes part of the platelet defect and complex activation of the platelets can cause thrombocytopenia. If transfusion has been massive, additional coagulation factors should be replaced with FFP, and cryoprecipitate will replace fibrinogen but will also improve the qualitative platelet defect.

Coagulation Inhibitors

Antibodies to specific coagulation proteins: Antifactor VIII antibodies are the most common inhibitors to a specific coagulation factor.

1. May occur with congenital hemophilia A
2. Nonhemophilia
- Elderly
- Postpartum (usually 3–12 months after delivery)
3. Diagnosis
- Demonstration of inhibition of APTT and factor VIII: No correction with addition of normal citrated plasma
- Quantified in Bethesda units, a confusing unit that is best thought of as the amount of inhibitor required to reduce the factor VIII activity in a volume of plasma by 50%.
- Low levels of inhibitor are fewer than 5 Bethesda units.
- High level inhibitors are more than 5 Bethesda units.
4. Treatment of acquired factor VIII inhibitors includes the use of prednisone 100 mg to 1 g daily, with or without other immunosuppressives such as cyclophosphamide. The higher the titer of the inhibitor, the less likely a complete response will occur and the greater the risk of fatality. For acute bleeding, plasmapheresis may be effective in

Table 1. Differences between disseminated intravascular coagulation (DIC) and primary fibrinogenolysis

	Acute DIC	Fibrinogenolysis
Platelet count	Low	Usually normal
Fibrinogen	Low	Low
Factor V	Low	Low
Factor VIII	Low	Normal to moderately Decreased
Protamine sulfate test	Positive	Negative
Euglobulin clot lysis time	Normal	Short
Fibrinogen degradation products (FDP)	None to large amounts	Very large amounts

lowering the antibody titer. Antifactor V antibodies are rare, but a flurry of cases occurred in the late 1980s with the use of topical bovine thrombin containing small amounts of bovine factor V. Antibodies with varying degrees of cross-reactivity with human factor V developed and, in some cases, caused fatal bleeding disorders.

Nonspecific inhibitors:
Lupus-type anticoagulants (LACs): The most common inhibitor encountered in clinical practice is the so-called **lupus inhibitor.** This inhibitor appears to be directed against a combination of a coagulation protein epitope and β_2-microglobulin and is enhanced by phospholipid. LAC typically prolongs the APTT. The combination of these epitopes causes a generalized *in vitro* inhibition of multiple coagulation factors. The titer of the anticoagulant is low and can be diluted, with apparent increasing activity of the coagulation factors with each dilution. They are associated with thrombosis, and hemorrhage is extremely rare except when associated with hypoprothrombinemia or severe thrombocytopenia. The exception to the thrombosis rule is the presence of apparent high-titer inhibition of multiple factors that apparently cannot be diluted out. Great caution must be used when dealing with such a pattern. LACs are in the family of antiphospholipid antibodies, which includes anticardiolipin antibodies that also are associated with thrombosis.

Therapy is with coumadin anticoagulation with minimum target international normalized ratio of 2.5 to 3.0 needed because of the *in vitro* effect of the LAC on the PT. Some investigators argue for low-molecular-weight heparin as standard therapy, but prolonged therapy is usually required, and long-term side effects remain problematic.

Thrombotic Disorders
Inherited Thrombotic Disorders
The well-defined congenital hypercoagulable disorders are clinically indistinguishable from one another, all characterized by predominantly venous events, which may range from peripheral venous events in the extremities to central nervous system thrombosis of the venous drainage system. Isolated arterial events are less likely to indicate one of these conditions, although the relatively high frequency of some of the disorders means that there is nearly a 1 in 20 chance of finding the condition serendipitously.

The most common inherited disorder is a point mutation in the factor V molecule (G1691A), rendering it resistant to degradation by APCs. This abnormality is termed APC resistance, and it is associated with 25% to 40% of recurrent venous thrombosis. The mutant factor V has full coagulant activity, but it has a prolonged half-life, resulting in a hypercoagulable state. One of the three sites where APC cleaves factor V is substituted, rendering it resistant to APC. The form of factor V that normally accelerates APC activity is formed after cleavage at arginine 506, and factor VIII inactivation is also slowed. The combination of factor V Leiden and other factors that increase the risk of thrombosis, such as estrogen therapy, has been shown to further increase the overall rate of thrombosis. There is significant ethnic variation of the prevalence of factor V Leiden, ranging from up to 5% of northern Europeans to extremely rare in Asian populations.

The second most common abnormality is an abnormality of the noncoding portion of prothrombin, G20210A, which results in a slight elevation of prothrombin (although not enough to be discernible by directly measuring prothrombin levels). The thrombotic risks of the combination of prothrombin 20210 and other prothrombotic states are multiplied.

Protein C and S deficiencies are present in about one in 300 persons and present in only 1% to 3% of persons with venous thrombosis. Protein C deficiency can be homozygous or heterozygous, with the homozygous state conferring a much higher rate of thrombosis. The homozygous form has been associated with neonatal purpura fulminans. Protein S deficiency may be of the total amount of protein S, the free form of protein S, or abnormal bioactivity.

Antithrombin, the first described deficiency, is rare, occurring in one in 2,000. The activity of antithrombin may be affected by concomitant heparin therapy, and the presence of an abnormal form with a normal antigen level makes the measurement of activity mandatory. Heparin binds to antithrombin, greatly increasing its anticoagulant affect by inhibiting thrombin and factor Xa.

The most common acquired risk factor for thrombosis is the presence of antiphospholipid antibodies (lupus anticoagulant), which can be associated with both venous and arterial thrombosis. The magnitude of risk is greatest with antithrombin deficiency and less with protein C, S, and APC resistance.

Laboratory Investigation of Thrombosis

The investigation of thrombosis has become more important with the recognition that mutable risk factors that may confer very strong probability of thrombosis recurrence. Testing for many thrombotic risk factors through DNA testing and plasma testing is now available through a number of reference laboratories.

Clot-based testing may identify APC resistance, the presence of lupus anticoagulant(s), protein C and S, and antithrombin deficiencies. The measurement of both activity as well as antigen levels should be performed because abnormal forms of the proteins may confer a decreased activity, even with normal antigen levels. Antigen testing alone is insufficient for detection of prothrombotic events. Both congenital and acquired antithrombin deficiencies occur, and the presence of heparin therapy may result in transient decreases of measured antithrombin levels. Therefore, the diagnosis of antithrombin deficiency may require confirmatory testing after recovery from the acute event. Free protein S should be measured because the balance between bound and free protein S may cause a prothrombotic state. Protein S activity remains a technically difficult assay, and it can be affected by the presence of other acute phase events, such as the severity of illness. DNA analysis can identify factor V and prothrombin mutations and determine heterozygosity or homozygosity states.

An elevated level of homocysteine from numerous enzyme abnormalities and nutritional deficiency increases the risk of both venous and arterial thrombosis. Elevated factor VIII and fibrinogen are identified as additional risk factors for thrombosis, but the magnitude of risk and the means of intervention are as yet unclear and should not be part of the routine thrombosis screening.

Treatment of Thrombosis and Thrombosis Risk

Venous thrombosis still has limited therapy with either heparin or vitamin K antagonists.

1. **Heparin and low-molecular-weight heparin (a fraction of the spectrum of heparin multimers):** Low molecular weight heparin has a more predictable pharmacokinetic profile than standard heparin and can be administered subcutaneously with predictable results and little monitoring. Standard heparin is associated with a higher rate of heparin-associated thrombocytopenia, a complication that appears to be mediated by antibodies directed against platelet factor 4 (PF4) complexed with heparin. There is also a more common mild thrombocytopenia, which may occur in as many as 15% to 20% of patients who are receiving standard heparin, that does not appear to be antibody mediated and occurs earlier during the course of heparin therapy. Both forms of heparin require the presence of antithrombin for the anticoagulant effect. The high-molecular-weight forms have some antiplatelet effect.

2. The family of **vitamin K antagonists** all inhibit the addition of a carboxyl group to glutamic acid, which confers calcium binding for localization of the coagulation reaction. In the presence of vitamin K antagonists, there are abnormal forms of the coagulation factors II, VII, IX, and X as well as proteins C and S. Because protein C and S, both naturally occurring anticoagulants, are also vitamin K dependent, it is a little confusing as to why the overall effect is anticoagulation, but the observation is indeed that of coagulation. In the presence of an inherited deficiency of protein C, however, there is an increased risk of the very rare side effect of warfarin-associated skin necrosis, a phenomenon of microvascular thrombosis that causes full-thickness necrosis of the skin in patchy distribution.

The most common side effect is bleeding associated with supratherapeutic levels of anticoagulation as measured by the PT. Initiation of therapy with the expected maintenance dose of the drug is the safest induction of the anticoagulated state. Loading doses should be avoided. Monitoring frequency is determined by the stability of the INR but should not be less frequent than every 3 to 4 weeks, even when equilibrium is reached. Any change in drug therapy or health should prompt more frequent assay of the INR.

Duration of Thrombosis Treatment
The presence of an inherited abnormality is not necessarily an indication for permanent anticoagulation. The presence of factor V Leiden or prothrombin 20210 mutations are sufficiently common that the relative risk for thrombosis overlaps with unity. The presence of two inherited thrombophilic conditions is more than additive and would be a reason to continue anticoagulation. The inheritance of protein C, S, or antithrombin deficiencies may need more prolonged therapy, although the rates of recurrence may not be substantially different from those in persons with venous thrombosis without identified abnormalities.

The longer the period of anticoagulation, the lesser the likelihood of recurrence, but the duration of anticoagulation must be balanced against the risk of therapy. That balance in a person with a single thrombotic event is 6 to 12 months of therapy. Other factors that must be considered with long-term anticoagulation therapy are age and other confounding medical problems.

Thrombosis Prevention
The presence of an inherited risk factor is managed by risk reduction. There is no indication for anticoagulation preceding the occurrence of a clinical event. Even if therapy had no associated risk, there would still be doubt as to its indication.

Certain additive risks should be modified, and pharmacologic estrogen should be carefully assessed in carriers of factor V Leiden because there is an additive effect of thrombosis beyond the approximately threefold risk that exists with estrogen alone. There is not sufficient risk to justify general screening for prothrombotic states before initiating estrogen therapy.

Elevated homocysteine levels may be treated with pharmacologic folate, 1 mg three times daily. Recent data suggest that there is low risk of thromboembolic events not anticoagulating a woman during pregnancy who has had a single prior thrombotic event. Anticoagulation is most appropriate during the postpartum period, when the risk is higher than it is during pregnancy.

Broad testing for prothrombotic states in the absence of symptoms or prior thromboembolic event is neither practical nor indicated at present. Symptom- and history-based evaluation and therapy are still the most appropriate.

Suggested Readings

Brill-Edwards P, Ginsberg J, Gent M, et al. Safety of withholding heparin in pregnant women with a history of venous thromboembolism. *N Engl J Med* 2000;343: 1439–1444.

Dahlback B. Activated protein C resistance and thrombosis: molecular mechanisms of hypercoagulable state due to FVR506Q mutation. *Semin Thromb Hemost* 1999; 25:273–289.

Dahlback B, Carlsson M, Svensson PJ. Familial thrombophilia due to a previously unrecognized mechanism characterized by poor anticoagulant response to activated protein C: prediction of a cofactor to activated protein C. *Proc Natl Acad Sci USA* 1993;90:1004–1008.

Kearon C, Gent M, Hirsh J, et al. A comparison of three months of anticoagulation with extended anticoagulation for a first episode of idiopathic venous thromboembolism. *N Engl J Med* 1999;340:901–907.

Kitchens CS. Disseminated intravascular coagulation. *Curr Opin Hematol* 1995;2: 402–406.

Liebman HA, Carfagno MK, Weitz IC, et al. Excessive fibrinolysis in amyloidosis associated with elevated plasma single-chain urokinase. *Am J Clin Pathol* 1992;98: 534–541.

Lockshin MD. Antiphospholipid antibody: nabies, blood clots, biology. *JAMA* 1997; 227:1549–1551.

Mann KG, van't Veer C, Cawthern K, et al. The role of the tissue factor pathway in initiation of coagulation. *Blood Coagul Fibrinolysis* 1998;9:S3–S7.

17. TRANSFUSION: BLOOD AND BLOOD COMPONENTS

Jerome L. Gottschall and Jay E. Menitove

General Considerations

Blood transfusion practices are slowly but steadily improving as greater physician awareness and new and safer products advance the field. Improved donor screening methods, better infectious disease tests, and continued attention to the risk versus benefits of transfusion help achieve this progress. Recent declines in the use of red cell and fresh frozen plasma (FFP) have recently reversed themselves to the point that there are now spotted blood shortages in the United States. Platelet transfusions continue to increase in response to more aggressive transplantation and oncology approaches. Despite concerns about the safety of blood and the institution of a number of new therapies, the need for an adequate and safe blood supply is greater than it has ever been (1).

Blood Donation

Blood bank regulations and guidelines are designed to deter donations from persons at risk of an adverse medical event following donation and to prevent donation of blood that may pose a risk to others. A donation of approximately 450 mL of whole blood may be made as often as every 8 weeks. Donation intervals for apheresis donors vary. Before donating blood, donors are asked a series of health history questions and questioned about behaviors that place them at risk for transfusion-transmitted infections such as hepatitis and human immunodeficiency virus (HIV). In addition, blood bank procedures require testing for hepatitis B surface antigen (HBsAg); antibodies against hepatitis C; HIV-1; HIV-2; human T-lymphotrophic viruses (HTLV-I, HTLV-II); hepatitis B core antigen; and a serologic test for syphilis. A new research test, nucleic acid testing (NAT), is now being performed on all blood donations for hepatitis C and HIV. This test is intended to shorten the window between infectivity and positivity to the standard serologic tests. A registry of deferred donors (i.e., a list of donors who are not eligible to donate because of medical history findings or laboratory test results) is used to prevent the collection or distribution of unsuitable units of blood. Following donation, whole blood is separated by centrifugation into various components, including red blood cells (RBCs, packed cells); platelet concentrates; FFP; and cryoprecipitate.

Autologous donation involves collection and subsequent reinfusion of a patient's own blood. The blood is obtained in three forms:

1. **Preoperative blood donation.** Optimally, preoperative collections should begin at least 2 weeks before a scheduled surgical procedure and can be repeated every 3 days, provided the patient's hemoglobin level remains above 11 g per deciliter. Patients scheduled for elective orthopedic and cardiovascular surgery are those most likely to benefit from autologous predonation. Only patients who would routinely have blood crossmatched for their surgical procedure should predeposit autologous blood. This is done to decrease the amount of autologous blood that is collected and not transfused. Recent national trends indicate a decrease in preoperative autologous blood donations.

2. **Perioperative blood salvage.** This procedure involves blood collected at the time of surgery. This blood then is anticoagulated, washed using semiautomated equipment, and reinfused or returned to the patient unwashed. Cell salvage is not performed if the operative field is contaminated with tumor or bacteria. Postoperative cell salvage involves the collection of defibrinated blood collected through catheters inserted into joint spaces, the mediastinum, and so on, that is filtered and reinfused.

3. **Normovolemic hemodilution.** Blood is removed immediately before surgery with simultaneous infusion of crystalloid or colloid solutions to replenish intravascular volume. Following surgery, the removed blood is reinfused. Use of intraoperative hemodilution is a growing procedure and one that is likely to be combined in the future with blood substitutes.

A **directed or designated donation** involves donors chosen by the patient, such as a family member or friends. Available data indicate that these donations, in general, are no safer than those provided by altruistically motivated volunteer donors.

Apheresis donations are expected to increase because of the ability to collect more than one type of product from one donation process. There is a growing trend to collect a number of blood products by the use of an apheresis technique using blood cell separators. Certain donors can now donate 2 U of RBCs by apheresis techniques and then will be deferred for 16 weeks instead of the normal 8 weeks. Apheresis technology allows the collection of a red cell and a platelet product at the same donation. This same technique allows collection of plasma as a separate product or in combination with a red cell or platelet product. In addition, one of the greatest uses of the apheresis technique using blood cell separators is the collection of a platelet concentrate containing a therapeutic dose of platelets obtained from a single donor. These products are donated as plateletpheresis or single-donor platelets (SDPs). If the donor was selected because his or her human leukocyte antigen (HLA) type was similar to that of the patient, the SDP is considered to be HLA matched. Cell separators also are used to collect granulocytes for transfusion by leukopheresis techniques and can be used in the collection of peripheral blood stem cells for autologous transplant and as a growing trend in allogeneic transplantation.

Expiration of Stored Blood Components
The basis of blood storage resolves around the anticoagulant-preservative solution, citrate, phosphate, dextrose (CPD), and the variations on this product. Citrate acts as the anticoagulant and the phosphate–dextrose as the preservative solution. Depending on the anticoagulant preservative solution used, RBCs may be stored for 21, 35, or 42 days at 1 to 6°C; whole blood may be stored for 21 or 35 days. Anticoagulant preservative solutions that contain dextrose, mannitol, and adenine in 100 mL of saline that can be added to the red cells extend the dating period to 42 days. Once added, these solutions reduce the hematocrit of the red cells to approximately 55% while improving flow characteristics similar to that of whole blood. RBCs or whole blood that is subjected to γ irradiation to prevent posttransfusion graft-versus-host disease has a limited shelf life of a maximum of 28 days after the irradiation but no longer than the originally assigned expiration date. Depending on the plastic container used to store platelet concentrates, the dating period of room temperature–stored random donor platelets varies between 72 hours and 5 days. Plateletpheresis components are stored at room temperature for either 24 hours or up to 5 days. Granulocyte concentrates are generally stored at room temperature for up to 24 hours. FFP and cryoprecipitate are stored at –18°C or colder for 1 year.

Effects of Storage on Blood Components
During the storage of RBCs, the pH, adenosine triphosphate (ATP), and 2,3-diphosphoglycerate (2, 3-DPG) levels fall. Plasma potassium levels increase, so that at the end of expiration, there is approximately a total of 8 to 10 mEq of potassium in each red cell product. Plasma hemoglobulin levels also increase slightly during storage but do not give the plasma a pinkish tinge. Posttransfusion hemoglobinuria does not occur as a result of hemolysis during storage. Irradiated RBCs have plasma potassium levels that are approximately 1.5 to 2 times higher than nonirradiated units. 2, 3-DPG levels decrease significantly during storage falling to 50% of initial levels by 7 days. Restoration of 2, 3-DPG occurs within 7 hours of transfusion. The most significant impact of platelets stored for 5 days is a slight increased risk of bacterial contamination as bacteria proliferate during storage. FFP has approximately normal levels of all coagulation factors, including the labile factors V and VIII.

Determination of Compatibility

Compatibility testing is performed for whole blood and RBC transfusions but not for FFP, cryoprecipitate, or platelet transfusion. FFP should be ABO compatible with the recipient's RBCs. In general, platelet concentrates should be ABO compatible, although it is not always possible to provide the product this way. Granulocyte concentrates contain RBCs and require compatibility testing.

Tests Performed

The ABO and Rh type is determined on both the patient's blood sample and the donor unit. The patient's serum is tested for the presence of "unexpected" RBC alloantibodies as part of the compatibility test called the *antibody screen*. It is important to determine whether unexpected alloantibodies are present because such antibodies may result in red cell hemolysis following transfusion.

Determination of Compatibility

Compatibility testing involves determining donor and recipient ABO and Rh types, performing the antibody screen for "unexpected" red cell alloantibodies and doing an actual cross-match between recipient serum and donor RBCs. In addition, all clerical and documentation procedures to ensure the blood will go to the correct patient must be complete. Blood is released for transfusion if the compatibility testing demonstrates that ABO and Rh types are compatible, no unexpected antibodies are present, and ABO incompatibility is not demonstrated. If "unexpected" alloantibodies are present, RBCs are selected that lack the antigen that the unexpected alloantibody is directed against. In a "STAT" administration situation, a fully cross-matched unit of blood can be ready to send to the floor in approximately 45 minutes from the time blood samples are received in the blood bank.

Options Available for Providing Blood in Emergency Situations

If blood is needed urgently in an acute emergency, type O RBCs (universal donor), usually Rh(D) negative, may be used prior to determining the patient's ABO type. Type-specific RBCs may be provided after the patient's ABO and Rh type are determined on a concurrent blood sample prior to the completion of the compatibility testing. As a general rule, approximately 1% of hospitalized patients and 10% of multiple transfused patients have alloantibodies (2). The physician ordering emergency blood must consider the possible benefit of transfusion against the risk of infusion of potentially incompatible blood. During emergency situations, as in all other situations, meticulous attention to proper identification of the attended recipient and proper labeling of the tube of blood obtained for compatibility testing is essential.

General Principles for Issuing and Transfusing Blood and Components

Identification

Before a unit of blood or component is released from the blood bank laboratory, a careful check is done to ensure that all the current tests were performed accurately. In addition, a check is done to ensure that any transfusion requirements (i.e., irradiation, leukoreduction) have been identified and the unit appropriately handled. At the bedside, positive identification of the recipient and the identification information on the blood container are required to ensure that the information identified on the container refers to the intended recipient. Most major hemolytic transfusion reactions occur because of a clerical error involving misidentification of a patient or the unit of blood assigned to the patient (3).

Equipment

Blood and components should be infused through a 19-gauge or larger needle; 23-gauge needles may be used for pediatric patients, however. All components must pass through a filter (routinely used filters have a pore size of approximately 170 µm).

Addition of Drugs and Solutions

Drugs or medications should not be added to the blood components. Normal saline may be added, however. Other solutions intended for intravenous use may be added provided they are approved for this use by the Food and Drug Administration (FDA) or documentation shows addition of the solution is safe and efficacious.

Infusion Rate

The infusion rate depends on the clinical situation. Routinely, one unit of red cells is infused over 2 to 3 hours but should not exceed 4 hours. If the patient's condition is such that more time is needed, some institutions will divide the unit into aliquots. If circulatory overload is a concern, the infusion rate of all blood products must be carefully monitored in association with the patient's clinical condition. Granulocyte transfusions should be infused within 4 hours. Cryoprecipitate must be infused within 6 hours of thawing or within 4 hours if the units are pooled.

Administration
Infusion of blood should start slowly at 5 mL per minute or less for the first 15 minutes. The patient should be observed closely throughout the transfusion with special emphasis during the early part of the transfusion. Severe reactions frequently occur within the first 50 mL of transfusion. If no complications occur, the flow can be increased. The same blood filter should not be used for more than 4 hours.

Blood Warmers
Blood warmers are indicated to decrease the risk of arrhythmias and cardiac arrest associated with rapid, massive infusion of cold blood. They also are used during exchange transfusion and in some patients with cold agglutinin disease. Blood should be warmed in conjunction with an approved warming device and should not be warmed to temperatures that cause hemolysis. Warmers must have an audible and visual alarm system. Blood that has been warmed but not used must be discarded. Blood bags must not be held under hot tap water, immersed in unmonitored water baths or heated in microwave ovens.

Blood Components
Whole Blood
  1. **Composition:** Whole blood contains RBCs, plasma proteins, stable clotting factors (reduced factor V and factor VIII) and 70 mL of anticoagulant-preservative solution. The hematocrit is approximately 35% to 40%. Platelets and granulocytes are nonviable. The dating period is 21 or 35 days, depending on the anticoagulant-preservative solution.
  2. **Indications:** Whole blood is indicated for patients who have a need for both oxygen-carrying capacity and intravascular volume replacement. It can be used in the setting of massive transfusion (*trauma*) and in surgical settings where blood loss is expected to be large, as in liver transplantation, and can be used in the setting of exchange transfusion.
  3. **Dose and infusion rate:** The dose and infusion rate depend on the clinical situation and are prescribed to stabilize the hemodynamic status.
  4. **Expected outcome:** The symptoms of decreased intravascular volume and anemia are expected to resolve. The hemoglobin and hematocrit levels may fluctuate in relationship to fluid shifts. In nonbleeding patients, 1 U of whole blood should increase the hematocrit by 3% and the hemoglobin by 1 g per deciliter.

Red Blood Cells
  1. **Composition:** Currently, the vast majority of RBCs are prepared from whole blood by centrifugation and supplemented with an additive solution containing 100 mL of saline and additional dextrose and adenine. The final hematocrit is about 55%, and the storage period is 42 days. The volume of RBCs with additive solutions is approximately 300 to 350 mL (55–64 g of hemoglobin). RBCs also can be collected in CPD or CPDA-1 anticoagulant preservative solutions that give them a 21- to 35-day expiration period. These products can have an approximate 250-mL volume and a hemocrit between 65% and 80% (55–64 g of hemoglobin).
  2. **Indications:** RBC transfusions are indicated when there is a need to increase oxygen-carrying capacity in anemic patients without a need for volume expansion. Such patients may have signs and symptoms of tachycardia, shortness of breath, pallor, fatigue, syncope, postural hypotension, angina, or cerebral hypoxia in conjunction with low hemoglobin–hematocrit levels. In the past, clinicians used a "transfusion trigger" or preset hemoglobin levels for determining the need for transfusion. This approach has been replaced by an emphasis on transfusion avoidance in the absence of signs or symptoms attributable to anemia. Transfusion is deferred until compensatory mechanisms become insufficient to alleviate the signs and symptoms of anemia. Patients with diseases that would respond to iron, vitamin B_{12}, folate, or in selected cases, erythropoietin

should be prescribed these medications before transfusion unless the patient's condition is unstable. Most patients generally tolerate hemoglobin concentrations of 7 to 9 g per deciliter without the need for transfusion. In some patients with cardiovascular disease, significant pulmonary disease, or cerebral vascular insufficiency or in some elderly patients, symptoms develop at higher hemoglobin levels (4–6).

3. **Dose and infusion rate:** The dose and infusion are determined by the clinical situation. In a stable setting, 1 U of blood is administered over 2 to 4 hours.

4. **Expected outcomes:** Symptoms of anemia should resolve following transfusion. The hematocrit should increase by 3% and the hemoglobin by 1 g per deciliter in non-bleeding adult patients for each unit of blood infused.

Leukocyte-reduced Red Blood Cells

1. **Composition:** At present, filtration is the most efficient method for removing leukocytes from RBCs. Adhesion or "third-generation" leukocyte reduction filters remove at least 99.9% of the leukocytes contained in RBC components. Prestorage (shortly after blood collection) is the growing method of producing leukocyte-reduced RBCs because this appears to provide the most reproducible quality product. Less efficient methods for removing leukocytes includes, bedside filtration, centrifugation, washing, or freezing RBCs and subsequently washing them. Leukocyte-reduced red cell components should contain at least 85% of the original red cells and should have a final leukocyte content of less than 5×10^6 white blood cells (WBC). Hypotensive reactions have been reported following infusion of blood passed through bedside leuko-reduction filters among patients receiving angiotensin-converting enzyme inhibitors.

2. **Indications:** Leukocyte-reduced RBCs have three clear indications: (a) prevention of nonhemolytic febrile transfusion reactions; (b) reduction in the occurrence of alloimmunization against HLA antigens in patients receiving multiple transfusions, such as those with acute leukemia or aplastic anemia (this was recently demonstrated in a large multicenter randomized, prospective, blinded study in the United States); and (c) prevention of posttransfusion cytomegalovirus (CMV) infection. It is apparent that CMV can reside in the leukocyte, and prevention of transmission of this virus by blood was demonstrated in multiple small studies and in a recent two-center study in the United States using leukocyte-reduced blood products. There is a growing trend in the United States toward "universal" prestorage leukocyte reduction of all blood products (7–9).

3. The **dose and infusion rate** are similar to that of RBC transfusions.

4. The **expected outcome** is similar to that of RBC transfusions in terms of providing oxygen-carrying content.

Washed Red Blood Cells

1. **Composition:** Washed RBCs are prepared by adding normal saline to RBCs or by using semiautomated machines to wash cells with saline and remove almost all the plasma; 90% to 99% of the residual leukocytes are removed by this process. The RBC volume is approximately 250 mL with a residual hematocrit of approximately 65% to 80% (55–64 g of hemoglobin) with the product being suspended in saline rather than plasma.

2. **Indications:** Plasma and plasma proteins, including immunoglobulin A (IgA), are implicated in the etiology of allergic and anaphylactic reactions. Because washing removes plasma, saline-washed red cells are used for patients with symptomatic anemia in whom prevention of recurrence of severe urticarial, allergic, or anaphylactic reactions is necessary.

3. The **dose and infusion rate** are similar to that of RBC transfusions.

4. The **expected outcome** is similar to that of RBC transfusions.

Frozen, Deglycerolized Red Blood Cells

1. **Composition:** In the presence of a cryoprotective agent, RBCs may be stored in the frozen state for up to 10 years at a temperature of at least –65°C. Following thawing, the cryoprotective agent is removed by saline washing and the product resuspended in normal saline.

2. **Indications:** Frozen RBCs are included in repositories of "rare" RBC units and are intended for patients who have alloantibodies directed against high-frequency red

cell antigens or who have multiple alloantibodies. Blood collected for autologous purposes, but not used because the surgical procedure is postponed, may be frozen as a means of extending the dating period.

3. The **dose and infusion rate** are similar to that of RBC transfusions.

4. The **expected outcome** is similar to that of RBC transfusions.

Irradiated RBCs

1. **Composition:** RBCs and other cellular components (i.e., platelet concentrates) are subjected to a minimum of 2,500 cGy gamma irradiation and are considered to be irradiated. RBCs may be stored for up to 28 days after irradiation but no longer than the original "expiration" date.

2. **Indications:** RBCs are irradiated with 2,500 cGy gamma irradiation to prevent posttransfusion graft versus host disease. Patients who are significantly immunosuppressed may be at risk for graft versus host disease following transfusion. Such patients include, but are not limited to, bone marrow transplant patients, both allogeneic and autologous; patients treated with high-dose chemotherapy such as acute leukemias, other malignant states treated with chemotherapy, patients with Hodgkin or non-Hodgkin lymphoma, congenital immunodeficiency disorders, low-birth-weight neonates; and those receiving intrauterine transfusion. Because of the rare occurrence of posttransfusion graft versus host disease when a blood relative donates as a directed donation, such units also are irradiated. Once the decision is made to irradiate blood products, all cellular blood products should be irradiated (10,11).

3. The **dose and infusion rate** are similar to that of RBC transfusion.

4. The expected outcome is similar to that of RBC transfusions.

Platelets

1. **Composition**

- **Random-donor platelets (RDPs):** Platelet concentrates are prepared by separating platelets from a single unit of whole blood so that a minimum of 5.5×10^{10} platelets are suspended in approximately 50 mL of plasma (1 U). Platelets should be separated from whole blood within 8 hours of collection. Depending on the container in which RDPs are stored, the shelf life varies from 3 to 5 days when stored at room temperature.

- **Pheresis–apheresis platelets** or single-donor platelets (SDPs): Platelets collected by apheresis techniques from a single donor, using blood cell separators, contain a minimum of 3.0×10^{11} platelets suspended in 200 to 400 ml of plasma. Apheresis platelets have a shelf life ranging from 24 hours to 5 days and are stored at room temperature. These products account for most platelet transfusions in the United States.

- **HLA-matched platelet concentrates:** If the donor of an apheresis platelet concentrate is selected because the donor's HLA type is matched to the recipient's HLA type (due to the development of alloimmunization to HLA antigens), the apheresis platelet product is considered to be an HLA-matched platelet component.

2. **Indications:** Use of platelet transfusions is indicated to control active bleeding or to prevent hemorrhage associated with a deficiency in platelet number or function. Platelets are used prophylactically to prevent bleeding when the platelet count is less than 10,000 to 20,000 per microliter in patients with hematologic malignancies or who are receiving chemotherapy. Patients who are undergoing minor surgical procedures or having a line placement may require the platelet count to be greater than 50,000 per microliter. Patients undergoing major surgical procedures may require platelet counts greater than 75,000 per microliter and those having neurosurgical procedures or eye procedures may require platelet counts greater than 100,000 prior to the procedure. There is a growing trend to reduce the prophylactic platelet transfusion "trigger" to counts as low as 5,000 to 10,000 per microliter in stable patients without significant hemorrhage (12–14).

- **RDPs and SDPs.** The indications for RDPs and SDPs are similar, that is, to control or prevent bleeding associated with thrombocytopenia or platelet dysfunction. As demonstrated in a recent multiinstitutional national trial, the incidence of refractoriness is similar when using either RDPs or SDPs in patients. Leukocyte reduction decreases the occurrence of alloimmunization.

- **HLA-matched platelets** obtained from single donors by apheresis techniques are used for patients who have an immunologic basis for refractoriness to platelet transfusion. That is, these patients develop no rise in platelet count following transfusion of platelets because of the development of antibodies to HLA antigens, and the use of HLA matched platelets may provide a significant benefit in this clinical setting. These platelets should not be used for patients considered refractory because of pathophysiologic processes (e.g., fever, sepsis, disseminated intravascular coagulation) (8,15).
- **Dose and infusion rate: RDPs.** The average adult platelet concentrate dose is one unit of RDP per 12 kilograms of body weight. There is a growing trend in the United States to define a standard "dose" of platelet concentrates. This standard varies among different institutions from 4 U, 6 U, or 8 U of platelet concentrates to be infused per transfusion episode. Platelet units usually are pooled into one bag by the transfusion service prior to issue. They should be infused within 4 hours at a rate that depends on the patient's ability to tolerate the volume. RDPs may be "volume reduced"; that is, the pooled RDPs undergo centrifugation that allow separation of platelets from the platelet poor plasma. Excess platelet poor plasma is removed, and the therapeutic dose then is concentrated into approximately 100 mL. Volume-reduced platelets are infused more rapidly than nonvolume-reduced platelets and must be infused within 4 hours of pooling.
- **Pheresis platelet-SDPs.** One SDP concentrate is considered a therapeutic dose, equivalent to 6 units of RDP. SDPs should be infused as rapidly as possible, depending on the patient's ability to tolerate the infused volume.
- **HLA-matched platelets.** The dose and infusion rate are similar to those of SDPs.

3. **Expected outcome:** Platelet transfusions should result in prevention or resolution of bleeding caused by thrombocytopenia or platelet dysfunction. As a general rule, platelet counts should be obtained 18 to 24 hours postinfusion. The average-sized adult who receives 1 U of RDP per 12 kg of body weight or one SDP dose should have a posttransfusion platelet increment of 30,000 to 50,000 µL. Patients who have smaller or no increment at 18 to 24 hours postinfusion should have platelet counts performed 10 to 60 minutes after the next platelet transfusion. If the 10- to 60-minute posttransfusion increment is minimal or not increased at all, the possibility of refractoriness caused by alloimmunization should be entertained. The patient then should be considered for HLA-matched platelet transfusions or crossmatched platelet concentrates. Poor posttransfusion platelet survival, in addition to being caused by alloimmunization, is often seen in conjunction with fever, sepsis, disseminated intravascular coagulation, and others. Patients in these settings are considered to be refractory on a nonimmunologic basis and are not expected to benefit from HLA-matched platelet transfusions. Patients who have life-threatening hemorrhage or who are bleeding following a major surgical procedure in association with thrombocytopenia may require larger platelet doses to be therapeutic. Currently, controversy is growing in the United States as to whether patients requiring prophylactic platelet transfusions would benefit more from repetitive small-dose platelet transfusions or be better off using extra high-dose platelet transfusions. Randomized, well-controlled studies to answer this issue have not yet been done (16).

4. **Special considerations:** Before the decision to transfused platelets is made, the underlying cause of thrombocytopenia should be considered:
- **Thrombocytopenia secondary to bone marrow failure.** The patients most likely to benefit from platelet transfusion are those who are thrombocytopenic on the basis of marrow failure as a result of chemotherapy, radiation therapy, or a myelophthisic condition.
- **Thrombocytopenia secondary to platelet destruction.** Patients who are thrombocytopenic because platelets are destroyed or consumed (e.g., idiopathic thrombocytopenic purpura, drug-induced immune thrombocytopenia, thrombotic thrombocytopenic purpura, and posttransfusion purpura) should not receive platelet transfusions unless there is a life-threatening hemorrhage. The recovery and survival of infused platelets are diminished in these conditions. Some physicians consider the use of platelet transfusions in the setting of thrombotic thrombocytopenic purpura a relative contraindication due to the potential of an adverse effect.

- **Thrombocytopenia secondary to an enlarged spleen.** In normal persons, approximately one third of endogenous platelets are sequestered or pooled in the spleen. In patients with splenomegaly, the percentage of sequestered platelets may be extremely high. These patients are unlikely to see as great an increase in the platelet increment following transfusion because most of the infused platelets will be sequestered in the spleen.
- **Dilutional thrombocytopenia.** Some patients who receive massive transfusions develop dilutional thrombocytopenia, that is, platelets are lost with hemorrhage and are not replaced by red cell or whole blood transfusions that are devoid of viable platelets. In these patients, platelet transfusions may be required to elevate platelet counts and to help maintain hemostasis.
- **ABO compatibility.** A and B antigens are expressed on platelet surface. It is preferable to provide platelet transfusions from donors whose ABO types are compatible with the recipient. When ABO-compatible platelets are not available (e.g., inventory considerations), ABO-incompatible platelet transfusions are provided. The posttransfusion platelet increment may be lower when ABO-incompatible platelets are given compared with ABO-compatible platelets. If the plasma is ABO incompatible with the patient, volume-reduced platelet transfusions should be considered because hemolytic reactions have been reported infrequently when blood group A or B patients have received group O platelets containing anti-A or Anti-B in the plasma (17).
- **Rh compatibility.** Rh antigens are not present on the platelet surface but are present on the trace amounts of red cells that contaminate platelet concentrates. For this reason, Rh-compatible platelet concentrates are always given to female children or women of childbearing age. Administration of Rh immune globulin should be considered for Rh-negative patients who receive platelets from Rh-positive donors, especially female children or women capable of childbearing.

Fresh Frozen Plasma

1. **Composition:** FFP is plasma that is separated from whole blood and frozen within 8 hours of collection and has normal levels of all clotting factors and anticoagulants. Three different types of FFP are available for transfusion: (a) Standard FFP is as just described. (b) Donor-retested FFP is plasma that is donated, frozen, and stored for 112 days. The donor then returns, and if all infectious disease testing is still negative, the original unit is released into the inventory. Donor-retested plasma has the value of closing the window period for the infectious diseases that are currently tested for [HIV, hepatitis C virus (HCV)]. (c) Pooled solvent detergent-treated plasma is frozen, and plasma has been sent to a commercial company to be treated by a solvent detergent process that will prevent the transmission of envelope viruses (i.e., HIV, HCV). The value of this product is that it will prevent transmission of any envelope virus by blood transfusion. It is a pooled product, and recipients are exposed to 1,500 to 2,500 donors with each transfusion of a unit of frozen plasma.

2. **Indications:** FFP is indicated to replenish clotting factors in patients with demonstrated deficiencies [i.e., prothrombin time or partial thromboplastin time greater than 1.5 times normal, international normalized ratio (INR) >1.6]. FFP is most commonly used in the setting of acquired coagulopathy, such as in patients with liver disease, DIC, or excess warfarin effect. FFP can reverse the effects of warfarin in patients who are actively bleeding or require emergency surgery and cannot wait the approximate 12 hours for vitamin K to become effective. FFP is also used to treat patients who are receiving massive blood transfusions and who have laboratory evidence of a dilutional coagulopathy. FFP is the preferred replacement fluid for patients undergoing therapeutic plasma exchange therapy for thrombotic thrombocytopenic purpura. Recent evidence suggests that FFP may provide a metalloprotease that is deficient in patients with thrombotic thrombocytopenic purpura. Cryo-poor plasma is a FFP variant in which the cryoprecipitable fraction [containing von Wilebrand factor (vWF) multimers] is removed. This product also has been used to treat patients with thrombotic thrombocytopenic purpura (TTP) (18,19).

3. **Dose and infusion rate:** The average adult dose is determined by the clinical situation and the underlying disease process. It is reasonable to administer plasma at

a dose of 10 to 15 mL per kilogram of body weight (2–4 U of FFP) followed by laboratory evaluation to determine responsiveness and to decide the interval between doses. The infusion rate is determined on the basis of the patient's clinical need and hemodynamic status. Plasma does not contain red cells, and therefore, cross-matching is not required. The ABO type of the donor should be compatible with the recipient. FFP is thawed at 37°C and must be transfused with 24 hours of thawing if used for coagulation factor replacement. Plasma can be thawed and maintained in the refrigerated state for up to 5 days, but there is some loss of coagulation factor V and a greater decrease in factor VIII.

4. **Expected outcomes:** Improvement of coagulation factor deficiency is expected as assessed by the prothrombin time (INR), partial thromboplastin time, or specific factor assays. Clinical improvement for most patients with TTP is expected.

Cryoprecipitate

1. **Composition:** Each bag of cryoprecipitate is prepared from 1 U of whole blood; the volume varies from 5 to 20 mL per bag. Each bag contains more than 80 U of factor VIII, vWF, more than 150 mg of fibrinogen, small amounts of factor XIII and fibronectin.

2. **Indications:** Cryoprecipitate is the only available source of fibrinogen in a concentrated form. At present, the major indication for the use of cryoprecipitate is fibrinogen replacement. The other significant use of cryoprecipitate is as fibrin sealant in certain surgical procedures. Cryoprecipitate is no longer used to treat patients with hemophilia A because new and safer factor VIII concentrates are available. Many physicians now treat von Willebrand's disease with factor VIII concentrates that contain high amounts of vWF and no longer use cryoprecipitate as the standard treatment. These concentrates have superseded the cryoprecipitate because they are subjected to viral inactivation procedures and are therefore safer products.

3. **Dose and infusion rate.** The dose is calculated on the basis of plasma volume. Most patients with fibrinogen levels of more than 125 mg per deciliter have an adequate amount of fibrinogen to form clot. Patients with fibrinogen levels below this may require fibrinogen replacement through the use of cryoprecipitate, depending on the clinical situation. In general, a dose of approximately 12 bags of cryoprecipitate should result in an increment of about 100 mg per deciliter of fibrinogen in a 70-kg adult. Cryoprecipitate usually is infused as rapidly as the patient's status can tolerate as determined by assessment of the hemodynamic status. Because the volume of plasma is small and no RBCs are present, compatibility testing is not required. Plasma ABO compatibility is preferred but not essential. Cryoprecipitate should be infused within 6 hours of the time it is thawed.

4. **Expected outcome:** Correction or prevention of bleeding is desired. Laboratory assessment of fibrinogen levels prior to infusion should be determined and then post-fibrinogen levels should again be ascertained to determine the effectiveness of therapy and the need and timing of future doses.

Granulocyte Transfusions

1. **Composition:** Granulocyte transfusions are obtained by apheresis technique and should contain a minimum of 1×10^{10} granulocytes. In the past, obtaining this number of granulocytes rarely resulted in an increment in the granulocyte count following transfusion and may have represented an inadequate dose of granulocytes for the clinical indications. Recently, using corticosteroids to stimulate the donor or a combination of steroids and granulocyte colony-stimulating factor (G-CSF) prior to apheresis technique has resulted in the ability to collect three to five times the number of granulocytes previously obtained. This has allowed for a significant rise in the granulocyte count following transfusion and possible greater survival of the granulocytes. Granulocyte concentrates also contain lymphocytes and RBCs. The presence of the RBCs necessitates that granulocyte transfusions undergo red cell cross-matching prior to infusion. The volume ranges from 200 to 400 mL (20).

2. **Indications:** Granulocyte transfusions are used infrequently because antibiotic therapy or G-CSF and granulocyte macrophage–colony-stimulating factor (GM-CSF) are effective in treating or preventing infectious complications associated with neutropenia. In general, granulocyte transfusion should be restricted to patients who have

an absolute granulocyte count of less than 500 per microliter, documented sepsis, or serious infection that is not responding to antibiotic therapy, and is expected to have a long period of neutropenia. The recent collection of high-dose granulocytes by using steroids or G-CSF have significant promise, but no large randomized, controlled trials have been done to demonstrate their effectiveness.

3. **Dose and infusion rate:** Granulocyte transfusions, prepared by apheresis technique, should be infused daily until no longer needed. They should be irradiated with 2500 cGy gamma irradiation. Granulocyte transfusions should be infused slowly over 1 to 4 hours. Premedication with antihistamines, acetaminophen, corticosteroids, or meperidine may be needed to prevent adverse reactions. If the patient is immunologically refractory to platelet transfusions, consideration should be given to obtaining granulocytes from HLA-matched donors. Because of a perceived adverse interaction between the infusion of granulocytes and amphotericin B therapy (acute pulmonary distress), granulocyte transfusions should be separated by a minimum of 4 hours from the amphotericin B therapy.

4. **Expected outcome:** With the higher dose of granulocyte concentrates, the WBC count will increase following granulocyte transfusions in adults. The clinical endpoint is improvement or resolution of the infection. In patients who respond to granulocyte concentrates, transfusions should be continued until resolution of the infection has occurred or restoration of the patient's own granulocyte production occurs.

Plasma-Derived Volume Expanders (Albumin and Plasma Protein Fraction)

1. **Composition:** Albumin is available in 5% and 25% solutions. In both solutions, 96% of the total protein is albumin. Plasma protein fraction is available in a 5% solution, of which at least 83% of the protein is albumin and no more than 17% is globulin. Both these products are heated for at least 10 hours at 60°C to inactivate contaminating viruses.

2. **Indications:** There remains controversy about the use of crystalloid versus colloid solutions in volume resuscitation. The volume of crystalloid solutions is two to three times that of a 5%-albumin solution to provide equal hemodynamic improvement. Albumin and plasma protein fractions are infused when the need to restore intravascular volume is urgent; for example, for 24 hours after thermal injury, following large volume paracentesis, for inducing diuresis in patients with nephrotic syndrome, and for patients undergoing therapeutic plasma exchange procedures. A recent review of randomized controlled clinical trials for critically ill patients showed no improvement in outcome in patients receiving albumin and raised the question of whether albumin may be harmful and have an increased rate of mortality compared with the use of other products in this setting (21,22).

3. **Dose and infusion rate:** The average adult dose depends on the clinical situation. The infusion rate depends on the clinical setting and can be more rapid if volume expansion is urgently required. Compatibility testing is not required. Sterile water should not be used to dilute 25% albumin as hemolysis has been associated with this.

4. **Expected outcome:** The outcome depends on the clinical situation for which albumin is infused.

Factor VIII Concentrates

1. **Composition:** Lyophilized factor VIII concentrates are available from several pharmaceutical companies and are prepared by various techniques. Factor VIII concentrates prepared from human plasma are subject to viral inactivation treatments to reduce or prevent the transmission of envelope viruses such as hepatitis B, C, and HIV. Such treatment does not inactivate hepatitis A or parvovirus. Recently, recombinant factor VIII products have come onto the market and are replacing human-derived factor VIII concentrates for the treatment of hemophilia A. In particular, all new patients are being placed on recombinant factor VIII products instead of the human-derived products because of the expected safety from an infectious point of view. Several human-derived factor VIII concentrates also contain adequate amounts of vWF to treat patients with von Willebrand disease. These products contain a relatively normal distribution of the high-molecular-weight factor VIII multimers. The number of units of factor VIII contained in each vial of factor VIII concentrates is stated on the product label. This is also so for those products used to treat von Willebrand's disease (19).

2. **Indications:** Factor VIII concentrates are indicated for the treatment of hemophilia A (antihemophiliac factor deficiency). If they contain an adequate amount of vWF, they can be used in the treatment of von Willebrand's disease.

3. **Dose and infusion rate:** The amount of factor VIII required depends on whether the treatment is prophylactic or for active bleeding or if bleeding has occurred, the extent and site of bleeding. For example, approximately 30% to 40% factor VIII levels are recommended to treat hemorrhage in joints, and approximately 100% factor VIII levels are appropriate for patients undergoing major surgery or suffering central nervous system injury. Infusion of 1 U of factor VIII per kilogram of body weight increases the factor VIII level by 2%. The infusion should occur at a rate as fast as tolerated and should be repeated every 12 hours to maintain adequate factor VIII levels necessary for hemostasis. The duration of therapy depends on the clinical setting.

4. **Expected outcome:** Hemostasis should occur as a result of increased levels of factor VIII or vWF. Laboratory assays should be done to determine the adequacy of response and to calculate the timing of the next dose.

Factor IX Concentrates

1. **Composition:** Factor IX concentrate is now available as a recombinant factor IX product. It is also available as an intermediate purity prothrombin complex concentrate and in a recent new human-derived highly purified coagulation factor IX concentrate. Recombinant factor IX concentrates are the product of choice for newly diagnosed patients with hemophilia B and for any previous patient who wishes to use this product. The amount of factor IX contained in the concentrates is stated on the product label.

2. **Indications:** Factor IX concentrates are used to treat patients with factor IX deficiency (hemophilia B or Christmas disease) who require treatment for hemarthrosis or minor or significant bleeding disorders. Activated prothrombin complex concentrates (FEIBA and Autoplex) are available to treat hemophilic patients with inhibitors to factor VIII. The use of these concentrates for this indication is decreasing now that recombinant factor VIIa is available for such treatment (19).

3. **Dose and infusion rate:** The dose is calculated on basis of the site of bleeding and the clinical condition of the patient. In general, infusion of 1 U of factor IX per kilogram of body weight increases the factor IX level by 1%. The infusion rate should be as fast as tolerated. A slightly higher dose is needed when recombinant factor IX is infused.

4. **Expected outcome:** Hemostasis should occur, and laboratory testing should be performed to determine the postinfusion factor IX level when appropriate. This will help in determining the time and amount of the next dose.

Antithrombin-III (AT-III) Concentrates

1. **Composition:** Heat-treated preparations of human-derived AT-III, lyophilized concentrates are available.

2. **Indications:** AT-III concentrates are used for patients with hereditary AT-III deficiency in connection with surgical or obstetric procedures or for therapeutic use for thromboembolic events (23) because it serves as an important antithrombotic plasma protein.

3. **Dose and infusion rate:** The dose should be designed to achieve postinfusion AT-III levels of approximately 120%. Subsequent doses should maintain levels of 80% to 120% and will need to be determined by measuring AT-III levels at periodic intervals.

4. **Expected outcome:** Prevention of thrombosis or recurrence of thrombosis should occur. AT-III concentrates also have been used in patients with acquired AT-III deficiencies who may have DIC or resistance to heparin therapy from AT-III deficiency. The efficacy of using AT-III concentrates in these conditions is not firmly established.

Immune Globulins

1. **Composition:** Intravenous and intramuscular immune globulin preparations are available. They should contain at least 90% immunoglobulin G (IgG) with subclasses in physiologic ratios that both maintain biologic activity against a variety of infectious agents and fix complement.

2. **Indications:** Intramuscular preparations are given to provide passive immune protection and to treat hypogammaglobulinemia. Intravenous preparations have been

used to treat a large number of disorders. These disorders include primary immuno-deficiencies and immunodeficiency in the acquired immunodeficiency syndrome (AIDS), to reduce the incidence of CMV in patients undergoing various forms of transplanta-tion, for selected patients with Kawasaki syndrome, Guillain-Barré syndrome, immune thrombocytopenic purpura, posttransfusion purpura, neonatal alloimmune thrombo-cytopenic purpura, pure red cell aplasia caused by parvovirus infection, and other diseases (24).

3. **Dose and infusion rate:** The dose depends on the underlying condition. For pa-tients with immune thrombocytopenic purpura, intravenous immune globulins are ad-ministered at doses of 2 g per kilogram of body weight in divided doses over 2 to 5 days.

4. **Expected outcome:** The outcome depends on the clinical condition for which immunoglobulins are prescribed. Adverse effects associated with immunoglobulin therapy include anaphylactic reactions in IgA-deficient patients, pyrogenic reactions, facial flushing, headache, myalgia, chills, nausea, hypotension, and tachycardia. Several intravenous gamma globulin preparations have been recently associated with the development of renal failure.

Rh Immune Globulin

1. **Composition:** Rh immune globulin is a human derived product containing anti-D antibodies against the major antigenic determinant of the Rh system.

2. **Indications:** Rh immune globulin is used as a prophylactic measure against the development of anti-D-mediated hemolytic disease of newborns and prevention of isoimmunization associated with transfusion of red cell products, such as a platelet con-centrates from an Rh-positive donor to an Rh-negative patient. Preparations designed for intravenous use have been used to treat patients with idiopathic thrombocytopenic purpura. It is used in this setting in patients who are Rh positive. Rh immune globulin for treatment of idiopathic thrombocytopenic purpura is not effective in Rh-negative pa-tients or in previously splenectomized patients.

3. **Dose and infusion rate:** One vial of intramuscular Rh immune globulin is given to prevent isoimmunization from exposure up to 15 mL of RBCs. It is standard to treat Rh negative pregnant women with Rh immune globulin at 28 weeks and following de-livery of an Rh-positive infant. The standard dose at this time is 300 µg of Rh immune globulin. Rh immune globulin is also used in the setting of miscarriage or bleeding associated with pregnancy when there is concern that there may be fetal to maternal hemorrhage.

4. **Expected outcome:** The outcome depends on the condition for which treatment is given. It has an outstanding record in preventing Rh isoimmunization to the D antigen.

Recombinant Factor VIIa (rFVIIa)

1. **Composition:** rFVIIa is a recently licensed product containing a recombinant activated factor VII as a lyophilized product.

2. **Indications:** rFVIIa is indicated to treat patients with hemophilia who have de-veloped inhibitors. Although not licensed for any other indication, clinical studies using rFVIIa in other bleeding situations are ongoing (25).

3. **Dose and infusion rate:** The exact dose has not been determined for all clinical situations for patients with inhibitors. In general, however, 90 micrograms per kilogram of body weight has been highly effective in treating minor and major bleeding episodes in these patients. The product can be infused as rapidly as necessary and repeated doses are frequently necessary.

4. **Expected outcome:** The expected outcome is a decrease in bleeding in patients with inhibitors.

Fibrin Sealants

1. **Composition and indication.** A recent new fibrin sealant called Tisseel was re-cently approved to help control bleeding in certain surgical situations. Tisseel is a pooled human blood product whose active ingredient is fibrinogen. It is used as a "fib-rin glue" to stop oozing from small blood vessels during surgery. The product comes as a freeze-dried preparation (26) and is applied locally at the site of hemorrhage.

2. **Dose:** The required dose of Tisseel depends on the size of the surface to be sealed or the defect in the blood vessel that needs closing.

3. **Expected outcome:** The outcome is a reduction in bleeding from the area that the fibrin sealant is applied.

New Blood Products of the Future
Numerous research studies are using cellular blood products, in particular lymphocytes, to treat patients with malignancies and certain viral illnesses. These products are still in the research stage but may become important blood products of the future.

Several oxygen-carrying blood substitutes are currently in clinical trials. These are either stroma-free hemoglobin solutions or a compound called perfluorocarbons. Although none of these products is yet licensed for use in the United States, it is anticipated that within the next several years some of these blood substitutes may be licensed. They are currently being studied in a number of settings where blood had been the standard therapy, such as in orthopedic surgery, cardiovascular surgery, and preoperative hemodilution. If and when these products are licensed, it will be important to know the indications, limitations, and adverse events associated with their use.

Adverse Reactions Associated with Transfusion

Transfusion reactions can be classified as acute or delayed, immunologic or nonimmunologic. Great strides have been made over the last years in reducing the infectious complications of blood transfusion. It is important to remember that there are other serious, sometimes fatal, reactions associated with blood transfusions that are not related to infectious diseases. Prevention of such adverse events has not been as successful as those for many of the serious infectious adverse consequences of blood transfusions. Thus, the use of blood when clinically indicated is an extraordinarily important responsibility of the transfusing physician. Clinicians must be aware of the alternatives to allogeneic transfusion, such as autologous blood, intraoperative cell salvage, hemodilution, use of hematopoietic growth factors, and pharmacologic agents that foster hemostasis.

Acute Transfusion Reactions
Acute hemolytic transfusion reaction: These reactions, which are among the most serious acute complications of blood transfusion, occur with a frequency of approximately 1 in 600 to 1 per 25,0000 components infused. Death associated with acute hemolytic transfusion reaction is associated most commonly with ABO incompatible blood (3).

The **clinical presentation** of acute hemolytic transfusion reaction is as follows. Hemolysis may be intravascular or extravascular. Antibodies such as anti-A, anti-B, anti-Kell, anti-Kidd, and anti-Fy[a] are associated with intravascular hemolysis by having the ability to activate complement through C9. Antibodies against the Rh system, such as anti-D and anti-E, do not activate complement and are associated with extravascular hemolysis. Both intravascular and extravascular hemolysis may occur within the same hemolytic transfusion reaction episode. Fever, or fever accompanied by chills, is the most common symptom of a hemolytic transfusion reaction. Nausea, vomiting, chest pain, wheezing, dyspnea, back pain, restlessness, and discomfort along the infusion site are other symptoms that occur less often. The most serious consequences associated with a hemolytic transfusion reaction are hypotension, renal failure, and DIC. In the unconscious or anesthetized patient, acute hemolytic transfusion reactions may be characterized only by bleeding at the surgical incision site or hemoglobinuria. Cytokine generation is thought to play an important role in the pathogenesis of hemolytic reactions.

The **laboratory testing** is done immediately after a hemolytic reaction is suspected; the infusion must be stopped, the patient attended to, a blood sample has been obtained for laboratory testing, and the blood bank or transfusion service has been notified. The floor should do a clerical check to ensure that the proper unit of blood was given to the proper patient. The transfusion service will repeat this clerical check to confirm that the appropriate unit of blood was issued to the correct patient. Evidence of a hemolytic transfusion reaction is sought by repeating the ABO blood type on a pretransfusion and posttransfusion blood sample and comparing the color of the serum or plasma from a pretransfusion with a posttransfusion blood sample. The presence of a pink or red color (hemolysis) in the post sample compared with the presample is evidence of a transfusion reaction. In addition, a direct antiglobulin test is performed to determine whether transfused red cells have become coated with immunoglobulin. A urine sample also should be examined for the presence of hemoglobin. If, following all these tests and checks, a hemolytic reaction is suspected, additional testing should be done. This includes repeating the cross-match and doing additional blood work, such as plasma-free hemoglobin, serum haptoglobin, bilirubin and lactate dehydrogenase (LDH) levels. Serious hemolytic transfusion reactions are preventable if appropriate time is taken to give assiduous attention to identification of the blood samples, donor units, and recipient and proper care when laboratory testing is performed.

Treatment:
1. Stop the transfusion.
2. Keep the intravenous line open with 0.9% normal saline.
3. Report the reaction to the transfusion service.
4. Check identification of donor unit and patient at the bedside.
5. Initiate symptomatic treatment to correct hypotension, control bleeding, and prevent acute tubular necrosis. Systolic blood pressure should be maintained. A diuretic such as furosemide (40–120 mg administered intravenously) should be administered to stimulate urine flow. Mannitol (20 g in 100 mL infused over 5 minutes) also has been used. Urine output should be maintained at 100 mL per hour or greater. If oliguria or anuria occurs, standard therapy for renal failure should be undertaken. The role of cytokine altering agents in these situations is unclear at this time.
6. Send blood bag and administration set to transfusion service.
7. Collect blood and urine samples and send to the laboratory for testing.
8. Document the transfusion reaction on the patient's chart.

Febrile nonhemolytic reactions are characterized by a posttransfusion temperature rise of 1°C or more in the absence of hemolysis or other defined cause. Similar reactions with lesser or no rise in temperature have been associated with chills and rigors, particularly in association with platelet transfusions. These reactions occur with a frequency of approximately 0.5% or more per component transfused.

Clinical presentation: Patients having febrile nonhemolytic transfusion reactions generally are asymptomatic during the early to middle part of the blood transfusion. Symptoms begin to develop near the end of the transfusion or shortly after the transfusion and are characterized by a rise in diastolic blood pressure, headache, chills, rigors, followed by a rapid rise in temperature and leukocytosis. The association of chills and rigors with platelet transfusions without fever is a common finding. Although disconcerting to the patient, febrile reactions usually respond to symptomatic therapy.

Laboratory testing: These reactions are caused by alloantibodies against granulocytes, lymphocytes, or platelets. In addition, they are associated with an increase in various cytokines during the storage of platelet concentrates, which can result in febrile reactions. When a red cell product is associated with these symptoms, the most important intervention is to stop the transfusion and rule out the possibility of a hemolytic transfusion reaction, since fever is the most common symptom of a hemolytic transfusion reaction. In general, additional tests are not done to determine the presence of WBC antibodies and the diagnosis is made on the absence of evidence of hemolysis in association with the clinical findings.

Treatment and prevention: Because fever is the most frequent presenting sign of a hemolytic or nonhemolytic febrile reaction, a hemolytic reaction cannot be distinguished on clinical grounds alone. For this reason, transfusion must be stopped when fever or a shaking chill occurs and should not be restarted. Most febrile nonhemolytic reactions are self-limited and are treated with orally administered antipyretics. Prevention of febrile reactions is accomplished by removing the WBCs from the blood product because many of these reactions are associated with antibodies against the transfused leukocytes. This is best accomplished by providing the patient with prestorage leukocyte-reduced blood products. At present, random donor platelet concentrates are not leukocyte-reduced until the time of the order for the product. This means they may have the ability to develop increased levels of cytokines associated with chill–rigor, febrile reactions; leukocyte reduction will not prevent these reactions. Pheresis platelets are generally leukocyte reduced at the time of collection and therefore usually not associated with cytokine reactions (7, 27).

Transfusion-related acute lung injury: This condition is characterized by the development of pulmonary infiltrates and noncardiogenic pulmonary edema. It is thought to occur as a result of passively transferred donor antibodies that react against recipient leukocyte antigens. This is an uncommon adverse transfusion event but one that many physicians are not aware of and may attribute to other causes.

Clinical presentation: Patients manifest fever, substernal chest pain, dyspnea, cyanosis, cough, blood-tinged sputum, and hypoxemia 1 to 4 hours after transfusion of whole blood, RBCs, FFP, platelet concentrates, or even cryoprecipitate. The heart size is normal, but bilateral diffuse pulmonary infiltrates are seen on chest radiographs. Left atrial and pulmonary wedge pressures are within normal limits and may even be low.

Treatment and prevention. Patients may require respiratory support and mechanical ventilation. Recovery usually occurs within 48 hours. Rarely, pulmonary edema is sufficient to result in intravascular hypovolemia and hypotension. If this occurs, patients will require fluid replacement rather than fluid restriction. Recurrence is prevented by identifying donors with antibodies leading to this complication and restricting future use of their blood (28).

Allergic reactions: These reactions range from urticaria and pruritus to severe anaphylactic reactions. Mild reactions may occur in as many as 1% to 3% of transfused patients, and severe reactions occur at a rate of approximately 1 in 150,000 components transfused.

Clinical presentation: Urticaria and pruritus occur without fever as a result of a reaction between a protein in donor plasma and corresponding antibodies in the recipient.

Laboratory testing. Because urticaria is not a sign of hemolysis, laboratory investigation for a transfusion reaction is not necessary. It is important, however, that such reactions be reported to the blood bank, so that they can be documented because recurrence of such reactions may require changes in blood product.

Treatment and prevention: Hives are treated with antihistamines. Patients with recurrent or severe urticarial reactions should receive blood components that have been saline washed to remove plasma.

Anaphylactic transfusion reactions occur predominantly among patients who are IgA deficient and are an extremely rare event with an estimate of 1 in 150,000 components transfused.

Clinical presentation: The general signs and symptoms of anaphylaxis are present and may include apprehension, a feeling of doom, chest or lumbar pain, facial and upper body flushing, generalized urticaria with pruritus, laryngeal or facial edema, bronchospasm, wheezing, dyspnea, hypotension, loss of consciousness, vomiting, and diarrhea.

Laboratory testing: No diagnostic tests are helpful prior to the transfusion. Patients who suffer an anaphylactic reaction should be tested for IgA levels and for the presence of antibodies directed against IgA.

Treatment and prevention: Treatment should be initiated promptly with epinephrine and careful clinical monitoring. If subsequent transfusions are required, red cells and platelets should be washed to remove plasma or should be obtained from an IgA-deficient donor if that is the cause. Plasma should also be obtained from IgA-deficient donors.

Hypervolemia: One of the most unrecognized complications of blood transfusion is the development of hypervolemia. Patients should be evaluated carefully prior to transfusion for their cardiac status and state of hydration. Patients who are at risk for hypervolemia should have their blood infused slowly over as long as 4 hours for 1 U of blood. It is important to note that blood contains a significant amount of sodium, with whole blood containing approximately 56 mEq sodium and packed red cells with additive solutions having 24–30 mEq of sodium per unit.

Nonimmune hemolysis: Rupture of transfused red cells may occur because of osmotic or mechanical stress if solutions other than normal saline or other approved solutions are added to red cells, if overheating occurs as a result of a malfunctioning blood warmer or if an infusion pump injures red cells. When hemolysis is suspected in a patient, these possibilities should always be considered in addition to immune-mediated hemolysis.

Complications of massive transfusion: Patients receiving massive transfusions often experience hypotension, tissue damage, and shock with concomitant complications. Massive transfusion, which is given under urgent circumstances frequently, has an associated increased risk of clerical errors.

Clinical presentation: Complications of massive transfusion include hemostatic defects, metabolic abnormalities, and hypothermia:

1. **Bleeding complications:** Microvascular bleeding associated with dilutional thrombocytopenia, dilutional coagulopathy or consumptive coagulopathies is a frequent complication of patients resuscitated with packed red cells or crystalloids or albumin-containing solutions or who have prolonged hypotension.

2. **Hypocalcemia:** Blood products contain citrate as the anticoagulant, and some patients transfused with massive amounts of blood can develop hypocalcemia. Patients who receive massive amounts of blood need to be monitored for the presence of impairment of cardiac performance. Hypothermia and acidosis exacerbate hypocalcemic symptoms.

3. **Hypokalemia:** Massive transfusion usually is associated with hypokalemia rather than hyperkalemia for a number of reasons.

4. **pH abnormalities:** Acidosis associated with hypoperfusion and tissue oxygen deprivation usually is reversed by transfusion and volume repletion. Citrate metabolism from the citrate in stored blood generates bicarbonate with resultant alkalosis rather than acidosis in patients who do not have prolonged hypotension.

5. **Hypothermia:** Infusion of cold blood leads to hypothermia and potentiates the myocardial depressant effects of hyperkalemia and hypocalcemia if they are present.

6. **Adult respiratory distress syndrome:** Although adult respiratory distress syndrome has been reported in the setting of massive transfusion, pulmonary insufficiency is more likely to be the consequence of injury to the upper abdomen or thorax rather than a result of infused microaggregates contained in stored blood.

Laboratory testing of the hemostatic state should be done on a periodic basis during massive transfusion and includes platelet count, prothrombin time (INR), partial thromboplastin times, and fibrinogen levels. Other hemostatic tests should be ordered only if indicated. Blood gas and electrolyte determinations should also be performed as needed.

Treatment of dilutional thrombocytopenia and dilutional coagulopathy should include replacement of platelets, coagulation factors, and fibrinogen through transfusion of platelet concentrates, FFP, and cryoprecipitate respectively. The need for these components should be based on results of laboratory tests and should not be given on an empirical basis or according to predetermined algorithms. Metabolic abnormalities should be treated appropriately when recognized. Blood warmers should be used in any patient undergoing massive transfusion in order to prevent hypothermia.

Bacterial sepsis: Although transfusion-related sepsis occurs infrequently, it is an extremely important complication of blood transfusion and has received increased attention for this reason. Both RBCs and platelet concentrates have been associated with bacterial contamination.

Clinical presentation: Chills or rigors often associated with nausea, vomiting, lethargy, and fever occur after infusion of 50 to 70 mL of blood. Patients may complain of pain in the abdomen or low back region or along the infusion site. Fever and hypotension subsequently develop and may progress to shock and disseminated intravascular coagulation (29,30).

Laboratory testing: Because such a reaction may not be totally distinguishable from a hemolytic transfusion reaction, the patient should be evaluated as previously described for hemolytic transfusion reaction. In addition, the blood transfusion should be immediately stopped, and an aliquot obtained from the remaining component should be examined for bacteria by Gram stain and a bacterial culture should be performed. A negative Gram stain does not rule out the possibility of a bacteria-contaminated blood product. Reactions caused by gram-negative bacteria often are exacerbated by the presence of endotoxin contained in the contaminated component.

Treatment: The symptom complex of chills shortly after the onset of a transfusion with subsequent development of fever and hypotension should raise clinical suspicion of transfusion-related sepsis. The blood transfusion should be stopped immediately. Gram stains and bacterial cultures should be performed and broad-spectrum antibiotics should be started. Supportive measures for maintaining blood pressure should be instituted promptly.

Delayed Transfusion Reactions

Delayed hemolytic transfusion reactions: These reactions are the result of alloantibody-mediated red cell destruction by antibodies that are not detected at the time pretransfusion testing is performed. The alloantibodies are generally secondary or anamnestic responses that manifest several days to 2 weeks after transfusion. Clinical reactions occur with a frequency of approximately 1 per 1,500 to 8,000 units transfused and are usually mild (31).

Clinical presentation: A delayed hemolytic transfusion reaction should be suspected when unexpected anemia develops in a patient with a history of a recent transfusion. Besides anemia, fever is the most common clinical symptom (75%). Jaundice (67%) and oliguria (17%) may occur. Most of these symptoms occur approximately 1 week after transfusion.

Laboratory testing: Patients should be evaluated with both a direct and indirect antiglobulin test. Implicated antibodies usually include Rh antibodies as well as antibodies directed against Kell, Kidd, and Duffy antigens. Delayed hemolytic transfusion reactions should be suspected in patients who have an unexplained fall in hematocrit following a blood transfusion and, in particular, in a patient who develops fever or clinical and laboratory evidence of hemolysis.

Treatment: Significant clinical consequences other than anemia and fever occur infrequently. Supportive therapy is indicated if serious complications such as oliguria occur.

Posttransfusion graft-versus-host disease: This rare complication is considered a result of infused viable lymphocytes present in a blood product that recognize and react against host tissues. The condition occurs when a blood product with viable T lymphocytes is given to a patient who is immunosuppressed. As previously noted, rare incidences have occurred when family members have directed their blood transfusion to another family member. The donor lymphocytes detect immunologic differences in the recipient, proliferate, and mount a cellular response against host tissues. Graft-versus-host disease has been reported after transfusion of whole blood, red cells, platelet concentrates, granulocyte transfusions, and fresh plasma (10).

Clinical presentation: Transfusion-associated graft-versus-host disease occurs 4 to 30 days after transfusion. It resembles the condition associated with bone marrow transplantation, but in this instance the bone marrow is involved additionally. Patients develop fever, erythema, diarrhea, liver function abnormalities, and bone marrow suppression marked by pancytopenia. Hepatomegaly and jaundice are common.

Laboratory testing: The diagnosis is made by performing a biopsy of the skin or gastrointestinal tract. In addition, DNA testing can be performed to determine whether the circulating lymphocytes show nonpatient types, presumably those of the blood donor.

Treatment and prevention: Treatment is usually unsuccessful, and mortality rates approach 90%. Prevention is the most effective therapy. Gamma irradiation of blood products (2,500 cGy) prevents lymphocyte proliferation but results in no or minimal damage to other cells.

Iron overload: This complication occurs in adult patients who receive 60 to 210 (mean, 120) units of blood. Endocrine, cardiac, and liver dysfunction occur. Iron chelation therapy is effective in decreasing and slowing the onset of organ dysfunction associated with iron overload (see Chapter 5).

Posttransfusion purpura: This uncommon syndrome manifests by profound thrombocytopenia that develops approximately 5 to 9 days after a blood transfusion. The exact pathogenesis still is not fully delineated. Other causes of thrombocytopenia, such as drug-induced thrombocytopenia, heparin-induced thrombocytopenia, and DIC must be excluded. Patients with this disorder develop an antibody to a platelet antigen that is not on their own platelets. The most common platelet-associated antigen that antibodies are directed against is the Pl^{A1} antigen. Treatment modalities include use of intravenous gamma globulin or therapeutic plasma exchange. Transfusion of Pl^{A1}-negative platelets to patients who have anti-Pl^{A1} antibodies is not successful.

Immunosuppressive effects of blood transfusion: Blood transfusion causes a downregulation of the immune system, with a number of immunologic parameters being downregulated. This finding has caused growing attention as to whether this has an adverse effect on patients receiving blood transfusions. A large number of articles have been published, both pro and con, addressing the issues of whether blood transfusion is associated with an increased frequency of tumor recurrence following tumor resection or with a higher incidence of postoperative infection following surgery. A small number of randomized controlled trials have been done to address this issue, but the results remain inconclusive. Some physicians are recommending leukocyte reduction of all blood products, suggesting that the leukocyte may be involved in the downregulation of the immune system. Removal of the leukocyte might be beneficial in preventing these potential complications (32,33).

Transfusion-transmitted Diseases

1. **Hepatitis:** Approximately 4 million persons in the United States are infected with hepatitis C, with about 10% (400,000) having been infected as a result of a blood transfusion. Remarkable advances have been made in the prevention of hepatitis C by blood transfusions since the discovery of the virus in the late 1980s. At present, the current estimated risk of posttransfusion hepatitis C infection is approximately 1 per 263,000 components transfused. Donor screening and testing procedures have reduced the risk of posttransfusion hepatitis B to approximately 1 per 63,000 to 1 per 233,000 components transfused.

2. **HIV infection:** More than 8,000 persons developed HIV infection from blood transfusion prior to development of testing in 1985. Since implementation of testing for HIV infectivity in blood donor units, only 47 cases of HIV infection have been reported in the last 15 years. Blood donors undergo extensive questions about risk factors for HIV and also undergo testing for antibodies against HIV-1, HIV-2, p24Ag, and now a new research nucleic acid test for HIV in an attempt to shorten the window period of infectivity. The current risk for acquiring HIV infection through blood product transfusion is approximately 1 per 1,000,000 units infused.

3. **Other retroviral infections:** HTLV-I and HTLV-II infections are transmitted by blood, but only by cellular containing components and not via FFP or cryoprecipitate. Tests are done on all blood donations to eliminate possible infectious units, and the current risk of these infections is extremely low (34).

4. **Cytomegalovirus (CMV):** Immunocompetent patients rarely have significant illnesses associated with transfusion-transmitted **(CMV)**. Certain patients, however, are at risk for the development of serious CMV infection following blood transfusion. Such patients include fetuses receiving intrauterine transfusions; premature infants smaller than 1,200 g of weight born to CMV-seronegative mothers; CMV-seronegative pregnant women receiving blood transfusions, which may place the fetus at risk; CMV-seronegative recipients of renal, heart, liver, lung, or bone marrow transplants. Posttransfusion CMV infection is prevented by providing blood products with a reduced risk of CMV infection (CMV safe). This is done by providing units of blood from donors that test seronegative for antibodies to CMV or by providing blood products that are leukocyte reduced using third-generation leukocyte reduction filters (9).

5. **Spirochete infection:** Syphilis is an unusual complication of blood transfusion because donors are tested and spirochetes are not viable after 24–96 hours at 4°C storage. Syphilis testing is still required on all donor units in the United States.

6. **Parasitic infections:** Transfusion-transmitted malaria occurs infrequently. Transfusion-associated babesiosis is a potentially fatal complication when occurring in immunocompromised, splenectomized, or elderly patients. Chagas disease (*Trypanosoma cruzi*) is associated with blood transfusion.

7. **Creutzfeldt–Jacob disease:** Much interest has recently centered around the potential for blood transfusion to transmit Creutzfeldt–Jacob disease. To date, there has

never been an instance when this disease has been transmitted by a blood transfusion. Blood-drawing institutions are required, however, to exclude certain persons who have a history of Creutzfeldt–Jakob disease in their family or a variant of Creutzfeldt–Jakob disease. Also, they are excluded as donors if they have lived in the United Kingdom for longer than 6 months since 1980–1996.

There is a great deal of active research currently ongoing in the United States and other parts of the world to develop methods that would essentially sterilize a blood product while maintaining the function of the product itself. It is potentially possible that in a few years blood products may be treated in such a way as to render them completely free of being able to transmit either bacterial or viral infections.

References

1. Wallace EL, Churchhill WH, Surgenor DM, et al. Collection and transfusion of blood and blood components in the United States, 1994. *Transfusion* 1998;38:625–635.
2. Walker RH, Linn DT, Hartrick MB. Alloimmunization following blood transfusion. *Arch Pathol Lab Med* 1989;113:254.
3. Linden JV, Paul B, Dressler KP. A report of 104 transfusion errors in New York State. *Transfusion* 1992;32:601–606.
4. American Society of Anesthesiologists Task Force on Blood Component Therapy. Practice guidelines for blood component therapy. *Anesthesiology* 1996;84:732–747.
5. Welch HG, Meehan KR, Goodnough LT. Prudent strategies for elective red blood cell transfusion. *Ann Intern Med* 1992;116:393–402.
6. Hebert PC, Wells G, Blajchman MA, et al. A multicenter, randomized, controlled clinical trial of transfusion requirements in critical care. *N Engl J Med* 1999; 340:409–417.
7. Dzik D, Aubuchou J, Jeffries L, et al. Leukocyte reduction of blood components: public policy and new technology. *Tranfus Med Rev* 2000;14:34–52.
8. The Trial to Reduce Alloimmunization to Platelets Study Group. Leukocyte reduction and ultraviolet B irradiation of platelets to prevent alloimmunization and refractoriness to platelet transfusions. *N Engl J Med* 1997;337:1861–1869.
9. Bowden RA, Slichter SJ, Sayers M, et al. A comparison of filtered leukocyte-reduced and cytomegalovirus (CMV) seronegative blood products for the prevention of transfusion associated CMV infection after marrow transplant. *Blood* 1995;86: 3598–3603.
10. Shivdasoaric RA, Anderson KC. Graft-versus-host disease. In: Petz LD, et al., eds. *Clinical practice of transfusion medicine*, 3rd ed. New York: Churchill Livingstone, 1998:931–946.
11. Moroff G, Leitman SJ, Luban NLC. Principles of blood irradiation, dose validation, and quality control. *Transfusion* 1997;37:1084–1092.
12. Beutler E. Platelet transfusions: the 20,000/microL trigger. *Blood* 1993; 81: 1411–1413.
13. Gruner J, Burger J, Shanz U, et al. Safety of stringent prophylactic platelet transfusion policy for patients with acute leukemia. *Lancet* 1991;338:1223–1226.
14. Pisciotto PT, Benson K, Hume H, et al. Prophylactic versus therapeutic platelet transfusion practices in hematology and/or oncology patients. *Transfusion* 1995; 35:498–502.
15. Friedberh RC, et al. Clinical and blood bank factors in the management of platelet refractoriness and alloimmunization. *Blood* 1993;81:3428–3434.
16. Norol F, et al. Platelet transfusion: a dose-response study. *Blood* 1998;92:1448–1453.
17. Mair B, Benson K. Evaluation of changes in hemoglobin levels associated with ABO-incompatible plasma in apheresis platelets. *Transfusion* 1998;38:51–55.
18. Contreras M and the British Committee for Standards in Hematology, Working Party of the Blood Transfusion Task Force. Guidelines for the use of fresh-frozen plasma. *Transfus Med* 1992;2:57–63.
19. Alving B, ed. *Blood components and pharmacologic agents in the treatment of congenital and acquired bleeding disorders*. Bethesda, MD: AABB Press, 2000.
20. Dale DC, Liles WC, Price TH. Renewed interest in granulocyte transfusion therapy. *Br J Haemotol* 1997;98:497–501.

21. Erstad B, Gales BJ, Rappaport WD. The use of albumin in clinical practice. *Arch Intern Med* 1991;151:901–911.
22. Cochrane Injuries Group Albumin Reviewers. Human albumin administration in critically ill patients: systematic review of randomized controlled trials. *BMJ* 1998;317:235–240.
23. Menache D, Grossman BJ, Jackson CM. Antithrombin III: physiology, deficiency, and replacement therapy. *Transfusion* 1992;32:580–588.
24. Ratko TA, Burnett DA, Toulke GE, et al. Recommendations for off-label use of intravenously administered immunoglobulin preparations. *JAMA* 1995;273: 1865–1870.
25. Hay CRM, Negrier C, Ludlam CA. The treatment of bleeding in acquired haemophilia with recombinant Factor VIIa: a multicenter study. *Thromb Haemost* 1997;78:1463–1467.
26. Radosevich M, Goubran HA, Burnouf T. Fibrin sealant: scientific rationale, production methods, properties, and current clinical use. *Vox Sang* 1997;92:133–143.
27. Heddle NM, Klama L, Meyer R, et al. A randomized controlled trial comparing plasma removal with white cell reduction to prevent reactions to platelets. *Transfusion* 1999;39:231–238.
28. Popovsky MA, Chaplin HC, Moore SB. Transfusion-related acute lung injury: a neglected, serious complication of hemotherapy. *Transfusion* 1992;32:589–592.
29. Tipple MA, et al. Sepsis associated with transfusion of red cells contaminated with Yersinia enterocolitica. *Transfusion* 1990;30:207–213.
30. Lee JH. Workshop on Bacterial Contamination of Platelets. CBER, FDA September 24, 1999. *http://www.fda.gov/cber/minutes/workshop-min.htm* (June 1, 2000).
31. Ness PM, et al. The differentiation of delayed serologic and delayed hemolytic transfusion reactions: incidence, long-term serologic findings, and clinical significance. *Transfusion* 1990:30:688–693.
32. Blajchman MA. Allogenic blood transfusion, immunomodulation and postoperative bacterial infection: do we have the answers yet? *Transfusion* 1997;37:121–125 [Editorial].
33. McAllister FA, Clark HD, Wells PS, et al. Perioperative allogeneic blood transfusion does not cause adverse sequelae in patients with cancer: a meta-analysis of unconfounded studies. *Br J Surg* 1998;85:171–178.
34. Centers for Disease Control and Prevention and the U.S.P.H.S. Working Group. Guidelines for counseling persons infected with human T-lymphotropic virus type I (HTLV-I) and type II (HTLV-II). *Ann Intern Med* 1993;118:448–454.

18. HEMATOLOGIC AND NEOPLASTIC ASPECTS OF HUMAN IMMUNODEFICIENCY VIRUS INFECTION

Mitchell D. Martin and George M. Rodgers

In addition to the significant immunologic, infectious, and neoplastic manifestations associated with human immunodeficiency virus (HIV) infection, hematologic abnormalities are also common. This chapter summarizes the incidence of HIV-associated hematologic manifestations, their laboratory evaluation and morphologic description, and clinical significance, as well as the current status of treatment for patients with these hematologic disorders. AIDS-related malignancies are reviewed as well. Basic immunologic aspects and therapy of HIV infection will not be reviewed.

General Consideration
Infection with HIV may be associated with a number of hematologic complications, some of which may result in significant clinical sequelae. The occurrence of cytopenias is a relatively common manifestation of HIV infection, related to bone marrow failure or decreased survival of all three cell lines derived from the hematopoietic stem cell. HIV infection may also be associated with significant co-morbidities such as opportunistic infection, malignancy, or medication side effects, which may result in coexisting hematologic abnormalities not directly attributed to viral load. A syndrome resembling classic thrombotic thrombocytopenic purpura (TTP) has been linked to HIV infection. Thrombotic events, often in association with acquired protein S deficiency or the lupus anticoagulant, have been reported. The development of highly active antiretroviral therapy (HAART) has changed the incidence and character of these complications, just as the spectrum of infectious manifestations of HIV have changed over the last several years.

Pathogenesis of Cytopenias
HIV-related Bone Marrow Suppression
Some evidence suggests that the hematopoietic progenitor cell is itself infected by HIV. This point is controversial; however, clearly the subsequent growth of the committed progenitor cells is abnormal. Likewise, the microenvironment of the marrow is abnormal as a result of infection of T cells and macrophages that are important in normal cell growth. Cytopenias also may result from the abnormal production of hematopoietic growth factors such as granulocyte colony-stimulating factor (G-CSF) and erythropoietin. Indirect modes of hematopoietic cell suppression such as production of autoantibodies, production of other humoral inhibitory factors, T-cell-mediated suppression of hematopoiesis, or production of inhibitory or stimulatory cytokines may also be contributory. Administration of effective antiretroviral therapy may result in an increase in circulating levels of total CD4+ T-cells and total white blood cells, including neutrophils, lymphocytes, and platelets. This phenomenon suggests that HIV-1 inhibits production of the hematopoietic progenitor cell and that viral suppression may be effective therapy for many of these patients.

Drug Effects
Drug-related hematopoietic toxicity is frequently observed in HIV patients. Zidovudine (ZDV) use was commonly associated with anemia in the 1980s, when the drug was used in doses greater than 600 mg per day. Neutropenia is less frequent and thrombocytopenia is very uncommon in patients using ZDV. Other nucleoside analogs, such as didanosine (ddI), zalcitabine (ddC), lamivudine (3TC), and stavudine (d4T), do not appear to have significant bone marrow toxicity. The protease inhibitors (indinavir, ritonavir, saquinavir, and nelfinavir) have little or no effect on hematopoiesis. Trimethoprim-sulfamethoxazole (TMP-SMX), commonly used for the prevention of *Pneumocystis* pneumonia, may result in megaloblastic anemia, leukopenia, and thrombocytopenia on the basis of folate deficiency in patients with poor nutritional status. Ganciclovir (GCV) produces leukopenia and thrombocytopenia in 40% to 48% of AIDS patients. Amphotericin

B is also frequently associated with hypochromic, normocytic anemia; renal toxicity may result in diminished erythropoietin production (Table 1).

Infection
Hematopoiesis may be depressed by several opportunistic infectious agents encountered in HIV infection. Viral pathogens commonly associated with cytopenias include the human cytomegalovirus (CMV) and B19 parvovirus. Pure red cell aplasia is classically associated with parvovirus B19 infection. A variety of bacterial pathogens, classically *Mycobacterium avium* intracellulare (MAI) and *M. avium* complex (MAC) may affect hematopoiesis. Additionally, systemic fungal infection may be associated with cytopenias.

Laboratory Manifestations
Anemia and Red Blood Cell Abnormalities
  1. **Incidence:** Anemia occurs in approximately 10% to 20% of patients at the initial presentation with HIV infection and is found in as many as 70% to 80% of HIV-infected

Table 1. Hematopoietic effects of drugs used in HIV patients

Drug	Activity/indication	Hematologic toxicity
Zidovudine	Nucleoside analog, antiviral	Anemia, neutropenia
Stavudine	Nucleoside analog, antiviral	Anemia, neutropenia
Lamivudine	Nucleoside analog, antiviral	Neutropenia, anemia
Saquinavir, ritonavir, indinavir	HIV protease inhibitors, antiviral	Minimal
Trimethoprim/ sulfamethoxazole	Antibiotic/pneumocystis pneumonia prophylaxis	Anemia/neutropenia, hemolytic anemia in G6PD deficiency
Dapsone	Antibiotic/pneumocystis pneumonia prophylaxis	Rare agranulocytosis, thrombocytopenia; hemolytic anemia in G6PD deficiency
Pentamidine	Pneumocystis pneumonia prophylaxis	Anemia, leukopenia, thrombocytopenia
Sulfadiazine	Toxoplasmosis	Leukopenia, thrombocytopenia (10%)
Clindamycin/ pyramethamine	Toxoplasmosis	Cytopenias (30%)
Ketoconazole, fluconazole, itraconazole	Candidiasis	Rare
Amphotericin B	Antifungal, cryptococcal meningitis	Anemia
Ganciclovir	Cytomegalovirus infection	Leukopenia, thrombocytopenia
Foscarnet	Cytomegalovirus infection	No significant toxicity
Rifampin, rifabutin	Mycobacterium avium-intracellulare	Rare thrombocytopenia
Acyclovir	Herpes simplex and zoster	No significant toxicity

G6PD, glucose-6-phosphate dehydrogenase; HIV, human immunodeficiency virus.

patients during the course of infection. Anemia is becoming less frequent since the advent of protease inhibitors and HAART. Early in the AIDS epidemic, the high incidence of anemia was often associated with high-dose ZDV. Anemia is now most commonly associated with advanced disease, and the Multicenter AIDS Cohort Study and other studies have identified anemia as an independent negative prognostic factor.

2. **Pathogenesis:** Anemia may result from direct bone marrow failure from HIV infection, opportunistic infection, drugs, vitamin deficiency (iron, B_{12}, folate), or an infiltrative neoplasm such as lymphoma or Kaposi sarcoma (KS). Increased red cell destruction may be caused by Coombs'-positive hemolytic anemia, TTP, disseminated intravascular coagulation (DIC), hemophagocytic syndrome, or the use of oxidative drugs in the setting of glucose-6-phosphate dehydrogenase deficiency (G6PD) (see Chapter 4).

3. **Red blood cell morphology:** Anemia in patients with advanced HIV disease is typically normochromic and normocytic but may be macrocytic when related to drug effects such as seen with ZDV or cytotoxic chemotherapy. A major morphologic finding on the peripheral blood smear is marked anisocytosis and poikilocytosis, which result in an increased red cell distribution width (RDW) as determined by the particle counter. Microcytosis is uncommon in the absence of bleeding, and macrocytosis is infrequent, except in patients being treated with ZVD. Approximately 70% of ZVD-treated patients develop macrocytosis after 2 weeks of therapy, and approximately 50% of these patients have a mean corpuscular volume (MCV) greater than 110 fl. Rouleaux formation has been noted in a minority of peripheral blood smears in patients with HIV infection and probably results from polyclonal hypergammaglobulinemia.

4. **Other laboratory results:** *Reticulocyte counts* are low when associated with bone marrow failure and high with increased red cell destruction. Red cell destruction is associated with elevated serum levels of *indirect bilirubin. Erythropoietin* levels may be decreased, providing important information for treatment options. *Antierythrocyte antibodies* are detected in some AIDS patients but also may be observed in asymptomatic HIV-infected patients. *Vitamin B_{12}* or *folate* deficiency due to malabsorption or malnutrition may produce megaloblastic anemia. Laboratory evaluation of the iron stores of patients with HIV infection usually is consistent with the anemia of chronic disease (*increased serum ferritin, decreased serum iron and transferrin*). *A positive Coombs' (direct antiglobulin) test* has been reported in 18% to 77% of HIV-infected patients, although the incidence of hemolysis is extremely low. This results from deposition of immunoglobulin G (IgG), complement, or both on the red blood cell membrane. The positive Coombs' test may simply be related to the *polyclonal hypergammaglobulinemia,* typically associated with HIV infection. Eluates prepared from IgG antiglobulin-positive cells in AIDS patients are typically nonreactive with reagent red cells, and the incidence of antiglobulin positivity is similar in both AIDS patients and non-AIDS patients with hypergammaglobulinemia. Significant hemolytic anemia appears to be uncommon. The incidence of *paraproteinemia* in HIV infection has ranged up to 45%. Paraproteins in these patients typically are not monoclonal, however, and represent a vigorous polyclonal antibody response to HIV antigens. Multiple myeloma and monoclonal gammopathy of unknown significance (MGUS) have only rarely been associated with HIV infection. Despite severe immunodeficiency, HIV-infected patients may become *alloimmunized* and may experience transfusion reactions.

Leukopenia and White Blood Cell Abnormalities

1. **Incidence and pathogenesis:** Neutropenia is reported in approximately 10% of patients with early HIV infection and in nearly 50% of persons with AIDS. The neutropenia is generally mild; however, it may become clinically significant when cytotoxic chemotherapy or other marrow suppressive agents such as ganciclovir are used. Antineutrophil antibodies are common, but they do not correlate with the presence of neutropenia. Decreased colony growth of the pluripotent stem cell has been implicated in the decreased production of granulocytes and monocytes. Decreased serum levels of G-CSF have been described in HIV-seropositive patients with afebrile neutropenia (<1,000 cells/μL). Persistent lymphopenia typically is associated with HIV infection. Myelosuppression related to drug therapy is commonly implicated in the development of leukopenia as well (Table 1).

2. **White blood cell morphology:** Evaluation of the peripheral blood smears of patients with AIDS and patients with acute HIV infection may reveal increased numbers

of atypical lymphocytes. Granulocytopenia in HIV infection may be accompanied by nuclear hyposegmentation. Large, vacuolated monocytes are a nonspecific finding. Morphologic evidence for an additional secondary diagnosis, including lymphoma or histoplasmosis, also may be detected by examining the peripheral blood smear.

3. **Risk for infection:** In a study of 62 HIV-infected patients with absolute neutrophil counts of 1,000 per microliter, 24% developed infectious complications. Factors associated with infection included more advanced HIV disease, neutropenia induced by chemotherapy or lymphoma, and the presence of a central venous catheter. Infections were less likely in patients who developed neutropenia associated with medication toxicity.

Thrombocytopenia
Thrombocytopenia occurs as the first sign or symptom in approximately 10% of patients infected by HIV and often prompts HIV testing. It will occur in approximately 40% of patients during the disease course. The major cause of thrombocytopenia in HIV infection is immune thrombocytopenic purpura (ITP).

1. **ITP:** Platelet-specific antibodies to the platelet membrane IIb/IIIa receptor on the platelet surface have been well described. Antibody-coated platelets are removed from the circulation by macrophages in the spleen. Bettaieb and colleagues demonstrated the presence of cross-reactive antibodies between the HIV-gp 160/120 antigen and the platelet surface antigen gp IIb/IIIa. Molecular mimicry between the HIV-gp 160/120 antigen and the platelet surface gp IIb/IIIa may be the operative mechanism of immune destruction in some cases of HIV-related ITP. Decreased platelet production may result from direct infection of the megakaryocyte by HIV, which exacerbates the degree of thrombocytopenia in HIV–ITP. Increased platelet production has been observed in patients with HIV–ITP treated with ZVD, supporting the hypothesis that direct infection of the megakaryocyte by HIV is a contributing factor. Most patients with HIV–ITP do not experience significant bleeding unless the platelet count drops below 10,000 to 20,000 per microliter.

2. **Other causes:** Thrombocytopenia may also result from platelet destruction in TTP, hemolytic uremic syndrome (HUS), and DIC. HIV infection is associated with an increased incidence of TTP and HUS. HIV-related TTP generally is associated with a milder course and better response to conventional therapy than classic TTP.

Coagulation Abnormalities in HIV Infection
Although numerous hematologic manifestations have been described in patients with HIV infection, only a few coagulation abnormalities have been noted consistently in these patients. An increase in autoantibodies to phospholipid–protein complexes and to coagulation proteins has been reported in a significant proportion of HIV patients, and protein S deficiency has been well-described.

Lupus Inhibitor
One major coagulation defect that does appear to be common in HIV infection is the **lupus inhibitor,** which is the antiphospholipid–protein antibody that impairs certain phospholipid-dependent coagulation assays. The lupus inhibitor usually is associated with an increased risk of thrombosis but not bleeding. Thrombotic events in HIV-infected patients with the lupus inhibitor are not common, however. The incidence of antiphospholipid antibodies in HIV infection is approximately 40% and is seen both in patients with opportunistic infection and in asymptomatic, seropositive patients. The lupus inhibitor usually is suspected in patients with a prolonged activated partial thromboplastin time (aPTT). Specific tests, such as the dilute Russell's viper venom time or the tissue thromboplastin inhibition test, are confirmatory. Patients with the lupus inhibitor, however, may exhibit excessive bleeding if the inhibitor is associated with thrombocytopenia, platelet dysfunction, or another coagulation defect.

Anticardiolipin Antibodies
Anticardiolipin antibodies constitute another group of autoantibodies that react with phospholipid antigens. These antibodies are commonly elevated in patients with HIV

infection. The presence of anticardiolipin antibodies may correlate with thrombocytopenia in this setting. Thrombosis is very uncommon in these patients.

Protein S
Protein S levels have been reported to be decreased in as many as 27% to 73% of HIV-infected adults. Approximately 10% to 12% of these patients have been reported to experience thrombotic complications.

Therapy of HIV-associated Hematologic Abnormalities
Anemia
Numerous causes for the development of anemia in HIV infection have been described and discussed herein. An inappropriate level of endogenous erythropoietin has commonly been observed in patients with bone marrow suppression related to HIV infection. Supplemental erythropoietin may decrease or eliminate red cell transfusion requirement, decrease fatigue, and improve quality of life. Patients with endogenous erythropoietin levels of 500 IU per liter or lower are expected to respond to erythropoietin, whereas those with endogenous levels greater than 500 U per liter are not. Erythropoietin is administered subcutaneously at a dose of 100 to 200 U per kilogram of body weight, three times weekly until normalization of the hemoglobin, then weekly at a dose necessary to maintain the desired hemoglobin concentration. Maximal responses may not be seen for 4 to 8 weeks, and may require erythrapoietin dosages up to 300 U per kilogram, three times weekly. Iron deficiency must be excluded prior to treatment with erythropoietin. Ferritin values should be maintained at least 100 mg/ml.

Parvovirus B19 infection must be considered in any HIV patient with pure red cell aplasia or persistent anemia. Treatment with standard immune globulin at a dose of 400 mg per kilogram daily for 5 to 10 days is associated with reticulocytosis, clinical improvement, and resolution of the anemia. Patients may have a relapse and require retreatment.

Neutropenia
Hematopoietic growth factors have been effective in the management of neutropenia associated with HIV infection. G-CSF has been shown to increase granulocyte counts in HIV patients with neutropenia due to cytotoxic chemotherapy, antiretroviral or antiinfective therapy. The initial dose is 1 microgram per kilogram of body weight daily, which is administered subcutaneously until the neutrophil count rises to an acceptable level (>1,000/μL), followed by dose titration up to a maximum of 10 microgram per kilogram daily. Once- or twice-weekly dosing is generally effective maintenance therapy. G-CSF does not enhance HIV replication *in vitro* or *in vivo*. GM-CSF administration will result in a dose-dependent increase in granulocytes, monocytes, and eosinophils. The suggested starting dose is 5 micrograms per kilogram daily for 5 to 7 days or 250 μg three times a week, then titrated to effect. Granulocyte macrophage–colony-stimulating factor (GM-CSF), 250 μg subcutaneously three times a week has been shown in a phase 3 randomized, placebo-controlled study to decrease opportunistic infection rates, increase CD4 counts, and have no significant effect on the viral load of HIV.

Both G-CSF and GM-CSF can increase the granulocyte number and function in patients who have become neutropenic on the basis of HIV, chemotherapy, or from the use of antiinfectious medications. These growth factors have decreased the duration of neutropenia and the extent of hospitalization of HIV patients who are receiving chemotherapy, and they appear to reduce the overall infectious morbidity and mortality of HIV patients who experience neutropenia from any cause.

Thrombocytopenia
The most common cause of thrombocytopenia in HIV patients is ITP. Serious bleeding episodes are uncommon in HIV–ITP. Antiviral therapy is effective in increasing the platelet count, suggesting a direct relationship between the viral load and thrombocytopenia. The HIV–ITP patient should first receive optimal antiviral therapy. Persistent, clinically significant thrombocytopenia may require additional therapy as discussed subsequently herein.

1. **Antiviral therapy alone** is often effective in increasing the platelet count in patients with HIV–ITP. The Swiss Group for HIV Studies was the first to demonstrate the effectiveness of ZDV therapy in HIV–ITP. At least 50% of patients with HIV-ITP treated with ZVD alone will experience a threefold increase in the platelet count. The more effective antiviral activity of the protease inhibitors, particularly when used in combination, may result in better response rates. Confirmatory trials are ongoing.

2. **Steroids:** The response of HIV–ITP to steroids is comparable to noninfected patients with ITP (80%–90%). Concern that steroid use could lead to further immunosuppression or promote growth of KS limits their use to very brief periods.

3. **High-dose intravenous gamma globulin** at a dose of 1,000 to 2,000 mg per kilogram daily is effective; however, response duration is brief, and this therapy is expensive. This is most often employed to elevate temporarily the platelet count for an invasive procedure or for emergent bleeding.

4. **Anti-Rh immunoglobulin** in nonsplenectomized, Rh-positive patients with HIV-ITP offers another effective mode of therapy. A typical dose of anti-Rh immunoglobulin is 25 µg per kilogram of weight administered intravenously over 30 minutes for two consecutive days; this is expected to produce an increase of the platelet count in 70% to 85% of Rh+ patients. Maintenance therapy of 13 to 25 µg per kilogram administered intravenously every 2 to 4 weeks may maintain the platelet count for extended periods. A subclinical hemolytic anemia is expected, with a typical drop in the hemoglobin by 1 to 2 g per deciliter. This therapy is not recommended for patients with hemoglobin levels below 10 g per deciliter.

5. **Vincristine** and **dapsone** may be effective agents in the management of HIV–ITP.

6. **Splenectomy** is effective management of HIV–ITP, with similar response rates as seen in non-HIV-infected patients with ITP; however, splenectomy has been associated with an increased risk of infection with encapsulated bacteria such as *Streptococcus pneumoniae* and *Haemophilus influenzae*. Patients should undergo appropriate vaccination prior to splenectomy, and this surgery is safest in patients who achieve an appropriate antibody response. Two prospective trials demonstrated no adverse effects on HIV disease progression following splenectomy for ITP.

7. **Thrombopoietin:** This megakaryocyte-specific growth factor has not been fully tested in HIV-infected patients but may prove effective. A large trial sponsored by the National Institutes of Health is ongoing and it is not yet commercially available for general use. However, IL-11 is available and used in AIDS patients.

Thrombotic Thrombocytopenic Purpura
Plasmapheresis will result in the complete remission of most patients with HIV–TTP. The disease course appears to be less severe in HIV–TTP compared with classic TTP. As in classic TTP, the goal of plasmapheresis is normalization of the LDH, renal function and platelet count with plasma exchange therapy. Platelet transfusion should be avoided unless clinically necessary. Patients with HIV and hemolytic uremic syndrome (HUS) appear to present with more severe immunologic deterioration, and the prognosis appears much worse than HIV–TTP. Life expectancy rarely exceeds 1 year after the diagnosis of HIV–HUS.

AIDS-Related Malignancies
Approximately 40% of all patients with AIDS will develop a malignancy sometime during the course of their illness. These cancers are not only a primary cause of death in some patients but also a source of considerable morbidity. In the current era of protease inhibitors and HAART, patients infected with HIV are surviving for longer periods of time, and many of these patients can be expected to develop malignancies.

Kaposi sarcoma (KS) is the most common tumor associated with HIV infection, developing in approximately 10% to 13% of homosexual men with AIDS in the United States and 1% to 2% of other HIV-infected persons.

1. **Etiology:** Human herpesvirus type 8 (HHV-8) has been found in more than 90% of AIDS–KS tumors as well as in classic KS, endemic African KS, and KS that occurs after organ transplant. It also has been identified in body cavity–based lymphoma and primary effusion lymphoma, multicentric Castleman disease, and angioimmunoblastic

lymphadenopathy with dysproteinemia (AILD) in the HIV-infected patient. The mechanism by which HHV-8 induces KS in susceptible persons is the subject of intense current investigations. Cutaneous KS is a lesion of the dermis comprised of a proliferation of aberrant vascular structures lined by abnormal-appearing, spindle-shaped endothelial cells and with extravasated erythrocytes and leukocytes within the structures.

2. **Clinical manifestations:** The manifestations of KS in patients with AIDS are variable and range from small, innocuous-looking, cutaneous lesions to symptomatic visceral tumors. These lesions may become disfiguring, disabling, or even life threatening. Just about every internal organ may be involved with KS, although it is rarely identified in the bone marrow or CNS.

3. **Treatment:** KS appears to be related to the state of the HIV infection. Therefore, all patients with AIDS–KS must have the HIV infection under optimal control. Local treatments, including cryotherapy, topical retinoic acid, intralesional chemotherapy, sclerosing agents, and local radiation, all can produce good local control of tumors. Patients with widespread symptomatic disease or life-threatening visceral involvement require prompt, cytoreductive treatment with one or more chemotherapeutic drugs. Interferon α (IFN-α) is active, generally administered at either 3 or 5 million units subcutaneously three times weekly, together with antiretroviral therapy. The two most frequently used combination chemotherapy regimens are Adriamycin, bleomycin, and vincristine (ABV) and bleomycin and vincristine (BV). Liposomal anthracycline (e.g., liposomal doxorubicin and liposomal daunorubicin) are also very effective in inducing tumor regression in KS. Clinical trials have shown that liposomal anthracycline used as a single agent can achieve a response rate equal to or better than the ABV combination regimen. As such, the liposomal anthracycline agents have become the first-line chemotherapy for AIDS–KS. Paclitaxel has been shown to produce responses in both chemotherapy-naive KS patients and patients with refractory tumors, including those refractory to liposomal anthracycline agents. Dosage is typically 100 to 135 mg/m^2 given intravenously over 3 hours every 3 to 4 weeks.

Non-Hodgkin lymphoma (NHL): The incidence of NHL is 60 times higher in persons with HIV infection than in the general population. The occurrence of lymphoma as a late manifestation of AIDS has increased as treatment of HIV and opportunistic infections has prolonged survival. As many as 20% of all cases of NHL in the United States are HIV-related. Although NHL currently constitutes approximately 3% of all initial AIDS-defining conditions, it accounts for as many as 12% to 16% of all AIDS-related deaths. Most patients present with advanced-stage, high- or intermediate-grade, B-cell lymphoma and have a high frequency of extranodal involvement. Most patients with AIDS-related lymphoma have advanced HIV disease. Median CD4 counts in patients with systemic lymphoma range from 100 to 200 cells/mm^2, whereas CD4 counts fewer than 50 cells/mm^2 are found in nearly all patients with primary CNS lymphoma.

1. **Etiology and risk factors:** AIDS-related NHL is believed to arise as a consequence of continued stimulation of B-cell proliferation as a result of HIV, Epstein–Barr virus (EBV), and other infections, all of which occur in the setting of profound T-cell immunodeficiency. Body cavity–based lymphoma/primary effusion lymphoma appears to be highly associated with HHV-8 and EBV. The disease appears to occur predominantly in males and may coexist with KS in patients with AIDS.

2. **Pathology:** More than 95% of AIDS-related NHL cases are of B-lymphocyte origin. Most AIDS–NHL tumors are high-grade types, including the immunoblastic and small noncleaved lymphomas. Diffuse large-cell lymphoma constitutes up to 30% of AIDS lymphomas. Advanced-stage disease is observed in most patients, with extranodal involvement reported in 60%–90% of patients in most series. Common sites of extranodal involvement include the CNS (occurring in approximately 30% of patients), gastrointestinal tract (25%), and bone marrow (25%). Essentially, any other site in the body can also be involved, including the rectum, soft tissue, oral cavity, lung, and heart.

3. **Prognostic factors:** Four factors have been shown to correlate most closely with survival in patients with systemic AIDS-related NHL:
- A history of opportunistic infection prior to the lymphoma
- CD4 count less than 100 cells/mm^2

- Karnofsky performance score below 70
- Stage IV disease, especially if due to bone marrow or meningeal involvement

The median survival for patients with one or more adverse prognostic features is approximately 4 to 5 months. For patients who lack these findings, median survival is typically 11 to 12 months. Patients with primary CNS lymphoma have an extremely poor prognosis, with a median survival of only 2 to 3 months despite therapy. This survival rate is far inferior to patients with primary CNS lymphoma not occurring in the setting of immunodeficiency. The prognosis for patients with primary effusion lymphoma is also poor, with a median survival of only 5 months.

4. **Treatment:** The mainstay of treatment for patients with systemic AIDS-related NHL is chemotherapy. As the likelihood of dissemination is great, AIDS patients who develop NHL must be assumed to have widespread disease at presentation and should be treated with systemic chemotherapy, even if dissemination is not confirmed on routine staging and evaluation. A randomized trial (ACTG 142) showed no differences between standard-dose m-BACOD (methotrexate, bleomycin, Adriamycin, cyclophosphamide, Oncovin, and dexamethasone) and reduced-dose m-BACOD with respect to complete response rate, time to disease progression, or overall survival. The major dose-limiting toxic effect of multiagent chemotherapy regimens is myelosuppression. Studies of m-BACOD or CHOP (cyclophosphamide, doxorubicin HCl, Oncovin, and prednisone) chemotherapy demonstrated that coadministration of myeloid hematopoietic growth factors enhanced patient tolerance of these regimens. CNS prophylaxis with either intrathecal cytarabine (Ara-C; 50 mg) or intrathecal methotrexate (10–12 mg) every week for four treatments has been shown to be effective in reducing the incidence of CNS relapse.

Cervical Carcinoma
Cervical carcinoma in the setting of HIV infection is recognized as an AIDS-defining malignancy. Cervical intraepithelial neoplasia (CIN) is also seen in association with HIV infection. Human papillomavirus (HPV) serotypes 16, 18, 31, 33, and 35 are the most oncogenic and have been associated with invasive cervical carcinoma and progressive dysplasia. Current screening recommendations call for women with HIV infection to have pelvic examinations and cytologic screening every 6 months. For women with invasive carcinoma, complete staging should be undertaken. This should include pelvic examination, computed tomography of the pelvis and abdomen, chest radiographs, and screening laboratory tests for hepatic and bone disease. HIV-infected women with cervical carcinoma typically present with more advanced disease and appear to have a more aggressive clinical course. Tumors are typically high-grade, with a higher proportion of lymph node and visceral involvement at presentation. Mean time to recurrence after primary treatment is short, and many patients have persistent disease after primary therapy. The same principles that guide oncologic management of the immunocompetent patient with cervical carcinoma are utilized in AIDS patients with this cancer.

Anal Carcinoma
Although anal carcinoma is not currently an AIDS-defining illness, the incidence of this tumor is increasing in the population at risk for HIV infection. HPV precursor lesions of anal intraepithelial neoplasia, have been found to be associated with HPV infection, typically with oncogenic serotypes, for example, types 16 and 18. For patients with squamous cell carcinoma of the anus, chemotherapy with mitomycin (Mutamycin, 10 mg/m² on day 1) and fluorouracil (1,000 mg/m² by continuous infusion on days 1–4) combined with radiation therapy can produce high rates of complete remission. Anal cancer can be controlled with chemotherapy and radiation therapy despite HIV infection. Patients who have CD4 counts below 200 cells/mm² appear to be more likely to experience severe toxicity and to require colostomy for salvage therapy.

Other Non-AIDS-Defining Malignancies
Case reports of other malignant tumors occurring in HIV-infected individuals include Hodgkin's disease, nonmelanomatous skin cancers, lung cancer, germ-cell tumors, myeloid or lymphoid leukemias, multiple myeloma, renal cell carcinoma, breast cancer, head and neck cancer, and leiomyosarcoma in pediatric patients.

1. **Hodgkin disease:** Male predominance, a higher prevalence of B-symptoms, and more extranodal disease on presentation are the main characteristics of Hodgkin disease in HIV patients. Chemotherapy is recommended for this group of patients. Standard treatments include ABVD (adriamycin, bleomycin, vinblastine, and dacarbazine) or ABVD alternating with MOPP (mechlorethamine, Oncovin, procarbazine, and prednisone).

2. **Nonmelanomatous skin cancers:** Basal cell carcinoma is more common than squamous cell carcinoma in the setting of HIV infection. The risk factors for the development of these tumors are the same as in the general population; namely, fair skin, history of sun exposure, and family history.

Suggested Readings

Abkowitz JL, Brown KE, Wood RW, et al. Clinical relevance of parvovirus B19 as a cause of anemia in patients with human immunodeficiency virus infection. *J Infect Dis* 1997;176:269–273.

Angel JB, High K, Rhame F, et al. Phase III study of granulocyte-macrophage colony-stimulating factor in advanced HIV disease: effect on infections, CD4 cell counts and HIV suppression. Leukine/HIV Study Group. *AIDS* 2000;14:387–395.

Bain BJ. Pathogenesis and pathophysiology of anemia in HIV infection. *Curr Opin Hematol* 1999;6:89–93.

Bettaieb A, Oksenhendler E, Duedari N, et al. Cross-reactive antibodies between HIV-gp120 and platelet gpIIIa (CD61) in HIV-related immune thrombocytopenic purpura. *Clin Exp Immunol* 1996;103:19–23.

Bussel JB, Haimi JS. Isolated thrombocytopenia in patients infected with HIV: treatment with intravenous gammaglobulin. *Am J Hematol* 1988;28:79–84.

De Angelis V, Biasinutto C, Pradella P, et al. Clinical significance of positive direct antiglobulin test in patients with HIV infection. *Infection* 1994;22:92–95.

de Larranaga GF, Forastiero RR, Carreras LO, et al. Different types of antiphospholipid antibodies in AIDS: a comparison with syphilis and the antiphospholipid syndrome. *Thromb Res* 1999;96:19–25.

Deeks SG, Smith M, Holodniy M, et al. HIV-1 protease inhibitors. A review for clinicians. *JAMA* 1997;277:145–153.

Demetri GD, Kris M, Wade J, et al. Quality-of-life benefit in chemotherapy patients treated with epoetin alfa is independent of disease response or tumor type: results from a prospective community oncology study. Procrit Study Group. *J Clin Oncol* 1998;16:3412–3425.

Durand JM, et al. Dapsone for thrombocytopenic purpura related to human immunodeficiency virus infection. *Am J Med* 1991;90:675.

Fuller A, Moaven L, Spelman D, et al. Parvovirus B19 in HIV infection: a treatable cause of anemia. *Pathology* 1996;28:277–280.

Gallant JE. Strategies for long-term success in the treatment of HIV infection. *JAMA* 2000;283:1329–1334.

Gringeri A, Cattaneo M, Santagostino E, et al. Intramuscular anti-D immunoglobulins for home treatment of chronic immune thrombocytopenic purpura. *Br J Haematol* 1992;80:337–340.

Groopman JE, Feder D. Hematopoietic growth factors in AIDS. *Semin Oncol* 1992; 19:408–414.

Harbol AW, Liesveld JL, Simpson-Haidaris PJ, et al. Mechanisms of cytopenia in human immunodeficiency virus infection. *Blood Rev* 1994;8:241–251.

Huang SS, Barbour JD, Deeks SG, et al. Reversal of human immunodeficiency virus type 1-associated hematosuppression by effective antiretroviral therapy. *Clin Infect Dis* 2000;30:504–510.

Henry DH, Beall GN, Benson CA, et al. Recombinant human erythropoietin in the treatment of anemia associated with human immunodeficiency virus (HIV) infection and zidovudine therapy: overview of four clinical trials. *Ann Intern Med* 1992;117:739–748.

Hymes KB, Greene JB, Karpatkin S. The effect of azidothymidine on HIV-related thrombocytopenia. *N Engl J Med* 1988;25;318:516–517.

Jacobson LP, Yamashita TE, Detels R, et al. Impact of potent antiretroviral therapy on the incidence of Kaposi's sarcoma and non-Hodgkin's lymphomas among HIV-1-infected individuals: Multicenter AIDS Cohort Study. *J Acquir Immune Defic Syndr Hum Retrovirol* 1999;21:S34–S41.

Kaplan LD, Straus DJ, Testa MA, et al. Low-dose compared with standard-dose m-BACOD chemotherapy for non-Hodgkin's lymphoma associated with human immunodeficiency virus infection: National Institutes of Allergy and Infectious Diseases AIDS Clinical Trials Group. *N Engl J Med* 1997;336:1641–1648.

Kravcik S, Toye BW, Fyke K, et al. Impact of *Mycobacterium avium* complex prophylaxis on the incidence of mycobacterial infections and transfusion-requiring anemia in an HIV-positive population. *Acquir Immune Defic Syndr Hum Retrovirol* 1996; 13:27–32.

Kuritzkes DR, Parenti D, Ward DJ, et al. Filgrastim prevents severe neutropenia and reduces infective morbidity in patients with advanced HIV infection: results of a randomized, multicenter, controlled trial. G-CSF 930101 Study Group. *AIDS* 1998; 12:65–74.

Landonio G, Cinque P, Nosari A, et al. Comparison of two dose regimens of zidovudine in an open, randomized, multicentre study for severe HIV-related thrombocytopenia. *AIDS* 1993;7:209–212.

Lord RV, Coleman MJ, Milliken ST. Splenectomy for HIV-related immune thrombocytopenia: comparison with results of splenectomy for non-HIV immune thrombocytopenic purpura. *Arch Surg* 1998;133:205–210.

Maiman M, Fruchter RG, Clark M, et al. Cervical cancer as an AIDS-defining illness. *Obstet Gynecol* 1997;89:76–80.

Meynard JL, Guiguet M, Arsac S, et al. Frequency and risk factors of infectious complications in neutropenic patients infected with HIV. *AIDS* 1997;11:995–998.

Mintzer DM, Real FX, Jovino L. Treatment of Kaposi's sarcoma and thrombocytopenia with vincristine in patients with the acquired immunodeficiency syndrome. *Ann Intern Med* 1985;102:200–202.

Munoz A, Schrager LK, Bacellar H, et al. Trends in the incidence of outcomes defining acquired immunodeficiency syndrome (AIDS) in the Multicenter AIDS Cohort Study: 1985–1991. *Am J Epidemiol* 1993;137:423–438.

Northfelt DW, Dezube JB, Thommes JA, et al. Pegylated-liposomal doxorubicin vs doxorubicin, bleomycin, and vincristine in the treatment of AIDS-related Kaposi's sarcoma: results of a randomized phase III clinical trial. *J Clin Oncol* 1998;16:2445–2451.

Palefsky JM, Holly EA, Ralston ML, et al. High incidence of anal high-grade squamous intra-epithelial lesions among HIV-positive and HIV-negative homosexual and bisexual men. *AIDS* 1998;12:495–503.

Stahl CP, Wideman CS, Spira TJ, et al. Protein S deficiency in men with long-term human immunodeficiency virus infection. *Blood* 1993;81:1801–1807.

Sullivan PS, Hanson DL, Chu SY, et al. Epidemiology of anemia in human immunodeficiency virus (HIV)-infected persons: results from the multistate adult and adolescent spectrum of HIV disease surveillance project. *Blood* 1998;91:301–308.

Sutor GC, Schmidt RE, Albrecht H. Thrombotic microangiopathies and HIV infection: report of two typical cases, features of HUS and TTP, and review of the literature. *Infection* 1999;27:12–15.

Toy PT, Reid ME, Burns M. Positive direct antiglobulin test associated with hyperglobulinemia in acquired immunodeficiency syndrome (AIDS). *Am J Hematol* 1985; 19:145–150.

Von Roenn JH, Krown SE. Management of AIDS-associated Kaposi's sarcoma: a multidisciplinary perspective. *Oncology* 1998;12(2; suppl 3):1–24.

Zauli G, Re MC, Davis B, et al. Impaired *in vitro* growth of purified (CD34+) hematopoietic progenitors in human immunodeficiency virus-1 seropositive thrombocytopenic individuals. *Blood* 1992;15;79:2680–2687.

19. AUTOLOGOUS AND ALLOGENEIC TRANSPLANTATION PROCEDURES FOR HEMATOLOGIC MALIGNANCIES

Hillard M. Lazarus

Hematopoietic stem cell transplantation involves the intravenous infusion of autologous or allogeneic stem cells collected from bone marrow, peripheral blood, or umbilical cord blood to reestablish hematopoietic function in patients with damaged or defective bone marrow or immune systems. This highly effective modality often can provide curative therapy for a varied group of malignant and nonmalignant disorders.

Background
Although a report in 1939 described the use of a small aliquot of sibling bone marrow for the treatment of aplastic anemia, significant advancements in transplantation science did not occur until the 1950s. At that time, two major preclinical observations advanced the field. First, rodents could be protected from the effects of lethal total body irradiation (TBI) by using marrow infusion. Second, many of the complexities of the histocompatibility system in animals were unraveled; this information ultimately led to understanding the human leukocyte antigen (HLA) system. Clinical advances led to the first successful transplants in the late 1960s, including an understanding of chemotherapeutic agents, progress in the blood banking and transfusion sciences, and the availability of new potent antibiotic agents. Few fields in medicine better illustrate the effective use of translational science into the clinical arena, a fact that culminated in the awarding of the Nobel Prize in medicine to E. Donnall Thomas for his pioneering work in human bone marrow transplantation. Estimates suggest that 30,000 to 40,000 transplants are performed yearly worldwide, and the number continues to increase by 10% to 20% per year. More than 20,000 people now have survived 5 years or longer after a hematopoietic stem cell transplant. Many of the recent sophisticated advances in transplant, including supportive care, are shown in Table 1.

Principles of Therapy
Myeloablative Therapy
Prior to hematopoietic stem cell transplant, patients usually are given extremely high doses of chemotherapy with or without radiation, referred to as *myeloablative treatment,* to eliminate the malignancy. Infusion of hematopoietic stem cells, for example, autologous or allogeneic stem cell transplantation, circumvents the problem of prolonged myelosuppression, permitting dose escalation to considerably higher dose levels. Marrow recovery, however, still takes many weeks and requires sophisticated supportive care until the effects of such therapy have lessened. Myeloablative transplants, the most common allogeneic transplant type, are a one-step approach. Higher chemotherapy doses result in greater kill of malignancy; stem cell infusion however, is essential to restore marrow function, which will not recover otherwise. Furthermore, when allogeneic cells are used, these immune cells may provide anticancer benefit in the form of graft-versus-tumor or leukemia. Unfortunately, allogeneic cells also can cause significant damage to the patient from the graft-versus-host disease (GVHD) complications. GVHD prophylaxis, using potent immunosuppressive therapy, must be given immediately before the transplant, continued for many months, and later slowly withdrawn.

Nonmyeloablative Therapy: Miniallografts (Two-step Approach)
In the first step, sufficient immunosuppressive therapy is given to allow donor cell engraftment to take place. Injury to the marrow and other organs is less than observed with a myeloablative regimen; visceral organs are less likely to be damaged, fewer infections occur, and less antibiotics and transfusions are required for support. Anticancer benefit, correspondingly, is much less than seen with a myeloablative state. A state of mixed chimerism results post transplant, that is, both donor and recipient hema-

Table 1. Advances in transplantation and supportive care

Agent/device	Utility	Example
Continuous-flow centrifugation	Apheresis product availability	Platelet transfusions, stem cell collection
Antiemetics	Prevent severe chemoradiation therapy-related nausea, vomiting	Ondansetron, granisetron
New antibacterial agents	Prevent/treat unusual infections	Linezolide (VRE)
Antiviral agents	Prevent/treat CMV infection	Ganciclovir, foscarnet
Antifungal agents	Prevent/treat *Aspergillus* sp infection	Fluconazole, FK463
Central venous catheters	Perform pheresis, venous access	Raaf hybrid catheter
Platelet transfusions	Prevent serious hemorrhage, reduce alloimmunization	UV light-treated, leukocyte-depleted
Anti-GVHD	Prevent/treat acute GVHD	Cyclosporine, tacrolimus, anti-T-cell monoclonal antibodies

CMV, cytomegalovirus; GVHD, graft-versus-host disease; UV, ultraviolet; VRE, vancomycin-resistant *Enterococcus*.

topoietic cells, exist in the host. The second step relies on the graft-versus-tumor effect. Prophylactic therapy to prevent GVHD is quickly withdrawn to allow donor immune cells to mediate graft-versus-tumor effects. If GVHD does not develop after withdrawal of prophylaxis, immunocompetent T cells and natural killer (NK) cells are obtained from the donor via leukapheresis and are infused to provide additional anticancer benefit. This adoptive immunotherapy or donor lymphocyte infusion (DLI) therapy has been most successful in preventing relapse or eliminating active disease in chronic myeloid leukemia (CML) and multiple myeloma patients who have low tumor burdens. The full effect of DLI therapy takes many months to manifest, and the effects appear to be significantly reduced in aggressive disease and in tumor types other than CML and multiple myeloma.

Patient Eligibility (Age and Functional Status)
Patients generally should be younger than 65 years for autologous transplants or "mini"allogeneic transplants and younger than 55 years for allogeneic (myeloablative) transplants. Patients with significant co-morbid illnesses (e.g., congestive heart failure, uncontrolled diabetes mellitus, active infection, renal insufficiency) generally are excluded from most types of transplant procedures, including nonmyeloablative transplants.

Preparative or Conditioning Regimens (Term for High-Dose Chemotherapy and Autologous or Allogeneic Myeloablative Transplants)
Therapy is dictated by the type of malignancy. The most common regimens involve high-dose cyclophosphamide 100 to 150 mg per kilogram of body weight given intravenously over several days, in association with TBI (1,000–1,320 cGy) given in four to six fractions (treatments) or with busulfan 12 to 16 mg per kilogram given intravenously or by mouth in divided dose over 4 days. Etoposide 1,200 to 2,400 mg/m^2 administered intravenously in divided dose over several days often is added. Other agents that have shown efficacy include carmustine (BCNU) 300 to 600 mg/m^2 in lymphoma, melphalan 140 to 225 mg/m^2 in lymphoma and multiple myeloma, and cytarabine 0.5 to 24 g/m^2 in leukemias and lymphoma.

Preparative or Conditioning Regimens (for Miniallogeneic Transplants)
Dual cytotoxic–immunosuppressive agents such as fludarabine 100 to 150 mg/m² administered intravenously, cladribine (2-CDA), or pentostatin, along with antithymocyte globulin 10 to 30 mg per kilogram intravenously often are given in combination with chemotherapeutic agents such as cyclophosphamide, busulfan, and melphalan.

Source of Graft
Hematopoietic stem cells can be collected for clinical use from several sources, including bone marrow, peripheral blood, umbilical cord blood, and rarely fetal liver. The donor sources include cells obtained from another person, known as an *allogeneic transplant*, an identical twin (*syngeneic transplant*), or self (*autologous transplant*). The choice of which type of transplant to perform is a complex decision that must be based on patient age, malignant disease type, overall health of the patient, and donor compatibility and health (Table 2).

Autotransplant
Candidates for autologous transplantation, in general, do not have histologically demonstrable malignancy in the blood or bone marrow. Whereas treatment-related morbidity and mortality rates are lowest with autografts, the major problem is relapse of tumor; this finding relates to the absence of graft-versus-tumor effect and reinfusion of occult tumor in the graft.

Allogeneic Transplants
Patients over the age of 50 years experience higher transplant-related morbidity and mortality rates with allogeneic grafts; this effect relates to the need for continuing immunosuppression after the transplant to prevent the development of GVHD (see section entitled **Complications**). Although a more toxic therapy than autografts, relapse rates are considerably lower from graft-versus-tumor effects, that is, immunologic attack on tumor by immunocompetent T cells and NK cells in the donor graft.

1. **Matched-sibling donors:** Successful transplants usually require a histocompatible donor, that is, a patient and donor who are "matched" at the major histocompatibility locus genes, located on chromosome 6. Histocompatibility is determined by using DNA extracted from blood samples and expressed as identity at the HLA-A, HLA-B, and

Table 2. Hematopoietic stem cell sources and transplant types

Donor type	Donor relationship	Comment
Autologous	Self	Lowest treatment-related mortality, highest relapse rate
Allograft: related		
HLA-identical	Sibling (6 of 6 HLA-A,B,DRB1 match)	Preferred allograft donor
haploidentical	sibling, parent, child (3 of 6 HLA-A,B, DRB1 match)	Requires massive CD34 number and T-cell depletion
Allograft: unrelated		
HLA-identical	Shares major (not minor) HLA antigens (5–6 of 6 HLA-A,B, DRB1 match)	Highest GVHD and rejection rates
Umbilical cord blood	Shares some major HLA antigens (3–4 of 6 HLA-A,B, DRB1 match)	Lower GVHD incidence but slowest marrow recovery

GVHD, graft-versus-host disease; HLA, human leukocyte antigen.

DRB1 loci (6 antigen match, because each complex is inherited from each parent and expressed codominantly). ABO red blood cell (RBC) antigens are not expressed on stem cells, and ABO incompatibility is not an exclusion for conducting an allograft (but blood banking issues still are important, see later discussion). Depending on family size, individual patients have approximately a 30% chance of having a sibling-matched donor as expressed by the following equation: The probability of having a donor = $1 - [0.75]^n$ where n = the number of potential sibling donors. A histocompatible sibling is the preferred allogeneic donor because the use of such grafts is associated with the lowest incidence of severe (grade III–IV) GVHD (about 40%) and the lowest failure-to-engraft rates (about 1%–2%).

2. **Alternative donors:** Matched unrelated (phenotypically identical to the patient). Various procurement agencies (i.e., registries such as the National Marrow Donor Program in the United States and other registries worldwide) provide hematopoietic cells from altruistic donors. DNA samples from these donors have been cataloged and can be located by computer searches; often many weeks to months are required to secure a donor. Severe (grade III–IV) GVHD (40%–80% incidence) and failure to engraft (up to 10%) represent significant, persistent problems with this alternative approach, making it less desirable.

3. **Alternative donors:** Haploidentical family members (i.e., parent, child, sibling). Donors can be approached without the need for a registry. Such stem cell products must contain many more stem cells (to overcome host rejection and facilitate engraftment). These grafts must be manipulated *in vitro* to reduce the number of immunocompetent T cells to lessen the likelihood and severity of GVHD.

4. **Alternative donors:** Umbilical cord blood units. Such units are cryopreserved in approximately 100-mL aliquots, frozen, and stored in large banks. Umbilical cord blood transplants are hampered by the smaller number of hematopoietic cells available. Until recently, most transplants were performed in children. In adults, using this small number cell inoculum results in a higher incidence of engraftment failure and much slower time to marrow recovery (i.e., median time to neutrophil count 500/μL in adults is 4 weeks). Such transplants, however, are associated with a lower incidence and severity of GVHD because of infusion of immunologically naive cells; as a result, the degree of matching between donor and recipient may be reduced from six to three or four of six HLA-A, HLA-B, and DRB1 antigens (Table 3).

Procurement of Stem Cells

Bone Marrow Harvest
Formerly, hematopoietic cells were collected with the patient under general or spinal anesthesia in the operating room. This approach is now used much less often.

Stem Cell Collection
Hematopoietic stem cells circulate in blood and can be identified and quantified using flow cytometry (cells express the CD34 antigen). Administration of recombinant hematopoietic growth factors (filgrastim, sargramostim combinations) to patients or donors results in the release of marrow stem cells into the peripheral blood, which can be collected from the veins of the patient or donor. Apheresis instruments, similar to those used for collecting platelet concentrates from volunteer donors for transfusions, are used in an ambulatory setting. Using this technique, during a 3- to 4-hour period, about 1 log more hematopoietic progenitors can be collected than a bone marrow harvest. Furthermore, the need for general anesthesia and a sterile operating room is eliminated. This process, known as *mobilization of stem cells,* may be enhanced in patients destined for autografts in which exposure to cytotoxic drugs such as cyclophosphamide plus hematopoietic growth factor therapy will cause the release of more than tenfold more primitive hematopoietic progenitors into the circulation than recombinant cytokines alone.

The risk-to-benefit ratio is as follows: The use of blood rather than bone marrow as the source of hematopoietic stem cells results in the collection of more cells and more rapid marrow recovery, that is, 2 weeks versus 4 weeks for neutrophil, platelet, and RBC counts. In the allograft setting, the incidence and severity of acute GVHD do not differ significantly between blood and marrow, but chronic GVHD rates appear to be increased.

Table 3. Comparison autologous versus allogeneic hematopoietic stem cell transplantation

Drawback	Autologous transplant	Allogeneic transplant
Upper age limit for candidates (yr)	60–70	50–55
Major difficulty of transplant	Collecting sufficient stem cells free of tumor	Locating HLA-matched sibling or alternative donor
Chemoradiation organ damage	+ – ++	+ – ++
Opportunistic infection	+	++ – ++++
Bleeding complications	+	+
Engraftment delay/failure	+	++ – +++
Tumor cell re-infusion	+ – +++	——
Graft-versus-host disease	+/–	++ – ++++
Tumor relapse	++ – +++	+ – ++
Second-degree myelodys-plastic syndrome, acute leukemia	+	+
Solid tumors, lymphoma (EBV)	+/–	+

EBV, Epstein–Barr virus lymphoproliferative disorder.

Storage of Stem Cells

Stem cells can be infused intravenously shortly after collection or, more frequently, after freezing using cryoprotectants such as dimethyl sulfoxide (5%–10% final concentration) with or without pentastarch (6% final concentration). Umbilical cord blood units are collected from the placenta (after delivery of the newborn infant) via cannulation of one of the umbilical vessels by withdrawing 50 to 100 mL into a syringe containing an anticoagulant and nutrient media. Such collections then are frozen. Samples of all products are tested for infectious contamination and analyzed for hematopoietic progenitor cell content.

Manipulation of Stem Cell Grafts

These techniques often require sophisticated laboratories and highly trained technical personnel and are often quite expensive.

1. **ABO incompatible allogeneic transplants:** Remove of isoagglutinins (minor compatibility) or RBCs (major incompatibility) from the donor graft to prevent hemolysis in the recipient.

2. **T-cell depletion in the allogeneic transplant setting:** Immunocompetent donor T cells may be removed using a variety of methods to reduce or eliminate the possibility for the development of GVHD. Although such a strategy often is effective in lowering the morbidity and mortality rates of GVHD, removal of these accessory cells may be associated with an increase in engraftment failure in up to 10% of transplants (loss of T-helper cells, which facilitate engraftment). Furthermore, T-cell depletion results in increased relapse rates compared with T-replete grafts because the removal of cytotoxic T cells eliminates the potential for a graft-versus-malignancy effect.

3. **In vitro purging in autografts:** Tumor cells can be detected by using sophisticated means such as tumor clonogenic assays, flow cytometry, or polymerase chain reaction. Using gene-marking techniques, occult tumor cells in the infused graft may contribute to relapse; removal methods include the following:

- Chemical and immunologic: 4-hydroperoxycyclophosphamide or mafosfamide (cyclophosphamide derivatives) chemotherapy *in vitro* kills residual autologous tumor cells; normal stem cells are injured, resulting in slower or incomplete engraftment.
- Positive selection of CD34$^+$ cells: Commercial instruments can be used to remove the desired cells by using solid-phase anti-CD34-monoclonal antibodies.
- Negative selection: Anticancer monoclonal antibodies can be used to remove tumor cells, leaving stem cells in the graft.

Complications and Specific Therapies
Prolonged, Severe Pancytopenia
Severe (<500/μL but often <100/μL) and prolonged (up to 4 weeks) neutropenia is frequent after a transplant and invariably requires the use of empiric broad-spectrum antibacterials until recovery of neutrophil count. Often empiric antifungal therapy with amphotericin B, liposomal amphotericin B, fluconazole, or other agents are administered if unexplained fever persists during neutropenia despite the use of broad-spectrum antibacterials. Antiviral therapy usually is given as prophylaxis (acyclovir in autografts and ganciclovir in allografts). Serious infections such as pneumonia, bacteremias, fungemias, and viremias may occur in up to 50% of transplants, more frequently in matched-unrelated and mismatched transplants than autografts and sibling-matched allografts and are the major contributor to the mortality associated with these procedures. Recombinant hematopoietic growth factors (filgrastim 5–10 μg/kg daily administered subcutaneously, sargramostim 250 μg/m^2 daily administered subcutaneously) begun shortly after stem cell infusion usually enhances the time to blood neutrophil recovery.

Severe thrombocytopenia requires prophylactic transfusions for platelet counts less than 10,000 per microliter, but for bleeding episodes or surgical procedures, the target may exceed 50,000 per microliter. Bleeding may occur despite platelet transfusions as a result of visceral organ injury from chemotherapy (gastritis, pneumonitis) or infection (adenovirus-induced hematuria in urinary bladder).

Severe anemia requires frequent RBC transfusions; recombinant erythropoietin 30,000 to 60,000 U per week administered subcutaneously in divided dose sometimes is used after stem cell infusion to enhance erythroid recovery.

Graft-Versus-Host Disease
This syndrome occurs when the immunocompetent T cells and NK cells in the donor graft recognize host antigens as foreign targets and mediate a reaction. GVHD occurs very frequently in the allograft setting. On the other hand, by several mechanisms, GVHD rarely can occur in the autologous and syngeneic settings. GVHD may cause significant morbidity and mortality and has been divided into acute and chronic forms (Table 4).

1. **Acute GVHD:** To avoid the effects of acute GVHD, patients are given potent immunosuppressives immediately before and for many months after transplant. The most commonly used agents are cyclosporine or tacrolimus (FK506), usually in association with a few days of methotrexate. Some centers prefer corticosteroids for a protracted period rather than "short-course" methotrexate therapy. Alternatively, the donor graft may be treated *in vitro* to remove the effector cells, which mediate the acute GVHD reaction. This technique, known as *T-cell depletion,* can be accomplished by using density gradients, monoclonal antibodies, or other means. In the absence of T-cell depletion of the graft, most adults develop acute GVHD despite prophylaxis using immunosuppressives. Anti-GVHD therapy includes high-dose corticosteroids, antithymocyte globulin, and anti-T-cell monoclonal antibodies. More recently, immunosuppressives such as pentostatin have been used. A clinical grading system (grade 0–4) identifies extent of clinical organ involvement (skin, liver, gastrointestinal tract), which usually correlates with patient outcome.

2. **Chronic GVHD:** This syndrome, which resembles connective tissue disorder like scleroderma, may develop as a continuation of active acute GVHD (*progressive*), occurs after successful clearing of acute GVHD (*quiescent*), or it may appear without antecedent acute GVHD (*de novo*). The target organs are more widespread than acute

Table 4. Comparison acute and chronic graft-versus-host disease (GVHD)

Variable	Acute GVHD (grade 2–4)	Chronic GVHD
Incidence	40%–70% HLA-sibling matched >75% mismatched related, or matched-unrelated donor	35%–50%
Usual onset after transplant	20–100 days	>100 days
Effector cells	Preformed donor T and NK cells	Donor stem cells maturing into T cells under influence host thymus
Target cells	Epithelial cells	Mixed epithelial and mesenchymal cells
Organs involved	Skin, GI tract, liver	Skin, GI tract, liver, musculoskeletal, lungs, eyes, salivary glands

GI, gastrointestinal; NK, natural killer.
Actual percentages are age- and disease state-dependent.

GVHD; chronic GVHD is more likely to develop in older patients and in recipients of donor grafts obtained from peripheral blood rather than from bone marrow. Successful prophylaxis strategies have not been developed, and therapy includes prednisone, mycophenolate mofetil, phototherapy, and thalidomide. Development of thrombocytopenia or hyperbilirubinemia implies a grave prognosis. A grading system identifying limited or extensive disease, based on the degree of involvement of skin, liver, or other affected organs, correlates with prognosis. Onset of chronic GVHD, however, is associated with fewer relapses, indicative of a graft-versus-tumor effect.

Graft Rejection
1. **Definition:** Donor cells fail to regenerate within the recipient (rejection, or failure to engraft).
2. **Incidence:** One percent to 2% in sibling-matched allografts; appreciably higher in the setting of matched-unrelated donor transplants, aplastic anemia diagnosis, the use of T-cell depletion techniques on the donor graft, infusion of lower numbers of hematopoietic stem cells (i.e., umbilical cord blood grafts in adults), or nonmyeloablative transplants.
3. **Mechanisms** include the failure of immunosuppressive agents to inactivate host immune system (host-versus-graft), inadequate numbers of donor stem cells or facilitator cells infused, drug injury to marrow, or viral infections such as cytomegalovirus (CMV) or human herpesvirus (HHV-6 or HHV-8).

Pulmonary Complications (Interstitial Pneumonitis)
1. **Allografts:** Frequently fatal syndrome often caused by viral infections (CMV)
   - Characterized by fever, infiltrates, hypoxemia, and acute respiratory distress syndrome (ARDS).
   - Lowered incidence using antiinfective prophylaxis; often treatment is effective with ganciclovir or foscarnet, plus intravenous immune serume globulin (IVIG).
2. **Autografts:** Sometimes termed *diffuse alveolar hemorrhage* (due to significant bleeding with bronchoalveolar lavage)
   - Lung injury due to TBI or pulmonary toxins (BCNU).
   - Often responds to many weeks of high-dose corticosteroid therapy.

Hepatic Venoocclusive Disease
1. **Definition:** Jaundice, tender hepatomegaly, unexplained weight gain or ascites
2. **Mechanism:** Direct injury from high-dose chemotherapy or chemoradiation therapy within the first month after allograft or autograft

3. **Histology:** Progressive and concentric occlusion of lumina of small intrahepatic veins, hepatocyte necrosis in centrilobular area, leading to portal hypertension, and hepatic failure

4. **Risk factors:** History of previous hepatocellular disease, certain preparative regimens, advanced patient age, presence of GVHD, type of GVHD prophylaxis, poor performance status at transplant, use of match-unrelated or mismatched donor grafts

5. Ursodiol (ursodeoxycholic acid) 300 mg administered orally, three times daily before beginning preparative regimen, lowers the incidence. Some researchers believe that continuous infusion heparin prophylaxis lowers the incidence. Therapy generally is unsatisfactory, although there are encouraging reports regarding the use of defibrotide.

Disease Indications and Stage/Pretreatment History

Late-onset Problems
Secondary Acute Leukemias, Solid Tumors, and Myelodysplastic Syndromes
These conditions are disease and regimen dependent; onset is months or years after transplant, with increased incidence after TBI (Table 5).

Late Infections (Bacterial, Viral, Fungal)
1. Onset months to many months after transplant
2. Usually after allografts in association with GVHD, or GVHD therapy; occasionally occur in autografts after posttransplant immunotherapy
3. Vaccinations strongly recommended (pneumococcus, *Hemophilus influenza* b, hepatitis B, poliovirus, diphtheria/tetanus, influenza)

Future Directions
Improved Patient Selection
Patient selection can be improved by identifying and treating malignancies at high risk for recurrence using newer prognostic guides (e.g., International Age-Adjusted Index in non-Hodgkin lymphoma, International Performance Scoring in myelodysplastic syndrome, Hasenclever–Diehl Classification in Hodgkin disease, poor-risk cytogenetics in leukemia, and others) and excluding poor-risk patients or those unlikely to benefit from transplant.

Improved Preparative Regimens
1. **Goals:** To reduce treatment-related morbidity and mortality and reduce relapses
2. **Approach:** Incorporate selective agents [monoclonal antibodies such as rituximab (anti-B cell), Campath-1H (anti-CD52), ^{131}I-anti-CD45 (antihematopoietic tissue), ^{90}Yt-or ^{131}I-anti-CD20 (anti-B cell) and gemtuzumab ozogamicin anti-CD33 (anti-AML)]
3. Incorporation of pharmacokinetic modeling (optimizing individual patient doses)

Incorporation of New-generation Hematopoietic Growth Factors
For example, FLT3-ligand, thrombopoietin can be used to enhance the collection of hematopoietic stem cells.

Improved GVHD Prevention and Therapy Agents
1. Monoclonal antibodies, blocking peptides
2. Suicide gene insertion to eliminate GVHD effector cells

*Ex Vivo Expansion Hematopoietic Progenitor Cells
(Enhanced Hematopoietic Recovery)*
Cytokine- and stromal cell-mediated expansion is a current example.

Reduced Costs
The use of ambulatory setting therapy could be used to a greater extent.

Posttransplant Minimal Residual Disease Therapy
1. Enhanced antiinfective vaccines: prevent late infections
2. Effective antitumor therapies

Table 5. Anticipated patient outcome using autologous and sibling-matched allogeneic transplants in malignant disorders in adult patients

Disease	Stage/state	Allograft	Autograft	Comment(s)
AML	1st CR	40%–60% cure	40%–50% cure	Allografts higher TRM; autografts higher relapse
AML	2nd CR	20%–40% cure	20%–30% cure	
AML	1° refractory	10% cure	Rarely performed	
ALL	1st CR	40%–60% cure	40%–50% cure	Worse results in Ph¹+ pts
ALL	2nd CR	20%–40% cure	20% cure	
CML	1st chronic phase	60%–70% cure	40%–50% PFS	Best results within 1st year after diagnosis
CML	Accelerated phase	30% cure	Rarely performed	
CML	Blast crisis	10% cure	Rarely performed	
CLL	Relapsed responders	40%–50% PFS	40%–50% PFS	Highly-selected patients
MDS	Untreated	40%–50% cure	Not performed	Long-term outcome uncertain; highly-selected patients
NHL	Relapsed responders	30%–50% cure	30%–50% cure	Highly selected patients, usually younger
NHL	1st CR at high-risk for relapse	50%–60% cure	60%–80% cure	
NHL	1° refractory	20% cure	20% cure	
HD	Relapsed responders	20%–25% cure	40%–50% cure	High TRM in allografts
HD	1° refractory	Rarely performed	30%–40% PFS	
Multiple myeloma	Stable/responders, low-volume disease	30%–50% PFS	30%–50% PFS	High TRM in allografts

AML, acute myeloid leukemia; ALL, acute lymphoblastic leukemia; Ph¹+, Philadelphia chromosome positive (t[9;22] ALL); CML, chronic myeloid leukemia; CLL, chronic lymphocytic leukemia; MDS, myelodysplastic syndrome; NHL, non-Hodgkin's lymphoma; HD, Hodgkin disease; 1st CR, first complete remission; 2nd CR, second complete remission; 1° refractory, primary refractory disease; PFS, progression-free survival; TRM, treatment-related mortality.

- Anticancer monoclonal antibody therapies
- Dendritic cell therapy/antitumor vaccines
- Apoptosis-inducing and antiangiogenesis therapies (i.e., thalidomide therapy in multiple myeloma)

Suggested Readings

Andre M, Henry-Amar M, Blaise D, et al. Treatment-related deaths and second cancer risk after autologous stem-cell transplantation for Hodgkin's disease. *Blood* 1998; 92:1933.

Armitage JO. Bone marrow transplantation. *N Engl J Med* 1994;330:827.

Attal M, et al. A prospective, randomized trial of autologous bone marrow transplantation and chemotherapy in multiple myeloma. *N Engl J Med* 1996;335:91.

Aversa F, et al. Treatment of high-risk acute leukemia with T-cell-depleted stem cells from related donors with one fully mismatched HLA haplotype. *N Engl J Med* 1998; 339:1186.

Carella AM, et al. Mini-allografts: ongoing trials in humans. *Bone Marrow Transplant* 2000;25:345.

Cassileth PA, et al. Chemotherapy compared with autologous or allogeneic bone marrow transplantation in the management of acute myeloid leukemia in first remission. *N Engl J Med* 1998;339:1649.

Curtis RE, et al. Solid cancers after bone marrow transplantation. *N Engl J Med* 1997;336:897.

Desikan R, et al. Results of high-dose therapy for 1000 patients with multiple myeloma: durable complete remissions and superior survival in the absence of chromosome 13 abnormalities. *Blood* 2000;95:4008.

Duell T, et al. Health and functional status of long-term survivors of bone marrow transplantation: EBMT Working Party on Late Effects and EULEP Study Group on Late Effects. European Group for Blood and Marrow Transplantation. *Ann Intern Med* 1997;126:184.

Gahrton G, et al. Allogeneic bone marrow transplantation in multiple myeloma. *N Engl J Med* 1991;325:1267.

Gajewski JL, et al. Bone marrow transplants from HLA-identical siblings in advanced Hodgkin disease. *J Clin Oncol* 1996;14:572.

Glucksberg H, et al. Clinical manifestations of graft-versus-host disease in human recipients of marrow from HLA-matched sibling donors. *Transplantation* 1974;18:295.

Grimwade D., et al. The importance of diagnostic genetics on outcome in AML: analysis of 1,612 patients entered into the MRC AML 10 trial. *Blood* 1998;92:2322.

Hasenclever D, Diehl V. A prognostic score for advanced Hodgkin's disease. *N Engl J Med* 1998;339:1506.

Hoelzer D. Treatment of acute lymphoblastic leukemia. *Semin Hematol* 1994;31:1.

International Non-Hodgkin's Lymphoma Prognostic Factors Project. A predictive model for aggressive non-Hodgkin's lymphoma. *N Engl J Med* 1993;329:987.

Kernan NA, et al. Analysis of 462 transplants from unrelated donors facilitated by the National Marrow Donor Program. *N Engl J Med* 1993;328:593.

Lazarus HM, et al. Autotransplants for Hodgkin disease in patients never achieving remission: a report from the Autologous Blood and Marrow Transplant Registry (ABMTR). *J Clin Oncol* 1999;17:534.

Lazarus HM, Vogelsang GB, Rowe JM. Prevention and treatment of acute graft-versus-host disease: the old and the new: a report from the Eastern Cooperative Oncology Group (ECOG). *Bone Marrow Transplant* 1997;97:577.

Leiper AD. What is in store after stem-cell transplantation? *Lancet* 1999;353:1544.

Lowenberg B, Downing JR, Burnett A. Acute myeloid leukemia. *N Engl J Med* 1999; 341:1051.

Majolino I, et al. Peripheral-blood stem-cell transplantation versus autologous bone marrow transplantation in Hodgkin's and non-Hodgkin's lymphomas: a new matched-pair analysis of the European Group for Blood and Marrow Transplantation Registry Data. Lymphoma Working Party of the European Group for Blood and Marrow Transplantation. *J Clin Oncol* 1997;15:509.

Martin P, et al. Reproducibility in retrospective grading of acute graft-versus-host disease after allogeneic marrow transplantation. *Bone Marrow Transplant* 1998;21:273.

Popplewell L, Forman SJ. Allogeneic hematopoietic stem cell transplantation for acute leukemia, chronic leukemia, and myelodysplasia. *Hematol Oncol Clin North Am* 1999;13:987.

Rocha V, et al. Graft-versus-host disease in children who have received a cord-blood or bone marrow transplant from an HLA-identical sibling. *N Engl J Med* 2000;342: 1846.

Rowlings PA, et al. IBMTR severity index for grading acute graft-versus-host disease: retrospective comparison with Glucksberg grade. *Br J Haematol* 1997:97:855.

Santos GW. History of bone marrow transplantation. *Clin Haematol* 1983;12:611.

Schenkein DP, et al. A phase II multicenter trial of high dose sequential chemotherapy and peripheral blood stem cell transplantation as initial therapy for patients with high risk non-Hodgkin's lymphoma. *Biol Blood Marrow Transplant* 1997;3:210.

Singhal S, et al. Long-term outcome of adult acute leukemia patients who are alive and well 2 years after autologous blood or marrow transplantation. *Bone Marrow Transplant* 1999;23:875.

Thomas ED. Bone marrow transplantation: a review. *Semin Hematol* 1999;36 (Suppl 7):95.

Thomas ED, et al. Bone-marrow transplantation. *N Engl J Med* 1975;292:895.

van Besien K, et al. Allogeneic bone marrow transplantation for low grade lymphoma. *Blood* 1998;92:1832.

Appendix A. NORMAL HEMATOLOGIC PARAMETERS

Table A1. Normal hematologic parameters

Component	Conventional units			Factor	Recommended SI units		

Typical reference intervals

Component	Conventional units	Factor	Recommended SI units
Erythrocyte indices			
MCV	80–96 μ^3	1	80–96 fl
MCH	27–31 pg	1	27–31 pg
MCHC	32%–36%	0.01	Concentration fraction: 0.32–0.36
White blood cell differential (adult)	Mean % Range of absolute counts		Mean number fraction Range of absolute count
Segmented neutrophils	56% 1,800–7,000/μL	10^6	0.56 1.8–7.8 × 10^9/L
Bands	3% 0–700/μL	10^6	0.03 0–0.70 × 10^9/L
Eosinphils	2.7% 0–450/μL	10^6	0.027 0–0.45 × 10^9/L
Basophils	0.3% 0–200/μL	10^6	0.003 0–0.20 × 10^9/L
Lymphocytes	34% 1,000–4,800/μL	10^6	0.34 1.0–4.8 × 10^9/L
Monocytes	4% 0–800/μL	10^6	0.04 0–0.80 × 10^9/L
Hemoglobin A_2	1.5%–3.5% of total hemoglobin	0.01	Mass fraction: 0.015–0.035 of total hemoglobin
Hemoglobin F	<2%	0.01	Mass fraction: <0.02

Osmotic fragility

% NaCl	% Lysis Fresh	% Lysis 24 h at 37°C	% NaCl 171 / % Lysis 0.01	NaCl mmol/L	Lysed fraction Fresh	Lysed fraction 24 h at 37°C
0.2	—	95–100		34.2	—	0.95–1.00
0.3	97–100	85–100		51.3	0.97–1.00	0.85–1.00
0.35	90–99	75–100		59.8	0.90–0.99	0.75–1.00
0.40	50–95	65–100		68.4	0.50–0.95	0.65–1.00
0.45	5–45	55–95		77.0	0.05–0.45	0.55–0.95
0.50	0–6	40–85		85.5	0–0.06	0.40–0.85
0.55	0	15–70		94.1	0	0.15–0.70
0.60	—	0–40		102.6	—	0–0.40
0.65	—	0–10		111.2	—	0–0.10
0.70	—	0–5		119.7	—	0–0.05
0.75	—	0		128.3	—	0

continued

Platelet count	150,000–400,000/μL	10^6	0.15–0.4×10^{12}/L
Reticulocyte count	0.5–1.5%	0.01	Number fraction: 0.005–0.015
ESR (Westergren)			
Men <50 yr	<50 mm/h	1	<15 mm/h
Men >50 yr	<20 mm/h		<20 mm/h
Women <50 yr	<20 mm/h		<20 mm/h
Women >50 yr	<30 mm/h		<30 mm/h
Viscosity	1.4–1.8 times water	1	1.4–1.8 times water
Zeta sedimentation ratio	41–54%	0.01	Fraction: 0.41–0.54
Red cell volume			
Male	25–36 mL/kg body weight	0.001	0.020–0.036 L/kg body weight
Female	19–31 mL/kg body weight	—	0.019–0.031 L/kg body weight
Plasma volume			
Male	25–43 mL/kg body weight	0.001	0.040–0.050 L/kg body weight
Female	28–45 mL/kg body weight	—	0.040–0.050 L/kg body weight
Coagulation and hemostatic tests:			
Bleeding time			
Mielke template	2–8 min		2–8 min
Simplate	3–8 min		3–8 min
Antithrombin III			
Immunologic	21–30 mg/dL		210–310 mg/L
Functional	80–120%		0.8–1.2
Clot retraction	40–94% of serum extruded in 1 h at 37°C		
Euglobulin clot lysis time	Clot lysis between 2 and 4 h at 37°C		
Factor assays (procoagulant)	0.5–1.5/U/mL		0.5–1.5
Factor VIII antigen (Factor VIIIR:Ag; Laurel)	0.5–1.5 U/mL		0.5–1.5

Table A1. (*continued*).

Component	Conventional units	Typical reference intervals	
		Factor	Recommended SI units
Ristocetin cofactor (Factor VIIIR: RCoF)	0.5–1.5 U/mL		0.5–1.5
Factor XIII (screening test)	Clot insoluble in 5M urea at 24 h		
Fibrinogen	200–400 mg/dL		2–4 g/dL
Fibrinogen split products	10 µg/dL		10 mg/L
PTT	Depends on phospholipid reagent used, typically 60–85 s		
Activated PPT	Depends on activator and phospholipid reagents used, typically 20–35 s		
Plasminogen			
Immunologic	10–20 mg/dL		100–200 mg/L
Functional	2.2–4.2 CTA U/mL		
Prothrombin time	Depends upon thromboplastin reagent used, typically 9.5–12 s		
Thrombin time	Depends upon concentration of thrombin reagent used, typically 20–29 s		
Whole blood clot lysis time	None in 24 h		

CBC			
Hematocrit			Volume fraction: 0.40–0.54
Male	40–54%	0.01	0.38–0.47
Female	38–47%		
Hemoglobin		0.155	
Male	13.5–18.0 g/dL		2.09–2.79 mmol/L
Female	12.0–16.0 g/dL		1.86–2.48 mmol/L
Red cell count			
Male	$4.6–6.2 \times 10^6/\mu L$	10^6	$4.6–6.2 \times 10^{12}/L$
Female	$4.2–11.0 \times 10^3/\mu L$	10^6	$4.5–10.0 \times 10^9/L$

CBC, complete blood count; CTA, committee on thrombotic agents; ESR, erythrocyte sedimentation rate; MCH, mean corpuscular hemoglobin; MCHC, mean corpuscular hemoglobin concentration; MCV, mean corpuscular volume; PTT, partial thromboplastin time; SI, international system of units.

All percentages are multiplied by 0.01 to give fraction.

From Henry JB. *Todd-Sanford-Davidsohn clinical diagnosis and management of laboratory methods*, 17th ed. Philadelphia: WB Saunders, 1984:1444–1445, with permission.

Table B1. Bone marrow differential counts during infancy, childhood, and adulthood[a]

	0–24 mo	1 wk	1 mo	3 mo	6 mo	12 mo	1–4 yr	4–12 yr	Adult
Myeloblasts	0.3 (0–1)	1.2 (0.4–1.9)	2.5	0.4	0.7	0.3	0.5 (0–1.2)	0.9 (0.75–1.1)	0.9 (0.3–5.0)
Promyelocytes	1.0 (0.5–1.5)	1.8 (1.0–2.5)	4.5	1.6	2.6	1.1	1.6 (0.6–3.5)	1.9 (1.8–2.1)	3.3 (1–8)
Myelocytes	1.6 (0.6–2.4)	4.3 (2.5–7.2)	5.4	1.5	4.8	2.1	1.6 (0–3.7)	10.5 (2.4–18.7)	12.7 (8–16)
Metamyelocytes	2.0 (0.7–3.0)	5.5 (3.1–9.1)	6.9	2.0	6.2	2.7	2.1 (0–4.8)	13.4 (3.1–23.8)	15.9 (9–25)
Bands	19.0 (13–23)	22.9 (17–32)	33.2 (14–52)	8.3	15.7	11.7	16.3 (4–31)	13.9 (7–20)	12.4 (9–15)
Segmented neutrophils	23.3 (9.6–39)	22.0 (8.7–30.2)	5.8 (4.0–7.6)	8.1 (3.7–11.5)	10.6	29.8 (11.0–48.5)	25 (9.6–66.9)	13.9 (9.7–14.6)	7.4 (3–11)
Eosinophils	1.3 (1–3)	2.9 (1.9–5.3)	6.0	3.9	3.2	1.9	2.9 (0–4.6)	4 (5–7)	3.1 (1–5)
Basophils	<0.1 (0–0.2)	<0.1 (0–0.2)	2.5 (0–5)	0.1	0.2	0	0.2	0.2 (0.2–1.8)	<0.1 (0–0.2)
Pronormoblasts	1.6 (0.4–2.5)	0.8 (0.4–1.1)	1.3	0.3	0.2	0.4	0.7 (0–1.4)	1.0 (0.2–2.5)	0.6 (0.2–1.3)
Normoblasts	37.8 (21–54)	19.1 (12–25)	13.9	18.4 (13–24)	10.4	5.9 (2.4–9.5)	22.2	23.4 (19–29)	25 (18–36)

continued

Table B1. (*continued*).

	0–24 mo	1 wk	1 mo	3 mo	6 mo	12 mo	1–4 yr	4–12 yr	Adult
Lymphocytes	6.1 (3.7–8.0)	14.5 (9.5–19)	12.1 (4–20)	51	37.2	27.6 (24–31)	22.0 (11–29)	24.3 (14–28)	16.2 (11–23)
Monocytes	5.3 (2.0–7.3)	5.2 (3–10)	6.8	5.0	8.0	3.4 (0–7)	6.1	6.3 (2–12)	0.3 (0–0.8)
Plasma cells	—	0.2 (0–0.2)	—	—	0.2	0.2	0.2 (0–0.4)	0.8 (0.6–0.9)	1.3 (0.4–3.9)
Myeloid: erythroid ratio	1.24	2.91	3.83	1.40	3.83	3.9	2.5	2.71	1.5–3.3

[a] First number is the *mean* (percentage). The *range* (percentage) is represented by the numbers in parentheses.
From Miller DR, et al. *Blood diseases of infancy and childhood*, 5th ed. St. Louis: Mosby–Year Book, 1984. Data from Gairdner D, Marks J, Roscoe JD. Blood formation in infancy. IV. The early anaemias of prematurity. *Arch Dis Child* 1955;30:203; Glaser K, Limarzi LR, Poncher HG. Cellular composition of the bone marrow in normal infants and children. *Pediatrics* 1950;6:789; Kalpaktsoglou PE, Emery JL. The effect of birth on the haemopoietic tissue of the human bone marrow: a biological study. *Br J Haematol* 1965;11:453; Lichtenstein A, Nordenson NG. Studies on bone marrow in premature children. *Folia Haematol* 1939;63:155; Shapiro LM, Bassen FA. Sternal marrow changes during the first week of life: correlation with peripheral blood findings. *Am J Med Sci* 1941;202:341; and Sturgeon P. Volumetric and microscopic pattern of bone marrow in normal infants and children. II. Cytologic pattern. *Pediatrics* 1951;7:642, with permission.

Appendix C. **COMPLEMENT ACTIVATION**

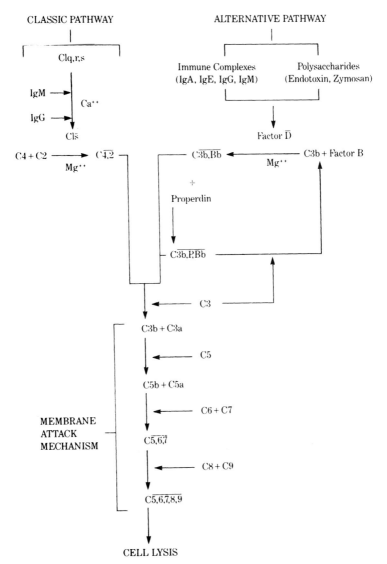

From Pittiglio DH. *Modern blood banking and transfusion practices.* Philadelphia: F.A. Davis, 1983.

Table D1. Schilling test: interpretation of excretion values[a]

Condition	B$_{12}$ alone	B$_{12}$ with intrinsic factor	After antibiotics
Normal	>8%	—	—
Pernicious anemia	<8%	>8%	—
Blind loop syndrome	<8%	No change	>8%
Malabsorption	Usually <8%	No change	No change
Absence of ileum or ileal fistula	<8%	No change	No change

[a] A third phase with human intrinsic factor may be necessary to demonstrate increase.
Source: B. H. Hyun and G. H. Salazar (directors), Bone Marrow Examination (workshop). American Society of Clinical Pathologists Meeting, New Orleans, Oct. 24–30, 1987.

Appendix E. HEMOGLOBIN-OXYGEN EQUILIBRIUM CURVE

Determination of P_{50}. The P_{50} is the P_{O_2} at which the hemoglobin is half saturated with oxygen. Since the fraction oxyhemoglobin (HbO_2) scale may not be perfectly normalized, the Y-axis values actually recorded for deoxygenation, and oxygenation must be used to calculate the midpoint. The hemoglobin-oxygen equilibrium curve indicates a 1.0 value for deoxygenation and a 101.5 value for oxygenation. The midpoint of this curve on the Y-axis is 51.25, which establishes a P_{50} of 27 mm Hg.

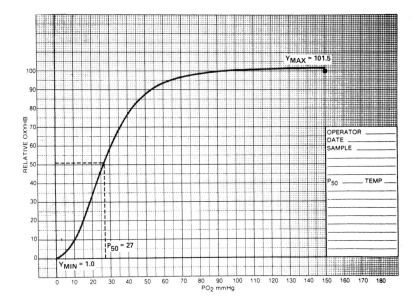

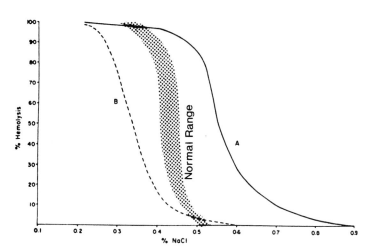

FIG. F-1. Normal and abnormal osmotic fragility curves, plotted from photoelectric data obtained by Dacie's method. A. Increased osmotic fragility. B. Decreased osmotic fragility. (From Miale JB, *Laboratory medicine: hematology*, 6th ed. St. Louis: Mosby-Year Book, 1982, with permission.)

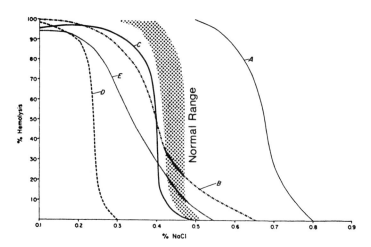

FIG. F-2. Osmotic fragility of erythrocytes by Dacie's method. A. Hereditary spherocytosis. B. Thalassemia major. C. Thalassemia minor. D. Hb E disease. E. Hb E-thalassemia. (From Miale JB, *Laboratory medicine: hematology*, 6th ed. St. Louis: Mosby-Year Book, 1982, with permission.)

Table F1. Patterns of autohemolysis with and without added
glucose or adenosine triphosphate (ATP)

Disease	Unmodified	Glucose added	ATP added[a]
Hereditary spherocytosis	+ + to ++++	±	±
Triosephosphate isomerase deficiency	++	±	±
G6PD deficiency	++	+	+
Unstable hemoglobinopathy	++	+	+
Hexokinase deficiency	++	+	+
Pyruvate kinase deficiency	++	++	0
Glutathione reductase deficiency	++	++	0
2,3-Diphosphoglycerate mutase deficiency	++	++	0
Isoimmune hemolytic disease	0	0	0
Acanthocytosis[b]	++	±	±
Thalassemia	0	0	0
Paroxysmal nocturnal hemoglobinuria (PNH)	++	++	?
Paroxysmal cold hemoglobinuria (PCH)	++[c]	++	++
Stomatocytosis	++[d]	±	±
Elliptocytosis (hemolytic)	++	±	±

G6PD, glucose-6-phosphate dehydrogenase.
[a] Of doubtful value because of acid pH.
[b] Autohemolysis inhibited by normal serum.
[c] After sensitization of erythrocytes at refrigerator temperature.
[d] At 37°C; no hemolysis at 4°C.
From Miale JB. *Laboratory medicine: hematology,* 6th ed. St. Louis: Mosby–Year Book, 1982:587, with permission.

Table F2. Osmotic fragility of erythrocytes in various diseases

Disease	Initial hemolysis (% saline ± 1 SD)	Complete hemolysis (% saline ± SD)	Remarks
Normal	0.44 ± 0.02	0.32 ± 0.02	
Hereditary spherocytosis	0.68 ± 0.14	0.46 ± 0.10	Abnormal in all cases; initial hemolysis may occur in 0.85% saline solution
Acquired hemolytic anemia	0.52 ± 0.04	0.42 ± 0.04	Abnormal in most cases; degree varies with severity
Hemolytic disease caused by A-B-O incompatibility	0.50 ± 0.02	0.40 ± 0.02	Abnormal in many cases; degree varies with severity
Hemolytic anemia caused by Rh incompatibility	0.60 ± 0.06	0.40 ± 0.04	Abnormal in many cases; degree varies with severity
Hemolytic anemia cause by drugs	0.50 ± 0.04	0.40 ± 0.04	Abnormal in most cases during onset, may be normal in later stages
Pernicious anemia	0.48 ± 0.04	0.36 ± 0.02	Occasionally very abnormal; normal in most cases
Congenital nonspherocytic hemolytic anemia	0.44 ± 0.02	0.32 ± 0.02	Fragility may be increased after blood is incubated
Elliptocytosis, asymptomatic	0.44	0.32	
Elliptocytosis with hemolytic anemia	0.50	0.32	
Thalassemia	0.38 ± 0.04	0.20 ± 0.06	Complete hemolysis may not be achieved until salt concentration of 0.1% is reached
Sickle cell anemia	0.36 ± 0.02	0.20 ± 0.04	Abnormal in all cases
Sickle cell trait (S/A)	0.44 ± 0.04	0.32 ± 0.04	Always normal
Hb C disease	0.34	0.22	Abnormal in almost all cases
Erythremia	0.40 ± 0.02	0.28 ± 0.02	Not a constant finding
Iron-deficiency anemia	0.38 ± 0.02	0.28 ± 0.02	Typical in severe anemia; not common otherwise
Obstructive jaundice (severe)	0.36 ± 0.02	0.28 ± 0.04	Decreased fragility usually noted in severely jaundiced patients

From Miale JB. *Laboratory medicine: hematology*, 6th ed. St. Louis: Mosby-Year Book, 1982:584, with permission.

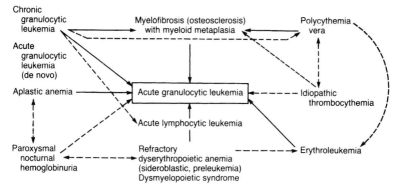

$\rightarrow$ = frequent; $\longrightarrow$ = infrequent. (Modified from Hyun BH, Salazar GH [directors]. Bone Marrow Examination [workshop]. American Society of Clinical Pathologists Meeting. New Orleans: Oct. 24–30, 1987.)

Table H1. Morphologic features of acute myelogenous leukemia according to FAB classification

M1 Myeloblastic leukemia without maturation
  Nongranular blasts
  1 or more distinct nucleoli
  Auer rods, reddish granules

M2 Myeloblastic leukemia with maturation
  Maturation promyelocyte and beyond >50% myeloblasts and promyelocytes
  Nucleoli present
  Variable amount cytoplasm/Auer rods
  All stages granulocytes present
  Abnormalities in mature granulocytes

M3 Hypergranular promyelocytic leukemia
  Most cells abnormal promyelocytes
  Nucleus varies in size and shape
  Nucleus often bilobed
  Cytoplasm packed with large granules
  "Bundles" of Auer rods
  Variable number of disrupted cells

M4 Myelomonocytic leukemia
  Both granulocytic and monocytic differentiation in PB and BM
  >20% promonocytes
    and monocytes in BM or PB
  Cytochemistry usually needed

M5a Monocytic leukemia—poorly differentiated
  Large blasts in marrow; sometimes blasts in blood
  Lacy delicate chromatin
  One or more nucleoli
  Abundant basophilic cytoplasm
  Pseudopods or buds
  Rare reddish granules
  Some promonocytes

M5b Monocytic leukemia—differentiated
  Monoblasts, promonocytes and monocytes
  Percentage of monocytes in PB greater than in marrow
  Promonocytes predominant in marrow
  Large cerebriform nucleus
  Nucleoli
  Less basophilic cytoplasm
  Greyish ground-glass appearance
  Fine azurophilic granules

M6 Erythroleukemia
  Erythroblasts >50% BM
  Bizarre morphology
  Multiple nuclear lobulation
  Multiple nuclei
  Nuclear fragments
  Giant forms
  Megaloblastic features
  Increased myeloblasts; promyelocytes
  Auer rods
  Abnormal megakaryocytes

M7 Megakaryocytic leukemia (added at a later date to the original FAB classification)

BM, bone marrow; PB, peripheral blood; FAB, French–American–British classification.
Modified from Bell A, Hippel T, Goodman H. The use of cytochemistry and FAB classification in leukemia and other pathological states. *Am J Med Tech* 1981;47:451–453; and Bennett JM, et al. Criteria for the diagnosis of acute leukemia of megakaryocyte lineage (M7): a report of the French–American–British cooperative study. *Ann Intern Med* 1985;103:460–462, with permission.

Table H2. Morphologic features of acute lymphocytic
leukemia according to FAB classification

FAB class	Cell size	Nucleus	Cytoplasm
L1	Small cells	Round, occasional cleft or fold	Usually scanty Slight to moderate basophilia
	Homogenous	Homogenous, finely dispersed chromatin Nucleoli not visible or small	
L2	Large cells Heterogeneous	Fine to coarse chromatin Clefts, folds, indenta-tions, 1 or more nucleoli	Often abundant Variable basophilia
L3	Large cells Homogeneous	Oval to round Dense, finely stippled chromatin 1 or more prominent nucleoli	Moderately abundant Intensely basophilic Prominent vacuoles

FAB, French–American–British classification.
Modified from Bell A, Hippel T, Goodman H. The use of cytochemistry and FAB classification in leukemia and other pathological states. *Am J Med Tech* 1981;47:451–452, with permission.

Table H3. Proposed WHO classification of myeloid neoplasms

Myeloproliferative diseases
  Chronic myelogenous leukemia, Philadelphia chromosome positive
    (t(9;22) (q34;q11),BCR/ABL)
  Chronic neutrophilic leukemia
  Chronic eosinophilic/hypereosinophilic syndrome
  Chronic idiopathic myelofibrosis
  Polycythemia vera
  Essential thrombocythemia
  Myeloproliferative disease, unclassifiable
Myelodysplastic/myeloproliferative diseases
  Chronic myelomonocytic leukemia
  Atypical chronic myelogenous leukemia
  Juvenile myelomonocytic leukemia
Myelodysplastic syndromes
  Refractory anemia
    With ringed sideroblasts
    Without ringed sideroblasts
  Refractory cytopenia (myelodysplastic anemia) with multilineage dysplasia
  Refractory anemia (myelodysplastic syndrome) with excess blasts 5q-syndrome
  Myelodysplastic syndrome, unclassifiable
Acute myeloid leukemia
  AMLs with recurrent cytogenetic translocations
  AML with t(8;21)(q22;q22), AML 1 (CBF-α)/ETO
  Acute promyelocytic leukemia (AML with (15;17)(q22;q11-12) and variants,
    PML/RAR-α)
  AML with abnormal bone marrow eosinophils (inv(16)(q13q22) or
    T(16;16)(q13;q11), CBFβ/MYH11X)
  AML with 11q23 (MLL) abnormalities
AML with multilineage dysplasia
  With prior myelodysplastic syndrome
  Without myelodysplastic syndrome
AML and myelodysplastic syndromes, therapy-related
  Alkylating agent-related
  Epipodophyllotoxin-related (some may be lymphoid)
  Other types
AML not otherwise categorized
  AML minimally differentiated
  AML without maturation
  AML with maturation
  Acute myelomonocytic leukemia
  Acute monocytic leukemia
  Acute erythroid leukemia
  Acute megakaryocytic leukemia
  Acute basophilic leukemia
  Acute panmyelosis with myelofibrosis
  Acute biphenotypic leukemias

AML, acute myelogenous leukemia; MLL, mixed lineage leukemia; WHO, World Health
Organization.

Table I1. Cytochemical reactions in normal and abnormal blood cells

Cell	Peroxidase	Sudan	Periodic acid-Schiff (PAS)	Alkaline phosphatase
Normal				
Myeloblast	Neg.	Neg.	Neg.	Neg.
Progranulocyte	++++	++++	++	±
Myelocyte	++++	++++	++++	±
Metamyelocyte	++++	++++	++++	+
Adult neutrophil	++++	++++	++++	+ to ++++
Eosinophil	++++	++++	Neg. to +	Neg.
Basophil	Neg.	++++	Neg. to +	Neg.
Lymphocyte	Neg.	Neg.	Neg.[a]	Neg.
Monocyte	± to ++	± to +	± to +	Neg.
Megakaryocyte	Neg.	±	++++	Neg.
Platelet	Neg.	±	++++	Neg.
Normoblast	Neg.	Neg.	Neg.	Neg.
Abnormal				
Leukemic lymphoblast	Neg.	Neg.	+ to +++[b]	Neg.
Myelomonocytic cell	Neg. to +++[c]	Neg. to +++[c]	Neg. to +++[c]	Neg.
Monocytic (histiocytic) leukemic cell	Neg. to ±	Neg. to ±[c]	Neg. to +	Neg.
Leukemic myeloblast	Neg.	Neg.[d]	±	Neg.
Erythroleukemic cell	Neg.	Neg.	+++	Neg.
Lymphocyte in chronic lymphocytic leukemia	Neg.	Neg.	+ to +++	Neg.
Auer bodies	++++	++++	Neg.	Neg.

[a] A few normal lymphocytes may show fine to medium-sized PAS-positive inclusions.

[b] PAS-positive inclusions are coarse.

[c] Varies with maturity; blasts are negative, whereas more mature cells are positive.

[d] Mitochondria may stain faintly.

From Miale JB, *Laboratory medicine: hematology,* 6th ed. St. Louis: Mosby-Year Book, 1982:206, with permission.

Appendix J1. Cytochemical reactions: esterase

Cell	NAS-DC	NAS-DA	NAS-DAF	α-NB
Myeloblast (normal)	Neg.	Neg.	Neg.	+
Myeloblast, leukemic	++++	++++	++	Neg.
Auer bodies	++++	++++	++	+
Progranulocytes	++++	++++	++++	+
Neutrophil, adult	+++	+++	+++	+
Basophil	+	+	+	Neg.
Eosinophil	Neg.	+	+	+
Monocyte	+	+++	0 to +	+++
Lymphocyte	Neg.	Neg.	Neg.	Neg.
Plasma cell	Neg.	+	Neg.	++
Myelomonocytic leukemia	+ to ++	+ to ++	+ to ++	+
Monocytic leukemia	+ to +++	+ to +++	Neg.	+++
Erythroleukemia	+++	+++	+++	++
Acute lymphocyte leukemia	Neg.	Neg.	Neg.	Neg.

NAS-DC, naphthol ASD chloroacetate; NAS-DA, naphthol ASC acetate; NAS-DAF, NAS-DA reaction from inhibition by fluoride; α-NB, α-naphthyl butyrate.
From Miale JB, *Laboratory medicine: hematology,* 6th ed. St. Louis: Mosby–Year Book, 1982:210, with permission.

Table K1. Cytochemical reactions in the acute leukemias (FAB classification)

Reaction	M1	M2	M3	M4	M5	M6	L1,2,3[a]
Peroxidase	+	+++	+++	+++	+	+ to ++[b]	Neg.[c]
Sudan black B	+	+++	+++	+++	+	+ to ++[b]	Neg.
NASDA	+	+++	+++	+++	+++	+ to ++[b]	Neg.
Fluoride inhibition	No	No	No	Variable	Yes	No	—
PAS	+	+	+	++	++	+	+ + to +++
Lysozyme[d]	Neg.	Low	Low	Intermediate	High	Low	Neg.

FAB, French–American–British.

NASDA, naphthol ASD chloroacetate; PAS, periodic acid-Schiff reaction.

+ = positive in a few cells; ++ = more than 25% of cells are positive; +++ = 50% or more of cells are positive.

[a] T-cell acute lymphocytic leukemias often show acid phosphatase positivity in the Golgi region. Diffuse acid phosphatase reactivity is characteristic of myeloblasts.

[b] Depending on the number of granulocytes.

[c] Arbitrarily, when more than 3% of the blasts are peroxidase positive, the disease is classified as other than acute lymphocytic leukemia.

[d] In serum or urine.

From Miale JB, *Laboratory medicine: hematology,* 6th ed. St. Louis: Mosby–Year Book, 1982.

Table L1. Platelet organelles and constituents

Organelle	Constituent	Function
Dense bodies	Calcium Adrenaline Noradrenaline Inorganice phosphate Adenosine triphosphate Adenosine diphosphate Phospholipids Pyrophosphate Antiplasmin (α_2-AP) Serotonin	Activates platelets Vasoconstrictor
Alpha granules	Fibrinogen Fibronectin Factor VIII R:Ag Factor V β-Thromboglobulin Mitogenic factor (growth factor)	Induces vascular smooth muscle proliferation
Lysosomes	Acid hydrolases	
Dense tubular system	Peroxidase Ca^{2+}	Shape change Aggregation Release Glycogenolysis Oxygen burst Arachidonic acid release

From Pittiglio DH, et al. *Treating hemostatic disorders—a problem-oriented approach.* Washington, DC: American Association of Blood Banks, 1984:13, with permission.

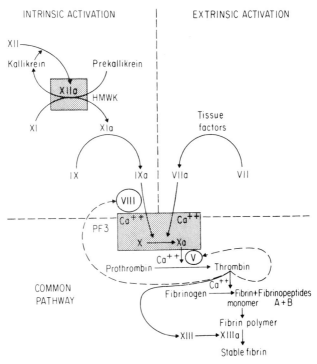

☐ = Cofactors; HMWK = high-molecular-weight kininogen; PF3 = platelet factor 3. (From Hoffbrand AV, Pettit JE. *Essential hematology*, 2nd ed. Oxford: Blackwell, 1984:199.)

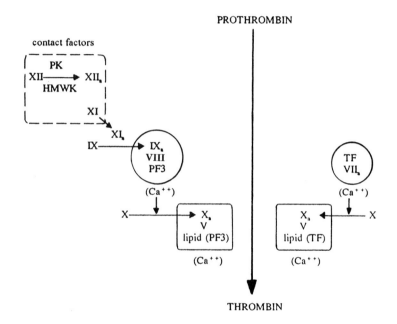

Coagulation schema as previously conceived with the activated partial thromboplastin time (aPTT) for the "intrinsic" system and the quick prothrombin time for the "extrinsic" system.

Table O1. Summary of blood components

Component	Content	Indications for use	Amount of active substance per unit	Volume (mL)	Shelf-life of product	Dosage effect
Concentrated red blood cells (CRC); packed red blood cells (Prbc)	70%–80% red cells, some white blood cells and platelets or their degradation products	Increase red blood cell mass for symptomatic anemia and hemorrhagic shock	175–280 packed red blood cell mass	250–350	ACD—21 days; CPD—21 days; CPDA—1–35 days	Increases Hct 3%
Leukocyte-poor red blood cells (LPrbc)	Red blood cells, some plasma, and white blood cells (at least 70% removed)	Increase red blood cell mass and reduce febrile reactions due to leukocyte antibodies	140–240 mL blood cell mass	200–300	Closed system; ACD, CPD—21 days; CPDA—1–35 days; Open system: 24 h	Increases Hct 3%
Washed red blood cells	Red blood cells	Same as above more effective in preventing febrile nonhemolytic reactions	200 mL packed red blood cell mass	200	Open system: 24 h	Increases Hct 3%
Frozen-thawed deglycerized red blood cells	Red blood cells, no plasma	Increase red cell mass, prevent sensitization to HLA antigens; prevent febrile or anaphylactic reactions to white blood cells, platelets, and proteins (IgA); provide rare blood storage	180 mL packed red blood cells	180	Frozen—3 yr Thawed—24 h	Increases Hct 3%

continued

Table O1. (continued).

Component	Content	Indications for use	Amount of active substance per unit	Volume (mL)	Shelf-life of product	Dosage effect
Leukocyte concentrates	White blood cells, platelets	Granulocytopenia with marked sepsis (neutrophils <500 μL) unresponsive to appropriate antibiotics	>1.0×10^{10} granulocytes	200–600	24 h	Cannot be determined
Platelet concentrates (PC)^a	Platelets, some red cells, some white cells and plasma	Bleeding due to thrombocytopenia or thrombocytopathy; Platelet disorders, DIC, massively transfused (6–8 U per 20 CRC transfused)	At least 5.5×10^{10} platelets	30–65	72–120 h room temperature (20–24°C) depending on container. 48 h (1–6°C)	Increases platelet count 5–8,000 per concentrate
Platelet concentrate (single donor)	Platelets, white cells, plasma	Platelet disorders, alloimmunized patients refractory to random-donor platelets	>3×10^{11}	300–500	24 h	Adult 30,000–60,000 μL
Fresh-frozen plasma (FFP)	Plasma, all coagulation factors, no platelets	Treatment of multiple coagulation disorders, massively transfused (2 U per 10 CRC transfused)	0.7–1.0 U of factors II, V, VII, VIII, IX, X, XI, XII, XIII, 500 mg fibrinogen	220–250	Frozen—1 yr Thawed—6 h	Increase of 20%–30% in coagulation factor activity/dose of 10–15 mL of plasma per kg body weight)

Component	Composition	Indications	Content	Volume (mL)	Storage	Dosage
Cyroprecipitated AHF (CYRO)	Fibrinogen factor VIII:C, factor XIII, von Willebrand's factor, fibronectin	Factor VIII deficiency (hemophilia A); von Willebrand's disease; factor XIII deficiency; fibrinogen deficiency; situation associated with consumption of fibrinogen	80 U factor VIII:C 200 mg fibrinogen (usually given every 15–20 h) 20%–30% of factor XIII present in initial unit 40%–70% of von Willebrand's factor present in initial unit	10–25	Frozen—1 yr (−18°C or below) Thawed—6 h. If entered or pooled—4 h	Increase of 50–100 U of factor VIII per unit of cryoprecipitate given (approximately 10-mL volume)
Purified AHF concentrate[b]	Factor VIII:C	Factor VIII deficiency (hemophilia A)	Stated on label	25	Dated period	1 U VIII/kg body wt = increase of factor VIII level 2%
Factor IX complex	Factors II, VII, IX, X	Factor IX deficiency (Christmas disease); some II, VII, and X deficiencies	Stated on label	25	Dated period	1 U IX/kg body wt = increase of factor IX level 1.5%
Single-donor plasma (SDP)	Plasma, no labile factors	Plasma volume expansion; stable clotting deficiencies	Plasma proteins, including clotting stable factors	225–250	Frozen—5 yr (−18°C)	
Albumin (5%; 25%)	96% albumin, 4% globulins (α-β)	Plasma volume expansion	12.5 g albumin	50 or 250	3 yr at room temperature 5 yr at 2–8°C	
Plasma protein fraction (PPF)[c]	83% albumin, 17% globulins	Plasma volume expansion	12.5 g, includes albumin and 17% α- and β-globulin	250	3 yr at room temperature 5 yr at 2–8°C	

continued

Table O1. (continued).

Component	Content	Indications for use	Amount of active substance per unit	Volume (mL)	Shelf-life of product	Dosage effect
Immune serum globulin	Gamma globulin, IgG antibody	Disease prophylaxis or attenuation agammaglobulinemia	16.5 g IgG/dL	Varies with patient's weight and indication	3 yr	
IV immune serum globulin	Gamma globulin, IgG antibody	Maintenance treatment of patients who are unable to produce sufficient amounts of IgG antibodies	50 mg IgG/mL	Varies with patient's weight and indication	1 yr	
Hepatitis B immune globulin	Gamma globulin, anti-HBS	Post exposure prophylaxis to HbsAg	90% Ig	Varies with patient's weight	3 yr	
Rho(D) immune globulin	Gamma globulin, anti-Rho(D)	Prevention of Rho(D) sensitization	300 µg IgG anti-Rho(D)	1.0–2.0	3 yr	
Plasma substitutes	Electrolytes and macromolecular substances	Blood volume expansion	N/A	As stated	N/A	
Antithrombin III concentrates (AT-III)	Antithrombin III DIC and other thrombotic disorders		(Investigational) 500 µ/10 mL			

ACD, antihemophilic factor; DIC, disseminated intravascular coagulation; Hct, hematocrit; HLA, human leukocyte antigen; IgG, immunoglobulin G; ITP, idiopathic thrombocytopenia purpura.

[a] Contraindicated in ITP (due to immune mediated destruction) and DIC (if intravascular clotting has not been controlled).

[b] Hemophilia patients with circulating anticoagulants (inhibitors) fail to respond to treatment with AHF. A hematologist should be consulted. Treatment consisting of prothrombin complex concentrates or possibly plasmapheresis may be implemented.

[c] Contraindicated in patients undergoing cardiopulmonary bypass or those suffering from congestive heart failure or increased blood volumes.

Modified from Pittiglio DH, et al. *Treating hemostatic disorders—A problem-oriented approach.* Washington, DC: American Association of Blood Banks, 1984:37–39, with permission.

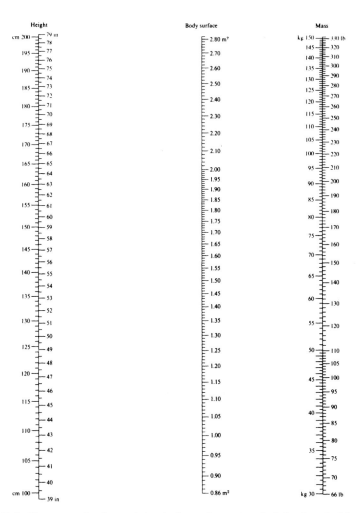

FIG. P-1. Nomogram for determining body surface area of adults from height and mass. (From Lenter C, ed. *Geigy scientific tables*, 8th ed. Basel, Switzerland: Ciba-Geigy, 1981;1:227.)

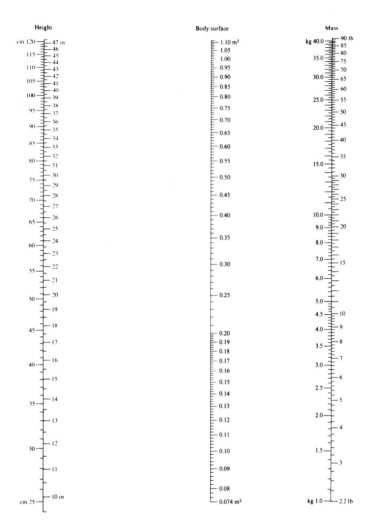

FIG. P-2. Nomogram for determining body surface of children from height and mass. (From Lentner C, ed. *Geigy scientific tables*, 8th ed. Basel, Switzerland: Ciba-Geigy, 1981;1:226.)

Appendix Q. **GROWTH FACTORS AND HEMATOPOIETIC DIFFERENTIATION**

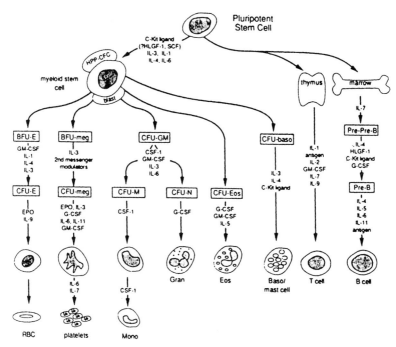

Hematopoietic differentiation. Schema plus assays. BFU-E = erythroid burst-forming cell; CFU-E = erythroid colony-forming cell; CFU-GM = granulocyte-macrophage colony-forming unit; CFU-meg = megakaryocyte colony-forming cell; HPCC = high proliferative potential cell; LTCIC = long-term culture initiating cell. (From *MKSAP in the subspeciality of hematology: book 1: syllabus and questions* developed by the American Society of Hematology and the American College of Physicians. Philadelphia: American College of Physicians, 1994:19.)

SUBJECT INDEX

Note: *f* denotes a figure; *t* denotes a table.

A

ABO compatibility
  in allogenic stem cell transplantation, 403
  with blood transfusions, 370–371, 376
ABVD chemotherapy, for Hodgkin disease, 304,
    305*t*–306*t*
  advanced, 309, 310*t*, 311, 314
Acetaminophen, methemoglobinemia from, 141, 141*t*
Acetanilid, methemoglobinemia from, 141, 141*t*, 148*t*
Aconitase, in iron metabolism, 18
F-Actin, in hemolytic anemia, 91*f*, 92
Activated lymphocytes, 281, 293
Activated partial thromboplastin time (APTT),
    359–360
Acute infectious lymphocytosis, 281–283
Acute leukemia(s)
  cytochemical reactions in, 432*t*
  epidemiology of, 214, 215*f*
  etiology of, 81, 83, 214
  lymphoblastic. *See* Acute lymphoblastic leukemia
  myelogenous. *See* Acute myelogenous leukemia
  platelet disorders with, 192*t*, 193
  promyelocytic, 221
  relapses of, 220, 226
  treatment of, 226
Acute lymphoblastic leukemia (ALL)
  classifications of, 224, 428*t*–429*t*
  immunophenotypic analysis of, 224–225
  incidence of, 214, 215*f*
  prognosis of, 223
Acute myelogenous leukemia (AML)
  classification of, 217, 427*t*
  clinical features of, 215–216
  complications of, 223
  genetics of, 214, 218
  with Hodgkin disease, 303, 313–314
  immunophenotypic analysis of, 218
  incidence of, 214, 215*f*
  infections with, 221–222
  laboratory features of, 216–217
  from myelodysplasia, 205–206, 209–210, 212
  prognostic factors of, 218, 220
  stem cell origin of, 214–215
  supportive care for, 220–223
  treatment of, 218–222
Acute promyelocytic leukemia (APL), 221
Acyclovir, hematopoietic effects of, 390*t*
Adenosine deaminase deficiency, 293–294
Adenosine triphosphate (ATP), osmotic fragility and,
    423*t*
Adherence
  immune, in hemolytic disorders, 106, 108
  in neutrophilia, 168*t*, 169
  as platelet process, 180, 181*f*
Adrenal cortical hypersecretion, erythrocytosis with,
    75, 85
Adult T-cell leukemia, 234*t*, 237
Agammaglobulinemias, 286–287
Aggregation
  in neutrophilia, 168*t*, 169
  as platelet process, 180, 181*f*
Agnogenic myeloid metaplasia (AMM)
  clinical features of, 198
  diagnosis of, 32, 197–198
  pathogenesis of, 197, 200*t*
  prognosis of, 198, 200
  treatment of, 200–201
AIDS-related malignancies, 394–397

Albumin, transfusion guidelines for, 378, 439*t*
Alcoholism and alcohol consumption
  apparent polycythemia with, 87
  folate deficiency with, 46*t*, 48, 50
  hereditary hemochromatosis and, 118, 123
  iron-overload disorders from, 118, 123
Alder-Reilly anomaly, of neutrophils, 156, 168
Alimentary tract disorders, iron-deficiency anemia
    from, 22*t*, 23
Alkaline phosphatase, in cytochemical reactions, 430*t*
Alkylating agents
  indications for, 233, 261, 268
  myelodysplastic syndrome from, 208
Allergic reactions
  hematologic mechanisms of, 6, 173, 174*t*
  to iron dextran, 37
  to transfusions, 383
Alloantibodies, activation of, 181, 188
Alloantibody-induced immune hemolytic anemia,
    109
Allopurinol, for acute lymphoblastic leukemia, 226
All trans-retinoic acid therapy (ATRA), acute
    leukemia from, 221
Alpha-like globin gene cluster, in hemoglobin, 138,
    139*f*
Aminoglycosides, for acute myelogenous leukemia,
    221
Amphotericin B
  for acute myelogenous leukemia, 222
  hematopoietic effects of, 389–390, 390*t*
Amyloidosis
  characteristics of, 262–263
  classification of, 263, 264*t*
  clinical features of, 263–264, 268
  diagnosis of, 263, 265, 268
  dialysis-associated, 264*t*, 269
  familial, 264*t*, 269
  pathogenesis of, 263
  primary, 263–268, 264*t*, 267*f*
  secondary, 263, 264*t*, 268–269
Anaerobic metabolism disorders, in hemolytic ane-
    mia, 92, 94, 95*f*
  pathobiology of, 100–103
Anagrelide
  for essential thrombocythemia, 202–203, 202*t*
  for polycythemia vera, 82–83, 197, 199*t*
Anal carcinoma, AIDS-related, 396
Analgesics, indications for, 63*t*, 144
Anaphylactic reaction/shock
  from iron dextran, 37
  to transfusions, 383
Androgens, exogenous
  erythrocytosis with, 75, 85
  indications for, 64, 114, 116, 165, 200, 211
Anemia(s). *See also* specific type
  aplastic, 61–72, 62*t*, 65, 158
  of chronic disease, 54–61
  with eosinophilia, 175
  Fanconi's, 64, 158
  hemolytic, 90–117, 147
  HIV-related, 62, 62*t*, 390–391, 393
  iron-deficient, 17–39
  iron overload associated with, 123–124, 134
  megaloblastic, 39–54, 161, 187
  with multiple myeloma, 257
  refractory, 32, 206, 207*t*
  Schilling test for, 420
  sideroblastic, 123–124, 134

445